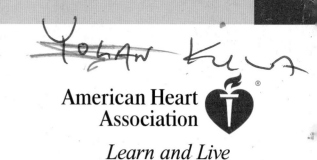

American Heart Association

Learn and Live

D0701589

ACLS
Resource Text

FOR INSTRUCTORS AND EXPERIENCED PROVIDERS

Editor

John M. Field, MD
Senior Science Editor

Senior Managing Editor

Erik S. Soderberg, MS

Special Contributors

Mary Ann Cooper, MD
Peter J. Kudenchuk, MD
Julie A. Linick, ELS
David Szpilman, MD
Carolyn M. Zelop, MD

ACLS Subcommittee 2006-2008

Laurie J. Morrison, MD, MSc, Chair
Terry L. Vanden Hoek, MD, Immediate Past
   Chair, 2005-2006

Robert W. Neumar, MD, PhD
Henry R. Halperin, MD, MA
Edward C. Jauch, MD, MS
Steven D. Kronick, MD, MS
Mark S. Link, MD
Graham Nichol, MD, MPH
Charles W. Otto, MD, PhD
Wanchun Tang, MD
Roger D. White, MD

Acknowledgements

Todd J. Crocco, MD
Elamin M. Elamin, MD
Louis Gonzales, BS, NREMT-P
David G. Sherman, MD

ISBN 978-0-87493-541-7

To find out about any updates or corrections to this text, visit *www.americanheart.org/cpr* and click on the "Course Materials" button.

Contents

Contents

Chapter 15:
Life-Threatening Electrolyte
and Acid-Base Abnormalities 381

Contents

Preface

Welcome to the *Advanced Cardiovascular Life Support Resource Text for Instructors and Experienced Providers (ACLS Resource Text)*. The *ACLS Resource Text* serves two purposes. First, the text is organized to allow you to understand in more depth the material you will teach to your students and will practice when caring for patients. Second, it will allow you to be an excellent team leader and mentor for others.

- **Part 1** expands on information presented in the *ACLS Provider Manual*. This part gives rationale, background information, and supplementary data on basic ACLS core material. It is intended to arm ACLS instructors with the material to understand and explain the ACLS core information. Experienced providers are expected to possess the depth of background knowledge reviewed in this part.

- **Part 2** provides additional and advanced ACLS material to increase your depth of understanding for more complicated and special resuscitation situations. If you are an ACLS instructor, this material will enrich your knowledge and prepare you to be an exceptional team leader for your patients and mentor for your students. If you are an experienced provider student, this material is *required reading* before taking the ACLS Experienced Provider Course (ACLS EP Course). The ACLS EP Course is an advanced interactive and case-based course that requires you to have mastered this information before entering the course. The ACLS EP Course has no lecture material and depends on you to have acquired the knowledge presented in this text *before* you participate with your colleagues in an interactive learning process *facilitated* by our most experienced ACLS instructors.

Experienced providers are expected to possess the depth of background knowledge reviewed in Part 1 of this text. The advanced material will further develop your understanding and skills to go beyond the basic resuscitation concepts. This material and the ACLS EP Course will give you the opportunity to

- Understand in depth the ACLS core material. This will make you a better team leader, experienced provider, or both.

- Identify prearrest situations and intervene with *rapid response interventions* targeted at preventing the cardiac arrest and stabilizing the patient.

- Prepare you to better answer the question, What may have caused this arrest that will require therapy or interventions different from or beyond those in the BLS and ACLS algorithms?

- Stabilize patients after a cardiopulmonary emergency and stabilize them for additional evaluation and interventions.

Look for the boxes on the next page as you read the text. They will identify important material for you, provide discussion and answers to frequently asked questions, and highlight important changes or information reviewed in the *2005 American Heart Association Guidelines for Cardiopulmonary Resuscitation and Emergency Cardiovascular Care (2005 AHA Guidelines for CPR and ECC)*.

Critical Concept	Information in this box highlights important concepts critical to patient care. This information serves as a cornerstone for an assessment or action.
FYI Guidelines 2005	Information in this box emphasizes important material from the *2005 AHA Guidelines for CPR and ECC.*
Foundation Facts	Information in this box identifies basic information that serves as a foundation for the principles and practice of ACLS and Emergency Cardiovascular Care. Pay special attention to these facts as they are cornerstones critical to successful outcomes.
FAQ Frequently Asked Question	Information in this box asks an FAQ identified by students, instructors, course directors, and AHA National Center staff in courses, pilots, and rollouts. If you or someone in your class has a question, look here first. Many questions may be frequently asked. Read the adjoining text. This will summarize the rationale and background information to help answer the question or will provide additional resources.
Rapid Response Interventions for the Medical Emergency Team (MET) or Rapid Response Team (RRT)	Look for these key assessments and actions in Part 2 of this text. Remember, one of your goals as an experienced provider is to prevent an arrest if the opportunity exists. These key points will highlight important aspects of assessment, action, or intervention to possibly prevent an arrest. One of the original EP concepts was *If you knew 10 minutes before an arrest that _____ , how would you intervene to prevent arrest or now change the resuscitation approach?*

For More Information

References

The *ACLS Resource Text* is lightly referenced with suggested reading, key references, landmark trials, and important meta-analyses. For more detailed references refer to the *2005 AHA Guidelines for CPR and ECC.*

Introduction to Advanced Cardiovascular Life Support

This Chapter

- **No ACLS survival without high-quality BLS**
- **Team resuscitation and the ACLS course**
- **Science behind the guidelines**

Is There Incremental Benefit With ACLS?

Advanced cardiovascular life support (ACLS) instructors face an important and difficult new challenge—training their students to function as a team, implementing and integrating both basic and advanced life support. The *2005 American Heart Association Guidelines for Cardiopulmonary Resuscitation and Emergency Cardiovascular Care (2005 AHA Guidelines for CPR and ECC)* reviewed evidence that the majority of people do not survive cardiac arrest, few people receive CPR and fewer receive high-quality CPR.[1] One study evaluating the benefit of out-of-hospital ACLS found no additional advantage of ACLS, raising questions about current-day quality and benefit of ACLS interventions.[2] To analyze these findings a "back-to-basics" evidence review refocused on the essentials of CPR—links in the Chain of Survival—and the integration of basic life support (BLS) with ACLS. The experts who participated concluded that high

survival rates from out-of-hospital sudden cardiac death are possible and share several common elements:

1. Training of knowledgeable healthcare providers
2. Planned and practiced response
3. Rapid recognition of sudden cardiac arrest
4. Prompt provision of bystander CPR
5. Defibrillation within 5 minutes of collapse

When trained persons implement these elements early, ACLS has the best chance of producing a successful outcome. If the patient remains in cardiac arrest despite early interventions, two key elements of ACLS are now thought to provide optimal outcome, serving as a cornerstone and matrix for survival:

1. High-quality chest compressions delivered with minimal interruption
2. A team approach to the integration of BLS and ACLS care

BLS Essentials for ACLS Healthcare Providers

The updated ACLS algorithms target minimal interruption in chest compressions as a major goal. Several important changes in BLS and ACLS allow for integration of this recommendation.

Compression-Ventilation Ratio

No human data has identified the optimal compression-ventilation ratio for CPR for patients of all ages. To be

FYI **Guidelines 2005**	ACLS is optimized when a team leader effectively integrates CPR and minimal interruption of high-quality chest compressions with advanced life support strategies.
	There is no question that high-quality advanced cardiovascular life support depends on high-quality basic life support.

effective, CPR must provide adequate coronary and cerebral blood flow during resuscitative efforts. Interruptions in chest compressions lower coronary perfusion pressure and decrease rates of survival from cardiac arrest.[3] In the first minutes of sudden cardiac arrest (SCA) due to ventricular fibrillation (VF), ventilation does not appear to be as important as chest compressions, and the ventilation rate needed to maintain a normal ventilation-perfusion ratio during CPR is much smaller than normal because pulmonary blood flow is low. Mathematical and animal models have shown that matching of pulmonary blood flow and ventilation might be more appropriate at compression-ventilation ratios higher than 15:2.[4] To achieve optimal compression rates and reduce the frequency of interruptions in compressions, a universal compression-ventilation ratio of 30:2 is recommended for all adults in cardiac arrest when an advanced airway is not in place.

Compression First vs Shock First for VF SCA

Recent data challenges the standard practice of providing defibrillation first to every patient with VF, particularly when more than 4 to 5 minutes has elapsed from collapse to healthcare provider intervention. But there was insufficient data to recommend CPR before defibrillation for all patients of VF SCA. Later in this text you will learn about the phases of cardiac arrest and the optimal timing for interventions. Consensus recommendations provide for the use of defibrillation immediately or early and a period of CPR when CPR, defibrillation, or ACLS is delayed or prolonged.

- Lay healthcare providers should use the AED as soon as it is available.
- Emergency medical services (EMS) healthcare providers may give 5 cycles (or about 2 minutes) of CPR before attempting defibrillation for treatment of out-of-hospital VF or pulseless ventricular tachycardia (VT) when the EMS response (call-to-arrival) interval is greater than 4 to 5 minutes or EMS responders did not witness the arrest.

1-Shock vs 3-Shock Sequence for Attempted Defibrillation

The *ECC Guidelines 2000*[5] recommended the use of a so-called "stacked" sequence of up to 3 shocks, **without** interposed chest compressions, for the treatment of VF/pulseless VT. Although no studies in humans or animals specifically compared the 1-shock defibrillation strategy with the 3-stacked-shock sequence, other evidence created the tipping point for a change from a 3-shock sequence to 1 shock followed immediately by CPR. After VF is terminated almost all patients demonstrate a nonperfusing rhythm initially (pulseless electrical activity or asystole) for several minutes. The 3-shock recommendation was based on the low first-shock efficacy of *monophasic* damped sinusoidal waveforms and efforts to decrease transthoracic impedance with delivery of shocks in rapid succession. Modern biphasic defibrillators have a high first-shock efficacy (defined as termination of VF for at least 5 seconds after the shock), averaging more than 90% so VF is likely to be eliminated with 1 shock. If 1 shock fails to eliminate VF, the VF may be of low amplitude, and the incremental benefit of another shock is low. In such patients immediate resumption of CPR, particularly effective chest compressions, is likely to confer a greater value than an immediate second shock.

Experts recommend that healthcare providers resume CPR, beginning with chest compressions, *immediately after attempted defibrillation*. Healthcare providers should not interrupt chest compressions to check circulation (eg, evaluate rhythm or pulse) until after 5 cycles (about 2 minutes) of CPR.

Vasopressors, Antiarrhythmics, and Sequence of Actions During Treatment of Cardiac Arrest

No placebo-controlled study has shown that any medication—vasopressor or antiarrhythmic drug—given routinely at any stage during human cardiac arrest increases rate of survival to hospital discharge. Given this

---

FAQ **How long is CPR delivered before shock?** **Should a period of CPR be routinely provided for all in-hospital patients?**	Data is presently insufficient to determine 1. The ideal duration of CPR before attempted defibrillation 2. If this recommendation should be applied to in-hospital cardiac arrest 3. The duration of VF at which time healthcare providers should switch from defibrillation first to CPR first

FAQ **Can a rhythm and pulse check be performed after defibrillation?**	Pulse and rhythm checks are not recommended immediately after defibrillation. In specific instances, a physician team leader may modify the resuscitation sequence for particular purposes with attention to minimal interruption in chest compressions. When performed, interruption of chest compressions, including the performance of a rhythm and pulse check, should take no longer than 10 seconds. Pulse checks are performed only if an organized rhythm is present.
	Almost all patients have a nonperfusing rhythm for a period of time after successful shock—they are in PEA or asystole. The administration of a vasopressor agent would be indicated, and chest compressions are needed to deliver the drug to the central circulation. One study found that 80% of patients were in PEA/asystole and 20% remained in VF.
If a rhythm and pulse check is not performed after shock administration, is drug administration harmful?	Administration of amiodarone after the next shock would not be indicated if the post-conversion rhythm is PEA or asystole but: 1. The interruption in chest compressions to determine the rhythm is potentially harmful and could reduce chances of a successful outcome 2. Amiodarone administration is associated with improved survival to hospital admission but recall that the effects of an agent are not observed until the *next* cycle of rhythm assessment because chest compressions are needed to move the agent into the central circulation. So shock success initially is independent of amiodarone effect. While it may be that amiodarone facilitates shock conversion of VF during arrest, improved survival to hospital admission could also be due to prevention of rearrest independent of VF shock conversion.
	In balance, no drug has been demonstrated to improve survival to hospital discharge, but interruption of chest compressions will definitely decrease chance of survival as well.

lack of documented effect of drug therapy in improving long-term outcome from cardiac arrest, the sequence for CPR deemphasizes drug administration and reemphasizes basic life support.

Coordination of Shock-Drug Sequence

To minimize interruptions in chest compressions for administration of drugs, the *2005 AHA Guidelines for CPR and ECC* recommend that healthcare providers resume CPR beginning with chest compressions *immediately* after a shock, without an intervening rhythm (or pulse) check. Vasopressors or antiarrhythmics can be administered just before, or at the same time as, a rhythm check. The drug will be circulated by the CPR that immediately follows the shock.

Healthcare providers should practice coordination of CPR and shock delivery so that when a shock is indicated, it can be delivered as soon as possible after chest compressions are stopped and healthcare providers are "cleared" from contact with the patient.

Team Leader and Team Resuscitation

The ACLS Healthcare Provider Course emphasizes the development of team roles, participation, and skills. Your role as an ACLS instructor involves student supervision and mentorship beyond instruction and testing in algorithms and interventions. Fully prepared ACLS healthcare providers can function as team members within their scope of practice. Many will be team leaders. Both roles require knowledge of team skills and practice as team players to ensure continuation of effective BLS and timely integration of appropriate ACLS skills (Figure 1).

FYI **Drug Administration Deemphasized**	No placebo-controlled study has shown that any medication—vasopressor or antiarrhythmic drug—given routinely at any stage during human cardiac arrest increases rate of survival to hospital discharge.

Critical Concept	Studies have shown that a reduction in the interval between compression and shock delivery by as little as 15 seconds can increase the predicted shock success.

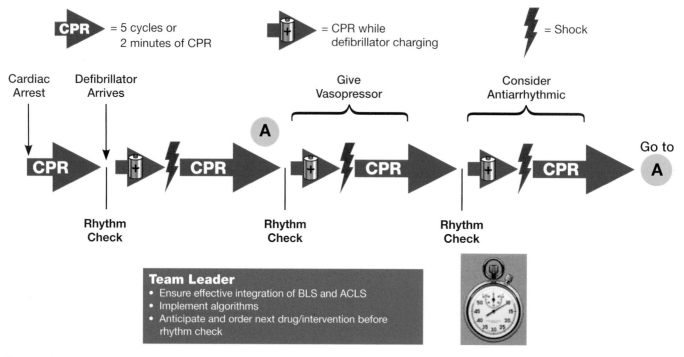

Figure 1. Integration of high-quality continuous CPR with minimal interruption is essential for optimal resuscitation and return of spontaneous circulation. The team leader anticipates and coordinates interventions that minimally interrupt CPR with team members.

Although Part 1 of this text will generally follow the *ACLS Healthcare Provider Manual,* remember that team leaders and members use common clinical interventions across a variety of scenarios and resuscitation situations. In Part 2 instructors will advance basic ACLS knowledge and integrate their ACLS team with three other concepts— prevention of cardiac arrest, unique or special interventions during arrest, and postarrest management.

Although we typically think of the "code blue" or cardiac arrest team, two other teams may potentially impact patient survival, the medical emergency team (MET) and the intensive care unit (ICU) team. A team leader may also need to coordinate a smooth transition of care or timely involvement of multidisciplinary specialists to impact survival when a life-threatening cardiopulmonary situation occurs (Figure 2).

Medical Emergency Team

Many in-hospital patients may demonstrate clinical deterioration before cardiac arrest occurs. This is the ideal time for an intervention to prevent cardiac arrest. Early detection and treatment of a life-threatening condition potentially could prevent cardiac arrest and improve outcomes. Many hospitals have implemented a rapid response system that uses a MET and an interdisciplinary approach to respond to generally unanticipated life-threatening emergencies. In many situations METs will need advanced life support skills and share common ground with cardiac arrest teams.

A rapid response system generally has 4 components:

1. A protocol and activation criteria for the team
2. The MET
3. An interdisciplinary leadership team
4. A quality assurance component for process evaluation and improvement

Cardiac Arrest Team

Cardiac arrest teams have become synonymous with advanced cardiac life support. For this reason it is important to emphasize the crucial role of basic life support

Critical Concept
 	
Survival to Hospital Discharge
	Survival from cardiac arrest means survival to hospital discharge neurologically intact. Three key stages occur:
	
	  1. Prearrest intervention if possible
	  2. Resuscitation from cardiac arrest
	  3. Postarrest management

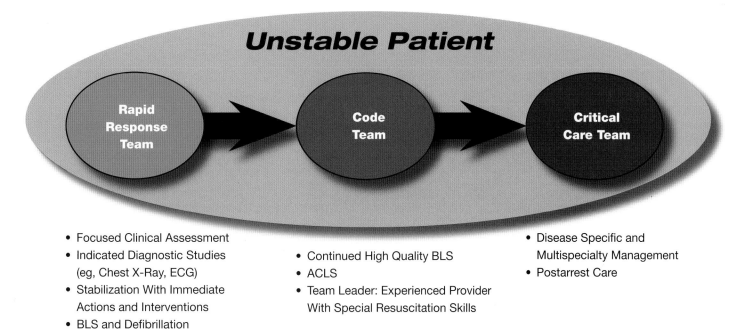

Unstable Patient

Rapid Response Team → Code Team → Critical Care Team

- Focused Clinical Assessment
- Indicated Diagnostic Studies (eg, Chest X-Ray, ECG)
- Stabilization With Immediate Actions and Interventions
- BLS and Defibrillation

- Continued High Quality BLS
- ACLS
- Team Leader: Experienced Provider With Special Resuscitation Skills

- Disease Specific and Multispecialty Management
- Postarrest Care

Figure 2. Management of life-threatening emergencies requires integration of multidisciplinary teams that can involve rapid response teams, cardiac arrest teams, and intensive care specialties to achieve survival of the patient. Team leaders have an essential role in coordination of care with team members and other specialists.

as the turnkey of advanced life support. ACLS clinical interventions include

- High-quality BLS, most importantly chest compressions
- A systematic approach to advanced life support
- An effective, experienced, and knowledgeable team leader

ACLS—The Systematic Approach

The "systematic approach of ACLS" refers to the BLS Primary and ACLS Secondary ABCD Surveys mnemonic.[6] This approach trains ACLS healthcare providers to review systematically each of 8 steps and to perform an "assess" action plus a "manage" action at each step. The approach is covered extensively in the *ACLS Provider Manual*.

ICU Team and Postarrest Care

When ACLS has been successful, resuscitation of the patient continues into the intensive care or specialty unit. This phase of resuscitation is equally important and may determine the success of a patient's surviving a life-threatening crisis or cardiac arrest. The ICU team must address the ultimate cause of cardiac arrest and treat complications that are often multisystem in nature and multidisciplinary in scope.

Initial objectives of postresuscitation care are to

- Optimize cardiopulmonary function and systemic perfusion, especially perfusion to the brain
- Transport the patient of out-of-hospital cardiac arrest to the hospital Emergency Department and continue care in an appropriately equipped critical care unit
- Try to identify the precipitating causes of the arrest
- Institute measures to prevent recurrence
- Institute measures that may improve long-term, neurologically intact survival

After Return of Spontaneous Circulation

The immediate objective of postarrest care is the reestablishment of effective perfusion of organs and tissue. After return of spontaneous circulation, the ACLS healthcare provider must consider and treat the cause and consequences of the arrest. In most cases the acidemia associated with cardiac arrest improves spontaneously when adequate ventilation and perfusion are restored. But restoration of blood pressure and improvement in gas exchange do not ensure survival and functional recovery. Significant myocardial stunning and hemodynamic instability can develop, requiring vasopressor support, with most postarrest deaths occurring during the first 24 hours.

The ACLS healthcare provider should assess the patient frequently, treat abnormalities of vital signs or cardiac arrhythmias, and request studies that will further aid in the evaluation of the patient. It is important to identify and treat any cardiac, electrolyte, toxicologic, pulmonary, and neurologic precipitants of arrest. It is helpful to review the H's and T's mnemonic to recall factors that may contribute to cardiac arrest or complicate resuscitation or postresuscitation care: hypovolemia, hypoxia, hydrogen ion (acidosis), hypo-/hyperkalemia, hypoglycemia, hypothermia, toxins, tamponade (cardiac), tension pneumothorax, thrombosis (coronary or pulmonary), and trauma.

After initial assessment and stabilization of airway, ventilation, and circulation, transfer the patient to a special care unit for observation, continuous monitoring, and further therapy. Personnel with appropriate training and resuscitation equipment must accompany the patient during transport to the special care unit.

Science Behind the Guidelines— Why Do They Change?

Evidence-based medicine defines a practice that uses a drug, intervention, or strategy based on levels of evidence and consensus opinion. The knowledge developed in the ACLS Provider Course and *ACLS Provider Manual* represents this international process in action through the 2000 and 2005 Consensus Conferences. In an open process experts evaluated evidence for key questions and historical ACLS treatment (Table 1). These experts gathered and ranked the evidence (Table 2), and then expert panels and committees made a class of recommendation based on this evidence (Table 3). This international consensus on science was published in 2005[7] and serves as the science foundation for guidelines published by many member councils of the International Liaison Committee on Resuscitation (ILCOR).[8] This process is a continual one and will repeat every 5 years. In this way new science can be incorporated into both AHA and ILCOR guidelines, and questions generated by evidence review will lead to new research and better recommendations with improved outcome. In addition, new clinical experiences may well confirm the promise of new developments. Members of the AHA ECC Committee and various subcommittees are always prepared to perform an expedited review of important new published scientific evidence in order to determine if the new evidence is sufficient to change the recommended resuscitation guidelines.

Table 1. Evidence Evaluation Process

Step	Activity	Results
1	Gather evidence using explicit inclusion and exclusion criteria determined in advance. Briefly summarize excluded studies.	Move included studies to step 2.
2	Establish a level of evidence for each accepted scientific study (Table 2).	Move studies with the most relevant and higher-level evidence to step 3. Briefly summarize excluded studies.
3	Critically appraise the quality of studies with the most relevant and higher-level evidence; determine the direction and magnitude of their conclusions. Sort studies by "level-quality-direction" (Table 3).	Move studies in the most powerful cell (or cells) in the evidence-sorting matrix to step 4. Explain major reasons for excluding other studies.
4	Establish the final class of recommendation by consensus debate. Describe the match between the final class of recommendation and the minimum acceptable criteria for that class (see Table 3).	• Presentations and panel discussions at Evidence Evaluation Conference • More presentations and debate at Guidelines Conference • Virtually continuous consensus discussions by experts • Final editorial review by International Editorial Board, Science Product Development Panel, ECC Committee and Subcommittees

Table 2. Levels of Evidence: Definitions

Evidence Level	Definition
1. Positive randomized, controlled trials (RCTs) (P<.05)	A prospective RCT. Conclusions: new treatment significantly better (or worse) than control treatment.
2. Neutral RCTs (NS)	An RCT. Conclusions: new treatment no better than control treatment.
3. Prospective, nonrandom	Nonrandomized, *prospective* observational study of a group that uses new treatment; *must* have a control group for comparisons.
4. Retrospective, nonrandom	Nonrandomized, *retrospective* observational study; one group used new treatment; *must* have a control group for comparisons.
5. Case series	Series of patients received new treatment in past or will receive in future; watch to see what outcomes occur; no control group.
6. Animal studies	Studies using animals or mechanical models.
7. Extrapolations	Reasonable extrapolations from existing data or data gathered for other purposes; quasi-experimental designs.
8. Rational conjecture, common sense	Fits with common sense; has face validity; applies to many non–evidence-based guidelines that "made sense." No evidence of harm.

Table 3. Classes of Recommendation: Evidence-Based Classification of Therapeutic Interventions in CPR and ECC

1. Search for Evidence: Locates the Following	2. Consensus Review by Experts: Intervention Is Placed in Following Class	3. Interpretation of This Class of Recommendation When Used Clinically
Minimum evidence required for a Class I recommendation • Level of evidence: 1 or more RCTs • Critical assessment: *excellent* • Results: homogeneous, consistently positive, and robust	***Class I: Excellent*** *Definitely recommended* Supported by **excellent** evidence Proven efficacy and effectiveness	**Class I** interventions are always acceptable, proven safe, and definitely useful.
Minimum evidence required for a Class IIa recommendation • Level of evidence: higher • Number of studies: multiple • Critical assessment: *good to very good* • Weight of evidence/expert opinion: more strongly in favor of intervention than Class IIb • More long-term outcomes measured than Class IIb • Results: positive in majority of studies • Observed magnitude of benefit: higher than Class IIb	***Class IIa: Good to very good*** *Acceptable and useful* ***Good/very good*** evidence provides support ***Note:*** "Contextual" factors: In addition to level of evidence, these additional factors are considered in making final class of recommendation. Contextual factors include small magnitude of benefit, high cost, educational and training challenges, large difficulties in implementation, and impractical, unfavorable cost-benefit ratios.	**Class IIa** interventions are acceptable, safe, and useful. • Considered standard of care: reasonably prudent physicians can choose • Considered ***intervention of choice*** by majority of experts • Often receive AHA support in training programs, teaching materials, etc *"Contextual" or "mismatch" factors may render an intervention Class IIa in one context and Class IIb in another (see* ***Note***).

(continued)

Table 3. *(Continued)*

1. Search for Evidence: Locates the Following	2. Consensus Review by Experts: Intervention Is Placed in Following Class	3. Interpretation of This Class of Recommendation When Used Clinically
Minimum evidence required for a Class IIb recommendation • Level of evidence: lower/intermediate • Number of studies: few • Critical assessment: *fair or poor* • Weight of evidence/expert opinion: less in favor of usefulness/efficacy • Outcomes measured: immediate, intermediate, or surrogate • Results: generally, not always, positive	***Class IIb: Fair to good*** *Acceptable and useful* ***Fair to good*** evidence provides support Contextual/mismatch factors should not be used to avoid the trouble and expense of adopting new but clinically beneficial interventions.	**Class IIb** interventions are acceptable, safe, and useful. • Considered within "standard of care": reasonably prudent physicians can choose • Considered *optional or alternative interventions* by majority of experts
Evidence found but available studies have one or more shortcomings • Promising but low level • Fail to address relevant clinical outcomes • Are inconsistent, noncompelling, or report contradictory results • May be high level but report conflicting results	***Class Indeterminate*** *Preliminary research stage* Available evidence insufficient to support a final class decision Results promising but need additional confirmation Evidence: no harm, but no benefit No recommendation until further evidence is available	Interventions classed *Indeterminate* can still be recommended for use, but reviewers must acknowledge that research quantity/quality fall short of supporting a final class decision. Do not use *Indeterminate* to resolve debates among experts, especially when evidence is available but experts disagree on interpretation. *Indeterminate* is limited to promising interventions.
Positive evidence completely absent *or* **Evidence strongly suggests or confirms harm**	***Class III: Unacceptable, no documented benefit, may be harmful*** *Not acceptable, not useful, may be harmful*	Interventions are designated as **Class III** when evidence of benefit is completely lacking or studies suggest or confirm harm.

RCT indicates randomized, controlled trial.

References

1. Wik L, Kramer-Johansen J, Myklebust H, Sorebo H, Svensson L, Fellows B, Steen PA. Quality of cardiopulmonary resuscitation during out-of-hospital cardiac arrest. *JAMA*. 2005;293:299-304.

2. Stiell IG, Wells GA, Field B, Spaite DW, Nesbitt LP, De Maio VJ, Nichol G, Cousineau D, Blackburn J, Munkley D, Luinstra-Toohey L, Campeau T, Dagnone E, Lyver M. Advanced cardiac life support in out-of-hospital cardiac arrest. *N Engl J Med*. 2004;351:647-656.

3. Kern KB, Hilwig RW, Berg RA, Sanders AB, Ewy GA. Importance of continuous chest compressions during cardiopulmonary resuscitation: improved outcome during a simulated single lay-healthcare provider scenario. *Circulation*. 2002;105:645-649.

4. Babbs CF, Kern KB. Optimum compression to ventilation ratios in CPR under realistic, practical conditions: a physiological and mathematical analysis. *Resuscitation*. 2002;54:147-157.

5. American Heart Association in collaboration with International Liaison Committee on Resuscitation. Guidelines 2000 for Cardiopulmonary Resuscitation and Emergency Cardiovascular Care: International Consensus on Science, Part 3: Adult Basic Life Support. *Circulation*. 2000;102(suppl I):I22-I59.

6. Cummins RO. The systematic ACLS approach. In: Cummins RO, Field JM, Hazinski MF, eds. *ACLS Provider Manual*. Dallas: American Heart Association; 2001:7-18.

7. ECC Committee, ECC Subcommittees, and ECC Task Forces; and Authors of Final Evidence Evaluation Worksheets 2005 International Consensus on Cardiopulmonary Resuscitation and Emergency Cardiovascular Care With Treatment Recommendations Conference. *Circulation*. 2005;112:b2-b5.

8. 2005 American Heart Association Guidelines for Cardiopulmonary Resuscitation and Emergency Cardiovascular Care. *Circulation*. 2005;112:IV-1-IV-203.

Chapter 2

Sudden Cardiac Death: Strategies for Survival—Integration of BLS and ACLS

This Chapter

- *Why people die suddenly*
- *Using a chain for survival*
- *Strengthening the weak links in the chain*
- *Closing the chain for the future*

Sudden cardiac death (SCD) is the most dramatic presentation of acute coronary ischemia and a major public health problem in most developed countries today. Cardiovascular disease accounts for approximately 50% of deaths. One third to one half of these are sudden and occur in the community. In 20% SCD is the first, last, and only symptom. Trends in the incidence of SCD parallel coronary artery disease and atherogenic risk factors, particularly cigarette smoking. Accordingly the incidence of sudden death has been declining in countries with decreasing rates of coronary artery disease. From 1950 to 1999 nonsudden coronary heart disease deaths in the United States decreased by 64% and SCD fell by 49%.[1] This decrease, the complexity of the problem, and recent therapeutic innovations have led to a false sense of security and progress.

Who Dies Suddenly?

Definition

Previous studies and reviews of sudden death and cardiac arrest have been limited by the lack of uniform definitions. In general the clinical event is sudden and by consensus occurs less than 1 hour from onset of symptoms. Instantaneous sudden death refers to the lack of premonitory symptoms and immediate collapse. To address problems of definition, a panel of international experts[2] developed consensus guidelines for the classification, definition, and reporting of sudden death and cardiac arrest. Cardiac arrest is now defined as "cessation of cardiac mechanical activity, confirmed by the absence of detectable pulse, unresponsiveness, and apnea, or agonal, gasping respirations."

Etiology

The etiology of atraumatic sudden death and the underlying and associated conditions are numerous and diverse. In general they can be separated into coronary atherosclerotic and nonatherosclerotic causes, noncoronary cardiac disease, and noncardiac disorders (Figure 1). Acute coronary syndromes (see Chapter 10) are the most common cause in the adult experiencing sudden death. However, pulmonary, vascular, and central nervous system events occur in 15% to 30% of cases and are often

FAQ	Cardiac arrest is defined as cessation of cardiac mechanical activity, confirmed by
What is cardiac arrest?	- Absence of detectable pulse - Unresponsiveness - Apnea, or agonal, gasping respirations

unsuspected and underdiagnosed. An underlying condition may be the cause of the cardiac arrest and serve as a trigger for sudden death. For example, hypoxia due to many causes may exacerbate or cause coronary ischemia, resulting in cardiac arrest. The success of resuscitation and the ultimate outcome of patient survival in many instances depend on rapid identification and treatment of an underlying condition when possible. These concepts are discussed in detail in Part 2 of this text.

Deaths Due to Coronary Artery Disease

Atherosclerotic coronary artery disease is by far the most common condition associated with SCD. Predisposing risk factors closely parallel those for coronary disease in general. These include male sex, age, cigarette smoking, hypertension, hyperlipidemia, and left ventricular hypertrophy. In several studies smoking had a particularly strong relationship to the risk of sudden death.

It is difficult to accurately estimate the percentage of sudden deaths due to cardiac causes because many studies use the term *presumed cardiac etiology* in the absence of autopsy confirmation. In developed countries

the underlying cause of sudden death in the majority of cases is coronary artery disease. Autopsy studies have shown that 60% to 75% of SCDs are due to coronary artery disease (Figure 2) and acute coronary syndromes (Table 1); the remainder are largely due to cardiomyopathy and valvular heart disease. Most adult patients with sudden death have multivessel coronary disease, and they often have previous infarction as an associated finding even in the absence of prior history of myocardial infarction. The demographics of SCD are changing, and chronic congestive heart failure accounts for an increasing percentage of patients with sudden death. In these patients an old myocardial infarct can serve as a focus for electrical instability and cause fatal arrhythmias. One third of patients with congestive heart failure die from acute coronary syndromes, which are undiagnosed or underdiagnosed in patients dying suddenly.[3]

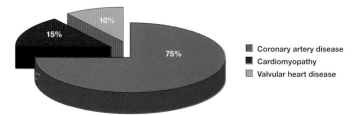

Figure 2. Major underlying etiologies of sudden cardiac death.

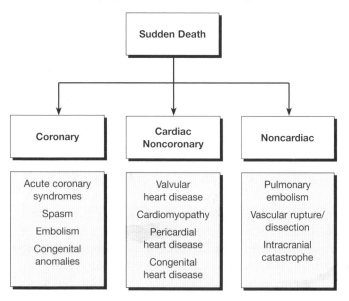

Figure 1. Classification of sudden death. Three general classes of sudden death occur. Those due to coronary heart disease are attributable largely to acute coronary syndromes. Others forms of cardiac noncoronary death occur. Hypertrophic obstructive cardiomyopathy is the most common cause in young adults. Several noncardiac causes are often unsuspected, including pulmonary embolism.

Cardiac Pathology	Clinical Syndrome (Examples)
Unstable plaque	Asymptomatic; acute coronary syndrome
Intraluminal occluding thrombus	Acute myocardial infarction
Old myocardial infarct(s)	CHF; ventricular arrhythmias
Dilated cardiomyopathy	Congestive heart failure

Table 1. Pathologic findings and clinical syndromes in sudden cardiac death. A ruptured or unstable coronary plaque is found in the majority of adults dying suddenly of cardiac causes. Chronic congestive heart failure accounts for an increasing percentage of patients with sudden death. In these patients an old myocardial infarct can serve as a focus for electrical instability, causing fatal arrhythmias.

<table>
<tr><td>FYI

Most Common Cause of SCD in Adults</td><td>A ruptured or unstable coronary plaque is found in the majority of adults who die suddenly of cardiac causes. Plaque rupture is the most common unstable plaque in the majority of patients. In others, plaque erosion occurs. Rarely, other causes such as a coronary spasm, embolism, and dissection occur.</td></tr>
</table>

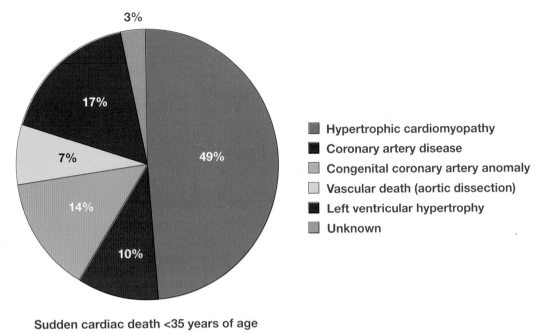

Sudden cardiac death <35 years of age

- Hypertrophic cardiomyopathy
- Coronary artery disease
- Congenital coronary artery anomaly
- Vascular death (aortic dissection)
- Left ventricular hypertrophy
- Unknown

Figure 3. Causes of sudden cardiac death in patients with identified structural heart disease. In this series hypertrophic cardiomyopathy accounted for the largest number of deaths in young persons.

Perhaps the most catastrophic presentation of SCD is in a child or healthy young adult. A review of the literature lists numerous causes for this tragedy, which fortunately is rare. Maron et al[4] were among the first to attempt to categorize the underlying etiologies (Figure 3). Hypertrophic cardiomyopathy, the presence of left ventricular hypertrophy, and congenital anomalies of the coronary arteries are found when a structural abnormality of the heart is identified. Other conditions, such as right ventricular dysplasia and idiopathic prolongation of the QT interval, have been defined and added to the growing list. In active young military recruits, an anomalous coronary artery and premature coronary artery disease were the most common causes of death when an identified cause was present. Myocarditis and hypertrophic cardiomyopathy were the next most common significant causes. Often no structural heart disease is found in women.[5,6] In young women and many patients without structural heart disease, cardiac arrhythmias, many with molecular etiologies, are thought to be the trigger for SCD.[7]

Strategies for Prevention and Treatment

A comprehensive strategy should be designed to modify risk factors, identify patients at high risk, and urgently treat patients with sudden death. Populations trained in cardiopulmonary resuscitation (CPR) and a highly skilled and rapidly responding emergency medical services (EMS) system are essential for survival of the patient with cardiac arrest. Survival, however, is low, and many patients have advanced disease at the time of cardiac arrest. A strategy for primary and secondary prevention must be part of any public health policy if long-term goals are to be realized. Patients at high risk of sudden death should be identified and survivors of sudden death extensively evaluated and treated as part of a postarrest management plan.

Primary Prevention

A major objective for decreasing mortality from sudden death is to reduce the incidence of coronary disease through measures targeted at decreasing risk factors for atherosclerosis and acute coronary syndromes. This is called primary prevention. Ultimately primary prevention has the greatest potential for epidemiologic curtailment of the disease. The major correctable risk factors are cigarette smoking, hypertension, hyperlipidemia, diabetes, and obesity. There is also evidence to implicate a sedentary lifestyle and lack of exercise as contributors to risk.

High-Risk Intervention

Many patients with known malignant arrhythmias, coronary artery disease, prior myocardial infarction, cardiomyopathy, and other structural heart diseases who are at very high risk for SCD can be identified. Modalities and treatment can now be individually applied to reduce the risk of a fatal coronary event. Coronary revascularization, targeted pharmacologic therapy, and automatic antitachycardia and defibrillatory devices are available for prevention and treatment of patients with sudden death syndromes.

The Chain of Survival

Who Has Survived?

Many living wills in effect today request that continued and extraordinary life support be limited or withheld if there is not a reasonable expectation that a patient can return to the prior state and quality of life. This ultimate goal is rarely witnessed by initial healthcare providers, who focus on surrogates for quality of life along a treacherous and complicated path to recovery. These intermediate goals are linked together, providing the maximum potential for patient quality of life. They include

- Return of spontaneous circulation (ROSC)
- Survival to hospital admission (for out-of-hospital arrest)
- Survival to hospital discharge neurologically intact

Evidence-based evaluation of clinical care and research often defines one of these intermediate goals as an end point. But it must be remembered that the goal of treatment is the patient's return to a reasonable functional state and quality of life acceptable to the patient and family.

ECC Chain of Survival

Emergency Cardiovascular Care

Emergency cardiovascular care (ECC) includes all responses necessary to deal with sudden and often life-threatening events affecting the cardiovascular, cerebrovascular, and pulmonary systems. ECC specifically includes

1. Recognition of the early warning signs of heart attack and stroke
2. Provision of immediate basic life support (BLS) at the scene when necessary

3. Provision of rapid advanced cardiovascular life support (ACLS) at the scene and treatment and stabilization en route to the emergency department (ED)
4. Transfer to a hospital where definitive care can be provided

Adult Chain of Survival

When cardiac arrest occurs, a series of events and critical interventions must occur as rapidly as possible to achieve the greatest potential for survival. If one critical action is neglected or delayed, survival is unlikely. These events are linked together in a chain of survival. They include

- Early recognition of the emergency and activation of EMS or the local emergency response system: "phone 911"
- Early bystander CPR
- Early delivery of a shock with a defibrillator
- Early advanced life support followed by postresuscitation care delivered by healthcare providers

Most patients with sudden cardiac arrest (SCA) demonstrate ventricular fibrillation (VF) at some point in their arrest, and resuscitation is most successful if defibrillation is performed within the first 5 minutes after collapse. Because the interval between a call to EMS and arrival of EMS personnel at the patient's side is typically longer than 5 minutes, achieving high survival rates depends on a public trained in CPR and on well-organized public access defibrillation programs. In this situation the most important link in the community is the layperson, who has the responsibility to activate the EMS system and initiate BLS. The best results of lay provider CPR programs have occurred in controlled environments with trained, motivated personnel and an automated external defibrillation program.[8,9]

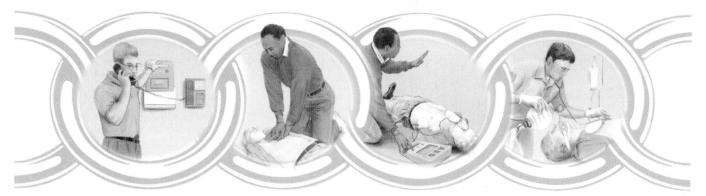

Figure 4. Links in the ECC Chain of Survival: early access to EMS, early CPR, early defibrillation, and early ACLS.

Critical Concept *Survival Goal for Cardiac Arrest*	• The goal in treating cardiac arrest is the patient's return to a prior normal functional state and survival neurologically intact with a quality of life acceptable to the patient and family. • Other goals achieved by the resuscitation team are intermediate goals and only surrogates for survival.

Foundation Facts

FIRST LINK

Early Access to EMS

Early recognition of the emergency and activation of the EMS or local emergency response system:

- *Phone 911 or activate the local emergency response system.*

The First Link: Early Access to EMS

Early access encompasses the events initiated after the patient's collapse until the arrival of EMS personnel prepared to provide care. Recognition of early warning signs, such as chest discomfort and shortness of breath, enables patients or bystanders to activate the emergency response system before collapse. This early recognition is the key component of the early access link.

The following events, each of which must occur rapidly, make up the early access link:

- Early identification of the patient's collapse or signs of emergency by someone who activates the system
- Rapid notification (usually by telephone) of the emergency medical dispatcher (EMD)
- Rapid recognition by the EMD of a potential cardiac arrest or emergency
- Immediate initiation of an EMS response (BLS-level and ACLS-level personnel respond simultaneously)
- Rapid directions, as needed, to guide EMS responders to the patient
- Determination by the EMD of the need for dispatcher instruction for CPR or defibrillation (see below)
- Rapid arrival of properly equipped EMS responders at the scene plus a short "interval to locate" and arrive at the patient's side
- Immediate assessment and management of the cardiac arrest

EMDs and the EMS System

Rapid emergency medical dispatch has emerged as a critical component of the early access link.[10] All EMS dispatch systems must be able to immediately answer all emergency medical calls, quickly determine the nature of the emergency, identify the nearest appropriate EMS responder unit, dispatch the unit to the scene in less than 1 minute on average, and provide critical information to EMS responders about the location and nature of the emergency.

Key Ingredient: Area-Wide, Dedicated Emergency Telephone Number

Use of a 3-digit dedicated emergency telephone number has simplified and shortened access to emergency assistance. Providing emergency response service through a dedicated number is highly recommended and should be a top priority for all communities. The 3 digits "911" are seldom used outside the United States. Websites are available for travelers to access international emergency numbers of more than 200 countries.

Sophisticated telecommunication systems make it possible for EMDs to identify the location and telephone number of the incoming call. Termed *enhanced 911* (E-911) in the United States, this feature requires a software and hardware upgrade. Cellular telephone calls to EMDs in some areas may pose a problem because the location of only the connecting cell tower can be identified. EMS systems can add features such as a global positioning system to telephone and cellular networks to enable tracking of calls from cellular phones. These systems have made rapid improvements in recent years, allowing expansion of rapid EMS dispatch.

Early Access by EMS Responders

EMS systems that implement a rapidly responding first tier of personnel trained to provide early defibrillation and a second tier of ACLS-level responders have consistently reported the highest rates of survival to hospital discharge.[11] The success or failure of the EMS responder system depends on 3 performance variables:

1. **Interval from activation of EMS units to arrival at the emergency premises.** Communities shorten this interval by adding response vehicles, placing response vehicles at strategic locations, and improving traffic paths. Multitiered systems seem to have the fastest response intervals because they have more first-responder units, usually consisting of firefighters, with or without advanced life support training. Communities that experience travel intervals greater than 5 to 6 minutes cannot meet the national goal to provide CPR and first shock within 5 minutes of the emergency call. Providing rapid EMS response in rural areas with smaller populations remains a challenge.

2. **Interval from arrival at the emergency premises to arrival at the patient's side (patient-location interval).** Few studies have reported the interval required to locate the patient, but locating the patient can be a source of significant delays to care in urban areas. Some EMS experts in large urban areas use the

term "vertical response time,"[12] which means delays such as waiting for elevators and climbing stairs.

3. **Early arrival with the proper range of ACLS skills and equipment.** The first responders involved in every EMS response to a possible cardiac arrest should be equipped with a defibrillator, oxygen, and proper airway management equipment.[13]

The Second Link: Early CPR

Many review articles have compiled results of studies that consistently confirm the value of bystander-initiated CPR started immediately after the patient's collapse.[14-16] The probability of survival to hospital discharge can double when bystanders initiate early CPR.[16]

Despite the value of early initiation of CPR by a trained layperson, no research has confirmed a method that increases the probability that a witness actually will start CPR. Randomized community intervention trials, such as sending out a short CPR training video, direct mail campaigns, home visits by nurses and CPR trainers, and targeting relatives of high-risk persons, do not seem to increase the likelihood that CPR will be performed or EMS will be called.

EMD-Assisted CPR

Dispatchers should receive appropriate training in providing prearrival CPR instructions to callers. Dispatcher CPR instructions increase the likelihood of bystander CPR being performed, but it is not clear if prearrival instructions increase the rate of survival from SCA.

In the late 1980s EMS leaders developed the highly successful concept of *prearrival instructions* that the EMD gives to the caller during a 911 call.[17] As the EMD learns more about the nature of the emergency, she offers advice or instructions to the caller about what to do until EMS responders arrive. This concept of prearrival instructions from trained EMDs has been embraced internationally, and improved outcomes have been documented.

Researchers from Seattle-King County, Washington, have developed and validated EMD-assisted CPR instructions.[18] Such EMD-assisted CPR instructions have been translated into more than 10 languages, and they are standard practice for EMD centers around the world in many international systems.

The Third Link: Early Defibrillation

Any community that can achieve earlier defibrillation may improve its rate of survival from cardiac arrest because early defibrillation is the only link in the Chain of Survival that is both necessary and can be sufficient (when the defibrillation results in ROSC).[19] The 3 links of early access, early CPR, and early ACLS cannot improve survival without early defibrillation in patients suffering from a VF cardiac arrest. In contrast, early defibrillation alone can achieve remarkable survival rates, as demonstrated by placement of automated external defibrillators (AEDs) in commercial airplanes,[20-22] gambling casinos,[23] and terminals of major airports.[22,24] When an AED or defibrillator is not immediately available, however (see below), a period of high-quality CPR may incrementally improve survival.

The Principle of Early Defibrillation

The principle of early defibrillation states that every emergency vehicle that responds to potential cardiac arrest patients or transports patients at risk for cardiac arrest should be equipped with a defibrillator and staffed with emergency personnel trained and permitted to use this device. The world's major resuscitation organizations, including the American Heart Association (AHA),[13,25-27] European Resuscitation Council,[28,29] and International Liaison Committee on Resuscitation,[30] have all endorsed this principle.

The widespread effectiveness and demonstrated safety of the AED have made it the defibrillator of choice for nonprofessional responders. Community lay rescuer AED programs, which place AEDs in the hands of nontraditional but trained providers, have improved rates of survival to hospital discharge among police departments,[31-35] on commercial aircraft,[20,22] and in casinos[23] and many other locations.[26,27] For more information on Community lay rescuer programs, see the AHA Scientific Statement, http://circ.ahajournals.org/cgi/reprint/CIRCULATIONAHA.106.172 289v1.

Reports of unsuccessful early defibrillation initiatives, by police in Indiana[36] and firefighters in Tennessee,[37] teach a valuable lesson. If personnel hesitate or fail to use their AED, survival will not increase.[38]

EMD-Assisted Defibrillation

Interest in public defibrillation programs and in-home use of AEDs by family and friends of patients at high risk for cardiac arrest has increased during the past several years. This interest has stimulated the intriguing question of EMD-assisted AED use. Research by Doherty et al[39] in Seattle-King County, Washington, has confirmed that dispatcher-assisted defibrillation can be achieved easily and implemented effectively across large EMS systems.

The "voice prompt" audio instructions that all AEDs provide has furnished the key to success. EMDs can take an AED orientation or course to become familiar with operation of an AED. Upon receiving a 911 call from a location that has an AED (information that is available to the EMD in areas with enhanced 911), the EMD instructs the caller to bring the AED and the telephone close to the patient. The dispatcher simply listens with the provider to the voice prompts of the AED, and together they work through the directions.

The Fourth Link: Early ACLS

Early ACLS provided by paramedics at the scene is another critical link in the management of cardiac arrest. EMS systems should have sufficient staff to provide at least one responder trained in ACLS. Because of the difficulties in treating cardiac arrest in the field, additional responders should be present when possible. In systems with survival rates of more than 20% for patients with VF, response teams usually have a minimum of 2 ACLS providers plus 2 BLS personnel at the scene.[40,41] Most experts agree that 4 responders (2 trained in ACLS and 2 trained in BLS) provide the most effective team for resuscitation of cardiac arrest patients. Although not every EMS system can attain this level of response, every system should actively pursue this goal. Typically in-hospital response teams have additional members on a "code" team. The ACLS course also emphasizes the major role of a team leader in the direction, coordination, and integration of good continued BLS (mainly high-quality uninterrupted chest compressions).

Strengthening the Links in the Chain of Survival

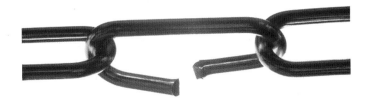

Team Leader and Team Concept

The ACLS Provider Course emphasizes the team concept and team leader. This important revision followed the identification of a critical need to integrate the links in the Chain of Survival, especially basic and advanced life support interventions. Correct priorities for basic and advanced life support are the responsibility of the team leader.

During cardiac arrest basic CPR and early defibrillation are of primary importance, and drug administration and placement of an advanced airway are of secondary importance. Few drugs used in the treatment of cardiac arrest are supported by strong evidence. After provision of CPR and early defibrillation, providers can establish intravenous access, consider drug therapy, and insert an advanced airway. Advanced life support interventions are performed with minimal interruption of CPR, especially chest compressions.

Foundation Facts **FOURTH LINK** **Early ACLS**	Early ACLS followed by postresuscitation care delivered by healthcare providers.

Foundation Facts **Minimal Interruption of Chest Compressions**	• During cardiac arrest basic CPR and early defibrillation are of primary importance, and drug administration is of secondary importance. • Advanced life support interventions are performed with minimal interruption of CPR, especially chest compressions.

Critical Concept **CPR BEFORE and AFTER Shock**	• When performed immediately after collapse from VF SCA, CPR can double or triple the patient's chance of survival. • When performed immediately after shock, CPR can convert nonperfusing to perfusing rhythms.

Integration of CPR and AED

CPR is important both before and after shock delivery. When performed immediately after collapse from VF SCA, CPR can double or triple the patient's chance of survival.[11,42] CPR should be provided until an AED or manual defibrillator is available. After about 5 minutes of VF with no treatment, outcome may be better if shock delivery (attempted defibrillation) is preceded by a period of CPR with effective chest compressions that deliver some blood to the coronary arteries and brain.[43,44] CPR is also important immediately after shock delivery. Many patients demonstrate asystole or pulseless electrical activity for several minutes after defibrillation, and CPR can convert these rhythms to a perfusing rhythm.[45]

Integration of CPR and Drug Administration

There is no longer emphasis on the need to follow each drug with a period of CPR or to assess rhythm before drug administration. Drugs may be administered during the rhythm check, but the timing of drug delivery is less important than the need to minimize interruptions in chest compressions. The drug can be administered while the rhythm is checked, immediately before shock delivery, in a Drug–Rhythm Check/Shock–CPR sequence (repeated as needed). The previous recommendations resulted in too many interruptions in chest compressions.

Rhythm checks when performed should be very brief. If a drug is administered during the rhythm check (or immediately before—or after—a shock), it will be circulated by the CPR that immediately follows the shock. After drug delivery and 5 cycles (about 2 minutes) of CPR, analyze the rhythm and be prepared to deliver another shock immediately if indicated.

Integration of CPR and Advanced Airway

Insertion of an advanced airway may interrupt CPR for prolonged periods. Providers must be aware of the risks and benefits of insertion of an advanced airway during a resuscitation attempt. Because insertion of an advanced airway may require interruption of chest compressions for many seconds, the provider should weigh the need for compressions against the need for an advanced airway. The risks and benefits are affected by the condition of the patient and the provider's expertise in airway control. If adequate ventilations are being provided by bag-mask ventilation, there is no urgency to place an advanced airway. Specifically, placement of an advanced airway is no longer viewed as a "routine" early task of the resuscitation team. Providers may defer insertion of an advanced airway until the patient fails to respond to initial CPR and defibrillation attempts or demonstrates ROSC.

FAQ **Why is there no rhythm check before drug administration?**	• Drugs may be administered during the rhythm check, but the timing of drug delivery is less important than the need to minimize interruptions in chest compressions. • After a shock almost all patients have a nonperfusing rhythm requiring a period of chest compressions. • Almost all patients have persistent VF or a nonperfusing rhythm after a shock is administered. A pulse or rhythm check in these cases provides no additional information and only delays resumption of high-quality chest compressions.

FYI **Guidelines 2005**	Providers may defer insertion of an advanced airway until **1.** The patient fails to respond to initial CPR and defibrillation attempts or **2.** Demonstrates ROSC
FAQ **When is an advanced airway inserted or required?**	• The provider should weigh the need for compressions against the need for an advanced airway • The risks and benefits are affected by – The condition of the patient – The provider's expertise in airway control – The ability to ventilate the patient with a bag-mask device

The In-Hospital Chain of Survival

The Chain of Survival has been a successful metaphor for analysis of out-of-hospital cardiac arrest, and it applies well to in-hospital cardiac arrest. The 4 links have features for in-hospital cardiac arrest that are analogous to those for an out-of-hospital emergency. The in-hospital early access link involves witnessing an emergency and activating the in-hospital response system. The in-hospital early CPR link is fulfilled at once, often by the witness or by the many other personnel who arrive in response to the emergency. The in-hospital early ACLS link is provided by the code team, the personnel who arrive from various locations after being summoned by a hospitalwide loudspeaker announcement or by radio-controlled pager.

Early defibrillation, however, has turned out to be a weak link and a significant problem for many hospitals. Some hospitals have been reluctant to acquire AEDs for in-hospital use.[46,47] This reluctance has led to collapse-to–first shock intervals in some larger hospitals as long as those seen in out-of-hospital settings.[47]

Important Additional Links in the Chain of Survival

Remember, survival is return of the patient to a prior state or acceptable quality of life. Prevention of cardiac arrest is the primary goal when possible. In addition, resuscitation of the patient does not end with successful termination of cardiac arrest, spontaneous return of circulation, or admission to the ED or critical care unit. Horizontal integration of 2 other links complete the chain at the beginning and end, defining comprehensive and optimal patient care.

Medical Emergency Teams and Rapid Response System

In hospital many patients have prodromal or warning signs and symptoms before actual cardiac or pulmonary arrest. Ideally prevention of a cardiac arrest before it occurs and treatment of the underlying condition will produce the best outcome. Many hospitals have created rapid response teams (RRTs) and medical emergency teams (METs) within a rapid response system (RRS) to quickly respond to patients at risk for cardiopulmonary arrest. METs studied so far usually consist of a physician and nurse with critical care experience. The team is available at all times, with nurses and other hospital staff available to activate the team based on specific criteria following implementation of an education and awareness program. In some studies a reduction or trend toward fewer cardiac arrests and intensive care unit (ICU) admissions has been observed.[48,49] One study in 23 hospitals, however, found no difference in a composite end point of cardiac arrest, unexpected death, and unplanned ICU admission.[50] Further research is needed to define the critical details of implementation, effectiveness, and intervention for METs and RRSs.

Postarrest Care and Continuing Resuscitation to Survival

Postarrest care has significant potential to decrease early mortality caused by hemodynamic instability and multiorgan failure and later mortality or morbidity resulting from brain injury. This section summarizes our evolving understanding of the hemodynamic, neurologic, and metabolic abnormalities encountered in patients who are resuscitated from cardiac arrest.

The initial objectives of postarrest care are to

- Optimize cardiopulmonary function and systemic perfusion, especially perfusion to the brain
- Transport the patient with out-of-hospital cardiac arrest to the hospital ED and continue care in an appropriately equipped critical care unit
- Try to identify the precipitating causes of the arrest
- Institute measures to prevent recurrence
- Institute measures that may improve long-term, neurologically intact survival

Closing the Links

The Challenge for Every Community and Every Hospital: How to Improve Survival

Quality Assessment, Review, and Translational Science

Every EMS system and hospital should perform continuous quality improvement (CQI) and assess their resuscitation interventions and outcomes through a defined process of data collection and review. There is now widespread consensus that the best way to improve either community or in-hospital survival from SCA is to start with the standard "quality-improvement model" and then modify that model according to the Chain of Survival metaphor. Each link in the chain comprises structural, process, and outcome variables that can be examined, measured, and recorded. System managers can quickly identify gaps that exist between observed processes and outcomes and local expectations or published "gold standards."

The National Registry of Cardiopulmonary Resuscitation

To prevent or intervene successfully in cardiac arrest, more data about in-hospital arrests is needed. In addition, in-hospital quality assurance systems require ongoing assessment of process and outcome for cardiac arrest. To aid and accomplish this effort, the AHA ECC Programs established a task force to develop the National Registry of Cardiopulmonary Resuscitation (NRCPR). The NRCPR program supports individual hospitals in conducting review, quality-assurance, and quality-improvement projects relating to resuscitation in the individual hospital. Today the registry is the largest repository of information on in-hospital cardiopulmonary arrest and has published initial findings.[51] The registry has great practical value for establishing the resuscitation performance level for an individual hospital. That step can be followed by projects to improve the quality of resuscitation attempts and increase survival. In addition, the NRCPR database allows researchers to query HIPPA-compliant aggregated data to answer investigator-initiated research questions. This database has resulted in

defining important outcomes and benchmarks for clinical care and research initiatives. Examples of current NRCPR-related publications are

- Survival From In-Hospital Cardiac Arrest During Nights and Weekends. *JAMA.* 2008; 299:785-792. Mary Ann Peberdy, Joseph P Ornato, G Luke Larkin, R Scott Braithwaite, T Michael Kashner, Scott M Carey, Peter A Meaney, Liyi Cen, Vinay Nadkarni, Amy Praestgaard, Robert A. Berg for the NRCPR Investigators.

- Delayed Time to Defibrillation and Survival After In-Hospital Cardiac Arrest. *N Engl J Med.* 2008; 358:9-17. Paul S Chan, Harlan M Krumholz, Graham Nichol, Noah Jones, Brahmajee K Nallamothu, for the National Registry of Cardiopulmonary Resuscitation Investigators.

- Increasing Amiodarone Use in Cardiopulmonary Resuscitation: An Analysis of the National Registry of Cardiopulmonary Resuscitiaton. *Crit Care Med* 2008; 36:126-130. Tessie W October, Charles L Schleien, Robert A Berg, Vinay M Nadkarni, Marilyn C Morris; for the National Registry of Cardiopulmonary Resuscitation Investigators.

- Higher survival rates among younger patients after pediatric intensive care unit cardiac arrests. *Pediatrics.* 2006;118:2424-2433. Peter Meaney, Vinay Nadkarni, E F Cook, Marcia Testa, Mark Helfaer, William Kaye, Gregory Larkin, Robert Berg, for the American Heart Association National Registry of Cardiopulmonary Resuscitation Investigators.

- Effect of hospital characteristics on outcomes from pediatric cardiopulmonary resuscitation: a report from the National Registry of Cardiopulmonary Resuscitation. *Pediatrics.* 2006;118:995-1001. Aaron J Donoghue, Vinay Nadkarni, Michael Elliott, Dennis Durbin, for the American Heart Association National Registry of Cardiopulmonary Resuscitation Investigators.

- Outcomes of in-hospital ventricular fibrillation in children. *N Engl J Med.* 2006;354:2328-2339. Ricardo A Samson, Vinay M Nadkarni, Peter A Meaney, Scott M Carey, Marc D Berg, and Robert A Berg, for the

Critical Concept **Postarrest Resuscitation**	Resuscitation does not end with ROSC. Continued resuscitation, identification and treatment of the precipitating cause, and management of postarrest complications are crucial for successful outcome and rehabilitation of the patient.
FYI **Guidelines 2005**	Participants in the 2005 Consensus Conference strongly endorsed the position that all ECC systems should assess their performance through ongoing evaluation.

American Heart Association National Registry of Cardiopulmonary Resuscitation Investigators.

- First documented rhythm and clinical outcome from in-hospital cardiac arrest among children and adults. *JAMA.* 2006;295:50-57. Vinay Nadkarni, Gregory Larkin, Mary Ann Peberdy, Scott Carey, William Kaye, Mary Elizabeth Mancini, Graham Nichol, Tanya Lane-Truitt, Jerry Potts, Joseph Ornato, Robert A Berg, for the National Registry of Cardiopulmonary Resuscitation Investigators.

- When minutes count—the fallacy of accurate time documentation during in-hospital resuscitation. *Resuscitation.* 2005;65:285-290. William Kaye, Mary E Mancini, Tanya L Truitt.

- Cardiopulmonary resuscitation of adults in the hospital: a report of 14,720 cardiac arrests from the National Registry of Cardiopulmonary Resuscitation.

Resuscitation. 2003;58:297-308. Mary Ann Peberdy, William Kaye, Joseph P Ornato, Gregory L Larkin, Vinay Nadkarni, Mary Elizabeth Mancini, Robert A Berg, Graham Nichol, Tanya Lane-Truitt.

Translational Science—Bench to Bedside

Evidence-based guidelines are derived from a basic and clinical research structure designed to ask and investigate questions to improve clinical outcome. Many of these questions are initially investigated in the laboratory and then in well-designed clinical trials. This ongoing investigative process is part of the continual process that improves recommendations and eventually clinical outcome in an ongoing process (Figure 5). This process generates evidence that is reviewed by experts (Table 2) and then assigned a class of recommendation (Table 3). Periodically new evidence is reviewed and recommendations are updated.

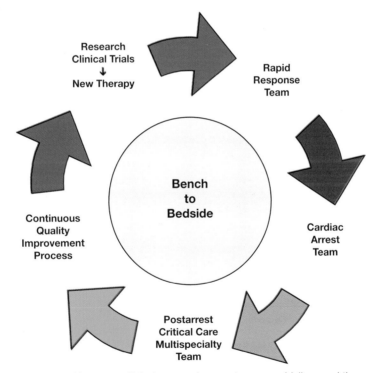

Figure 5. A continuous process evaluates and improves clinical care and generates new guidelines and therapy. Outcome data from cardiac arrest and periarrest periods is reviewed in a continuous quality-improvement process. Research and clinical initiatives are periodically reviewed in an evidence-based process. Experts then evaluate new therapy and make clinical and educational recommendations for patient care. The process is repeated and continual progress and improvement in care is generated.

FAQ **Why do guidelines and recommendations constantly change?**	An ongoing investigative process continually looks for interventions and strategies to improve outcome from cardiac arrest and emergency cardiovascular care. When some questions are answered, new ones may be generated. A process of evidence review and recommendations by international experts integrates science into treatment algorithms and strategies in a process of continuous quality improvement.

Table 2. Levels of Evidence

Evidence	Definition
Level 1	Randomized clinical trials or meta-analyses of multiple clinical trials with substantial treatment effects
Level 2	Randomized clinical trials with smaller or less significant treatment effects
Level 3	Prospective, controlled, nonrandomized cohort studies
Level 4	Historic, nonrandomized cohort or case-control studies
Level 5	Case series; patients compiled in serial fashion, control group lacking
Level 6	Animal studies or mechanical model studies
Level 7	Extrapolations from existing data collected for other purposes, theoretical analyses
Level 8	Rational conjecture (common sense); common practices accepted before evidence-based guidelines

Table 3. Applying Classification of Recommendations and Level of Evidence

Class I	Class IIa	Class IIb	Class III
Benefit >>> Risk	Benefit >> Risk	Benefit ≥ Risk	Risk ≥ Benefit
Procedure/treatment or diagnostic test/assessment should be performed/administered.	It is reasonable to perform procedure/administer treatment or perform diagnostic test/assessment.	Procedure/treatment or diagnostic test/assessment may be considered.	Procedure/treatment or diagnostic test/assessment should not be performed/administered. It is not helpful and may be harmful.

Class Indeterminate:
- Research just getting started
- Continuing area of research
- No recommendations until further research (eg, cannot recommend for or against)

References

1. Fox CS, Evans JC, Larson MG, Kannel WB, Levy D. Temporal trends in coronary heart disease mortality and sudden cardiac death from 1950 to 1999: the Framingham Heart Study. *Circulation*. 2004;110:522-527.

2. Cummins RO, Chamberlain DA, Abramson NS, Allen M, Baskett PJ, Becker L, Bossaert L, Delooz HH, Dick WF, Eisenberg MS, et al. Recommended guidelines for uniform reporting of data from out-of-hospital cardiac arrest: the Utstein style. A statement for health professionals from a task force of the American Heart Association, the European Resuscitation Council, the Heart and Stroke Foundation of Canada, and the Australian Resuscitation Council. *Circulation*. 1991;84:960-975.

3. Uretsky BF, Thygesen K, Armstrong PW, Cleland JG, Horowitz JD, Massie BM, Packer M, Poole-Wilson PA, Ryden L. Acute coronary findings at autopsy in heart failure patients with sudden death: results from the assessment of treatment with lisinopril and survival (ATLAS) trial. *Circulation*. 2000;102:611-616.

4. Maron BJ, Roberts WC, McAllister HA, Rosing DR, Epstein SE. Sudden death in young athletes. *Circulation*. 1980;62:218-229.

5. Eckart RE, Scoville SL, Shry EA, Potter RN, Tedrow U. Causes of sudden death in young female military recruits. *Am J Cardiol*. 2006;97:1756-1758.

6. Eckart RE, Scoville SL, Campbell CL, Shry EA, Stajduhar KC, Potter RN, Pearse LA, Virmani R. Sudden death in young adults: a 25-year review of autopsies in military recruits. *Ann Intern Med*. 2004;141:829-834.

7. Wever EF, Robles de Medina EO. Sudden death in patients without structural heart disease. *J Am Coll Cardiol*. 2004;43:1137-1144.

8. Caffrey SL, Willoughby PJ, Pepe PE, Becker LB. Public use of automated external defibrillators. *N Engl J Med*. 2002;347:1242-1247.

9. The Public Access Defibrillation Trial Investigators. Public-access defibrillation and survival after out-of-hospital cardiac arrest. *N Engl J Med*. 2004;351:637-646.

10. Clawson JJ. Emergency medical dispatching. In: Roush WR, Aranosian RD, Blair TMH, Handal KA, Kellow RC, Steward RD, eds. *Principles of EMS Systems*. Dallas, Tex: American College of Emergency Physicians; 1989:119-133.

11. Valenzuela TD, Roe DJ, Cretin S, Spaite DW, Larsen MP. Estimating effectiveness of cardiac arrest interventions: a logistic regression survival model. *Circulation*. 1997;96:3308-3313.

12. Becker LB, Ostrander MP, Barrett J, Kondos GT. Outcome of CPR in a large metropolitan area—where are the survivors? *Ann Emerg Med*. 1991;20:355-361.

13. Kerber RE. Statement on early defibrillation from the Emergency Cardiac Care Committee, American Heart Association. *Circulation*. 1991;83:2233.

14. Holmberg M, Holmberg S, Herlitz J. Effect of bystander cardiopulmonary resuscitation in out-of-hospital cardiac arrest patients in Sweden. *Resuscitation*. 2000;47:59-70.

15. Gallagher EJ, Lombardi G, Gennis P. Effectiveness of bystander cardiopulmonary resuscitation and survival following out-of-hospital cardiac arrest. *JAMA*. 1995;274:1922-1925.

16. Larsen MP, Eisenberg MS, Cummins RO, Hallstrom AP. Predicting survival from out-of-hospital cardiac arrest: a graphic model. *Ann Emerg Med*. 1993;22:1652-1658.

17. Carter WB, Eisenberg MS, Hallstrom AP, Schaeffer S. Development and implementation of emergency CPR instruction via telephone. *Ann Emerg Med*. 1984;13(pt 1): 695-700.

18. Eisenberg MS, Cummins RO, Litwin P, Hallstrom AP, Hearne T. Dispatcher cardiopulmonary resuscitation instruction via telephone. *Crit Care Med*. 1985;13:923-924.

19. Cummins RO, Ornato JP, Thies WH, Pepe PE. Improving survival from sudden cardiac arrest: the "chain of survival" concept. A statement for health professionals from the Advanced Cardiac Life Support Subcommittee and the Emergency Cardiac Care Committee, American Heart Association. *Circulation*. 1991;83:1832-1847.

20. O'Rourke MF, Donaldson E, Geddes JS. An airline cardiac arrest program. *Circulation*. 1997;96:2849-2853.

21. Page RL, Hamdan MH, McKenas DK. Defibrillation aboard a commercial aircraft. *Circulation*. 1998;97:1429-1430.

22. Page RL, Joglar JA, Kowal RC, Zagrodzky JD, Nelson LL, Ramaswamy K, Barbera SJ, Hamdan MH, McKenas DK. Use of automated external defibrillators by a US airline. *N Engl J Med*. 2000;343:1210-1216.

23. Valenzuela TD, Roe DJ, Nichol G, Clark LL, Spaite DW, Hardman RG. Outcomes of rapid defibrillation by security officers after cardiac arrest in casinos. *N Engl J Med*. 2000;343:1206-1209.

24. Robertson RM. Sudden death from cardiac arrest—improving the odds. *N Engl J of Med*. 2000;343: 1259-1260.

25. Cobb LA, Eliastam M, Kerber RE, Melker R, Moss AJ, Newell L, Paraskos JA, Weaver WD, Weil M, Weisfeldt ML. Report of the American Heart Association Task Force on the Future of Cardiopulmonary Resuscitation. *Circulation*. 1992;85: 2346-2355.

26. Nichol G, Hallstrom AP, Kerber R, Moss AJ, Ornato JP, Palmer D, Riegel B, Smith S Jr, Weisfeldt ML. American Heart Association report on the second public access defibrillation conference, April 17-19, 1997. *Circulation*. 1998;97:1309-1314.

27. Weisfeldt ML, Kerber RE, McGoldrick RP, Moss AJ, Nichol G, Ornato JP, Palmer DG, Riegel B, Smith SC. American Heart Association report on the Public Access Defibrillation Conference, December 8-10, 1994. Automatic External Defibrillation Task Force. *Circulation*. 1995;92:2740-2747.

28. Bossaert L, Callanan V, Cummins RO, Kloeck W, Chamberlain D, Carli P, Christenson J, Connolly B, Ornato J, Sanders A, Steen P. Early defibrillation: an advisory statement by the Advanced Life Support Working Group of the International Liaison Committee on Resuscitation. *Resuscitation*. 1997;34:113-114.

29. Bossaert L, Handley A, Marsden A, Arntz R, Chamberlain D, Ekstrom L, Evans T, Monsieurs K, Robertson C, Steen P. European Resuscitation Council guidelines for the use of automated external defibrillators by EMS providers and first responders: a statement from the Early Defibrillation Task Force, with contributions from the Working Groups on Basic and Advanced Life Support, and approved by the Executive Committee. *Resuscitation*. 1998;37:91-94.

30. Kloeck W, Cummins RO, Chamberlain D, Bossaert L, Callanan V, Carli P, Christenson J, Connolly B, Ornato JP, Sanders A, Steen P. Early defibrillation: an advisory statement from the Advanced Life Support Working Group of the International Liaison Committee on Resuscitation. *Circulation*. 1997;95:2183-2184.

31. White RD, Hankins DG, Bugliosi TF. Seven years' experience with early defibrillation by police and paramedics in an emergency medical services system. *Resuscitation*. 1998;39:145-151.

32. White RD, Asplin BR, Bugliosi TF, Hankins DG. High discharge survival rate after out-of-hospital ventricular fibrillation with rapid defibrillation by police and paramedics. *Ann Emerg Med*. 1996;28:480-485.

33. White RD, Vukov LF, Bugliosi TF. Early defibrillation by police: initial experience with measurement of critical time intervals and patient outcome. *Ann Emerg Med*. 1994;23:1009-1013.

34. Mosesso VN Jr, Davis EA, Auble TE, Paris PM, Yealy DM. Use of automated external defibrillators by police officers for treatment of out-of-hospital cardiac arrest. *Ann Emerg Med*. 1998;32:200-207.

35. Davis EA, Mosesso VN Jr. Performance of police first responders in utilizing automated external defibrillation on victims of sudden cardiac arrest. *Prehosp Emerg Care*. 1998;2:101-107.

36. Groh WJ, Newman MM, Beal PE, Fineberg NS, Zipes DP. Limited response to cardiac arrest by police equipped with automated external defibrillators: lack of survival benefit in suburban and rural Indiana—the police as responder automated defibrillation evaluation (PARADE). *Acad Emerg Med*. 2001;8:324-330.

37. Kellermann AL, Hackman BB, Somes G, Kreth TK, Nail L, Dobyns P. Impact of first-responder defibrillation in an urban emergency medical services system. *JAMA*. 1993;270: 1708-1713.

38. Sweeney TA, Runge JW, Gibbs MA, Raymond JM, Schafermeyer RW, Norton HJ, Boyle-Whitesel MJ. EMT defibrillation does not increase survival from sudden cardiac death in a two-tiered urban-suburban EMS system. *Ann Emerg Med*. 1998;31:234-240.

39. Doherty A, Damon S, Hein K, Cummins RO. Evaluation of CPR prompt and home learning system for teaching CPR to lay rescuers. *Circulation*. 1998;98(suppl I):I-410.

40. Jacobs I, Callanan V, Nichol G, Valenzuela T, Mason P, Jaffe AS, Landau W, Vetter N. The chain of survival. *Ann Emerg Med*. 2001;37(4 suppl):S5-S16.

41. Pepe PE, Bonnin MJ, Mattox KL. Regulating the scope of EMS. *Prehosp Disaster Med*. 1990;5:59-63.

42. Holmberg M, Holmberg S, Herlitz J, Gardelov B. Survival after cardiac arrest outside hospital in Sweden. Swedish Cardiac Arrest Registry. *Resuscitation*. 1998;36:29-36.

43. Cobb LA, Fahrenbruch CE, Walsh TR, Copass MK, Olsufka M, Breskin M, Hallstrom AP. Influence of cardiopulmonary resuscitation prior to defibrillation in patients with out-of-hospital ventricular fibrillation. *JAMA*. 1999;281:1182-1188.

44. Wik L, Hansen TB, Fylling F, Steen T, Vaagenes P, Auestad BH, Steen PA. Delaying defibrillation to give basic cardiopulmonary resuscitation to patients with out-of-hospital ventricular fibrillation: a randomized trial. *JAMA*. 2003;289:1389-1395.

45. Carpenter J, Rea TD, Murray JA, Kudenchuk PJ, Eisenberg MS. Defibrillation waveform and post-shock rhythm in out-of-hospital ventricular fibrillation cardiac arrest. *Resuscitation*. 2003;59:189-196.

46. Kaye W, Mancini ME, Giuliano KK, Richards N, Nagid DM, Marler CA, Sawyer-Silva S. Strengthening the in-hospital chain of survival with rapid defibrillation by first responders using

automated external defibrillators: training and retention issues. *Ann Emerg Med*. 1995;25:163-168.

47. Kaye W, Mancini ME. Improving outcome from cardiac arrest in the hospital with a reorganized and strengthened chain of survival: an American view. *Resuscitation*. 1996;31:181-186.

48. Bellomo R, Goldsmith D, Uchino S, Buckmaster J, Hart G, Opdam H, Silvester W, Doolan L, Gutteridge G. Prospective controlled trial of effect of medical emergency team on postoperative morbidity and mortality rates. *Crit Care Med*. 2004;32:916-921.

49. Buist MD, Moore GE, Bernard SA, Waxman BP, Anderson JN, Nguyen TV. Effects of a medical emergency team on reduction of incidence of and mortality from unexpected cardiac arrests in hospital: preliminary study. *BMJ*. 2002;324:387-390.

50. The MERIT study investigators. Introduction of the medical emergency team (MET) system: a cluster-randomised controlled trial. *Lancet*. 2005;365:2091-2097.

51. Peberdy MA, Kaye W, Ornato JP, Larkin GL, Nadkarni V, Mancini ME, Berg RA, Nichol G, Lane-Trultt T. Cardiopulmonary resuscitation of adults in the hospital: a report of 14720 cardiac arrests from the National Registry of Cardiopulmonary Resuscitation. *Resuscitation*. 2003; 58:297-308.

Chapter 3

Defibrillation

This Chapter

- **Shocking for life**
- **It is not just electricity—phases of cardiac arrest**
- **CPR first or shock first for best survival**
- **How defibrillators work if you need to know**

Defibrillation involves the delivery of electrical current through the chest and heart to depolarize myocardial cells and eliminate ventricular fibrillation (VF). The technique of delivering electrical current to the heart to terminate arrhythmias dates to Kouwenhoven, Zoll, and Lown over one-half century ago.[1] Initially the use of defibrillators was restricted to the operating suite. Now these devices are found in virtually all emergency medical services (EMS) systems and many large public buildings, and they can be used with minimal training. Defibrillation is a critical component of the Chain of Survival. But the use of a defibrillator alone does not guarantee success or survival.

Principle of Defibrillation

Definition

Ventricular fibrillation is the rhythm most often associated with survival. Time to defibrillation is critical and a major determinant of the outcome of resuscitation attempts. A defibrillator is a device that administers a controlled electrical shock to patients to terminate a cardiac arrhythmia, usually VF. Defibrillators are also used to terminate pulseless ventricular tachycardia (VT).

The technique of administering the electrical shock is usually referred to as *defibrillation* if the shock is used to successfully terminate VF. Defibrillators can be synchronized to an organized rhythm for shock delivery to perform *cardioversion* (eg, for atrial fibrillation, atrial flutter, or stable VT with pulses), and some then use the term *cardioverters*. Until recently all shocks were delivered externally, but now a device that can pace and perform defibrillation or cardioversion can be implanted in high-risk patients. These devices are called *automated implantable cardioverter/defibrillators*—or *AICDs* for short.

Defibrillatory shocks deliver massive amounts of electrical energy almost instantaneously over a few milliseconds. Passing between positive and negative defibrillatory paddles pressed against the chest or between adhesive pads placed on the chest, this electrical energy flows through the interposed, fibrillating heart (Figure 1). The split-second flow of current does not "jump-start" the heart. Instead the current flow totally depolarizes, or *stuns*, the entire myocardium, producing complete electrical silence, or *asystole*. This brief period of electrical silence allows

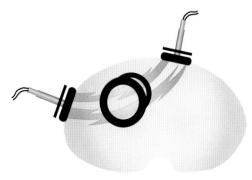

Figure 1. Current pathway through the chest and heart with placement of paddles (or pads) for defibrillation. Reproduced with permission from Ewy GA, Bressler R, eds. *Cardiovascular Drugs and the Management of Heart Disease*. New York, NY: Raven Press; 1982.[2]

<table>
<tr><td>

Foundation Facts

Time to Defibrillation: A Major and Critical Determinant of Survival

</td><td>

Ventricular fibrillation is the cardiac arrest rhythm most often associated with survival. Time to defibrillation is critical and a major determinant of the outcome of resuscitation attempts. But the use of a defibrillator alone does not guarantee success or survival.

• Integration of defibrillation with CPR, especially chest compressions, is crucial.

</td></tr>
</table>

<table>
<tr><td>

Critical Concept

</td><td>

The most critical interventions during the first minutes of VF or pulseless VT are immediate CPR with minimal interruption in chest compressions and defibrillation as soon as it can be accomplished.

</td></tr>
</table>

spontaneously repolarizing *pacemaking* cells within the heart to recover. The regular cycles of repolarization/depolarization of these pacemaker cells allow coordinated contractile activity to resume if the cells are not stunned or damaged.

Recipe for Success and Survival

The Scientific Evidence for Early Defibrillation

The most critical interventions during the first minutes of VF or pulseless VT are immediate CPR with minimal interruption in chest compressions and defibrillation as soon as it can be accomplished. A significant body of research supports the concept that defibrillation must be performed as early as possible for adult patients with sudden cardiac arrest (SCA):

• The most frequent initial rhythm in SCA is VF.

• The treatment for VF is electrical defibrillation.

• The probability of successful resuscitation diminishes rapidly as time to defibrillation increases.

• VF tends to convert to permanent asystole within a few minutes.

Evidence: Survival Before and After Early Defibrillation Programs

In the 1980s communities with no out-of-hospital ACLS services and defibrillation programs began to perform "before-and-after" studies. EMS systems invariably reported improved survival rates for cardiac arrest patients when the community added *any* type of program that resulted in earlier defibrillation (Table 1). Impressive results were reported from early studies in King County, Washington, where the odds ratio for improved survival (comparing the odds of survival after versus before the addition of an early defibrillation program) was 3.7,[3] and rural Iowa, where the odds ratio was 6.3.[4] That is, a person was about 4 to 6 times more likely to survive a VF arrest after institution of an early defibrillation program.

Evidence continued to accumulate during the 1980s; investigators reported positive odds ratios for improved survival of 4.3 in rural communities of southeastern Minnesota,[5] 5.0 in northeastern Minnesota,[6] and 3.3 in Wisconsin.[7]

When the survival rates were examined by the type of system deployed across larger geographic areas, that

Table 1. Effectiveness of Early Defibrillation Programs by Community

Location	% Survival Before Early Defibrillation		% Survival After Early Defibrillation		Odds Ratio for Improved Survival
King County, Wash	7	(4/56)	26	(10/38)	3.7
Iowa	3	(1/31)	19	(12/64)	6.3
Southeast Minnesota	4	(1/27)	17	(6/36)	4.3
Northeast Minnesota	2	(3/118)	10	(8/81)	5.0
Wisconsin	4	(32/893)	11	(33/304)	3.3

Values are percent surviving and, in parentheses, how many patients had ventricular fibrillation. Reproduced from Cummins.[8]

Table 2. Survival to Hospital Discharge From Cardiac Arrest by System Type: Data From 29 Locations*

System Type	Survival: All Rhythms (%)	Weighted Average (%)	Survival: Ventricular Fibrillation (%)	Weighted Average (%)
EMT only	2-9	5	3-20	12
EMT-D	4-19	10	6-26	16
Paramedic	7-18	10	13-30	17
EMT/paramedic	4-26	17	23-33	26
EMT-D/paramedic	13-18	17	27-29	29

*Values are the range of survival rates for all rhythms and ventricular fibrillation and the weighted average of each range. EMT indicates emergency medical technician; EMT-D, emergency medical technician-defibrilation. Reproduced from Eisenberg et al.[9]

same pattern emerged: the system organized to get the defibrillator there the fastest—independent of the arrival of personnel to perform endotracheal intubation and provide intravenous (IV) medications—achieved better survival rates (Table 2). If early defibrillation was combined with early advanced airway placement and IV medications, survival rates were even higher.

By the end of the 1980s evidence had confirmed the importance of each link in the Chain of Survival. Figure 2 illustrates this concept in a different way. The figure gives general estimates of survival among patients who receive different interventions ("links in the chain") at different intervals. Figure 2A shows what happens when the patient receives no CPR and delayed defibrillation is provided 10 minutes after collapse. A dismal survival rate of 0% to 2% is all that can be expected. Figure 2B shows an

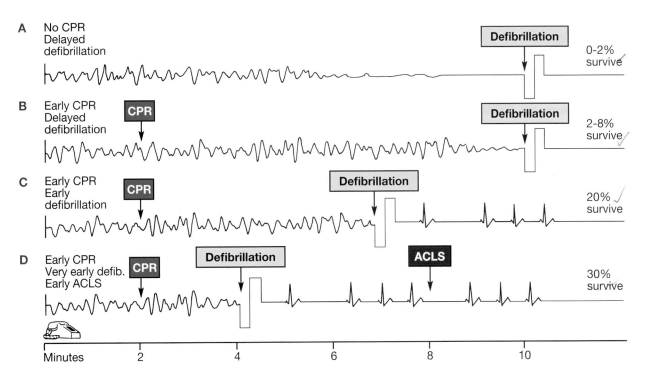

Figure 2. Estimated rates of survival to hospital discharge for patients with witnessed ventricular fibrillation arrest based on presence or absence of Chain of Survival links. **A**, No bystander CPR; defibrillation performed by advanced life support personnel, who arrive 10 minutes after call to 911. **B**, Bystander CPR at 2 minutes; defibrillation at 10 minutes after call to 911. **C**, Bystander CPR at 2 minutes; defibrillation at 7 minutes after call to 911 by emergency medical technicians-defibrillation. **D**, Bystander CPR at 2 minutes; public access defibrillation at 4 minutes after call to 911; ACLS interventions start at 8 minutes. Estimates are based on a large number of published studies, which are collectively reviewed by Eisenberg et al.[9,10]

The major determinant of survival in early studies was the interval between collapse and delivery of the first shock.

• It is now well established that the earlier defibrillation occurs, the better the prognosis.

improvement in survival to 2% to 8% because a witness started CPR 2 minutes after collapse, but early defibrillation was still missing. Figure 2C shows a jump in survival to 20% because the witness who called 911 started CPR and because this particular community had an early defibrillation program that delivered the first shock at 6 to 7 minutes. Figure 2D demonstrates what can occur with a very early public defibrillation program. The witness calls 911, starts CPR, and delivers the first shock, using an automated external defibrillator (AED), at 4 to 5 minutes.

Some EMS systems organized in this manner have reported survival rates as high as 30%, and studies of lay provider AED programs in airports and casinos and first-responder programs with police officers have demonstrated 49% to 74% survival from out-of-hospital witnessed VF SCA when immediate bystander CPR is provided and defibrillation occurs within 3 to 5 minutes of collapse. These high survival rates, however, are not attained in programs that fail to reduce time to defibrillation.

Time: The Major Determinant of Survival

The major determinant of survival in each study in Tables 1 and 2 was time, or more precisely, the interval between collapse and delivery of the first shock. It is now well established that the earlier defibrillation occurs, the better

the prognosis. Emergency personnel have only a few minutes after the collapse of a patient to reestablish a perfusing rhythm. CPR can sustain a patient for a short period, but it cannot directly restore an organized rhythm. Restoration of a sustained adequate perfusing rhythm requires defibrillation, which must be administered within a few minutes of the initial arrest, and advanced cardiac care provided in a timely manner.

The Contributions of a Witness and a Witness Who Performs CPR

Survival rates from cardiac arrest can be remarkably high if the event is witnessed. For example, when people in supervised cardiac rehabilitation programs suffer a witnessed cardiac arrest, defibrillation is usually performed within the first minutes after VF has occurred. In studies of cardiac arrest in this setting, approximately 90% of patients were resuscitated.[11,12] No other studies with a defined out-of-hospital population have observed survival rates this high.

When defibrillation is delayed, the critical factor determining survival is whether witnesses to the collapse perform effective CPR while waiting for the defibrillator. But CPR alone does not convert a heart in VF to a heart with a perfusing rhythm. This interaction between early defibrillation and early CPR is shown in Figure 3. This

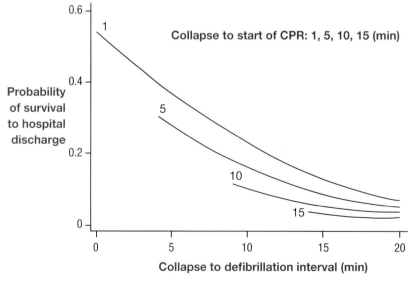

Figure 3. Effect of collapse-to-CPR interval and collapse-to-defibrillation interval on survival to hospital discharge. The graph displays the probability of survival to hospital discharge in relation to 4 intervals from collapse to start of CPR (1, 5, 10, and 15 minutes) and collapse to defibrillation (5, 10, 15, and 20 minutes). To determine the probability of survival for an individual patient, identify the curve indicating the interval collapse and CPR and then identify the point on that curve that corresponds to the interval from collapse to defibrillation (see horizontal axis). The probability of survival is then indicated on the vertical axis. Based on data from King County, Washington (N = 1667 witnessed VT/VF arrests),[13] and Tucson, Arizona (N = 205 witnessed VT/VF arrests).[14] Adapted from Valenzuela et al.[14]

figure illustrates the probability of survival in relation to the intervals from collapse to first shock and from collapse to start of CPR. The figure clearly shows that the sooner someone starts CPR and the sooner the defibrillator arrives, the better the outcome. It also shows how starting CPR early changes the slope of the defibrillation survival curve and "buys time" for the defibrillator to arrive. See the legend for more details.

The 3-Phase Model of Cardiac Arrest and New Recommendations

Successful Defibrillation From the Metabolic Perspective: "Using Up the Fuel"

Successful defibrillation depends on the electrical and metabolic state of the myocardium, the amount of myocardial damage that occurs during hypoxic arrest, the prior functional state of the heart, and the cause of VF. From a metabolic perspective VF depletes more of the cardiac energy stores—adenosine triphosphate (ATP)—per minute than does normal sinus rhythm. Prolonged VF will exhaust the energy stores of ATP in the myocardium, particularly in the cardiac pacemaker cells. The longer VF persists, the greater the myocardial deterioration as energy stores become exhausted. In a heart stunned into electrical silence by a defibrillatory shock, no spontaneous contractions will resume if the fibrillating myocardium has consumed all its energy stores. When ATP is depleted and cellular functions are disrupted, shocks are more likely to convert VF to asystole than to a spontaneous rhythm because no "fuel" remains to support spontaneous depolarization in the pacemaker tissues or the contracting myocardium. With depleted reserves of energy, any postshock *asystole* or *agonal rhythms* will be permanent, not temporary.

Delayed Defibrillation

For this reason VF of short duration is much more likely to respond to a shock delivered soon after VF starts. An important objective for resuscitation, and any effort to improve outcome, is to shorten the interval between the onset of VF and the first shock. In the *ECC Guidelines 2000* the American Heart Association (AHA) recommended that all patients who have a VF arrest out of hospital receive shocks in <5 minutes; a goal for patients who have an in-hospital VF arrest is <3 minutes.

Cobb et al[15] noted, however, that as more Seattle first responders were equipped with AEDs, survival rates from SCA unexpectedly fell. They attributed this decline to a reduced emphasis on CPR when defibrillation is delayed, and there is growing evidence to support this view. When VF causes cardiac arrest, 3 general phases of arrest occur: an electrical phase, a hemodynamic phase, and a

Phases of VF Cardiac Arrest

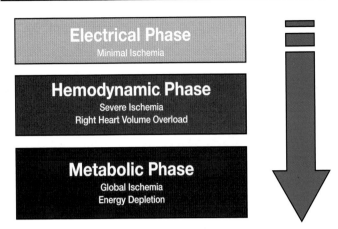

Figure 4. When cardiac arrest occurs due to ventricular fibrillation (VF), 3 phases can be proposed: an initial electrical phase, when early defibrillation is critical; a hemodynamic phase, when perfusion pressure to the heart and brain assume increasing importance; and a metabolic phase, when adenosine triphosphate is depleted and cellular damage and stunning are present. Adapted from Weisfeldt and Becker.[16]

metabolic phase (Figure 4).[16] Whether a shock is delivered immediately (during the early electrical phase) or after a brief period of CPR later during the hemodynamic phase may be one explanation for this observation. During the hemodynamic phase, a brief period of CPR may "prime the pump" and provide a small but important period of oxygen and energy substrate.

VF—Shock First or CPR First?

Witnessed Arrest and Defibrillator Immediately (or Rapidly) Available

When any provider witnesses an out-of-hospital arrest and an AED is immediately available on-site, the provider should use the AED as soon as possible. Healthcare providers who treat cardiac arrest in hospitals and other facilities with AEDs on-site should start immediate CPR and should use the AED/defibrillator as soon as it is available. This recommendation will provide immediate defibrillation during the electrical phase and possibly prolong the time period when immediate defibrillation has the best chance of success.

Unwitnessed Arrest or Defibrillator Not Immediately Available

When an out-of-hospital cardiac arrest is not witnessed by EMS personnel, the *2005 AHA Guidelines for CPR and ECC* recommend that EMS personnel may give 5 cycles (about 2 minutes) of CPR before checking the ECG rhythm and attempting defibrillation. This recommendation takes into account the delay inherent in the EMS call time and

- When any provider witnesses an out-of-hospital arrest and an AED is immediately available on-site, the provider should use the AED as soon as possible.
- Healthcare providers who treat cardiac arrest in hospitals and other facilities with AEDs on-site should provide immediate CPR and should use the AED/defibrillator *as soon as it is available.*
- When an out-of-hospital cardiac arrest is not witnessed by EMS personnel, EMS personnel may give about 5 cycles (about 2 minutes) of CPR before checking the ECG rhythm and attempting defibrillation.

response. Almost all patients treated out of hospital by EMS providers will be in the hemodynamic or metabolic phase of cardiac arrest.

Two studies showed that when EMS call-to-arrival intervals were 4 to 5 minutes or longer, patients who had received 1½ to 3 minutes of CPR before defibrillation had higher rates of initial resuscitation, survival to hospital discharge, and 1-year survival when compared with those who had received immediate defibrillation for VF SCA.[15,17] More evaluation is needed, however, because one randomized study found no benefit to CPR before defibrillation for non–paramedic-witnessed SCA.[18]

Automated External Defibrillators

The use of AEDs is discussed in detail in the BLS for Healthcare Providers Course. The ACLS Provider Course requires students to be proficient in 1-provider CPR and use of an AED. A brief summary and science update are included here to help you understand new recommendations and science as well as the integration of CPR with an AED into ACLS.

AEDs are sophisticated, reliable computerized devices that use voice and visual prompts to guide lay providers and healthcare providers to safely defibrillate VF SCA. Modified prototype AEDs that record information about the frequency and depth of chest compressions during CPR are being tested. If such devices become commercially available, AEDs may one day prompt providers to improve CPR performance and provide high-quality chest compressions with minimal interruption. An analysis of the VF waveform may also guide whether to perform CPR first or provide an immediate shock.

How Do AEDs Work?

Automated Rhythm Analysis

AEDs have microprocessors that analyze multiple features of the surface ECG signal that is displayed as a rhythm on a monitor. This signal is complex and includes frequency, amplitude, and some integration of frequency and amplitude, such as slope or wave morphology. Filters check for artifact such as QRS-like signals, radio transmission, or 50-cycle or 60-cycle interference as well as loose electrodes and poor electrode contact (Figure 5).

AEDs have been tested extensively, both in experiments using libraries of recorded cardiac rhythms and clinically in many field trials in both adults and children. They are extremely accurate in rhythm analysis. AEDs are not designed to deliver synchronized shocks and will not perform cardioversion (eg, for VT with pulses or supraventricular tachycardia [SVT]). AEDs will recommend a shock (non-synchronized) for monomorphic and polymorphic VT if the rate and R-wave morphology exceed preset values.

Lay Provider AED Programs

Since 1995 the AHA has recommended the development of lay provider AED programs to improve survival rates from out-of-hospital SCA. These programs have also been called public access defibrillation (PAD) programs. The goal of these programs is to shorten the time from onset of VF until CPR and shock delivery by ensuring that AEDs and trained lay providers are available in public areas where SCA is likely to occur. To maximize the effectiveness of these programs, the AHA has emphasized the importance of organization, planning, training, linking with the EMS

EMS system medical directors may consider implementing a protocol that would allow EMS responders to provide 5 cycles (about 2 minutes) of CPR before defibrillation of patients found by EMS personnel to be in VF, particularly when the EMS system call-to-arrival interval is >4 to 5 minutes.

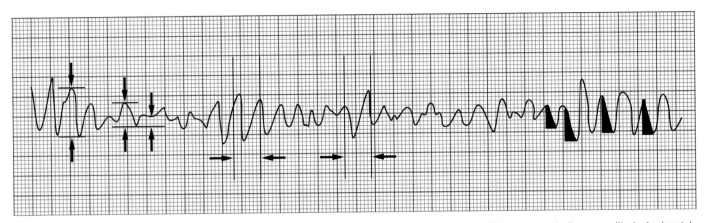

Figure 5. Features of the surface electrocardiogram analyzed by automated external defibrillators. Vertical arrows indicate amplitude, horizontal arrows indicate frequency, and black wedges indicate morphology.

system, and establishing a process of continuous quality improvement.

Improved Survival Using AED Programs

Lay provider AED public access defibrilation (PAD) programs will have the greatest potential impact on survival from SCA if programs are created in locations where SCA is likely to occur. In the PAD trial, programs were established at sites with a history of at least 1 out-of-hospital cardiac arrest every 2 years or where at least 1 out-of-hospital SCA was predicted during the study period (ie, sites having >250 adults over 50 years of age present for >16 h/d).[19] When time to defibrillation is not reduced, improved survival in AED programs is not observed.[20,21]

To be effective, AED programs need integration into an overall EMS strategy for treating patients in cardiac arrest. CPR and AED use by public safety first responders are recommended to increase survival rates for SCA. AED programs in public locations where there is a relatively high likelihood of witnessed cardiac arrest (eg, airports, casinos, sports facilities) are recommended. Because the improvement in survival rates in AED programs is affected by the time to CPR and to defibrillation, sites that deploy AEDs should establish a response plan, train likely responders in CPR and AED use, maintain equipment, and coordinate with local EMS systems. A process to evaluate AED use and integration into the EMS system is recommended for quality assurance and continuous improvement.

Approximately 80% of out-of-hospital cardiac arrests occur in private or residential settings.[22] To date no studies have documented the effectiveness of home AED deployment. Recently AEDs can be sold directly to the public. These sales may make AEDs much more common in the home, and studies are in progress to assess whether this may improve survival in this group of patients when arrests are witnessed.

Foundation Facts *Survival Using AED Programs*	Recommendations for AED programs: • Place AEDs in locations where SCA is likely to occur • Integrate with the local EMS system • No present documented value for in-home use • Not effective for asystole or nonperfusing rhythms
Critical Concept *AED Integration With EMS and Cardiac Care Systems*	Survival rates in AED programs are affected by • Time to CPR • Time to first shock Sites that deploy AEDs should • Establish a response plan • Train likely responders in CPR and AED use and regularly practice • Maintain equipment • Coordinate with local EMS systems • Develop a process of quality review and improvement

Suggested Components for AED Continuous Quality Improvement

Quality improvement efforts for lay rescuer AED programs should include both routine inspections and postevent data analysis (from AED recordings and responder reports) to evaluate the following elements:

- Emergency response plan, including accurate time intervals for key interventions (eg, collapse to shock or no shock advisory to initiation of CPR) and patient outcome
- Responder performance
- AED function, including accuracy of the ECG rhythm analysis
- Battery status and function
- Electrode pad function and readiness, including expiration date

AEDs are of no value for arrest not caused by VF/pulseless VT, and they are not effective for treatment of nonshockable rhythms that may develop after termination of VF. Nonperfusing rhythms are present in most patients after shock delivery, and CPR is required until a perfusing rhythm returns. For this reason AED providers should also be trained to support ventilation and circulation with CPR, especially high-quality chest compressions.

Manual Defibrillation

In the ACLS Provider Course some of you will instruct students in manual defibrillation and, most important, integration of manual defibrillation with ACLS interventions and CPR. This section discusses the background and technical aspects of manual defibrillation. Chapter 5 discusses integration of manual defibrillation and clinical application during cardiac arrest.

Energy, Power, Current, and Impedance—the Terms

Electrical Nomenclature

Successful defibrillation requires the delivery of enough energy to generate sufficient current flow through the heart to terminate VF, but the operator must avoid delivering excess current, which may cause significant myocardial damage. Myocardial damage or stunning may cause postarrest myocardial dysfunction. A few terms in basic electricity help with understanding defibrillation and these concepts (Table 3 and Figure 6). A defibrillatory shock passes a large flow of charged particles (electrons) through the heart over a brief period of time. This flow of electricity is called *current*, which is measured in *amperes*. The *pressure* pushing this flow of electrons is the electrical

potential, measured in *volts*. There is always a *resistance* to this flow of electrons, called *impedance*, measured in *ohms*. In short, electrons flow (*current, amperes*) with a *pressure (volts)* for a *period of time* (usually *milliseconds*) through a substance that has *resistance (impedance, ohms)*. A typical shock will terminate VF within 400 to 500 milliseconds of shock delivery.

Table 3. **Electrical Nomenclature and Equations to Help Understand Defibrillation**

Ohm's Law: the potential must overcome impedance or no electrons will flow (current):

Current (amperes) = Potential (volts) ÷ Impedance (ohms)

Power is a measure of the current flowing with a certain force:

Power (watts) = Potential (volts) × Current (amperes)

Energy is a measure of power delivered over a period of time:

Energy (joules) = Power (watts) × Duration (seconds)

OR

Energy (joules) = Potential (volts) × Current (amperes) × Duration (seconds)

Electrical Formulas

A series of formulas defines these relationships (Table 3 and Figure 6). The electrical *potential* (measured in *volts*) multiplied by *current* (measured in *amperes*) equals the *power* (measured in *watts*). One *watt* is the *power* produced by 1 *ampere* of *current* flowing with a *pressure* of 1 *volt*. This *power (watts)* sustained over a duration of *time (seconds)* determines the total *energy (joules)*.

What Really Defibrillates the Heart?

Although the defibrillator operator selects the shock energy (in joules), it is the current flow (in amperes) through the heart that actually defibrillates. Defibrillation is achieved by generating an amplitude of current flow and sustaining that flow for a time interval. Current amplitude, shock duration, and how the current amplitude changes over that interval interact in complex ways to determine how a given shock will defibrillate.

Scientific researchers in this area speak more precisely in terms of *current density* as the key to defibrillation. Current density is the ratio of the magnitude of current flowing through a conductor to the cross-sectional area perpendicular to the current flow; it is expressed as current flow per unit of area (amperes/cm^2). Current density is a concept that will help in understanding the differences in defibrillation efficacy among different types of waveforms, such as monophasic and biphasic, discussed later in this chapter. Current density, in part dependent on the selected shock dose, differs from the amount of current passing through the heart. This *fractional*

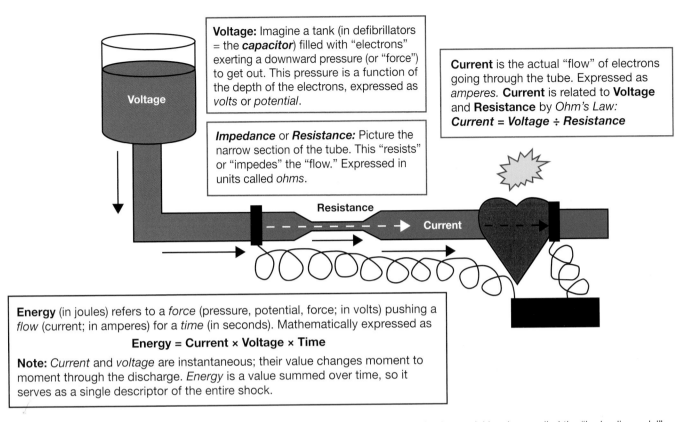

Voltage: Imagine a tank (in defibrillators = the *capacitor*) filled with "electrons" exerting a downward pressure (or "force") to get out. This pressure is a function of the depth of the electrons, expressed as *volts* or *potential*.

Current is the actual "flow" of electrons going through the tube. Expressed as *amperes*. **Current** is related to **Voltage** and **Resistance** by *Ohm's Law:* **Current = Voltage ÷ Resistance**

***Impedance* or *Resistance*:** Picture the narrow section of the tube. This "resists" or "impedes" the "flow." Expressed in units called *ohms*.

Energy (in joules) refers to a *force* (pressure, potential, force; in volts) pushing a *flow* (current; in amperes) for a *time* (in seconds). Mathematically expressed as

Energy = Current × Voltage × Time

Note: *Current* and *voltage* are instantaneous; their value changes moment to moment through the discharge. *Energy* is a value summed over time, so it serves as a single descriptor of the entire shock.

Figure 6. This sketch is a diagram depicting some basic principles of electricity. This physics model has been called the "hydraulic model" of electricity because it depicts the flow of electrons during electric current as the flow of water through a series of pipes. This model is a metaphorical memory aid only. It would be incorrect to think that the heart between 2 paddles in the figure has water flowing through it.

transmyocardial current is completely independent of the selected shock dose; it is determined more by pad or paddle position and thoracic anatomy.

Some of the nomenclature used in association with defibrillation can be confusing. Ventricular fibrillation is defined as chaotic, disorganized, and rapid depolarizations and repolarizations in multiple locations throughout the ventricles. Two types of VF have been reported, and both forms likely contribute to VF in humans. Recent terminology uses the term *wavelets* of VF. The term *defibrillation* (shock success) is typically defined as termination of VF for at least 5 seconds following the shock, and it should not be equated with resuscitation success. The dominant hypothesis of the mechanism of defibrillation holds that a shock totally depolarizes every myocardial cellular membrane. When the shock achieves this total electrical neutrality across most or all of the heart, VF is abolished and *defibrillation* has been achieved.

Foundation Facts **Shock Success**	• Termination of VF is not equivalent to return of spontaneous electrical complexes, cardiac contractions, and perfusing rhythm. • Return of spontaneous circulation is critical for resuscitation, but it is influenced by multiple factors besides the ability of a shock to terminate fibrillation.
Critical Concept **Transthoracic Impedance a Significant Variable**	• If transthoracic impedance is too high, a low-energy shock will not generate enough current to achieve defibrillation. • Stated another way, a shock with the energy set too low will leave the heart in VF; a shock with the energy set too high may leave the heart in asystole or atrioventricular block.

Reducing Transthoracic Impedance

To reduce transthoracic impedance, the defibrillator operator should follow these recommendations:

- If using handheld electrode paddles, press firmly. Self-adhesive monitor/defibrillator electrode pads are preferred; they do not require additional pressure.
- When using handheld electrode paddles, always apply an electrode gel or paste made specifically for defibrillation. Lack of a coupling material between electrodes and the chest wall creates high transthoracic impedance.
- Apply self-adhesive monitor/defibrillator electrode pads with firm pressure over the entire surface of the pads to achieve good adhesion. Self-adhesive pads are recommended for speed, safety, and consistency in training.
- Consider the respiratory phase, because a large tidal volume can increase impedance by moving the defibrillator paddles farther apart. Most patients will be in end-expiration when a shock is delivered because the person providing ventilations will stop when the patient is "cleared." Use firm paddle-to-chest contact pressure to ensure lower impedance and to seat the whole paddle into the skin, which will reduce paddle-to-paddle electrical current "arcing."
- Consider the presence of excessive chest hair. Poor electrode-to-chest contact and hair may produce significant air trapping between the electrode or paddle and the skin. This situation can result in high impedance, and the gaps produced by the hair and air pockets can lead to occasional current arcing. Although rare, in oxygen-rich environments such as critical care units, current arcing has been known to produce fires if an accelerant is present. Use of self-adhesive pads reduces the risk of arcing. It may be necessary to shave the area of intended pad placement.
- Do not use alcohol-based foams or gels; evaporation increases the chance of arcing and fires.
- Avoid placing the apex defibrillation electrode directly on the breast of female patients. This position can significantly increase transthoracic impedance. Ensure that the apex electrode is placed either lateral to or underneath the breast.

In the strictest sense, *success* for a shock that attempts defibrillation is simply removal of VF; it has nothing to do with return of spontaneous electrical complexes, cardiac contractions, and circulation. Although return of spontaneous circulation (ROSC) is a critical point in the resuscitation process, it is influenced by multiple factors besides the ability of a shock to terminate fibrillation.

Transthoracic Impedance

Ohm's Law defines a relationship between current, voltage, and impedance (Current = Voltage ÷ Impedance). A study of this relationship reveals that the operator can have more of a direct effect on transthoracic impedance than on any other aspect of defibrillation. Many factors determine transthoracic impedance. These factors affecting current transmission through the chest include energy selected, electrode size, quality of electrode-to-skin contact, number and time interval of previous shocks, electrode-skin coupling material, phase of ventilation, distance between electrodes (size of the chest), and electrode-to-chest contact pressure. Studies have established a wide range of normal for human transthoracic impedance (15 to 150 ohms); the average for an adult is about 70 to 80 ohms. If transthoracic impedance is too high, a low-energy shock will not generate enough current passing through the chest and heart to achieve defibrillation.

Defibrillation Waveforms and Energy Requirements for Defibrillation of VF

Defibrillation involves delivery of current through the chest and to the heart to depolarize myocardial cells and eliminate VF. The energy settings for defibrillators are designed to provide the lowest effective energy needed to terminate VF. Because defibrillation is an electrophysiologic event that occurs 300 to 500 milliseconds after shock delivery, the term *defibrillation* (shock success) is typically defined as termination of VF for at least 5 seconds following the shock. VF frequently recurs after successful shocks, but this recurrence should not be equated with shock failure.

Shock success using the typical definition of defibrillation should not be confused with resuscitation outcomes such as restoration of a perfusing rhythm (ROSC), survival to hospital admission, or survival to hospital discharge. Although resuscitation outcomes, including survival, may be affected by many variables in addition to shock delivery, defibrillation programs must strive to improve patient survival, not just shock success.

Defibrillation success, as defined and discussed above, depends on selecting an appropriate energy setting to generate a sufficient current density throughout the heart to defibrillate while causing minimal electrical injury. Electrical injury is important because it can cause postarrest myocardial dysfunction. Because the fractional transmyocardial current will affect the current density generated throughout the heart, positioning of the defibrillation pads or paddles is critically important (this topic is discussed in more detail later in this chapter).

- Successful defibrillation (shock success) is typically defined as termination of VF for at least 5 seconds following the shock.

- VF frequently recurs after successful shocks, but this recurrence should not be equated with shock failure.

A shock will not terminate the arrhythmia if the selected energy and the resulting transmyocardial current flow are too low, yet functional and histologic damage may result if the energy and current are too high.

Selection of the appropriate current will both reduce the need for multiple shocks and limit the myocardial damage per shock. Stated another way, a shock with the energy set too low will leave the heart in VF; a shock with the energy set too high may leave the heart in asystole or atrioventricular block. Although the relationship between body size and energy requirements for defibrillation has been hotly debated for decades, there is no fixed relationship. The critical relationships have to do with the fractional transmyocardial current (defined by the thoracic pathway between the 2 defibrillator electrodes and the position of the heart in that pathway) and the impedance to current flow from pad to pad. These relationships in combination determine the current density throughout the heart and thus the ultimate effect of the shock. In adults the body mass surrounding the thoracic current pathway plays only a minimal role.

Defibrillation Waveforms Overview

Modern defibrillators, including AEDs, deliver energy or current in *waveforms*. There are 2 broad categories of waveforms, monophasic and biphasic (Figure 7). Energy settings and their associated delivered current levels vary with the type of device and type of waveform. Monophasic waveforms (Figure 7A) deliver current in primarily one direction (polarity). Biphasic waveforms deliver current that flows in a positive direction for a specified duration. The current then reverses and flows in a negative direction for the remaining milliseconds of the electrical discharge (Figure 7B and 7C). The first phase of the biphasic waveform "prepares" the cell membrane for uniform depolarization when the second phase occurs.

Defibrillators can also vary the speed of both waveform rise and return to zero voltage point. A waveform that rises sharply and returns gradually is a *damped sinusoidal waveform* (Figure 7A and 7B). A waveform that rises sharply and then is cut off abruptly is a *truncated exponential waveform* (Figure 7C).

Biphasic waveforms were proven superior to monophasic waveforms when used in implantable defibrillators. The

mechanisms underlying the superiority and greater efficacy of biphasic waveforms are still a subject of scientific investigation and debate. The most salient characteristic of biphasic waveforms is their ability to defibrillate with a significantly lower myocardial current density than monophasic waveforms. This characteristic provides a distinct advantage in transthoracic defibrillation, where the factors affecting the biphasic truncated exponential

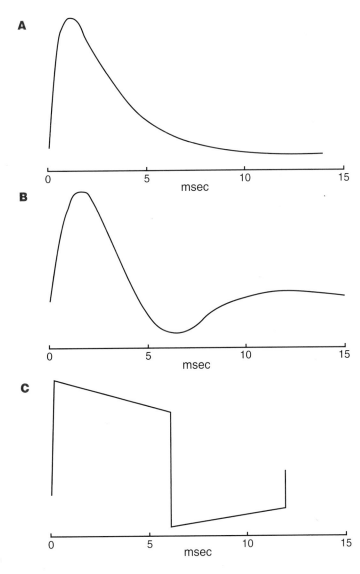

Figure 7. Voltage transition of three different defibrillation waveforms. **A,** Critically damped, sinusoidal monophasic; **B,** quasi-sinusoidal biphasic; and **C,** truncated exponential biphasic. Reproduced from Walcott et al.[23]

current density are either imprecise, such as pad position, or unknown, such as the exact intrathoracic anatomy or current pathways. No specific waveform (either monophasic or biphasic), however, is consistently associated with a higher rate of ROSC or rates of survival to hospital discharge after cardiac arrest.

Monophasic Waveform Defibrillators

Monophasic waveforms deliver current of one polarity (ie, direction of current flow). Monophasic waveforms can be further categorized by the rate at which the current pulse decreases to zero. The monophasic damped sinusoidal waveform returns to zero gradually, whereas the monophasic truncated exponential waveform abruptly returns to zero.

Monophasic waveform defibrillators are no longer being manufactured but are still in use. Most of these use monophasic damped sinusoidal waveforms. As noted above, no specific waveform (either monophasic or biphasic) is consistently associated with a greater incidence of ROSC or survival to hospital discharge rates after cardiac arrest. Research indicates, however, that when doses equivalent to or lower than monophasic doses

are used, biphasic waveform shocks are safe and effective for termination of VF.

Biphasic Waveform Defibrillators

Researchers have collected data from both out-of-hospital and in-hospital studies (electrophysiologic studies and AICD testing and evaluation). Overall this research indicates that lower-energy biphasic waveform shocks have equivalent or higher success for termination of VF than either damped sinusoidal or truncated exponential monophasic waveform shocks delivering escalating energy (200 J, 300 J, and 360 J) with successive shocks. No direct comparison of the different biphasic waveforms has been made.

The optimal energy for first-shock biphasic waveform defibrillation yielding the highest termination rate for VF has not been determined. Several randomized and observational studies have shown that defibrillation with biphasic waveforms of relatively low energy ($\leq$200 J) is safe and has equivalent or higher efficacy for termination of VF than monophasic waveform shocks of equivalent or higher energy. Until more is known, providers should consult the recommendations of the manufacturer of their biphasic defibrillator.

FYI
Some Principles and Relationships

1. Defibrillation is achieved by the flow of *current* for a certain duration through the heart, between the 2 defibrillator pads or paddles. To deliver enough current to defibrillate an average adult heart, roughly 30 to 40 amperes must be delivered to the *chest* (not necessarily the heart) for most monophasic waveforms. Biphasic waveforms require significantly less.
2. Current is markedly affected by impedance. Defibrillators are calibrated under the assumption that human chest impedance is 50 ohms. The more operators can do to reduce impedance, the more likely the shock will deliver enough current to achieve defibrillation.
3. A shock lasts approximately 5 to 20 milliseconds depending on the waveform, delivered against the estimated impedance of 50 ohms.
4. For a defibrillator to deliver a shock of the requisite 30 amperes against 50 ohms of impedance requires 1500 volts (Current × Impedance = Voltage). The shock is delivered over time, so think in terms of the energy required over time: 200 watts delivered for 1 second against 50 ohms of impedance would accomplish delivery of 30 amperes (200 watt-seconds = 200 joules).
5. For a shock that lasts only 4 to 5 milliseconds, for example, the defibrillator accomplishes the goal of 200 joules (200 watt-seconds) by actually delivering 45,000 watts! See the math below:

Voltage ÷ Impedance = *Current*

Current × Voltage = **Power (watts)**

Power × Time (duration) = Energy (joules or watt-seconds)

Example math:

1500 volts ÷ 50 ohms = 30 amperes

30 amperes × 1500 volts = 45,000 watts

45,000 watts delivered for 0.0044 second = 200 watt-seconds (joules)

Compensation for patient-to-patient differences in impedance may be achieved by changes in duration and voltage of shocks or by releasing the residual membrane charge (called *burping*). Whether there is an optimal ratio of first-phase to second-phase duration and leading-edge amplitude is unclear. It is unknown whether a waveform more effective for *immediate outcomes* (defibrillation) and *short-term outcomes* (ROSC, survival to hospital admission) results in better *long-term outcomes* (survival to hospital discharge, survival for 1 year). Given the high efficacy of all biphasic waveforms, other determinants of survival (eg, interval from collapse to CPR or defibrillation) are likely to supersede the impact of specific waveforms or energies.

Pads, Paddles, and Positions

Pad and Paddle Position

Placement of pads or paddles for defibrillation and cardioversion is an important but often neglected topic. Pads should be placed in a position that will maximize current flow through the myocardium. This fractional transmyocardial current affects the current density generated in the heart. It has been estimated that even with properly placed paddles, only 4% to 25% of the delivered current actually passes through the heart. The recommended placement is termed either *sternal-apical* or *anterior-apex* (Figure 8). The sternal (or anterior) electrode is placed to the right of the upper part of the sternum below the clavicle.

The apex electrode is placed to the left of the nipple with the center of the electrode in the *midaxillary line*. An acceptable alternative approach is to place one paddle anteriorly over the left apex (precordium) and the other posteriorly behind the heart, in the left infrascapular location. Either pathway will maximize current flow through the cardiac chambers.

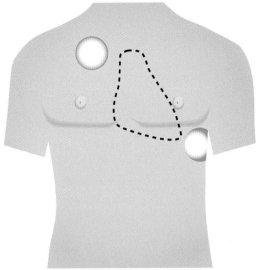

Figure 8. Recommended sternal-apex positions for placement of defibrillation paddles or adhesive defibrillation pads. Place the anterior electrode to the right of the upper sternum below the clavicle. Place the apex electrode to the left of the nipple with the center of the electrode in the midaxillary line.

Defibrillation Considerations for Patients With a Pacemaker or AICD

When performing cardioversion or defibrillation in patients with permanent pacemakers or AICDs, do not place the electrodes over or in close proximity to the device generator, because defibrillation can cause pacemaker malfunction. A pacemaker or AICD (indicated by a lump or scar) also may block some current to the myocardium during defibrillation, causing delivery of suboptimal energy to the heart.

Previous recommendations for electrode pads recommended placement of the pad at least 1 inch (2.5 cm) away from the device (Figure 9). Finally, because some of the defibrillation current flows down the pacemaker leads, permanent pacemakers and AICDs should be reevaluated after the patient receives a shock.

Foundation Facts **Pad and Paddle Position Is Important**	Placement of pads or paddles for defibrillation and cardioversion is an important but often neglected topic. Even with properly placed paddles, only 4% to 25% of the delivered current actually passes through the heart.

FYI **Guidelines 2005** **Recommended AED Pad Position**	• When using AED electrode pads, place them on the patient's bare chest in the conventional sternal-apical position. Place the right (sternal) chest pad on the patient's right superior-anterior (infraclavical) area and the apical (left) pad on the patient's inferior-lateral left chest, lateral to the left breast in the midaxillary line. • Other acceptable pad positions are placement on the lateral chest wall on the right and left sides (biaxillary) or placement of the left pad in the standard apical position and the other pad on the right or left upper back.

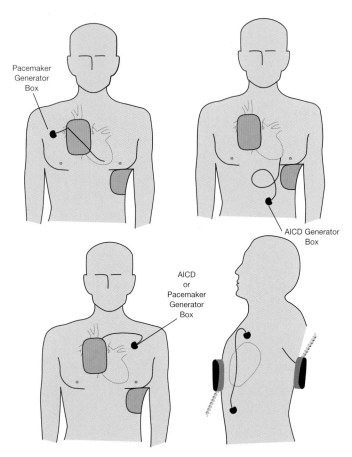

Pacemaker
Generator
Box

AICD Generator
Box

AICD
or
Pacemaker
Generator
Box

Figure 9. Suggested defibrillator paddle positions for patients with implanted pacemakers or automated implantable cardioverters/defibrillators (AICDs). Printed with permission from Medtronic Physio-Control.

A recent study evaluated the safety of external electrical cardioversion of atrial fibrillation in patients having a variety of permanent pacemakers and ICDs that had been implanted in either the right or left infraclavicular regions. Cardioversion electrodes were uniformly placed strictly in the anterior-posterior position (to the right of the sternum with the upper edge of the electrode at the 4th anterior intercostal space; and to the left of the patient's spine at the midscapular level posteriorly). In addition, the anterior

electrode was kept a minimum of 8 cm (approximately 3 inches) away from the implanted device. These precautions assured both a safe distance of shock electrodes away from the pacemaker or ICD and a shock direction that was perpendicular to the orientation of the implanted lead systems. Both biphasic and monophasic waveform escalating synchronized shocks were deployed ranging from 100 to 200 J and 200 to 360 J, respectively, including multiple shocks, if required, each separated by a 5-minute interval. No device or lead dysfunction resulting from cardioversion was observed in any patient.[24]

Placement of external shock electrodes in patients with an ICD is identical to those having a permanent pacemaker, described above. Some patients with older ICD systems may have epicardial defibrillation electrodes and an ICD generator implanted in the abdomen rather than a pectoral location. In this instance, external defibrillator electrodes may be placed in their traditional (right anterior to left anterolateral [at the heart apex]) positions, so long as each is a safe distance from the ICD generator, without the need for other special precautions. A theoretical concern in this instance is whether the epicardial defibrillator electrodes may insulate the heart from external shock and require higher energy settings in order to defibrillate successfully. In such instances, external cardioversion or defibrillation should default to using high energy settings.

If the patient has an AICD that is delivering shocks (ie, the patient's muscles contract like they do during external defibrillation), allow 30 to 60 seconds for the AICD to complete the treatment cycle before attaching a defibrillator. In general an AICD will likely have delivered its full complement of therapies within a few minutes of the patient's collapse. Thus, when encountering an unconscious, pulseless patient with an AICD, the most likely scenario is that the device has exhausted all of its therapies and failed to terminate the arrhythmia. All standard treatment measures should be initiated by providers, as though an implanted device were not present,

FAQ **Can defibrillation be performed with an implanted pacemaker or AICD?**	• When providing cardioversion or defibrillation for patients with permanent pacemakers or AICDs, do not place the electrodes over or close to the device generator, because defibrillation can cause pacemaker malfunction. • New information suggests that pads should be placed at least 3 inches away from the pacemaker or AICD device. Some manufacturers recommend placement 6 inches from the device when possible. • When possible anterior posterior pad placement is also preferred to minimize the chance of damage to the device, but placement of pads should not delay defibrillation.
FYI **AED and AICD Interactions**	Occasionally the analysis and shock cycles of AICDs and AEDs will conflict. Switching to a manual external defibrillator mode can circumvent such issues, once providers with rhythm recognition skills are on scene.

FYI: Cardiac Emergencies in Patients With an AICD: Assessment and Treatment

Effects of Magnet Application

- Suspends overdrive pacing for tachycardias
- Allows sensing and pacing if programmed for bradycardias
- Suspends detection and treatment of VF and VT
- Suspends functions only while magnet is in place
- Device programming head has same effect as magnet

	I. Cardiac arrest: patient in VF/VT	**II. Cardiac arrest: patient not in VF/VT**	**III. No cardiac arrest: patient not in VF/VT**
AICD: delivering shocks	**A.** Allow AICD to complete one treatment cycle: count to 60 seconds → if no shock → usual treatment; if shock → next step **B.** If shocks seem ineffective → apply magnet → treat per usual protocols	**A.** Apply magnet to inactivate AICD → treat per usual protocols	**A.** Apply magnet to inactivate AICD → treat per usual protocols
AICD: not charging, not firing	**C.** Treat per usual VF/VT arrest protocols	**B.** Treat per usual protocols	**B.** No problem

I. **Cardiac arrest: patient in presumed VF or VT:**

    A. If AICD is shocking and shocks *may be effective*:

        — Allow device to complete one treatment cycle (deliver 1 witnessed shock); then count to 60 seconds. If no shock occurs in 60 seconds, start CPR; follow usual treatment protocols.

        — If second shock occurs in <60 seconds, assume shocks are ineffective (see next step).

    B. If AICD is shocking but shocks *are ineffective (witnesses report multiple previous shocks)*:

        — Position magnet to turn off AICD.

        — Treat as if there is no AICD (ACLS VF/VT protocol).

    C. If AICD is *not shocking*:

        — Treat immediately as if there is no AICD (ACLS VF/VT protocol).

II. **Cardiac arrest: patient *not* in presumed VF or VT:**

    A. If AICD is shocking and *shocks are inappropriate*:

        — Position magnet to turn off AICD.

        — Treat as if there is no AICD (ACLS protocols).

    B. If AICD is *not shocking*:

        — Treat immediately as if there is no AICD (ACLS protocols).

III. **No cardiac arrest: patient *not* in VF or VT:**

    A. If AICD is shocking and *shocks are inappropriate* (eg, rhythm is SVT, atrial fibrillation, or atrial flutter; lead fracture or displacement):

        — Position magnet to turn off AICD.

        — Treat as if there is no AICD (ACLS protocols).

    B. If AICD is not shocking, there is no problem (shocks would be inappropriate); treat per ACLS protocols including external defibrillation. However, AICDs require the same precautions as those required for patients with pacemakers when external shocks are administered. In particular, providers should note where the AICD generator and leads are located and place external defibrillation electrodes accordingly. Though AICD generators, unlike pacemakers, are better protected from high-energy shock by specialized high-voltage circuitry, they are nonetheless susceptible to the same spectrum of damage. It is therefore advised by manufacturers, as with pacemakers, that defibrillator electrodes should be placed at least 6 inches away from the AICD when possible, and shocks should be administered perpendicular to the orientation of the AICD leads and the heart.

Occasionally the analysis and shock cycles of AICDs and AEDs will conflict. AICDs and AEDs both deploy automated arrhythmia detection algorithms. This can lead to "back-to-back" shocks should the AICD and AED simultaneously detect a shockable arrhythmia. In such instances, providers should recognize the sudden muscular contraction that identifies receipt of an AICD shock and, if possible, be prepared to inhibit AED shock delivery. In addition, AICDs deploy both bradycardia pacing and antitachycardia pacing, which can in theory mislead the AED detection algorithm as to the nature of the patient's rhythm. Switching to a manual external defibrillator mode can circumvent such issues, once providers with rhythm recognition skills are on scene.

Mistakes in Pad Position or Size

One of the most common errors in pad placement is to place the pads too close together. Figure 10A displays a cross-section of the heart and thorax showing how most of the current bypasses the heart when the paddles are placed too close together. Notice also that the sternal

paddle is indeed over the sternum, which blocks much of the current flow. In Figure 10B the apex paddle is in the proper position in the midaxillary line, which allows all the current to flow through the myocardium, achieving defibrillation.

An interesting manikin study from England supports the idea that improper placement of the apex pad or paddle is the most common positional error.[25] During a course on resuscitation techniques doctors were asked to place the 2 defibrillator paddles in the "proper" locations on the breastplate of a resuscitation training manikin. Figure 11 presents a composite "map" of all the locations selected by the 101 subjects. This map unequivocally shows how the doctors erred in paddle placement more than 90% of the time, placing the apex paddle too far anterior, well away from the recommended location near the axillary line. Look again at Figure 10B to see how, somewhat counterintuitively, moving the apex paddle *away* from the heart and toward the axillary line will lead to more effective defibrillatory shocks.

Safety During Operation of a Defibrillator

Providers should make sure that the pads are separate and not touching. Providers should also ensure that paste or gel has not smeared along the skin between the paddles. Smearing of the paste or gel may allow current to follow a superficial pathway (arc) along the chest wall, "missing" the heart. Self-adhesive monitor/defibrillator electrode pads are as effective as gel pads or paste, and they can be placed before cardiac arrest to allow for monitoring and then rapid administration of an initial shock when necessary.[26] As a result, self-adhesive pads should be used routinely instead of standard paddles. Remember that the principles discussed above for correct placement also apply to

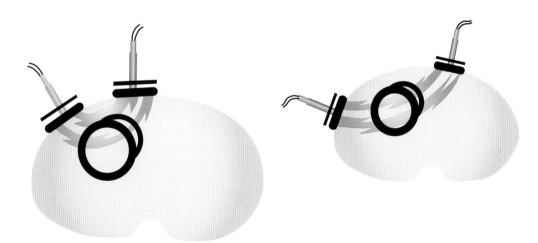

Figure 10. Pad positions. **A,** Current pathway when the paddles are placed too close together. **B,** A more optimal current pathway, achieved when the paddles are placed in the standard position. Reproduced with permission from Ewy GA, Bressler R, eds. *Cardiovascular Drugs and the Management of Heart Disease.* New York, NY: Raven Press; 1982.[2]

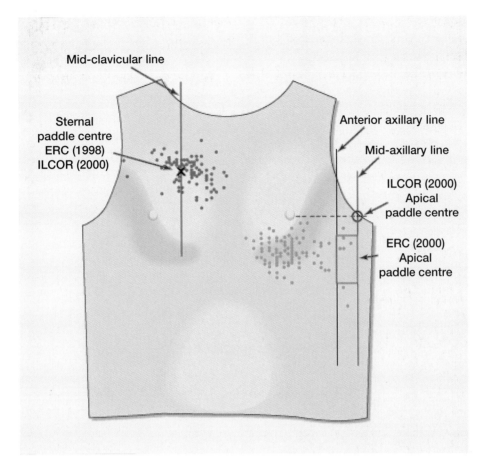

Figure 11. Anatomical position of center of sternal and apical defibrillation paddles placed by 101 doctors. Reproduced from Heames et al. *BMJ.* 2001;322:1393. With permission from the *BMJ* Publishing Group.[25]

pads. An improperly placed pad can decrease chances of successful defibrillation.

Do not place electrodes directly on top of a transdermal medication patch (eg, patches containing nitroglycerin, nicotine, analgesics, hormone replacements, or antihypertensives), because the patch may block delivery of energy from the electrode pad to the heart and may cause small burns to the skin. Remove medication patches and wipe the area before attaching the electrode pad.

If an unresponsive patient is lying in water or the chest is covered with water, remove the patient from the water and briskly wipe the chest dry before attaching electrode pads and attempting defibrillation. Defibrillation can be accomplished when a patient is lying on snow or ice.

Safety Concerns With a Patient AICD in Place

Unlike external defibrillation, which typically deploys 150 to 360 J, the maximum shock output from an ICD is only a fraction of this level and ranges from 30 to 40 J,

FYI *Guidelines 2005* *Pads or Paddles?*	Self-adhesive monitor/defibrillator pads should be used routinely *instead* of standard paddles. • Self-adhesive pads are as effective as gel pads or paste. • Self-adhesive pads can be placed before cardiac arrest to allow for monitoring and rapid administration of an initial shock when necessary.

FAQ *Can you defibrillate in snow or ice or if the patient is wet?*	• If the chest is covered with water, briskly wipe the chest dry before attaching electrode pads. • Defibrillation can be accomplished when a patient is lying on snow or ice.

depending on the manufacturer. However, approximately 20% of an AICD's shock voltage may reach the patient's surface. Such voltage is not sufficient to cause harm to providers or others who are in contact with the patient at the time of ICD shock but may nonetheless be felt by them. The voltage is sufficiently small that the provider is more likely to feel the effect of abrupt muscle contraction when the patient is shocked than the electrical impulse itself. However, the degree of discomfort felt depends on where and how the provider may be in contact with the patient at the time of shock. Transmission of shock from the patient to the provider requires a 2-point contact in order to complete the electrical circuit and a conductor (such as defibrillator paddle gel) that facilitates transmission of current between the patient and provider. Contact at only one location is unlikely to transmit shock to the provider unless in addition the provider and patient are grounded to one another (for example, both on a wet surface). For the typical "heel of hand" on the chest, with the second hand overlying the first, during CPR a relatively small single area is in contact with the patient and shock risk is minimal. In addition, providers who use protective gloves during resuscitation are insulated from the patient and are unlikely to experience shock unless the integrity of the glove has been compromised. As a rule, apart from the location where defibrillator electrodes are placed, the presence of an ICD should not alter the handling of the patient in cardiac arrest.

Fire Hazard and Prevention

Several case reports have described fires ignited by sparks from poorly applied defibrillator paddles in the presence of an oxygen-enriched atmosphere. Severe fires have been reported when ventilator tubing is disconnected from the endotracheal tube and then left adjacent to the patient's head, blowing oxygen across the chest during attempted defibrillation.

The use of self-adhesive defibrillation pads is probably the best way to minimize the risk of sparks igniting during defibrillation. If manual paddles are used, gel pads are preferable to electrode pastes and gels because the pastes and gels can spread between the 2 paddles, creating the potential for a spark. Do not use medical gels or pastes with poor electrical conductivity, such as ultrasound gel.

Providers should take precautions to minimize sparking during attempted defibrillation; try to ensure that defibrillation is not attempted in an oxygen-enriched atmosphere. When ventilation is interrupted for shock delivery, providers should try to ensure that oxygen does not flow across the patient's chest during defibrillation attempts.

Recommendations for Fire Prevention

Defibrillator fires in oxygen-enriched environments, although rare, are an unacceptable danger to patients and healthcare providers. A defibrillator fire requires 3 fire-critical ingredients; if any one is lacking, a fire cannot occur. Prevention of defibrillator fires is relatively simple: prevent a defibrillation error *or* prevent an oxygen supply error. See "Recommendations for Prevention" in Table 4.[27,28]

Proposals to routinely turn off or disconnect the oxygen supply immediately before defibrillation[28] have generated controversy,[29] primarily because supplying oxygen is considered a higher priority than instituting time-consuming steps simply to prevent fires.[30] Much of this controversy loses clinical relevancy when providers focus on proper defibrillation techniques to prevent an electrical arc from ever occurring. As noted in Table 4, oxygen flow should be turned off and airway adjuncts disconnected for patients at higher risk for electrical arc formation. All ACLS providers and instructors can help generate greater awareness of this danger. Most important, though, is the lesson that simply by performing resuscitation procedures properly and effectively, the problem of defibrillator-associated fires will remain rare.

Table 4. 3 Fire-Critical Ingredients: Common Errors That Supply Ingredients and Recommendations for Prevention

Required Ingredients	Ingredient Sources and Common Errors That Yield Ingredient	Recommendations for Prevention
1. **Agent for flame propagation**	• Fine surface body hair • Surface nap fibers on most fabrics • Fibers, dust, particulate matter suspended in the ambient air	• Move gown, pajamas from resuscitation area • Move bedding, drapes, curtains from immediate vicinity

2. **Oxygen-enriched atmosphere close to electrical arc** (*"vicinity of potential ignition point"*)	• Device for oxygen administration:
	  — Left connected to open oxygen source
	  — Placed close to defibrillation area
	     or
	  — Disconnected from oxygen source
	  — Open oxygen source directed close to defibrillation area
	• "Pockets" of high oxygen concentration allowed to collect close to defibrillation area
		• Always properly connect an airway adjunct to open oxygen supply lines
		• If oxygen is not properly connected to an airway adjunct or if the airway adjunct is not in use, then TURN OFF OXYGEN
		• If an airway device with oxygen flow must be set aside urgently, place it as far away from the chest as practical
		• Never let oxygen flow directly onto the chest surface during defibrillation
		• Consider turning off oxygen supply or disconnecting ventilation bag immediately before shock delivery
		• Always turn off and disconnect oxygen source in clinical scenarios with high risk of electrical arc (eg, irregular chest surface)

3. **Electrical arc** (*"source of ignition"*)	• Paddles not pushed evenly down against skin with force • Paddles "tipped" (paddle surface not parallel to skin surface) • No (or insufficient) conductive gel • Too much gel (smears across skin surface, contacting other paddle, ECG wires, or electrodes) • Hairy chest (pockets of air and gaps within hair between skin and paddles) • Irregular chest surface (eg, highly curved thorax, pectus excavatum, or depressed intercostal spaces between ribs secondary to cachexia) • Paddles or pads placed on or close to wires or monitoring electrodes • Adhesive pads for "hands-free" remote defibrillation dried out, folded, or not pressed down firmly • Adhesive metal "target pads" (on which paddles are placed): paddle overlaps edge of pad; pads dried out, folded, or not pressed down firmly • Prolonged resuscitations: gel rubs off; pads dry out	• Push paddles down firmly with at least 25 pounds of pressure • Make sure paddles are parallel to skin surface with no "tipping" or angles • Carefully apply sufficient conductive gel, specifically formulated for defibrillation, to cover paddle surface • Avoid excessive gel that spreads beyond the edges of the paddles • If excessive chest hair interferes with paddle-skin contact, clip or shave chest hair or consider extra gel (can sometimes fill in the spaces between skin, hair, and paddles) • For patients with an irregular chest surface, check carefully for gaps between paddle surface and skin • If gaps are not corrected by firmer paddle pressure, try kneading conductive gel into several 4" × 4" saline-moistened gauze pads; try defibrillation if "conductive gauze" bridges gaps • Avoid placing paddles or pads over or adjacent to ECG wires or electrodes • Make sure pads for "hands-free" defibrillation or metal "target" pads are not dried out, have no folds, and are at least the size of the defibrillator paddles (avoid overlap)

References

1. Kouwenhoven WB, Milnor WR, Knickerbocker GG, Chesnut WR. Closed chest defibrillation of the heart. *Surgery*. 1957;42:550-561.

2. Ewy GA. Ventricular fibrillation and defibrillation. In: Ewy GA, Bressler R, eds. *Cardiovascular Drugs and the Management of Heart Disease*. New York, NY: Raven Press; 1982:331-340.

3. Eisenberg MS, Cummins RO. Defibrillation performed by the emergency medical technician. *Circulation*. 1986;74(pt 2):IV9-IV12.

4. Stults K, Brown D, Schug V, Bean J. Prehospital defibrillation performed by emergency medical technicians in rural communities. *N Engl J Med*. 1984;310:219-223.

5. Vukov LF, White RD, Bachman JW, O'Brien PC. New perspectives on rural EMT defibrillation. *Ann Emerg Med*. 1988;17:318-321.

6. Bachman JW, McDonald GS, O'Brien PC. A study of out-of-hospital cardiac arrests in northeastern Minnesota. *JAMA*. 1986;256:477-483.

7. Olson DW, LaRochelle J, Fark D, Aprahamian C, Aufderheide TP, Mateer JR, Hargarten KM, Stueven HA. EMT-defibrillation: the Wisconsin experience. *Ann Emerg Med*. 1989;18:806-811.

8. Cummins RO. From concept to standard-of-care? Review of the clinical experience with automated external defibrillators. *Ann Emerg Med*. 1989;18:1269-1275.

9. Eisenberg MS, Horwood BT, Cummins RO, Reynolds-Haertle R, Hearne TR. Cardiac arrest and resuscitation: a tale of 29 cities. *Ann Emerg Med*. 1990;19:179-186.

10. Eisenberg MS, Cummins RO, Damon S, Larsen MP, Hearne TR. Survival rates from out-of-hospital cardiac arrest: recommendations for uniform definitions and data to report. *Ann Emerg Med*. 1990;19:1249-1259.

11. Van Camp SP, Peterson RA. Cardiovascular complications of outpatient cardiac rehabilitation programs. *JAMA*. 1986;256:1160-1163.

12. Fletcher GF, Cantwell JD. Ventricular fibrillation in a medically supervised cardiac exercise program: clinical, angiographic, and surgical correlations. *JAMA*. 1977;238:2627-2629.

13. Larsen MP, Eisenberg MS, Cummins RO, Hallstrom AP. Predicting survival from out-of-hospital cardiac arrest: a graphic model. *Ann Emerg Med*. 1993;22:1652-1658.

14. Valenzuela TD, Roe DJ, Cretin S, Spaite DW, Larsen MP. Estimating effectiveness of cardiac arrest interventions: a logistic regression survival model. *Circulation*. 1997;96:3308-3313.

15. Cobb LA, Fahrenbruch CE, Walsh TR, Copass MK, Olsufka M, Breskin M, Hallstrom AP. Influence of cardiopulmonary resuscitation prior to defibrillation in patients with out-of-hospital ventricular fibrillation. *JAMA*. 1999;281:1182-1188.

16. Weisfeldt ML, Becker LB. Resuscitation after cardiac arrest: a 3-phase time-sensitive model. *JAMA*. 2002;288:3035-3038.

17. Wik L, Hansen TB, Fylling F, Steen T, Vaagenes P, Auestad BH, Steen PA. Delaying defibrillation to give basic cardiopulmonary resuscitation to patients with out-of-hospital ventricular fibrillation: a randomized trial. *JAMA*. 2003;289:1389-1395.

18. Jacobs IG, Finn JC, Oxer HF, Jelinek GA. CPR before defibrillation in out-of-hospital cardiac arrest: a randomized trial. *Emerg Med Australas*. 2005;17:39-45.

19. Ornato JP, McBurnie MA, Nichol G, Salive M, Weisfeldt M, Riegel B, Christenson J, Terndrup T, Daya M. The Public Access Defibrillation (PAD) trial: study design and rationale. *Resuscitation*. 2003;56:135-147.

20. White RD. Early out-of-hospital experience with an impedance-compensating low-energy biphasic waveform automatic external defibrillator. *J Interv Card Electrophysiol*. 1997;1:203-208.

21. Groh WJ, Newman MM, Beal PE, Fineberg NS, Zipes DP. Limited response to cardiac arrest by police equipped with automated external defibrillators: lack of survival benefit in suburban and rural Indiana—the police as responder automated defibrillation evaluation (PARADE). *Acad Emerg Med*. 2001;8:324-330.

22. Becker L, Eisenberg M, Fahrenbruch C, Cobb L. Public locations of cardiac arrest: implications for public access defibrillation. *Circulation*. 1998;97:2106-2109.

23. Walcott GP, Walcott KT, Knisley SB, Zhou X, Ideker RE. Mechanisms of defibrillation for monophasic and biphasic waveforms. *Pacing Clin Electrophysiol*. 1994;17(pt 2):478-498.

24. Manegold JC, Israel CW, Ehrlich JR, Duray G, Pajitnev D, Wegener FT, Hohnloser SH. External cardioversion of atrial fibrillation in patients with implanted pacemaker or cardioverter-defibrillator systems: a randomized comparison of monophasic and biphasic shock energy application. *Eur Heart J*. 2007;28:1731-1738.

25. Heames RM, Sado D, Deakin CD. Do doctors position defibrillation paddles correctly? Observational study. *BMJ*. 2001;322:1393-1394.

26. Perkins GD, Roberts C, Gao F. Delays in defibrillation: influence of different monitoring techniques. *Br J Anaesth*. 2002;89:405-408.

27. ECRI. Defibrillation in oxygen-enriched environments. *Health Devices*. 1987;16:113-114.

28. ECRI. Fires from defibrillation during oxygen administration. *Health Devices*. 1994;23:307-309.

29. Lefever J, Smith A. Risk of fire when using defibrillation in an oxygen enriched atmosphere. *Medical Devices Agency Safety Notices*. 1995;3:1-3.

30. McAnulty GR, Robertshaw H. Risk of fire outweighed by need for oxygen and defibrillation. *J Accid Emerg Med*. 1999;16:77.

Chapter 4

Basic Airway Management: Integration of CPR With Ventilation, Airway and Circulatory Adjuncts

This Chapter

- **Who requires oxygen, when, and how much**
- **How to integrate ventilation with CPR and ACLS interventions**
- **Why less emphasis on advanced airway techniques**
- **How blood and oxygen move during CPR**
- **Optimizing blood flow during CPR**

Overview

Participants in the ACLS Provider Course learn to use a systematic approach to adult resuscitation based on the *BLS Primary Survey* and the *ACLS Secondary Survey*. Many of the topics covered in this chapter can be organized around the A (Airway) and B (Breathing) components of these surveys. Although the fit is not always perfect, this approach is often helpful. The ACLS Provider Course Respiratory Arrest Case discusses respiratory arrest with a pulse. This chapter also reviews essential airway management, ie, oxygenation and ventilation, in patients with cardiopulmonary emergencies and in cardiac arrest.

Advanced Airway Management for the Basic Provider

A major emphasis of the *2005 AHA Guidelines for Cardiopulmonary Resuscitation and Emergency Cardiovascular Care* is high-quality chest compressions with minimal interruption. There has been a decreased emphasis on early advanced airway insertion and increased emphasis on consideration of the risk-benefit ratio for the interruption of chest compressions to place an advanced airway. As a result, this chapter in specific and the ACLS Provider Course in general review and practice integration of CPR with advanced airway but no longer teach or practice placement of an advanced airway. An Advanced Airway Module is available for students who have an interest or use advanced airway placement in their scope of practice.

Providers must be aware of the risks and benefits of insertion of an advanced airway during a resuscitation attempt. Such risks are affected by the condition of the patient and the provider's expertise in airway control. Because insertion of an advanced airway may require interruption of chest compressions for many seconds, the need for uninterrupted compressions is weighed against the need for insertion of an advanced airway. Providers may defer insertion of an advanced airway until the patient

FAQ When is an advanced airway inserted?	Providers may defer insertion of an advanced airway until the patient fails to respond to initial CPR and defibrillation attempts or demonstrates ROSC. • Insertion of an advanced airway may require interruption of chest compressions for many seconds. • The need for uninterrupted compressions is weighed against the need for insertion of an advanced airway.

fails to respond to initial CPR and defibrillation attempts or demonstrates return of spontaneous circulation (ROSC).

Oxygenation and Ventilation

Overview—Objectives and Techniques of Respiratory Support

The major objectives of respiratory support are as follows:

BLS Primary A—Airway
- Provide supplementary oxygen.
- Ensure a patent and protected airway; use manual techniques as needed.
- Ensure a patent and protected airway; use simple, noninvasive airway adjuncts as needed.

BLS Primary B—Breathing
- Monitor the quality of oxygenation and ventilation with noninvasive devices.
- Provide positive-pressure oxygenation and ventilation with manual techniques or noninvasive airway devices when spontaneous breathing is inadequate or absent.

ACLS Secondary A—Airway
- Establish a patent and protected airway with invasive advanced airway devices.
- Confirm proper placement of these devices with both clinical and device confirmation techniques.

ACLS Secondary B—Breathing
- Provide effective positive-pressure oxygenation and ventilation through properly inserted advanced airway devices.
- Secure the advanced airway devices to prevent displacement.
- Monitor oxygenation and ventilation and tailor support as needed.

Cardiac or Respiratory Arrest?

The provider should quickly determine if the patient demonstrates spontaneous breathing efforts.

- Is the patient making spontaneous breathing efforts?
- Do these efforts appear adequate?
- If the efforts are inadequate, are the inadequate efforts caused by fatigue or one of the many causes of respiratory depression?

- If the patient is making spontaneous breathing efforts, is there evidence of partial or complete upper airway obstruction caused by foreign material, such as food, vomitus, or blood clots, or posterior displacement of the tongue or epiglottis?

Clues to Suspect Airway Obstruction

Significant partial upper airway obstruction typically causes noisy airflow during inspiration (stridor or "crowing") and cyanosis (late sign). Another sign of airway obstruction is use of accessory muscles, indicated by retractions of the suprasternal, supraclavicular, and intercostal spaces. If the patient is not making spontaneous breathing efforts, airway obstruction becomes more difficult to recognize. Occasionally, isolated bradycardia, secondary to occult hypoxemia, provides an early sign of airway obstruction. Recognize the presence of airway obstruction caused by the tongue and epiglottis.

If spontaneous breathing is absent or inadequate, provide positive-pressure ventilation with one of the following ventilation techniques described in this chapter:

- Mouth to mouth (with barrier protection)
- Mouth to mask
- Ventilation with a bag through a face mask, endotracheal tube, esophageal-tracheal Combitube, or laryngeal mask airway (LMA)

How to Assess the Need for Supplementary Oxygen and Ventilation

Providers must be able to accurately assess *oxygenation* and *ventilation* to detect and treat respiratory distress and failure. The 2 major functions of respiration are to achieve

- Oxygenation (oxygenate arterial blood)
  - Evaluate oxygenation with pulse oximetry
- Ventilation (remove carbon dioxide from venous blood)
  - Evaluate ventilation with capnography and capnometry

Oximetry—Basic Principles

To understand the clinical utility of oximetry—as well as its limitations and pitfalls—one must understand the physics involved in measurement and the clinical principles of

FAQ **What happened to the advanced airways in the ACLS Provider Course?**	The ACLS Provider Course no longer instructs students on the *insertion* of advanced airways. <ul><li>Emphasis is placed on optimal ventilation rates and the avoidance of large volumes.</li><li>With an advanced airway in place, emphasis is on good integration of CPR using the proper rate: 1 ventilation every 6 to 8 seconds.</li></ul>

adequate tissue oxygenation. Here too "treat the patient and not the number" is most important.

Basic Physics of Pulse Oximetry

The concentration of a substance in a fluid can be determined by its ability to transmit light. Oxygenated hemoglobin absorbs and reflects red and infrared light differently than nonoxygenated hemoglobin. Oxygenated hemoglobin in a pulsatile tissue bed primarily absorbs *infrared* light; reduced (nonoxygenated) hemoglobin in a pulsatile tissue bed primarily absorbs *red* light. In pulse oximetry red and infrared light are passed through a pulsatile tissue bed, and a photodetector captures any nonabsorbed light on the other side of the tissue bed. A microprocessor calculates the relative absorption of red and infrared light that occurred as it passed through the tissue bed and can determine the percentage of oxygenated and nonoxygenated hemoglobin present in that tissue bed. In this way the pulse oximeters calculate the *percent of hemoglobin that is saturated with oxygen (percent saturation, percent SO_2; percent SaO_2).* In the absence of abnormal hemoglobins, such as carboxyhemoglobin or methemoglobin, if the arterial oxygen saturation is greater than 70%, there should be no more than 3% variance between pulse oximetry and the arterial oxyhemoglobin saturation measured by co-oximeter used in arterial blood gas determinations. Studies have shown pulse oximetry to be an accurate and useful guide for patient care in the in-hospital setting as well as in the prehospital EMS setting,[1-4] including transport by rotary-wing aircraft.[5]

Hemoglobin and Tissue Oxygen Delivery

Analysis of arterial blood is an invasive procedure, and arterial blood gases are infrequently ordered, available, or clinically useful during cardiac arrest. *Pulse oximetry* was developed to provide a noninvasive, painless approximation of the percent of hemoglobin saturated with oxygen (percent SaO_2). During cardiac arrest pulse oximetry will not function (and should not be measured) because pulsatile blood flow is inadequate for measurement in peripheral tissue beds. But pulse oximetry is commonly used for monitoring patients who are not in arrest, because it provides a simple, continuous method of tracking oxyhemoglobin saturation. There are 3 major determinants of adequate tissue oxygenation:

1. There must be an adequate amount of oxygen to saturate the hemoglobin molecules.
2. There must be enough hemoglobin to carry adequate oxygen.
3. Cardiac output must be sufficient to deliver the saturated hemoglobin to peripheral tissues.

Arterial oxygen content is determined by the hemoglobin concentration and its saturation with oxygen. Normal pulse oximetry saturation, however, does not ensure adequate systemic *oxygen delivery* because it does not calculate the total oxygen content (O_2 bound to hemoglobin + dissolved O_2) *and* adequacy of blood flow (cardiac output).

Pulse Oximetry Precautions and Limitations

Pulse oximetry readings, even those that appear to be accurate, do not always correlate with cardiac output and

Foundation Facts	Normal pulse oximetry saturation does not ensure adequate tissue oxygenation. Tissue oxygen delivery is determined not only by hemoglobin saturation but also by • Total oxygen content (O_2 bound to hemoglobin + dissolved O_2) *and* • Adequacy of blood flow (cardiac output) to the peripheral tissues

Arterial oxygen content (mL of oxygen per dL of blood)	=	**Hemoglobin concentration (g/dL)**	×	**1.34 mL oxygen**	×	**Oxyhemoglobin saturation**	+	**(PaO_2 × 0.003)**

Normal oxygen content is 18 to 20 mL/dL of blood.

Measurement of the oxygen content is only part of the determination of effective oxygenation. The oxygen present needs to be delivered to the tissues for use. Peripheral cells need to be able to uptake and use oxygen for cellular metabolism. Oxygen delivery is defined by how much oxygen is present and how much of it is delivered to the body. Oxygen delivery is defined by the following equation:

Oxygen delivery	=	**Arterial oxygen content**	×	**Cardiac output**	**(× constant)**

Most commercially available pulse oximeters use 2 light-emitting diodes and a photodetector in a sensor. The 2 diodes emit a red and an infrared light. Oxygenated hemoglobin in the pulsatile tissue bed primarily absorbs infrared light, but reduced (nonoxygenated) hemoglobin in the pulsatile tissue bed primarily absorbs red light. A microprocessor in the unit determines the relative absorption of red and infrared light to calculate the percentage of oxygenated versus reduced (nonoxygenated) hemoglobin present in the tissue bed.

The light absorption of methemoglobin and carboxyhemoglobin is different from that of normal hemoglobin, so pulse oximeters will not accurately reflect total hemoglobin saturation in the presence of these 2 products.[6] With significant methemoglobinemia, pulse oximeters display an oxygen saturation of approximately 85%. With significant carboxyhemoglobinemia (such as occurs in carbon monoxide poisoning), the pulse oximeter will typically reflect the oxygen saturation of *normal* hemoglobin, not the percentage of hemoglobin bound to carbon monoxide. If these or other conditions affecting oxyhemoglobin saturation are present, arterial hemoglobin oxygen saturation must be determined by using co-oximetry.

oxygen delivery. When clinically evaluating a patient's cardiac output and oxygen delivery always assess systemic perfusion and be aware of the hemoglobin concentration. If cardiac output or hemoglobin concentration is low, oxygen delivery can be inadequate even if oxyhemoglobin saturation is normal.

Abnormal Hemoglobins (eg, Carbon Monoxide Poisoning)

The light absorption of carboxyhemoglobin (carbon monoxide) and of methemoglobin (cyanide) differs from that of normal hemoglobin, so carboxyhemoglobin and methemoglobin are *not* recognized by pulse oximeters. If these altered forms of hemoglobin are present, the SaO_2 calculated by the pulse oximeters will be falsely high because most pulse oximeters calculate the percent of *normal* hemoglobin that is saturated with oxygen rather than the percent of *total* hemoglobin that is saturated with oxygen. When you suspect the presence of carbon monoxide poisoning or methemoglobin toxicity, you should measure the oxyhemoglobin saturation with a co-oximeter (this requires arterial blood sampling).

Abnormal Conditions Affecting Pulse Oximetry

In several clinical situations abnormal or inaccurate oximetry readings may occur. In a large review of pulse oximeter devices, the major sources of error were finger thickness, hemoglobin level, skin color, and peripheral temperature.

- Motion artifact and low perfusion are the most common sources of SaO_2 inaccuracies. Motion artifacts can occur with patient transport, movement, twitching, and agitation.

- When the systolic blood pressure is low, oximetry becomes inaccurate because of decreased pulsatile flow, response time, or calibration characteristics of the instrument. Oximetry may also read falsely high when the SaO_2 is less than 70% or may become inaccurate when the hemoglobin level is very low (2 to 3 g/dL).
- Peripheral hypoperfusion from hypothermia, low cardiac output, or vasoconstrictive drugs may cause or increase inaccuracies.
- Very dark skin, fingernail polish, and fungal infections of the nails (onychomycosis) may cause spuriously low readings when digital monitors are used.

Safety Considerations

There are some safety precautions regarding use of the pulse oximetry equipment:

- Do not use oximetry probes with broken or cracked casings. Burns have been reported when the lights from the probes come into direct contact with the skin.
- Do not connect the probes from one manufacturer to base units made by another manufacturer.

Capnography and Capnometry

Detection of exhaled CO_2 is one of several independent methods of confirming endotracheal tube position. Given the simplicity of the exhaled CO_2 detector (waveform, colorimetry, or digital), it can be used as the initial method for detecting correct tube placement even in the patient in cardiac arrest. Detection of exhaled CO_2, however, is not infallible as a means of confirming tube placement, particularly during cardiac arrest. Evidence from a meta-analysis in adults[7] indicated a range of results:

- Sensitivity (percentage of correct endotracheal placement detected when CO_2 is detected): 33% to 100%

- Specificity (percentage of incorrect esophageal placements detected when no CO_2 is detected): 97% to 100%
- Positive predictive value (probability of endotracheal placement if CO_2 is detected): 100%
- Negative predictive value (probability of esophageal placement if no CO_2 is detected): 20% to 100%

The use of CO_2 detecting devices to determine the correct placement of other advanced airways (eg, Combitube, LMA) has not been adequately studied.

Basic Principles

The body eliminates CO_2 through *ventilation*. When blood passes through the lungs, CO_2 moves from the blood, across the alveolar capillary membrane into the alveoli, and then into the airways and is exhaled. Alveolar P_{CO_2} should be approximately equal to pulmonary venous, left atrial and arterial P_{CO_2}. If there is a good match of ventilation and perfusion in the lungs and if there is no airway obstruction, exhaled CO_2 should correlate well with arterial P_{CO_2}, and exhaled carbon dioxide can be used to estimate arterial carbon dioxide tension. CO_2 can be detected by either of 2 techniques:

- *Capnometry* is a *qualitative* method that detects the presence of CO_2 in exhaled air. *Colorimetric* capnometers are semiquantitative devices based on a chemical reaction between exhaled CO_2 and a chemical detector impregnated in a strip of paper. These devices are used to identify the presence or absence of a sufficient quantity of CO_2 to produce a color change at a point in time.
- *Capnography* devices are *quantitative* devices that measure the concentration of CO_2 using infrared absorption detectors. Carbon dioxide concentration is typically displayed by these devices as a continuous exhaled CO_2 concentration waveform with a digital display of end-tidal CO_2. This plot of CO_2 concentration against time is called a *capnograph*.

Capnometry

A carbon dioxide concentration of more than 2% will react with the chemical reagent in a colorimetric CO_2 detector and change the color. Most initial devices used a color change from purple to yellow (see Figure 2 on page 55). If the endotracheal tube is actually in the trachea, the CO_2 detector will turn yellow (Yellow = Yes, CO_2 is present = the

tube is in the trachea). In the *absence* of expired CO_2, the colorimetric indicator will remain purple (Purple = Problem). Healthcare providers commonly use this purple-to-yellow color change with a disposable device as a quick check to provide one method of device confirmation of the success (yellow) or failure (purple) of endotracheal intubation.[10]

The product insert for some commercially available semiqualitative colorimetric capnometers recommend that after intubation, 6 positive-pressure breaths be provided by hand or mechanical ventilation before attempting to identify exhaled CO_2. Six breaths will wash out any CO_2 that is present in the stomach or esophagus from bag-mask ventilation. Any CO_2 detected after 6 breaths can be presumed to be from the lungs.[8,9]

In patients weighing more than 2 kg with a perfusing rhythm (not in cardiac arrest), the sensitivity and specificity of colorimetric capnometry methods approaches 100% if 6

Color Change With Colorimetric Device—Know Your Device

The 2000 Guidelines for Advanced Cardiovascular Life Support (ACLS) and Pediatric Advanced Life Support (PALS), as well as associated training materials, offer examples of how colorimetric CO_2 detection devices work and suggest mnemonic schemes for interpretation. Those details were meant to help providers remember the significance of specific colors indicating the relative concentration of CO_2 present in the expired air. Some of the materials, for example, link the color purple with a sign of low CO_2 and yellow with high CO_2. New devices have been introduced on the market with new indicators and color schemes. The indicators in some commercially available devices respond to detection of increasing CO_2 concentration by transitioning in color using one of the following schemes:

- purple-to-yellow
- blue-to-yellow
- white-to-purple

Even more possibilities will likely appear on the market in the coming years. Clearly, any one mnemonic that relies on color will not fit all available devices.

Critical Concept *Check Colorimetric Device After 6 Breaths*	Six breaths will wash out any CO_2 that is present in the stomach or esophagus from bag-mask ventilation. - CO_2 detected after 6 breaths can be presumed to be from the lungs.

ventilations have been provided following intubation. This means that if the endotracheal tube is in the trachea of a patient with a perfusing rhythm, the colorimetric device will change color with few exceptions (see "False-Positive Results," below). If the tube is in the esophagus, there should be no CO_2 detected after 6 breaths, so a colorimetric CO_2 detector should remain unchanged.

False-Positive Results

When exhaled CO_2 is detected (positive reading for CO_2) in cardiac arrest, it is usually a reliable indicator of tube position in the trachea. *False-positive* readings (CO_2 is detected, but the tube is located in the esophagus) have been observed in animals that ingested large amounts of carbonated liquids before the arrest.[8]

A color change is generally a reliable indicator of the presence of carbon dioxide and endotracheal intubation. False-positive color changes are uncommon but can occur when the tip of the tube is in the supraglottic area rather than in the trachea. A false-positive result may also be possible following prolonged bag-mask ventilation.[8-10] This is why some manufacturers recommend that 6 ventilations should be provided after intubation and before the check for exhaled CO_2. Finally, if the colorimetric detector is contaminated with acidic gastric contents or acidic drugs, such as endotracheally administered epinephrine, a colorimetric detector may remain unchanged during the entire respiratory cycle.

False-Negative Results

False-negative results occur if the tube is in the trachea but the colorimetric indicator remains unchanged. A false-negative result is most often associated with cardiac arrest (see below). False-negative results may also occur with severe airway obstruction or pulmonary edema, which can impair CO_2 elimination so that inadequate CO_2 is detected in exhaled gas. Administration of an intravenous (IV) bolus of epinephrine in patients with cardiac arrest or very low cardiac output may transiently reduce pulmonary blood flow and reduce exhaled CO_2.

False-negative readings (in this context defined as failure to detect CO_2 despite tube placement in the trachea) may be present during cardiac arrest for several reasons. The most common explanation for false-negative readings during CPR is that blood flow and delivery of CO_2 to the lungs are low. False-negative results have also been reported in association with pulmonary embolus because pulmonary blood flow and oxygen delivery to the lungs are reduced. In addition, elimination and detection of CO_2 can be significantly reduced following an IV bolus of epinephrine[11] or with severe airway obstruction (eg, status asthmaticus) and pulmonary edema.[12,13] For these reasons, if CO_2 is not detected, we recommend that a second method be used to confirm endotracheal tube placement, such as direct visualization of the tube passing through the vocal cords with a laryngoscope or the esophageal detector device.

Capnography

Some *capnography devices* are infrared devices in which a light-emitting diode is used to measure the intensity of light transmitted across a short distance, usually the diameter of an endotracheal tube. The measured light absorption varies inversely with the concentration of CO_2 passing through the endotracheal tube. When attached to the end of an endotracheal tube, these infrared devices are called *mainstream capnometers*. These devices readily reveal low exhaled CO_2 indicative of esophageal intubation, and they can provide estimates of the adequacy of ventilation and the effectiveness of circulation during CPR.

Capnography devices provide a continuous readout of the concentration of CO_2. They are used to monitor the quality of ventilation in nonarrest patients. Because of their high degree of sensitivity to expired CO_2, however, capnographs can often detect a sufficient quantity of CO_2 to indicate the presence of a tracheal tube in the trachea even when cardiac arrest is present. Continuous capnography monitoring devices can identify and signal a fall in exhaled CO_2 consistent with tracheal tube dislodgment. This may be very helpful in emergencies.

Capnometry and Capnography in Cardiac Arrest

End-tidal CO_2 monitoring is a safe and effective noninvasive indicator of cardiac output during CPR and may be an early indicator of ROSC in intubated patients. During cardiac arrest CO_2 continues to be generated throughout the body. During cardiac arrest, however, there is little pulmonary blood flow, and the level of CO_2 in exhaled gas may be too low to produce a color change or a graphic exhaled CO_2 waveform. In such situations, when a colorimetric device is attached to the distal end of a properly placed tracheal tube, the color remains unchanged or the CO_2 level remains very low. Because the unchanged color and lack of exhaled CO_2 may also indicate that the tube has been placed in the esophagus, the healthcare provider must decide whether the lack of CO_2 indicates esophageal intubation or reflects the absence of blood flow to the lungs. The major determinant of CO_2 excretion is its rate of delivery from the peripheral production sites to the lungs. In the low-flow state during CPR, ventilation is relatively high compared with blood flow, so the end-tidal CO_2 concentration is low. If ventilation is reasonably constant, then changes in end-tidal CO_2 concentration reflect changes in cardiac output. Patients who are successfully resuscitated from cardiac

Confirmation of endotracheal tube placement requires both

- Clinical confirmation and
- A technique such as capnometry

arrest have significantly higher end-tidal CO_2 levels than patients who cannot be resuscitated. Capnometry can also be used as an early indicator of ROSC.

Administration of Oxygen

Overview—General Guidelines

Oxygen Administration During CPR

During CPR the purpose of ventilation is to maintain adequate oxygenation, but the optimal tidal volume, respiratory rate, and inspired oxygen concentration to achieve this are unknown. During the first minutes of sudden cardiac death due to ventricular fibrillation, the oxygen level in the blood remains high for several minutes after cardiac arrest. To improve oxygenation, healthcare providers should give 100% inspired oxygen ($FiO_2 = 1.0$) during basic life support and advanced cardiovascular life support as soon as it becomes available. High inspired oxygen tension will tend to maximize arterial oxygen saturation and, in turn, arterial oxygen content. This will help support oxygen delivery (Cardiac output × Arterial oxygen content) when cardiac output is limited. This short-term oxygen therapy does not produce oxygen toxicity.

Oxygen Administration for Acute Cardiac or Respiratory Distress

Oxygen administration is always appropriate for patients with acute cardiac disease or pulmonary distress. The following are some general guidelines for providing supplementary oxygen:

- For patients without respiratory distress: give oxygen at 4 L/min by nasal cannula.
- For patients with mild respiratory distress: give oxygen at 5 to 6 L/min.

- For patients with severe respiratory distress, acute congestive heart failure, or cardiac arrest: use a system that provides a high inspired oxygen concentration (near 100%).
- Titrate oxygen up or down according to PaO_2 or SaO_2.
- For patients with chronic obstructive pulmonary disease (COPD) known to be dependent on hypoxia-driven ventilation: Never withhold oxygen when needed. If there is concern about elimination of hypoxia-driven ventilation, you can provide low-dose supplementary oxygen via a 24% Venturi mask and titrate oxygen administration while monitoring the patient for signs of hypoventilation or apnea.
- In the most serious cases: Consider advanced airway devices, intubation, and 100% oxygen.

Oxygen Administration for Acute Coronary Syndromes

Oxygen is administered to all patients with overt pulmonary congestion or arterial oxygen saturation less than 90%. Short-term oxygen administration is beneficial for the patient with unrecognized hypoxemia or unstable pulmonary function. It is also reasonable to administer supplementary oxygen to all patients with suspected acute coronary syndromes (ACS) or possible ischemic-type pain for the first 6 hours. This rationale is supported by observations that even patients with uncomplicated myocardial infarction may be modestly hypoxic initially, presumably due to ventilation-perfusion mismatch. Supplementary oxygen limited ischemic myocardial injury in animal studies, and oxygen therapy to patients with ST-segment elevation myocardial infarction reduced the amount of ST-segment elevation, although no long-term mortality benefit has been demonstrated.

For patients without complications, excess oxygen can lead to systemic vasoconstriction, and no benefit in infarct reduction or mortality can be demonstrated. There is little justification to continue "routine" administration of oxygen beyond 6 hours.

When to Provide Supplementary Oxygen

During Cardiac Arrest

Mouth-to-mouth or mouth-to-mask rescue breathing (ventilation using exhaled air) can deliver only about 16% to 17% inspired oxygen concentration to the patient. Under ideal conditions this can produce an alveolar oxygen tension of 80 mm Hg. Hypoxia, however, is often associated with cardiac arrest, so healthcare providers should give supplementary 100% inspired oxygen ($FiO_2 = 1.0$) as soon as it is available:

- Tissue hypoxia develops as the result of low cardiac output and reduced peripheral oxygen delivery and results in a wide arteriovenous oxygen difference.
- Underlying respiratory problems may be associated with ventilation-perfusion abnormalities, causing hypoxia.
- Untreated tissue hypoxia leads to anaerobic metabolism, lactate production, and metabolic acidosis. Acidosis can blunt the beneficial effects of chemical and electrical therapy.
- Adequate arterial oxygen tension supports an adequate arterial oxygen saturation and adequate systemic oxygen delivery (O_2 Delivery = Arterial oxygen content × Cardiac output).

During Acute Cardiac Emergencies

Oxygen content and oxygen delivery are compromised during severe respiratory distress, acute congestive heart failure, or cardiac arrest. When this happens:

- Give oxygen at 4 L/min by nasal cannula to all patients with acute cardiac emergencies, even those without respiratory distress.
- Use a system that can provide a high inspired oxygen concentration (near 100%).

- Titrate oxygen according to the PaO_2 or oxygen saturation value.
- Identify potential for respiratory deterioration or compromise (eg, suspected aspiration of vomitus or suspected congestive heart failure).
- Intubate if respiratory failure is imminent or respiratory muscle fatigue develops.

During Acute Coronary Syndromes

In patients with acute myocardial infarction, supplementary oxygen has been shown to reduce both the magnitude and extent of ST-segment changes on the ECG in some patients, but no definite benefit from reduction in infarct size or mortality has been demonstrated.

- Provide oxygen at 4 L/min by nasal cannula for all patients with suspected ACS for the first 6 hours after onset of symptoms.
- Continue to provide oxygen beyond 6 hours for patients with continuing or recurrent ischemia, complicated infarcts, congestive heart failure, or arrhythmia.
- Continue oxygen therapy until the patient is clinically stable.

How to Provide Supplementary Oxygen

Healthcare providers and ACLS students should understand the oxygen delivery systems they use. The following description of oxygen systems will provide background information to allow you to answer questions that may be asked during the course about the use and delivery of oxygen. Selection of the appropriate method and device to supply oxygen requires clinical assessment and judgment. Although this is within the scope of an experienced provider, general guidelines are provided in Table 1.

Table 1. General Indications for Provision of Supplementary Oxygen

Pulse Oximetry Reading (Abnormal Hemoglobins *Absent**)	Interpretation	Indicated Intervention
95% to 100%	Desired range	*None* (except for cardiac patients, who need O_2 by nasal cannula at 4 L/min)
90% to <95%	Mild to moderate hypoxia	*Nasal cannula → face mask* (adjust O_2 flow rate [L/min] based on PaO_2 or SaO_2)
85% to <90%	Moderate to severe hypoxia	Face mask with O_2 reservoir → assisted ventilations
<85%	Severe to life-threatening hypoxia	Assisted ventilations → intubation

*Note: If abnormal hemoglobins are *present* (eg, carboxyhemoglobin or methemoglobin), the saturations listed represent saturation of total hemoglobin as measured by co-oximeter.

Check Oxygen Supply System (Cylinder or Piped Wall Oxygen)

Providers should be familiar with the oxygen delivery system as part of conscientious professional care, analogous to checking IV line continuity, ventilation connections, or the pathway from a defibrillator/monitor to the patient's chest. This familiarity will help *troubleshoot* possible problems with oxygen delivery. Mistakes can easily occur during emergencies if healthcare personnel are using equipment for the first time. Trained ACLS providers should be sure they are familiar with all emergency equipment *before* an emergency arises.

The following are essential components of the oxygen delivery system:

- Oxygen supply (cylinder or wall oxygen)
- Pressure gauge, flow meter, and valve handles to open the cylinder
- Tubing connecting the oxygen supply to the oxygen administration device
- Humidifier
- Oxygen administration device
- Patient

Devices Used to Deliver Supplementary Oxygen

Four devices are generally used to administer supplementary oxygen (Table 2):

1. Nasal cannula
2. Face mask
3. Face mask with oxygen reservoir
4. Venturi mask

Nasal Cannula

The nasal cannula (Figure 1A) is a low-flow oxygen administration system designed to add oxygen to ambient gas (room air) as the patient inspires. The inspired oxygen concentration depends on the oxygen flow rate through the cannula and the patient's tidal volume. For every 1 L/min increase in the oxygen flow rate (starting with 1 L/min), the inspired oxygen concentration increases by approximately 4% (Table 2). For patients with altered ventilation, the inspired oxygen concentration may vary widely.

Indications

- Patients with adequate spontaneous respiratory effort and airway protective mechanisms
- Patients with minimal respiratory or oxygenation problems
- Patients who find a face mask uncomfortable

Simple Oxygen Face Mask

A simple oxygen face mask delivers low oxygen flow to the patient's nose and mouth. Exhalation ports present on either side of the mask allow exhaled air to escape and allow the patient to entrain room air during inspiration. The oxygen concentration delivered to the patient will be reduced if the patient's spontaneous respiratory flow requirement is high, the mask is loose, or the oxygen flow into the mask is low. An oxygen flow rate of at least 6 L/min is needed to prevent rebreathing of exhaled CO_2 and to maintain increased inspired oxygen concentration. A flow rate of 6 to 10 L/min is recommended to deliver an inspired oxygen concentration of 35% to 60%.

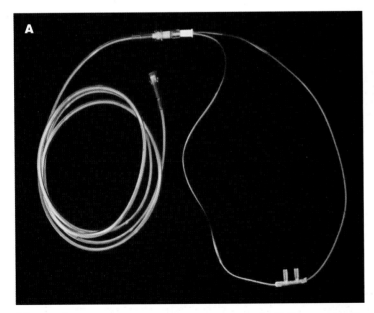
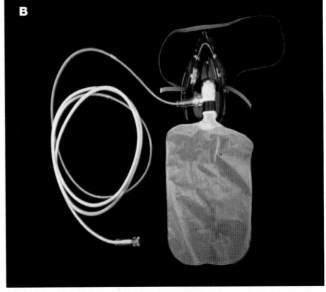

Figure 1. Airway adjunct devices. **A,** Nasal cannula. **B,** Face mask with oxygen reservoir.

Table 2. Delivery of Supplementary Oxygen: Flow Rates and Percentage of Oxygen Delivered

Device	Flow Rates	Delivered O_2*
Nasal cannula	1 L/min	21%-24%
	2 L/min	25%-28%
	3 L/min	29%-32%
	4 L/min	33%-36%
	5 L/min	37%-40%
	6 L/min	41%-44%
Simple oxygen face mask	6-10 L/min	35%-60%
Face mask with O_2 reservoir (nonrebreathing mask)	6 L/min	60%
	7 L/min	70%
	8 L/min	80%
	9 L/min	90%
	10-15 L/min	95%-100%
Venturi mask	4-8 L/min	24%-40%
	10-12 L/min	40%-50%

*Percentage is approximate.

Indications

- Patients with adequate spontaneous respiratory effort and airway protective mechanisms
- Patients with minimal respiratory or oxygenation problems
- Patients who find a nasal cannula uncomfortable

Face Mask With Oxygen Reservoir

A *partial rebreathing mask* consists of a face mask with an attached reservoir bag (Figure 1B). With this device, entrainment of room air is minimized so that it is possible to deliver a higher concentration of oxygen than is delivered with a simple face mask. During exhalation some exhaled air flows into the reservoir bag and combines with fresh oxygen. Since the initial portion of exhaled gas comes from the upper airway and is not involved in gas exchange, the oxygen concentration in the reservoir remains high. During inspiration the patient draws air from the fresh oxygen inflow as well as from the reservoir bag. If the oxygen flow rate is maintained above the patient's minute ventilation and the mask fits securely, an oxygen concentration of 50% to 60% can be provided.

A *nonrebreathing mask* consists of a face mask and a reservoir bag plus (1) a valve incorporated into one or both exhalation ports to prevent entrainment of room air during inspiration and (2) a valve placed between the reservoir bag and the mask to prevent flow of exhaled gas into the reservoir. Oxygen inflow is adjusted to prevent collapse of the reservoir bag. During inspiration the patient draws oxygen from the reservoir bag and the oxygen inflow. Each liter-per-minute increase in oxygen flow over 6 L/min will increase the inspired oxygen concentration by 10% (Table 2). Inspired oxygen concentrations near 100% can be achieved with an oxygen flow rate of 10 to 15 L/min with a well-sealed face mask.

Indications

- Patients who are seriously ill, responsive, spontaneously breathing, and require high oxygen concentrations
- Patients who may avoid endotracheal intubation if acute interventions produce a rapid clinical effect, such as patients with acute pulmonary edema, COPD, or severe asthma
- Patients who have relative indications for endotracheal intubation but have intact airway protective reflexes (cough and gag)
- Patients who have relative indications for endotracheal intubation but have physical barriers to immediate intubation, such as clenched teeth or head injury
- During preparation for intubation

Clinical Application

- Start oxygen flow at ≥6 L/min to avoid accumulation and rebreathing of exhaled air in the mask.
- Titrate oxygen flow rate as needed; a flow rate of 10 to 15 L/min will be required for maximum oxygen delivery.

Precautions

Patients who require the use of a face mask with an oxygen reservoir may have a diminished level of consciousness and may aspirate if vomiting occurs. Monitor the patient closely and be prepared to provide suction if vomiting develops.

Venturi Mask

The Venturi mask enables delivery of a reliable oxygen concentration of 24% to 50%. Oxygen under pressure is passed through a special oxygen outlet. The outlet creates a subatmospheric pressure that entrains a specific quantity of room air with the oxygen flow. The inspired oxygen concentration can be adjusted by changing the size of the oxygen outlet and the oxygen flow rate.

Indications

Because the Venturi mask offers more control over inspired oxygen concentration, it is most useful for patients who require precise control of inspired oxygen.

Patients with chronic hypercarbia (high level of carbon dioxide) and moderate to severe hypoxemia may theoretically develop respiratory depression if oxygen administration blunts their hypoxic respiratory drive.

Airway Management in Patients With Severe Trauma

Trauma poses special problems in airway control. In the patient with vertebral injury, excessive movement of the spine may produce or exacerbate a spinal cord injury. A possible spine injury is suspected based on other apparent injuries (multiple trauma, head or neck injury, or facial trauma) and the type and mechanism of injury (eg, motor vehicle crash, fall from a height). If suspected, appropriate immobilization precautions are taken until qualified personnel can evaluate the patient properly.

Techniques

Only providers experienced in these procedures should attempt them.

- The initial step in a patient with a suspected neck injury is chin lift or jaw thrust *without* head extension.
- If the airway remains obstructed, add head tilt slowly and carefully until the airway is open.

- Then stabilize the head in a neutral position. A trained provider should stabilize the patient's head during any airway manipulation to prevent excessive flexion, extension, or lateral movement of the head during airway control.
- Nasotracheal intubation is relatively contraindicated in a patient with facial fractures or fractures at the base of the skull. Direct orotracheal intubation becomes the technique of choice in such circumstances. A second provider is needed to provide manual immobilization of the head and neck during intubation attempts.

If the patient is breathing spontaneously and requires intubation but oral intubation is not possible, the experienced provider may attempt *"blind" nasotracheal intubation*. This technique, however, is rarely indicated and should be attempted only by personnel with experience in the technique. A second provider must provide head and neck immobilization during the intubation attempt to prevent reactive neck movement.

- Be prepared to provide immediate suctioning of the upper airway if necessary.
- When endotracheal intubation cannot be performed, experienced experts should achieve airway control using alternative airway devices or perform cricothyrotomy.

Integration of CPR and Advanced Airways

Avoid Forceful, Fast, and Full Ventilations

During CPR blood flow to the lungs is substantially reduced, so an adequate ventilation-perfusion ratio can be maintained with lower tidal volumes and respiratory rates than normal. Providers should not hyperventilate the patient (too many breaths or too large a volume). Excessive ventilation is unnecessary and is harmful because it increases intrathoracic pressure, decreases venous return to the heart, and diminishes cardiac output and survival.

Foundation Facts **Withhold Oxygen in Patients With COPD and Hypoxic Ventilatory Drive?**	- Never withhold oxygen from patients with respiratory distress because you suspect the patient depends on hypoxic ventilatory drive. - Administer 24% oxygen initially and observe the patient for respiratory depression. Titrate administered oxygen to the preferred oxyhemoglobin saturation or PaO_2.

- Excessive ventilation is unnecessary and is harmful because it increases intrathoracic pressure, decreases venous return to the heart, and diminishes cardiac output and survival.
- When an advanced airway has been inserted, be careful to avoid hyperventilation.

Continuous Ventilations With an Advanced Airway

When the patient has an advanced airway in place, 2 providers no longer deliver *cycles* of CPR (ie, compressions interrupted by pauses for ventilation). Instead the compressing provider gives continuous chest compressions at a rate of 100 per minute without pauses for ventilation. The provider delivering ventilation provides 8 to 10 ventilations per minute or 1 ventilation every 6 to 8 seconds. Providers should change compressor and ventilator roles approximately every 2 minutes to prevent compressor fatigue and deterioration in quality and rate of chest compressions. When multiple providers are present, they should rotate the compressor role about every 2 minutes.

Confirmation of Endotracheal Tube Placement

The 3 most important caveats for providers performing CPR after insertion of the advanced airway are

- Be sure the advanced airway is correctly placed (verify).
- Do not deliver *cycles* of CPR (ie, compressions interrupted by pauses for ventilation). Instead the compressor gives *continuous* chest compressions at a rate of 100 per minute without pauses for ventilation.
- Avoid delivering an excessive ventilation volume and rate because it can compromise venous return and cardiac output during CPR.

Be Sure the Airway Is in the Right Place!

Clinical Assessment to Confirm Tube Placement

Providers should perform a thorough assessment of endotracheal tube position immediately after placement. This assessment should not require interruption of chest compressions. Assessment by physical examination consists of visualizing chest expansion bilaterally and listening over the epigastrium (breath sounds should not be heard) and the lung fields bilaterally (breath sounds should be equal and adequate). If there is doubt about correct tube placement, use the laryngoscope to visualize the tube passing through the vocal cords. If still in doubt, remove the tube and provide bag-mask ventilation until the tube can be replaced.

Use of Devices to Confirm Tube Placement

ACLS providers should always use *both* clinical assessment and devices to confirm endotracheal tube location immediately after placement and each time the patient is moved. No study, however, has identified a single device as both sensitive and specific for endotracheal tube placement in the trachea or esophagus. All confirmation devices should be considered adjuncts to other confirmation techniques. There is no data to quantify the capability of devices to monitor tube position after initial placement.

Exhaled CO_2 Detectors

Detection of exhaled CO_2 is one of several independent methods of confirming endotracheal tube position (Figure 2). Given the simplicity of the exhaled CO_2 detector,

After an advanced airway is placed during CPR:

- Deliver ventilations at a rate of 8 to 10 ventilations per minute, or 1 ventilation every 6 to 8 seconds.
- Give continuous chest compressions at a rate of 100 per minute without pauses for ventilation.

Both clinical and device confirmation of the endotracheal tube are required:

- Always use both clinical assessment and devices to confirm endotracheal tube location immediately after placement.
- To exclude tube displacement, reconfirm placement each time the patient is moved.

it can be used as the initial method for detecting correct tube placement even in the cardiac arrest patient. Detection of exhaled CO_2, however, is not infallible as a means of confirming tube placement, particularly during cardiac arrest. (See "Capnography and Capnometry," above, and Table 3, below.)

Use of CO_2 detecting devices to determine the correct placement of other advanced airways (eg, Combitube, LMA) has not been adequately studied.

Esophageal Detector Devices

The esophageal detector device (EDD) consists of a bulb that is compressed and attached to the endotracheal tube (Figure 3). If the tube is in the esophagus (positive result for an EDD), the suction created by the EDD will collapse the lumen of the esophagus or pull the esophageal tissue against the tip of the tube, and the bulb will not reexpand. The EDD may also consist of a syringe that is attached to the endotracheal tube; the provider tries to pull the barrel

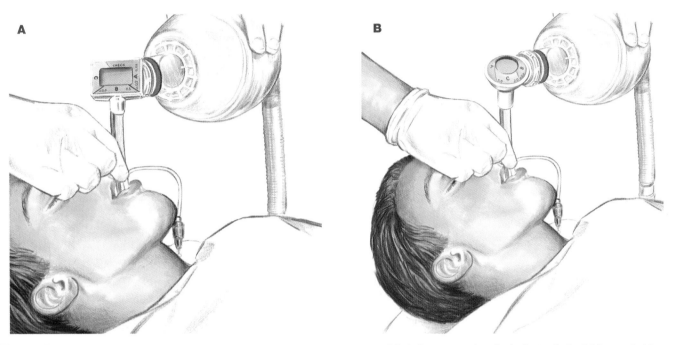

Figure 2. Confirmation of endotracheal tube placement. **A,** End-tidal colorimetric CO_2 indicator: purple color indicates lack of CO_2—probably in the esophagus. **B,** End-tidal colorimetric CO_2 indicators: yellow indicates the presence of CO_2 and tube in the airway. Note that CO_2 detection cannot ensure proper *depth* of tube insertion. The tube should be held in place and then secured once correct position is verified. Note that different manufacturers may use different colors.

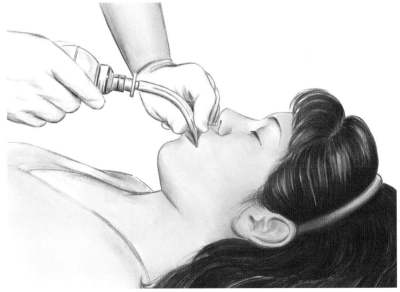

Figure 3. Esophageal detector bulb device: the aspiration technique. The tube should be held in place and then secured once correct position is verified.

of the syringe. If the tube is in the esophagus, it will not be possible to pull the barrel (aspirate air) with the syringe.

The EDD *is* highly sensitive for detection of endotracheal tubes that *are* misplaced in the esophagus (sensitive for esophageal placement). The EDD has poor specificity for endotracheal placement of the tube when patients are in cardiac arrest (Table 4). This can result in incorrect withdrawal of the endotracheal tube when, in fact, it is correctly placed. The EDD may yield misleading results

Table 3. Reasons for Misleading Results Using a Colorimetric End-Tidal CO_2 Detector

Colorimetric End-Tidal CO_2 Detector		
Reading	**Actual Location of ETT: Trachea**	**Actual Location of ETT: Esophagus (or Hypopharynx)**
CO_2 Detected Yellow (or as specified by manufacturer) (positive = CO_2 present)	*ETT in trachea* Proceed with ventilations.	*Reasons for apparent CO_2 detection despite tube in esophagus* Causes: Distended stomach, recent ingestion of carbonated beverage, nonpulmonary sources of CO_2. Consequences: Unrecognized esophageal intubation; can lead to iatrogenic death.
No CO_2 Detected Blue (or as specified by manufacturer) (negative = CO_2 absent)	*No CO_2 detection with tube in trachea* Causes: Low or no blood flow state (eg, cardiac arrest); any cardiac arrest with no, prolonged, or poor CPR. Consequences: Leads to unnecessary removal of properly placed ETT. Reintubation attempts increase chances of other adverse consequences.	*No CO_2 detection and tube is not in trachea (ie, tube is in esophagus)* Causes: Provider has inserted ETT in esophagus/hypopharynx. A life-threatening adverse event has occurred. Consequences: Provider recognizes ETT is not in trachea; properly and rapidly identified; tube is removed at once; patient is reintubated.

ETT indicates endotracheal tube.

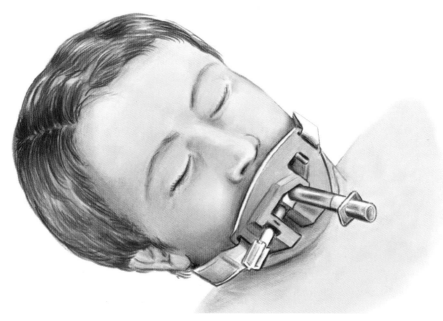

Figure 4. Endotracheal tube holder, adult.

Table 4. Reasons for Misleading Results Using an Esophageal Detector Device

Esophageal Detector Device		
Reading	**Actual Location of ETT: Esophagus**	**Actual Location of ETT: Trachea**
Consistent With Tube in Esophagus Bulb does not refill or refills slowly (>10 seconds × 2), or syringe cannot be aspirated, suggesting that tip of ETT is in esophagus.	*Device suggests tube in esophagus when it is in esophagus* Causes: Provider has inserted tube in esophagus/hypopharynx. A life-threatening adverse event has occurred. Consequences: Rescuer correctly recognizes ETT is in esophagus; ETT is removed at once; patient is reintubated.	*Device suggests tube in esophagus when it is in trachea* Causes: Secretions in trachea (mucus, gastric contents, acute pulmonary edema); insertion in right main bronchus; pliable trachea (morbid obesity, late-term pregnancy). Consequences: Leads to unnecessary removal of properly placed ETT. Reintubation attempts increase chances of other adverse consequences.
Consistent With Tube in Trachea Bulb fills immediately or syringe can be aspirated, suggesting that ETT is in trachea	*Results suggest that tube is NOT in esophagus (ie, that it is in trachea) when tube IS in esophagus* Causes: • Conditions that cause increased lung expansion (eg, COPD, status asthmaticus). • Conditions that fill stomach with air (eg, recent bag-mask ventilation, mouth-to-mask or mouth-to-mouth breathing). • Conditions that cause poor tone in esophageal sphincter or increased gastric pressure (late pregnancy). Consequences: Unrecognized esophageal intubation can lead to death.	*Results suggest that tube is NOT in esophagus (ie, that it is in trachea) when it IS in trachea* Esophageal detector device indicates ETT is in trachea. Proceed with ventilations.

ETT indicates endotracheal tube; and COPD, chronic obstructive pulmonary disease.

in patients with morbid obesity, late pregnancy, or status asthmaticus, or when there are copious endotracheal secretions, because with these conditions the trachea tends to collapse. Because of poor sensitivity and specificity, use of the EDD should be considered as just one of several independent methods for confirmation of correct endotracheal tube placement. There is no evidence that the EDD is accurate for the continued monitoring of endotracheal tube placement.

Secure the Airway

After inserting the advanced airway and confirming correct placement, the provider should record the depth of the tube as marked at the front teeth and secure it. Because there is significant potential for endotracheal tube movement with head flexion and extension, ongoing monitoring of endotracheal tube placement is essential during transport, particularly when the patient is moved from one location to another. Providers should verify correct placement of all advanced airways immediately after insertion and whenever the patient is moved.

Secure the endotracheal tube with tape or a commercial device (Figure 4). Backboards, commercial devices for securing the endotracheal tube, and other strategies provide an equivalent method for preventing accidental tube displacement when compared with traditional methods of securing the tube (tape). These devices may be considered during patient transport. After tube confirmation and fixation, obtain a chest x-ray (when feasible) to confirm that the end of the endotracheal tube is properly positioned above the carina. A chest x-ray is never used as a primary method for confirmation of endotracheal tube position.

Airway Adjuncts and Advanced Airways

Oropharyngeal Airways

Maintain a Patent Airway Using Adjuncts

Oropharyngeal airways should be reserved for use in unconscious (unresponsive) patients with no cough or gag reflex. They should be inserted only by persons trained in their use. Incorrect insertion of an airway can displace the tongue into the hypopharynx, causing airway obstruction. Although studies have not specifically considered the use of advanced airways in arrest, airways may aid in the delivery of adequate ventilation with a bag-mask device by preventing the tongue from occluding the airway.

The oropharyngeal airway is a single-use, disposable plastic device that

- Holds the tongue away from the posterior wall of the pharynx
- Facilitates suctioning of the pharynx
- Prevents the patient from biting and occluding an endotracheal tube

The 2 common types of oropharyngeal airway are the Guedel device, which is tubular, and the Berman device, which has side channels. Oropharyngeal airways should be available in various sizes for use in infants, children, and adults. To estimate the size, place the airway against the patient's face. When the flange is at the lips, the tip of the airway should be just cephalad to the angle of the mandible. The millimeter size reflects the distance from the flange to the tip:

- Large adult: 100 mm (Guedel size 5)
- Medium adult: 90 mm (Guedel size 4)
- Small adult: 80 mm (Guedel size 3)

Indications

- The patient is spontaneously breathing.
- The patient is *obtunded/unconscious* (in danger of mechanical upper airway obstruction from a flaccid tongue and relaxed hypopharyngeal structures).
- The patient has *lost airway protective reflexes* (cough/gag reflex).

Technique

Use a rigid pharyngeal suction tip (Yankauer) to clear the mouth and pharynx of secretions, blood, or vomitus.

- Turn the airway so that it enters the mouth either inverted or on its side.
- As the airway transverses the oral cavity and approaches the posterior wall of the pharynx, rotate the airway into proper position (Figure 5).
- Alternatively, use a tongue depressor to move the tongue downward before inserting the airway. Be careful not to obstruct the airway with the tongue.

Complications

Successful use of the oropharyngeal airway without complications requires adequate initial training, frequent practice, and timely retraining.

- If the oropharyngeal airway is too long, it may press the epiglottis against the laryngeal entry, causing complete airway obstruction.
- If the oropharyngeal airway is inserted incorrectly or is too small, it may push the tongue posteriorly into the hypopharynx, aggravating upper airway obstruction.
- The patient's lips and tongue can be lacerated if they are caught between the teeth and the oral airway.
- Attempts to insert the airway in a patient with intact cough and gag may stimulate vomiting and laryngospasm.

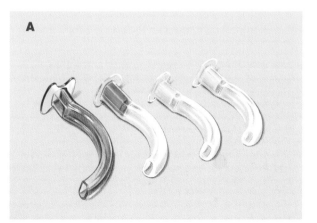
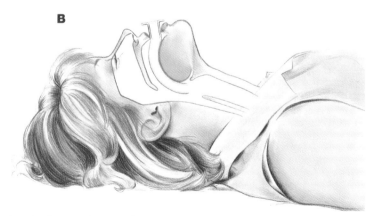

Figure 5. Oropharyngeal airways. **A,** Four oropharyngeal airway devices. **B,** One oropharyngeal airway device inserted.

Nasopharyngeal Airways

The nasopharyngeal airway (Figure 6) is an uncuffed tube made of soft rubber or plastic. Nasopharyngeal airways are useful in patients with airway obstruction or those at risk for development of airway obstruction, particularly when conditions such as a clenched jaw prevent placement of an oral airway. No studies exist on the use of this device in patients in cardiac arrest, but the nasopharyngeal airway may be used in patients with an obstructed airway to facilitate delivery of ventilations with a bag-mask device.

Nasopharyngeal airways are better tolerated than oral airways in patients who are not deeply unconscious. Airway bleeding can occur in up to 30% of patients following insertion of a nasopharyngeal airway. Rarely, inadvertent intracranial placement of a nasopharyngeal airway may occur in patients with basilar skull fractures. Nasopharyngeal airways should be used with caution in patients with severe craniofacial injury.

Adult Sizes

- The millimeter size of the nasopharyngeal tube indicates internal diameter of the tube; the larger the internal diameter, the longer the tube.
- The proper tube length is estimated by the distance from the tip of the nose to the tragus of the ear. Tubes with the following inner diameters are recommended:

  - Large adult: 8 to 9 mm (32 to 36 F)
  - Medium adult: 7 to 8 mm (28 to 32 F)
  - Small adult: 6 to 7 mm (24 to 28 F)

Insertion Technique

- Lubricate the appropriate size airway with a water-soluble lubricant or anesthetic jelly.
- Gently insert the airway close to the midline, along the floor of the nostril, into the posterior pharynx behind the tongue.

- If you encounter resistance, slightly rotate the tube to facilitate insertion at the angle of the nasal passage and nasopharynx.
- Maintain head tilt; maintain anterior mandible displacement by chin lift or, if necessary, jaw thrust (without head extension if possible cervical spine injury).

Complications

Successful use of the nasopharyngeal airway without complications requires adequate initial training, frequent practice, and timely retraining.

- If the nasopharyngeal tube is *too long,* the tube may injure the epiglottis or vocal cords or may cause bradycardia through vagal stimulation. If assisted ventilation is required, the tube will facilitate air entry into the esophagus, causing gastric inflation and possible hypoventilation.
- If the patient has an intact cough and gag reflex, tube insertion may provoke laryngospasm and vomiting.
- Insertion of the tube may injure the nasal mucosa, causing bleeding. Aspiration of a clot into the trachea is possible.
- Insertion of a nasopharyngeal tube stimulates excessive secretions that may require suctioning.
- If adequate spontaneous respirations do not resume after 15 to 30 seconds, the tube may be malpositioned or obstructed. If this occurs, remove the tube and reattempt proper placement.
- If the patient has occult basilar skull fractures or previous maxillofacial surgery, insertion of a nasopharyngeal tube is contraindicated because a tear in the dura may enable the tube to enter the brain.

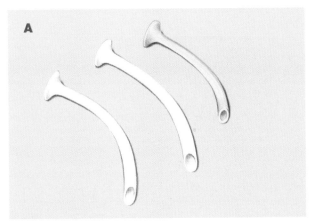
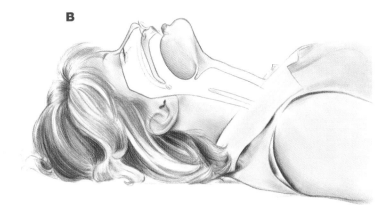

Figure 6. Nasopharyngeal airways. **A,** Three nasopharyngeal airway devices. **B,** One nasopharyngeal airway device inserted.

Optimizing Cardiac Output With Airway and Circulatory Adjuncts

Blood Flow During CPR

CPR provides blood flow to vital organs until more definitive care, such as defibrillation, can be provided or effective circulation established. Cardiac output and perfusion pressures achieved with CPR vary considerably among individual patients and providers. Many patients have very poor perfusion during CPR.[14,15] Circulatory adjuncts or changes in CPR technique that improve blood flow or perfusion pressures may improve the likelihood of successful resuscitation for some patients in cardiac arrest.

The Heart Is the Pump

In 1960 Kouwenhoven, Jude, and Knickerbocker described successful closed-chest compressions.[16] They theorized that compressions displace the sternum downward and squeeze the heart between the sternum and the vertebral bodies of the spine. In this cardiac pump mechanism, compression of the heart between the sternum and spine forces blood into the arterial system. The cardiac valves prevent retrograde blood flow.

The Thorax Is the Pump

In the thoracic pump mechanism, chest compressions generate increased intrathoracic pressure, which is transmitted to the great vessels in the chest and to the extrathoracic arteries, establishing a pressure gradient between the arterial and venous systems. Transmission of the increased intrathoracic pressure into the venous system is prevented by the venous valves and the much greater capacitance of the venous system. The pressure gradient between the arterial and venous systems causes venous return to the thorax during chest relaxation. During chest relaxation retrograde blood flow from extrathoracic arteries supplies blood to the coronary bed (Figure 7).

Data from animal and human studies first suggested the intrathoracic pressure mechanism during CPR. In canine experiments chest compressions produced no differences in cardiac arterial-venous pressure, suggesting that the heart was not squeezed directly. Furthermore, in humans, rapid coughing, which produces blood flow by cyclical variations in intrathoracic pressure, has been reported to help patients in the cardiac catheterization suite maintain consciousness during brief episodes of ventricular

A **Cardiac Compression Pump**

Compression

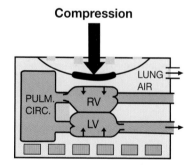

B **Intrathoracic Pressure Pump**

Compression

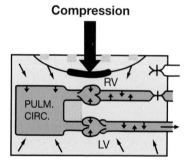

Relaxation

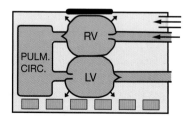

Relaxation

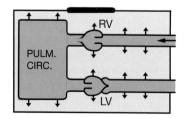

Figure 7. Theoretical mechanisms of blood flow during CPR. **A,** The cardiac compression pump model proposes that chest compression squeezes the heart between the sternum and the spine, forcing blood into the systemic circulation. Relaxation "siphons" blood from the venous system. **B,** The intrathoracic pressure pump model proposes that increased intrathoracic pressure generated with compression "squeezes" the thoracic contents. Blood flows into the extrathoracic arterial system, but venous valves and the increased capacitance of the venous system prevent transmission of pressure. With relaxation, intrathoracic pressure falls, producing an antegrade venous pressure gradient and venous return. As blood "refluxes" from the extrathoracic great vessels into the chest, coronary perfusion occurs. Modified from Halperin et al[17] with permission.

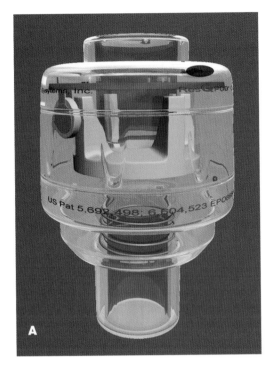
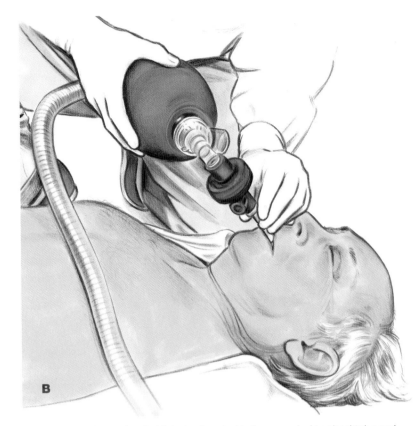

Figure 8. A, The impedance threshold device (ResQPod™). **B,** The impedance threshold device inserted between end of tracheal tube and bag-valve device.

tachycardia. In patients with a flail chest, blood flow is poor until the sternum is stabilized.

Heart or Thorax?

Direct pressure measurements of arterial and intrathoracic pressures have provided conflicting evidence for these mechanisms. Similarly measurements of cardiac dimensions and mitral valve position during CPR with cardiac ultrasound are inconclusive. The precise mechanism of blood flow from chest compressions remains a subject of controversy. It is likely that some components of each mechanism are operative during the dynamic physiologic conditions of resuscitation.

Perfusion is determined by 2 major factors: *cardiac pumping action* and *vascular resistance*. Adjuncts that improve cardiac pump function during CPR directly increase coronary and cerebral perfusion. Adjuncts that increase peripheral vascular resistance indirectly increase vital organ perfusion by shunting blood from the peripheral to the central circulation.

How CPR Adjuncts Work

Several different adjuncts to circulation have been evaluated, but they are beyond the scope of the ACLS Provider Course. One, however, is currently being evaluated

in clinical trials and serves as an example of how the basic principles of high-quality CPR and the physiology of blood flow during cardiac arrest can be optimized in a clinical setting.

Impedance Threshold Device (Circulatory Adjunct Device)

The impedance threshold device (ITD) (Figure 8) uses a valve that limits air entry into the lungs during chest recoil between chest compressions. It is designed to reduce intrathoracic pressure and enhance venous return to the heart. In essence, when used properly it "siphons" blood into the chest and may improve cardiac output during cardiac arrest.

How It Works

By preventing passive inspiration during chest recoil, the impedance threshold valve helps sustain negative intrathoracic pressures that enhance refilling of the thorax and heart and thus cardiac output with the ensuing chest compression. Although increased long-term survival rates have not been documented, when the ITD is used by trained personnel as an adjunct to CPR in intubated adult cardiac arrest patients, it can improve hemodynamic parameters and ROSC.

In recent reports the ITD has been used during conventional CPR[18,19] with an endotracheal tube or face mask. Studies suggest that when the ITD is used with a face mask, it may create the same negative intratracheal pressure as use of the ITD with an endotracheal tube if providers can maintain a tight face mask seal.[20]

The Science

Animal studies have shown that intermittent inspiratory impedance improves coronary perfusion pressure, arterial pressure, tracheal CO_2, and blood flow (both myocardial and cerebral) when added to standard CPR or active compression-decompression (ACD) CPR. One clinical study has shown improved hemodynamics as measured by levels of end-tidal CO_2. Several experimental studies and 1 small clinical trial have shown no negative effects with use of the ITD.

Potential benefit in patients who receive standard CPR remains under investigation. In 2 studies[20,21] of 610 adults in cardiac arrest in the out-of-hospital setting, use of ACD-CPR plus the ITD was associated with improved ROSC and 24-hour survival rates when compared with use of standard CPR alone. A randomized study of 230 adults documented increased admission to the intensive care unit and 24-hour survival[18] when an ITD was used during standard CPR in patients in cardiac arrest (pulseless electrical activity only) in the out-of-hospital setting. The addition of the ITD was associated with improved hemodynamics during standard CPR in 1 clinical study.[19]

References

1. Carlson KA, Jahr JS. An update on pulse oximetry. Part II: limitations and future applications. *Anesthesiol Rev*. 1994;21:41-46.

2. Aughey K, Hess D, Eitel D, Bleecher K, Cooley M, Ogden C, Sabulsky N. An evaluation of pulse oximetry in prehospital care. *Ann Emerg Med*. 1991;20:887-891.

3. Bota GW, Rowe BH. Continuous monitoring of oxygen saturation in prehospital patients with severe illness: the problem of unrecognized hypoxemia. *J Emerg Med*. 1995;13:305-311.

4. Brown LH, Manring EA, Kornegay HB, Prasad NH. Can prehospital personnel detect hypoxemia without the aid of pulse oximeters? *Am J Emerg Med*. 1996;14:43-44.

5. Valko PC, Campbell JP, McCarty DL, Martin D, Turnbull J. Prehospital use of pulse oximetry in rotary-wing aircraft. *Prehospital Disaster Med*. 1991;6:421-428.

6. Wahr JA, Tremper KK. Noninvasive oxygen monitoring techniques. *Crit Care Clin*. 1995;11:199-217.

7. Li J. Capnography alone is imperfect for endotracheal tube placement confirmation during emergency intubation. *J Emerg Med*. 2001;20:223-229.

8. Sum Ping ST, Mehta MP, Symreng T. Accuracy of the FEF CO2 detector in the assessment of endotracheal tube placement. *Anesth Analg*. 1992;74:415-419.

9. Ornato JP, Shipley JB, Racht EM, Slovis CM, Wrenn KD, Pepe PE, Almeida SL, Ginger VF, Fotre TV. Multicenter study of a portable, hand-size, colorimetric end-tidal carbon dioxide detection device. *Ann Emerg Med*. 1992;21:518-523.

10. Chow LH, Lui PW, Cheung EL, Jong HR, Yang TC, Chen YC. Verification of endotracheal tube misplacement with the colorimetric carbon dioxide detector during anesthesia. *Chung Hua I Hsueh Tsa Chih*. 1993;51:415-418.

11. Cantineau JP, Merckx P, Lambert Y, Sorkine M, Bertrand C, Duvaldestin P. Effect of epinephrine on end-tidal carbon dioxide pressure during prehospital cardiopulmonary resuscitation. *Am J Emerg Med*. 1994;12:267-270.

12. Ward KR, Yealy DM. End-tidal carbon dioxide monitoring in emergency medicine. Part 2: clinical applications. *Acad Emerg Med*. 1998;5:637-646.

13. Hand IL, Shepard EK, Krauss AN, Auld PA. Discrepancies between transcutaneous and end-tidal carbon dioxide monitoring in the critically ill neonate with respiratory distress syndrome. *Crit Care Med*. 1989;17:556-559.

14. Paradis NA, Martin GB, Rivers EP, Goetting MG, Appleton TJ, Feingold M, Nowak RM. Coronary perfusion pressure and the return of spontaneous circulation in human cardiopulmonary resuscitation. *JAMA*. 1990;263:1106-1113.

15. Sanders AB, Ogle M, Ewy GA. Coronary perfusion pressure during cardiopulmonary resuscitation. *Am J Emerg Med*. 1985;3:11-14.

16. Kouwenhoven WB, Jude JR, Knickerbocker GG. Closed-chest cardiac massage. *JAMA*. 1960;173:1064-1067.

17. Halperin HR, Tsitlik JE, Guerci AD, Mellits ED, Levin HR, Shi AY, Chandra N, Weisfeldt ML. Determinants of blood flow to vital organs during cardiopulmonary resuscitation in dogs. *Circulation*. 1986;73:539-550.

18. Aufderheide TP, Pirrallo RG, Provo TA, Lurie KG. Clinical evaluation of an inspiratory impedance threshold device during standard cardiopulmonary resuscitation in patients with out-of-hospital cardiac arrest. *Crit Care Med*. 2005;33:734-740.

19. Pirrallo RG, Aufderheide TP, Provo TA, Lurie KG. Effect of an inspiratory impedance threshold device on hemodynamics during conventional manual cardiopulmonary resuscitation. *Resuscitation*. 2005;66:13-20.

20. Wolcke BB, Mauer DK, Schoefmann MF, Teichmann H, Provo TA, Lindner KH, Dick WF, Aeppli D, Lurie KG. Comparison of standard cardiopulmonary resuscitation versus the combination of active compression-decompression cardiopulmonary resuscitation and an inspiratory impedance threshold device for out-of-hospital cardiac arrest. *Circulation*. 2003;108:2201-2205.

21. Plaisance P, Soleil C, Lurie KG, Vicaut E, Ducros L, Payen D. Use of an inspiratory impedance threshold device on a facemask and endotracheal tube to reduce intrathoracic pressures during the decompression phase of active compression-decompression cardiopulmonary resuscitation. *Crit Care Med*. 2005;33:990-994.

Chapter 5

Pulseless Arrest: VF/VT

This Chapter

- **Proper priorities for arrhythmias associated with pulseless arrest**
- **Why only 1 shock at a time now?**
- **Amiodarone or lidocaine again?**
- **Epinephrine or vasopressin, or vasopressin or epinephrine?**

Overview

Four rhythms produce pulseless cardiac arrest: ventricular fibrillation (VF), rapid ventricular tachycardia (VT), pulseless electrical activity (PEA), and asystole. PEA is not a single rhythm but can be any organized rhythm without a detectable pulse. Survival from these arrest rhythms requires both immediate basic life support (BLS), early defibrillation if indicated, prioritized advanced cardiovascular life support (ACLS), and postresuscitation care.

The foundation of ACLS care is continued good BLS care, beginning with prompt, high-quality bystander CPR and, for VF/pulseless VT, attempted defibrillation within minutes of collapse. For victims of witnessed VF arrest, prompt bystander CPR and early defibrillation can significantly increase the chance of survival to hospital discharge. In comparison, typical ACLS therapies, such as insertion

of advanced airways and pharmacologic support of circulation, have not been shown to increase the rate of survival to hospital discharge. This chapter details the initial general care of a patient in VF (or pulseless VT) cardiac arrest and provides an overview of the ACLS Pulseless Arrest Algorithm (Figure 1).

Access for Medications: Correct Priorities

During cardiac arrest basic CPR and early defibrillation are of primary importance, and drug administration is of secondary importance. Few drugs used in the treatment of cardiac arrest are supported by strong evidence. After provision of CPR and early defibrillation, ACLS providers can establish intravenous (IV) access, administer drug therapy, and then consider insertion of an advanced airway, providing bag-mask ventilation is effective.

Advanced Airway Adjuncts: Correct Priorities

ACLS providers must be aware of the risks and benefits of insertion of an advanced airway during a resuscitation attempt. Such risks are affected by the condition of the patient and the provider's expertise in airway control. Because insertion of an advanced airway may require interruption of chest compressions for many seconds, the ACLS team leader should weigh the need for compressions against the need for insertion of an advanced airway. If adequate ventilations can be achieved with a bag-mask

---

Critical Concept	*After* provision of CPR and attempts at early defibrillation if needed, ACLS providers can
Priorities in Cardiac Arrest	• Establish IV access • Administer drug therapy • Consider insertion of an advanced airway

device, the team leader may defer insertion of an advanced airway until the patient fails to respond to initial CPR and defibrillation attempts or demonstrates return of spontaneous circulation (ROSC).

Defibrillation Plus CPR: A Critical Combination[1]

The important and central contribution of early CPR and early defibrillation to improving the outcome from VF/pulseless VT is now a foundation for resuscitative efforts. In comparison, clinical trials have demonstrated only a small magnitude of benefit from vasopressor and antiarrhythmic therapy.

Early defibrillation is critical to survival from sudden cardiac arrest (SCA) for several reasons:

1. The most frequent initial rhythm in witnessed SCA is VF.
2. The treatment for VF is electrical defibrillation.
3. The probability of successful defibrillation diminishes rapidly over time.
4. VF tends to deteriorate to asystole within a few minutes.[2]

Effect of CPR on ROSC

Overall, CPR can double or triple[3] survival from witnessed SCA at any interval from collapse to defibrillation. For every minute that passes between collapse and defibrillation, survival rates from witnessed VF SCA decrease 7% to 10% if no CPR is provided.[2] When bystander CPR is provided, the decrease in survival rates is more gradual and averages 3% to 4% per minute from collapse to defibrillation.[2,4]

Effect on Neurologic Outcome

If bystanders provide immediate CPR, many adults in VF can survive with intact neurologic function, especially if defibrillation is performed within about 5 minutes after SCA.[5] CPR also provides a small amount of blood flow that may maintain some oxygen and substrate delivery to the heart and brain,[6] extending the window of time during which defibrillation can occur. CPR prolongs VF, keeping it from deteriorating into asystole.[7,8]

So CPR First or Shock First?

Delays to the start of *either* CPR or defibrillation can reduce survival from SCA. In the 1990s some predicted that CPR could be rendered obsolete by the widespread development of community automated external defibrillator (AED) programs. But Cobb et al[9] noted that as more first responders in Seattle were equipped with AEDs, survival rates from SCA unexpectedly fell. They attributed this decline to reduced emphasis on CPR. Although several factors may contribute to this observation, there is growing evidence to support an association between decreased survival rates and a reduced priority on CPR. So should you do CPR first or defibrillate first?

If an AED or Defibrillator Is **Immediately Available**

When any provider witnesses an arrest and a defibrillator is *immediately* available on-site, use the defibrillator as soon as possible. Otherwise provide immediate CPR and use the AED or defibrillator as soon as it is available. This correlates with using the defibrillator during the electrical phase of cardiac arrest (see Chapter 3, Figure 4).

If an AED or Defibrillator Is **Not Immediately Available**

If an arrest is not witnessed, consider giving 5 cycles (about 2 minutes) of CPR (30 compressions: 2 ventilations) before checking the ECG rhythm and attempting defibrillation. In studies of adult out-of-hospital VF SCA, patients in the hemodynamic phase of VF cardiac arrest (after the electrical phase) who received 1½ to 3 minutes of CPR before defibrillation had increased rates of initial resuscitation, survival to hospital discharge, and 1-year survival when compared with those who received immediate defibrillation.[5,9]

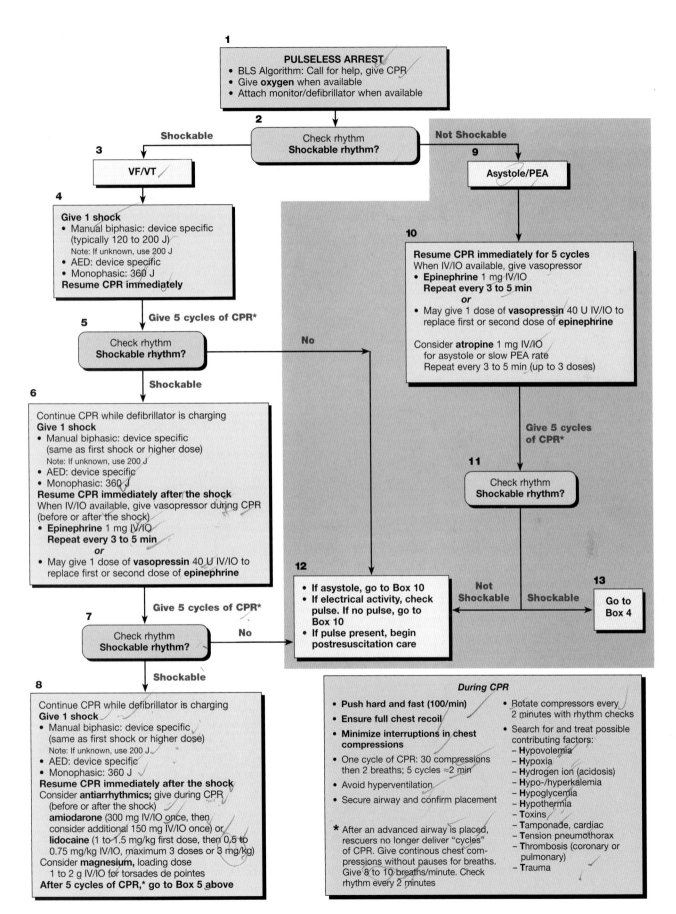

Figure 1. ACLS Pulseless Arrest Algorithm. Left Side of Algorithm VF/VT.

FYI

Guidelines 2005

Emergency medical services (EMS) system medical directors may consider implementing a protocol that would allow EMS responders to provide 5 cycles (about 2 minutes) of CPR before defibrillation when EMS personnel find patients in VF, particularly when the EMS system call-to-response interval is >4 to 5 minutes.

- At the present time there is no evidence to evaluate CPR before defibrillation for in-hospital cardiac arrest.

Ventricular Fibrillation—The Importance of Early Recognition

VF is the single most important rhythm for the ECC provider to recognize. In VF multiple areas within the ventricles display marked variation in depolarization and repolarization (Figure 2). There is no organized ventricular depolarization. Some have described VF as "myocardial chaos." The ventricles do not contract as a unit, and they produce no effective cardiac output. The initial, specific treatment for VF and pulseless VT is always immediate electrical defibrillation.

Coarse Versus Fine VF—Significance of VF Frequency

When myocardial ischemia or infarction causes SCA, it is most often through the mechanism of VF. The terms *coarse* and *fine* have been used to describe the amplitude of the waveforms in VF (Figures 2 and 3). *Coarse* VF generally indicates VF that has been present only a short time, usually less than 3 to 5 minutes. High-amplitude, *coarse* VF requires significant levels of high-energy adenosine triphosphate (ATP) to persist. If the heart receives defibrillatory shocks before these energy stores are exhausted, spontaneous, organized contractions are more likely to resume after the myocardial "stunning" from a direct-current shock. The presence of *fine* VF that resembles asystole indicates "old" or "exhausted" VF. Often considerable delay—and no CPR—have followed patient collapse; high-energy phosphate stores and myocardial

oxygen are depleted, and postshock resumption of spontaneous circulation becomes very unlikely.

The *power* or *frequency spectrum* of VF is now the focus of continuing investigation as a possible way to predict whether the outcome of a defibrillatory shock will be *postshock ROSC, postshock asystole,* or *persistent VF*. This information could potentially be integrated with new knowledge about CPR and the hemodynamic phases of CPR. Providers could be prompted to continue with CPR for longer periods or to start other interventions before attempting defibrillation if informed by an AED or defibrillator that a shock is more likely to produce asystole. A complex analysis of central frequency, peak power frequency, spectral flatness, and energy has already achieved high levels of discrimination between rhythms that when shocked are followed by ROSC and rhythms that when shocked are followed by asystole.

Shock One Time! Then Immediately Resume CPR

A significant change in the *2005 AHA Guidelines for CPR and ECC* was the elimination of the 3-shock sequence for VF. There are no studies evaluating a 1-shock versus a 3-shock protocol in humans. But frequent or long interruptions in precordial chest compressions for rhythm analysis or rescue breathing[10,11] are associated with postresuscitation myocardial dysfunction and reduced survival rates. In addition, interruption in chest compressions is associated with a decreased probability of

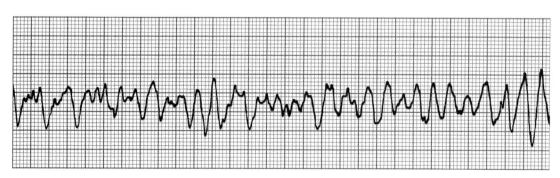

Figure 2. Coarse ventricular fibrillation. Note high-amplitude waveforms, which vary in size, shape, and rhythm, representing chaotic ventricular electrical activity. The ECG criteria for VF are as follows: (1) QRS complexes: no normal-looking QRS complexes are recognizable; a regular "negative-positive-negative" pattern (Q-R-S) cannot be seen. (2) Rate: uncountable; electrical deflections are very rapid and too disorganized to count. (3) Rhythm: no regular rhythmic pattern can be discerned; the electrical waveforms vary in size and shape; the pattern is completely disorganized.

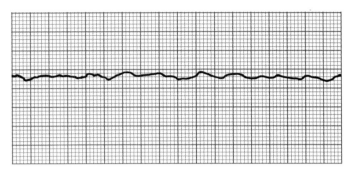

Figure 3. Fine ventricular fibrillation. In comparison with Figure 2, the amplitude of electrical activity is much reduced. Note the complete absence of QRS complexes. In terms of electrophysiology, prognosis, and the likely clinical response to attempted defibrillation, adrenergic agents, or antiarrhythmics, this rhythm pattern may be difficult to distinguish from that of asystole.

FAQ **Will resumption of CPR provoke VF if an organized rhythm is present?**	Concern that chest compressions might provoke recurrent VF in the presence of a postshock organized rhythm does not appear to be warranted. • When VF/pulseless VT is present, 1 shock is delivered and CPR is immediately resumed, beginning with chest compressions. • After 5 cycles (about 2 minutes) of CPR, the AED or ACLS provider should analyze the cardiac rhythm and deliver another shock if indicated.

conversion of VF to another potentially perfusing rhythm. Rhythm and pulse checks are also thought to contribute significantly to interruptions in chest compressions.[12] Concern that chest compressions might provoke recurrent VF in the presence of a postshock organized rhythm does not appear to be warranted.[13]

Another cause of delay with AEDs is the time between delivery of the first shock and delivery of the first postshock compression. When 3 shocks were given previously, this delay averaged up to 37 seconds. This delay is difficult

to justify considering the first-shock efficacy of >90% now being reported for current biphasic defibrillators. If 1 shock fails to eliminate VF, the incremental benefit of another shock is low, and resumption of CPR beginning with chest compressions is likely to confer a greater benefit than another shock. This fact, combined with the data from animal studies documenting harmful effects from interruptions to chest compressions, suggests that a 1-shock scenario plus immediate CPR without rhythm or pulse checks is reasonable.

Critical Concept **Benefit of 1-Shock Sequence**	**Resume CPR Immediately After Shock** If 1 shock fails to eliminate VF, the incremental benefit of another shock is low, and resumption of CPR is likely to confer a greater benefit than another shock. • The first-shock efficacy of current biphasic defibrillators is >90%.

FAQ **Why was first-shock energy (monophasic) increased?** **Is immediate replacement of monophasic defibrillators recommended?**	Experts weighed the potential negative effects of a high first-shock energy versus the negative effects of prolonged VF: • The consensus was that providers using monophasic AEDs should give an initial shock of 360 J. • This single dose for monophasic shocks is designed to simplify instructions to providers; it is not a mandate to recall monophasic AEDs for reprogramming or to replace monophasic defibrillators.

Rationale for Increase in First-Shock Energy for Monophasic Defibrillators

First-shock efficacy for a monophasic shock is lower than first-shock efficacy for a biphasic shock. Although the optimal energy level for defibrillation using any of the monophasic or biphasic waveforms has not been determined, a recommendation for higher initial energy when using a monophasic waveform was evaluated by experts at the 2005 Consensus Conference, who considered the potential negative effects of a high first-shock energy versus the negative effects of prolonged VF. The consensus was that providers using monophasic AEDs should give an initial shock of 360 J; if VF persists after the first shock, second and subsequent shocks of 360 J should be given. This single dose for monophasic shocks is designed to simplify instructions to providers; it is not a mandate to recall monophasic AEDs for reprogramming. If the monophasic AED being used is programmed to deliver a different first or subsequent dose, that dose is acceptable.

Persistent, Refractory, Recurrent, and Shock-Resistant VF?

Except for shocks from implantable defibrillators, it is unusual for a single shock to immediately return VF to a perfusing rhythm. In fact, this situation is uncommon, and almost all postshock rhythms are nonperfusing. After a shock VF may be persistent, refractory to subsequent shocks, or recurrent after successful termination of VF.

- *Persistent or shock-resistant VF:* VF that persists after a defibrillatory shock
- *Refractory VF:* VF that persists after shocks, adrenergic agents, airway control, and antiarrhythmics
- *Recurrent or intermittent VF:* VF that recurs after 5 seconds following elimination (definition of successful defibrillation) or returns after an intervening restoration of a spontaneous perfusing rhythm

These distinctions are intended to remind clinicians to consider broader differential diagnoses and alternative or additional therapeutic strategies.

Vasopressors and Antiarrhythmics
Little Success

Because defibrillation is the definitive therapy for VF, vasopressors and antiarrhythmic agents should be given only when defibrillation and CPR are ineffective and VF or pulseless VT persists. The ACLS Pulseless Arrest Algorithm (Figure 1) directs providers to administer a vasopressor and consider antiarrhythmia therapy after shocks and CPR fail to restore a perfusing rhythm. This chapter discusses persistent VF/VT. The next chapter reviews asystole and PEA. For patients with shock-refractory arrhythmias, providers should consider pharmacologic therapies sooner rather than later because the likelihood of benefit, if any, declines rapidly with increasing duration of VF. Amiodarone is the only agent shown to improve survival to hospital admission.

Remember, priority is given to high-quality CPR with minimal interruption rather than to detailed rhythm analysis, pulse evaluation, and debate about drug administration.

- To date no placebo-controlled trials have shown that administration of any vasopressor or antiarrhythmic agent at any stage during management of pulseless VT, VF, PEA, or asystole increases the rate of neurologically intact survival to hospital discharge. There is evidence, however, that the use of vasopressors may improve initial ROSC.

- In addition, there is no evidence that any antiarrhythmic drug given routinely during human cardiac arrest increases survival to *hospital discharge*. Amiodarone, however, has been shown to increase short-term survival to hospital admission when compared with placebo or lidocaine.

FAQ *Should I use a fixed dose or escalating dose for repeat biphasic shocks?*	At the time the *2005 AHA Guidelines for CPR and ECC* were published, no information was available, so no recommendation was made for fixed or escalating *repeat biphasic* doses when VF persists. Research continues, and a recently published study[14] found that an escalating dose was associated with more VF termination but not increased survival. More research is needed and continuing.
Foundation Facts *Vasopressors and Antiarrhythmics*	To date no placebo-controlled trials have shown that administration of any vasopressor or antiarrhythmic agent given at any stage during management of pulseless VT, VF, PEA, or asystole increases the rate of neurologically intact survival to *hospital discharge*.

Vasopressors

Epinephrine or vasopressin are administered when VF or pulseless VT persists despite CPR and shock. Epinephrine hydrochloride produces beneficial physiological effects in patients during cardiac arrest, primarily because of its α-adrenergic receptor–stimulating (ie, vasoconstrictor) properties.[15] The α-adrenergic effects of epinephrine can increase myocardial and cerebral perfusion pressure during CPR.[16] The value and safety of the β-adrenergic effects of epinephrine are controversial because they may increase myocardial work and reduce subendocardial perfusion.[17] Vasopressin is a nonadrenergic peripheral vasoconstrictor that also causes vasoconstriction but lacks β-adrenergic side effects.[18,19]

Why Vasopressors?

Adrenergic and nonadrenergic vasopressors increase aortic diastolic pressure, which increases coronary perfusion pressure. During cardiopulmonary arrest coronary perfusion pressure produced by CPR becomes the major determinant of successful resuscitation.[20] Cerebral perfusion pressure becomes the major determinant of successful neurologic resuscitation.[21]

Abnormal cardiac output and distribution and compromised oxygen delivery to tissues may be present before a cardiac arrest. Almost certainly they will be present during and immediately after a cardiac arrest. When cardiac output falls before or during cardiac arrest, peripheral vascular resistance initially increases in an attempt to compensate for the fall in mean arterial pressure. However, a measurable blood pressure (or palpable peripheral pulse during CPR) does not necessarily mean that cardiac output and peripheral perfusion are adequate. Remember, blood pressure is only a surrogate measure of cardiac function. Also, a measurable cardiac output does not necessarily mean that tissue oxygen delivery and oxygen uptake and utilization at the cellular level are adequate. Oxygen delivery may be also be compromised by a decrease in hemoglobin concentration, in arterial oxygen tension, or in cardiac output. Distribution of blood flow and use of oxygen may be compromised in patients with diseases such as sepsis.

Mechanism of Action
Cardiovascular Adrenergic Receptors
Receptor Physiology: Signal Transduction

A *receptor* is a molecule or molecular complex that interacts with a stimulus called an *agonist*. Agonists are mediators such as hormones or neurotransmitters that bind selectively to a receptor, inducing a series of cellular changes that produce a biological response.

Autonomic (sympathetic) agonists in the cardiovascular system include epinephrine, released from the adrenal gland, and norepinephrine, released from adrenergic nerve terminals. When these agonists activate receptors, a second (intracellular) messenger alters intracellular calcium concentration. In muscle cells this increase of intracellular calcium interacts with the contractile apparatus of the cell, producing the biologic effect of a muscle contraction. The following diagram illustrates this sequence:

Process of Signal Transduction

Agonist (eg, epinephrine):

- Leads to receptor binding and activation

- Which causes an increase in intracellular calcium concentration

- Which causes an interaction with cell contractile apparatus

- Which produces a biologic effect (muscle contraction)

Foundation Facts **Blood Pressure Is Only a Substitute for Cardiac Output and Myocardial Function**	Blood pressure is only a surrogate measure of cardiac function:
	• A measurable blood pressure (or palpable peripheral pulse during CPR) does not necessarily mean that cardiac output and peripheral perfusion are adequate.
	• A measurable cardiac output does not necessarily mean that tissue oxygen delivery and oxygen use are adequate.
	Cardiac output (CO) = Heart rate × Stroke volume
	Blood pressure = CO × Systemic vascular resistance

Adrenergic Receptors

Adrenergic receptors regulate cardiac, vascular, bronchiolar, and gastrointestinal smooth muscle tone.[22] The major classes of adrenergic receptors are

- α-Adrenergic (α_1 and α_2) receptors
- β-Adrenergic (β_1 and β_2) receptors
- Dopaminergic (DA) receptors

α-Adrenergic (α_1 and α_2) Receptors

α-Adrenergic receptors predominantly regulate vascular smooth muscle tone and are important during resuscitation and the postarrest period. When α-adrenergic agonists stimulate vascular α-receptors, vasoconstriction occurs. This increases blood pressure during hypotension and cardiac arrest. The potency of the major α-adrenergic agonists (catecholamines) is as follows:

Norepinephrine	++++
Epinephrine	+++
Isoproterenol	++
Phenylephrine	+

α-Adrenergic receptors are also located in myocardial muscle cells, and stimulation of these receptors increases cardiac inotropic (force of contraction) function. This α-adrenergic inotropic effect, however, is not as significant as the β_1-adrenergic effect on myocardial function. The β_1-adrenergic effect increases myocardial oxygen requirements and is not beneficial during ischemia.

β-Adrenergic (β_1 and β_2) Receptors

There are several types of β-adrenergic receptors. β_1 and β_2 are the most important:

- β_1-Adrenergic receptors are the β-adrenergic receptors of the heart. They are concentrated in the sinus node and ventricles. β_1-Adrenergic receptors are excitatory. When agonists stimulate these receptors, the heart responds with an increase in rate plus an increase in strength of contractility.

- β_2-Adrenergic receptors are the β-adrenergic receptors of the rest of the body. These receptors in the periphery are counterregulatory. They oppose α-adrenergic vasoconstriction, leading to vasodilation.

Dopaminergic (DA) Receptors

Dopaminergic receptors are located in smooth muscle cells in the cerebral, coronary, renal, and splanchnic vascular beds. Dopaminergic receptors are also present in proximal renal tubular cells and in the pituitary gland. Activation of dopaminergic receptors in the smooth muscle cells results in cerebral, coronary, renal, and splanchnic vasodilation. Activation of the dopaminergic cells in the proximal renal tubular cells results in inhibition of sodium ion reabsorption from tubular fluid, so renal sodium excretion increases. Activation of pituitary dopaminergic receptors modulates thyroid and prolactin hormone release. The most significant effect of dopaminergic receptor activation is increased blood flow to the cerebral, coronary, renal, and splanchnic circulations.[23]

Adrenergic Agonists and Vasoactive Drugs: Pharmacologic Effects

The clinical effects of a specific dose of adrenergic agonists may vary widely from patient to patient because the pharmacokinetics (relationship between drug dose and plasma concentration) and pharmacodynamics (relationship between plasma concentration and clinical effects) of these agents are influenced by a wide variety of factors. For example, the class of receptor, drug distribution factors, the large variety of drugs and hormones that influence the receptors, and the potential physical effects of receptor stimulation all play a role in how these agents work in an individual patient. The Table presents the overlapping effects of the adrenergic agonists. Note that most vasoactive drugs affect several types of adrenergic receptors (β_1, β_2, α, and DA). The receptors are affected by varying degrees of *receptor selectivity* (ie, the *binding affinity* of agonists for one type of receptor over another).

| **Foundation Facts** **Drug Dosing and Patient Variability** **Titrate to Effect— One Dose Does Not Fit All Patients and May Vary at Times in Each Patient** | The clinical effects of a specific dose of adrenergic agonists may vary widely from patient to patient because of the pharmacokinetics and pharmacodynamics of these agents:

 • Pharmacokinetics: relationship between drug dose and plasma concentration
 • Pharmacodynamics: relationship between plasma concentration and clinical effects

 Perform serial evaluations for all patients who receive adrenergic agonists to monitor the effects of these agents. |

Other factors that contribute to the net effect of these drugs include

- Receptor density (a variety of clinical conditions influence the number of receptors present on the cell surface) and function (may be affected by activation of other receptors and other body processes)
- Parasympathetic nervous system
- Vasoactive platelet–mediated products such as thromboxane A_2 and prostacyclin
- Endothelial function (dysfunction may cause paradoxical responses to vasodilating stimuli)
- Loss of vasodilating substances such as endothelium relaxing factor

Bottom Line: Table

The interaction of a drug with receptors is complex. It varies from person to person and is further influenced by disease states, drug dose, drug distribution, receptors, and whether the patient is in cardiac arrest.

The ACLS provider should recognize that clinical response to adrenergic vasoactive drugs is variable, so these drugs must be titrated at the bedside with close observation of patient response. The Table is an attempt to simplify the clinical selection of vasoactive drugs. This table summarizes the major receptor sites of each drug and the net effect each agent has on arterial constriction or dilation, heart rate and contractility, bronchial constriction, potential for arrhythmias, and renal blood flow. Careful selection of agents, dose titration, and serial monitoring of patients are essential.

Epinephrine in Cardiac Arrest
Pharmacology

Epinephrine is a natural catecholamine with both α- and β-adrenergic agonist activity. The beneficial effects of epinephrine during cardiac arrest come from its α-adrenergic effects. During resuscitation epinephrine increases peripheral vasoconstriction and improves coronary artery perfusion pressure. As a result, stimulation of α-adrenergic receptors during CPR increases myocardial and cerebral blood flow.[16] Stimulation of the β-adrenergic receptors results in increased heart rate, contractility, and conduction velocity.

Table. Adrenergic Receptor Subtypes: Anatomic Location, Response to Activation, and Effects of Selective Adrenergic Agonists

Receptors	α_1	β_1	β_2		Dopaminergic
Receptor location	*Arteries*	*Heart*	*Arteries*	*Bronchi*	*Kidney*
Response to receptor activation	Constriction	Increased heart rate, contractions, and AV conduction	Dilation	Dilation	Dilation of renal vasculature
	←————————— Epinephrine —————————→				
	←——— Norepinephrine ———→				
		←——— Isoproterenol ———→			
		Dobutamine*			
	Dopamine (at high or "vasopressor" doses) ←————→	**Dopamine** (at moderate or "cardiac" doses) ←————→			**Dopamine** (at low, formerly "renal," doses) ←————→

*Note: Dobutamine has theoretical α-adrenergic agonist effects, but a major metabolite of dobutamine **inhibits** α-adrenergic receptors. In addition, any α-adrenergic effects are balanced by minimal activation of β_2-adrenergic receptors. These complex interactions of dobutamine result in net β_1-adrenergic effects.

Epinephrine—Double-Edged Sword

Both beneficial and toxic physiologic effects of epinephrine administration during CPR have been shown in animal and human studies.[24-26] Epinephrine produces significant renal vasoconstriction even at very low doses, causing decreased renal blood flow and urine output.[7] It increases heart rate by increasing the spontaneous depolarization rate of the sinoatrial node. The refractory periods of some cardiac conduction and myocardial cells can be decreased, and these effects may increase the likelihood of arrhythmias and contribute to a hyperadrenergic state after resuscitation. Epinephrine does increase coronary artery blood flow, but its β-adrenergic effects increase myocardial work and reduce subendocardial perfusion. The net effect may be a greater increase in oxygen demand than oxygen delivery to the myocardium.

Overall epinephrine makes VF more responsive to direct-current shock. Although epinephrine has been used universally in resuscitation, there is a paucity of evidence to show that it improves outcome in humans.

Mechanism of Action

IV administration of epinephrine can increase

- Systemic vascular resistance
- Systolic and diastolic blood pressures
- Electrical activity in the myocardium
- Coronary and cerebral blood flow
- Strength of myocardial contraction
- Myocardial oxygen requirements
- Automaticity

Indications

- **Cardiac arrest:** VF and pulseless VT unresponsive to initial shocks, asystole, and PEA
- **Symptomatic bradycardia:** After other measures (atropine, dopamine, and transcutaneous pacing) have failed
- **Severe hypotension:** Low blood pressure from shock, although its effects on myocardial oxygen demand may limit its usefulness in adults with coronary artery disease (see Part 2 of this text: ACLS for Experienced Providers)

- **Anaphylaxis, severe allergic reactions:** Combine with large fluid volume administration, corticosteroids, and antihistamines (see ACLS for Experienced Providers)

Dose

Origin of Standard (1 mg) Epinephrine Dose

For the last 2 decades researchers and clinicians have attempted to determine the optimal dose of epinephrine for CPR. The "standard" dose of epinephrine (1 mg) is not based on body weight. Historically a standard dose of 1 mg epinephrine was used in operating rooms for intracardiac injections.[24-26] Surgeons observed that 1 to 3 mg of *intracardiac* epinephrine was effective in restarting the arrested adult heart. When these and other experts first produced resuscitation guidelines in the 1970s, they assumed that 1 mg of *intravenous* epinephrine would work similarly to 1 mg of *intracardiac* epinephrine without any adjustment for patient weight.

The Dose-Response Curve of Epinephrine

The dose-response curve of epinephrine was investigated in a series of animal experiments during the 1980s. This work showed that epinephrine produced the optimal response in the range of 0.045 to 0.2 mg/kg. From these studies it seemed that higher doses of epinephrine were required to improve hemodynamics and achieve successful resuscitation, particularly as the duration of cardiac arrest increased. Many clinicians began to extrapolate from these studies to empirically use higher doses of epinephrine. Optimistic case series and retrospective studies began to appear in the late 1980s and early 1990s.

Standard Versus High or Escalating Dose of Epinephrine?

It is appropriate to administer a 1-mg dose of epinephrine intravenously/intraosseously (IO) every 3 to 5 minutes during cardiac arrest despite the paucity of evidence in humans. Higher doses were previously used and advocated by some clinicians, but evidence has accumulated that higher doses have no incremental benefit and may be harmful in some patients. Initial or escalating high-dose epinephrine has occasionally improved initial ROSC and early survival rates. But in 8 randomized clinical studies involving >9000 cardiac arrest patients, high-dose epinephrine produced no improvement in survival to hospital discharge rates or neurologic outcomes when compared with standard doses, even in subgroups initially given high-dose epinephrine.[27,28]

FAQ	High- or escalating-dose epinephrine is no longer recommended.
Are high or escalating doses of epinephrine still recommended?	- Initial or escalating high-dose epinephrine has occasionally improved initial ROSC and early survival rates, but - High-dose epinephrine has produced no improvement in survival to hospital discharge rates or neurologic outcomes when compared with standard doses, even in subgroups initially given high-dose epinephrine.

In theory higher doses may have the potential to cause harm. Careful laboratory studies corroborate both beneficial and harmful physiologic effects and outcomes. High-dose epinephrine may improve coronary perfusion and increase vascular resistance to promote initial ROSC during CPR. But these same effects may lead to increased myocardial dysfunction and occasionally a severely toxic hyperadrenergic state in the postresuscitation period. Higher doses may be indicated to treat specific problems, such as β-blocker or calcium channel blocker overdose, as discussed in Part 2 of this text.

Vasopressin in Cardiac Arrest

Vasopressin is a nonadrenergic peripheral vasoconstrictor that also causes coronary and renal vasoconstriction.[19,29] Two large randomized controlled human trials[30,31] have failed to show an increase in rates of ROSC or survival when vasopressin (40 U, with the dose repeated in 1 study) was compared with epinephrine (1 mg, repeated) as the initial vasopressor for treatment of cardiac arrest. In the multicenter trial involving 1186 out-of-hospital cardiac arrests with all rhythms, a post hoc analysis of patients with asystole showed significant improvement in survival to hospital discharge but not neurologically intact survival when 40 U (repeated once if necessary) of vasopressin was used as the initial vasopressor compared with epinephrine (1 mg, repeated if necessary). Because the effects of vasopressin have not been shown to differ from those of epinephrine in cardiac arrest, 1 dose of vasopressin 40 U IV/IO may replace either the first or second dose of epinephrine in the treatment of pulseless arrest.

Pharmacology

Arginine vasopressin is a naturally occurring hormone, also known as antidiuretic hormone. Endogenous vasopressin levels in patients undergoing CPR are significantly higher in patients who survive than in patients who have no ROSC. This finding stimulated interest in evaluation of vasopressin as a vasoconstrictor during cardiac arrest. It was hypothesized that vasopressin might be beneficial as well as avoid the harmful physiologic effects of epinephrine.

After a short duration of VF, vasopressin administration during CPR has been shown to increase

- Coronary perfusion pressure
- Vital organ blood flow
- Median frequency of VF
- Cerebral oxygen delivery

Mechanism of Action

In higher doses than needed for its antidiuretic action, vasopressin is a nonadrenergic peripheral vasoconstrictor. Vasopressin causes vasoconstriction by directly stimulating smooth muscle V_1 receptors. A potential advantage is that vasopressin does not increase myocardial oxygen consumption during CPR because it has no β-adrenergic activity. The half-life of vasopressin in animal models with intact circulation is 10 to 20 minutes, which is longer than the half-life of epinephrine during CPR.

Consider an Antiarrhythmic Agent

When high-quality CPR, shocks, and a vasopressor have failed to terminate pulseless VF or VT, the use of antiarrhythmic agents can be considered. However, there is no evidence that any antiarrhythmic drug given routinely during human cardiac arrest increases survival to hospital discharge. Amiodarone has been shown to increase short-term survival to hospital admission when compared with placebo or lidocaine. A cautious attitude toward routine administration of antiarrhythmics to VF patients now pervades all discussions of antiarrhythmics for VF. This guarded approach has solidified further in light of repeated confirmation that simply performing CPR or defibrillation just 1 or 2 minutes earlier confers more benefit to the patient than has been reported for antiarrhythmic agents. This caution becomes much stronger whenever the

Foundation Facts **Guidelines 2005**	Because the effects of vasopressin have not been shown to differ from those of epinephrine in cardiac arrest, either vasopressin or epinephrine can be used as the initial vasopressor during cardiac arrest. • One dose of vasopressin 40 U IV/IO may replace either the first or second dose of epinephrine in the treatment of pulseless arrest.
FAQ **Must you wait 10 to 15 minutes before giving epinephrine after vasopressin?**	A vasopressor is given every 3 to 5 minutes during cardiac arrest. • One dose of vasopressin 40 U may replace either the first or second dose of epinephrine. • Epinephrine is administered 3 to 5 minutes after the dose of vasopressin if there is a continuing need for a vasopressor.

preparation and administration of an antiarrhythmic pose a risk of postponing or interrupting CPR or defibrillation.

Vasopressin and Epinephrine Sequential Administration

Several questions have arisen on the use of epinephrine and vasopressin after updated guidelines and algorithms:

- Can vasopressin be substituted for epinephrine in pulseless arrest?
- If vasopressin is used, can epinephrine be given after it?
- When should epinephrine be given after vasopressin is administered?

The *ECC Guidelines 2000*[32] recommended only 1 dose of vasopressin and noted that the half-life of vasopressin in animal models with intact circulation was 10 to 20 minutes, compared with the shorter half-life of epinephrine. Because no data on the subsequent use of epinephrine in humans existed, the guidelines noted that epinephrine could be resumed if after *5 to 10 minutes* there was no response to vasopressin.[32] This recommendation was given a Class Indeterminate status and was based on no data. Since the publication of the *ECC Guidelines 2000,* additional data has become available. In one study[31] patients were given 2 doses of vasopressin or epinephrine at 3-minute intervals. If patients were unresponsive to the study drug, then a dose of epinephrine could follow 2 doses of epinephrine or vasopressin at the physician's discretion. Although not a predefined group, patients receiving epinephrine after vasopressin with this dosing regimen had an increased rate of ROSC (but not intact neurologic survival). The authors raised the possibility of a positive interaction between these vasopressors, a point for further investigation. Overall, outcome was no different in this trial than in other studies, so the guidelines expert panel recommended that 1 dose of vasopressin could be substituted for the first or second dose of epinephrine. The dosing schedule recommended in the guidelines is, in fact, a lower cumulative dose of epinephrine than in the Wenzel et al study[31] (2 doses of epinephrine before vasopressin).

Principles of Pharmacologic Treatment of VF

Defibrillatory and Antifibrillatory Pharmacology

Antifibrillation Drugs: How They *Might* Work

For patients in VF arrest, providers administer the drugs during VF. Research in animals has concluded that the fibrillating myocardium receives no blood flow in the absence of CPR. Effective CPR must be performed to deliver drug therapy to the myocardium. Even with CPR, coronary blood flow is severely compromised (at no more than 15% to 25% of normal). In theory some drug-myocardium interaction occurs between attempted defibrillatory shocks in persistent VF. When a subsequent shock completely depolarizes the heart, there is a brief period of electrically *silent* asystole. During these few seconds of asystole before VF resumes, it is assumed that the antiarrhythmic drug in the tissues accomplishes 2 unlikely tasks:

- Selective suppression of myocardial action potentials related to fibrillation
- Selective facilitation of myocardial action potentials related to coordinated contractions

Antiarrhythmic Agents: Little Support From Human Research

Antifibrillatory drugs have not been shown to improve survival to hospital discharge in any animal or human study. Historically lidocaine has been the drug most often used as an antifibrillatory agent, having entered VF/pulseless VT resuscitation protocols decades ago via empirical reasoning. Over years of use lidocaine acquired a "grandfather" status. Lacking human evidence of any long-term or short-term efficacy from lidocaine administration in VF cardiac arrest or pulseless VT, experts at the International Guidelines 2000 Conference ranked lidocaine as Class Indeterminate, and this classification was continued by experts at the 2005 Consensus Conference.

Improvements in Short-Term but Not Long-Term Outcomes

Studies to date of antiarrhythmic drugs for VF/pulseless VT arrest have been able to detect outcome differences for only short-term outcomes, such as ROSC or

Critical Concept | Administration of antiarrhythmics for persistent VF should not take priority over established interventions such as uninterrupted high-quality CPR and attempts at defibrillation.

admission alive to the hospital. Observed improvements in intermediate outcomes have not translated into observed improvements in longer-term outcomes. A confounding variable effecting drug benefit on hospital discharge rates is the consistently high in-hospital mortality rate among those who experience sudden death and then survive to hospital admission, as well as the lack of a comprehensive postresuscitation management plan and cardiovascular evaluation. Historically, virtually every longitudinal study of out-of-hospital sudden death observes an in-hospital death rate of about 50% among admitted patients. Because of this high in-hospital mortality rate, it is methodologically difficult to demonstrate small but genuine benefits from out-of-hospital interventions. These issues are discussed in more detail in the FYI box "Intermediate vs Long-Term Outcomes."

Interventions to Consider Must Never Delay Definitive Interventions Shown to Affect Long-Term Outcome

Administration of antiarrhythmics for persistent VF should not take priority over established interventions such as uninterrupted high-quality CPR and attempts at defibrillation. So there is an important caveat to the use of any antifibrillatory agent. Intravenous administration of drugs outside the hospital requires time and personnel. The team leader should direct these decisions and should ensure minimal interruption in chest compressions and anticipate sequential drug dosing.

When the established benefits of defibrillation and high quality chest compressions are balanced against the uncertain long-term benefits of antiarrhythmic agents, a clear choice emerges: *never delay the definitive benefits of defibrillation to attempt to provide the questionable long-term benefits of antiarrhythmics.* Equally clear is the corollary that for patients with VF refractory to repeated defibrillation attempts, proceed expeditiously with use of pharmacologic interventions because any beneficial effect decreases rapidly with time.

Antiarrhythmics to Consider for VF/VT: Amiodarone

Intravenous amiodarone is the preferred treatment for shock-refractory VF when an antiarrhythmic agent is thought to be indicated. Lidocaine is an acceptable alternative when amiodarone is unavailable. In patients with shock-refractory cardiac arrest due to incessant or recurrent VF or pulseless VT, administration of amiodarone after repeated transthoracic shocks and epinephrine has been associated with a significantly improved immediate outcome of ROSC and a significantly improved intermediate outcome of admission alive to the hospital. At the Guidelines 2000 Conference, only one prospective clinical trial, the ARREST trial,[33] had been published and was available for evidence evaluation (see the Relevant Research box for a condensed abstract). Amiodarone received a Class IIb recommendation for use in persistent or recurrent VF/pulseless VT.

FYI

Intermediate vs Long-Term Outcomes

Which Outcome Should We Assess for Efficacy of Sudden Death Therapy? Short-Term Survival to Hospital Admission With Amiodarone?

Survival to hospital discharge is the definitive and final goal for resuscitation and treatment interventions. Other, intermediate goals used in clinical trials have included termination of VF, ROSC, and admission to hospital alive. Past resuscitation studies of amiodarone, lidocaine, and biphasic waveform defibrillation, to name just a few, have observed significant differences between immediate and intermediate outcomes. But these differences disappear when longer-term outcomes are examined.

Emphasis on survival to discharge is a matter of straightforward, clinical epidemiology based on hard-core scientific principles. Although short-term outcomes can guide clinical trials, only patient survival and return to the community is the final and ultimate goal. To accept intermediate outcomes without examining long-term outcomes would violate widely accepted principles of clinical investigation. A medication or medical intervention may result only in more people admitted to the hospital, not in more survivors leaving the hospital. Though a challenging standard to fulfill, **improved survival to hospital discharge** is the proper resuscitation outcome to examine before making recommendations for human interventions and strategies for survival.

Amiodarone may be administered for VF or pulseless VT unresponsive to CPR, shock, and a vasopressor (Class IIb). An initial dose of 300 mg IV/IO can be followed by 1 dose of 150 mg IV/IO.

The Evidence

More than a decade ago, data from a small European trial suggested that amiodarone may be more effective than lidocaine in improving short-term outcome from cardiac arrest. In a large series of patients with nonarrest VT unresponsive to lidocaine, procainamide, or bretylium, the response rate for amiodarone was 40%. In a head-to-head, randomized, controlled trial, amiodarone and bretylium were found to be equally effective in reducing recurrent, hemodynamically significant ventricular tachyarrhythmias in patients who did not respond to lidocaine and procainamide. The incidence of significant hypotension, however, was much lower with amiodarone.

Results from the ARREST and ALIVE trials are presented and discussed in this chapter (see Relevant Research boxes).

Disadvantages

Disadvantages of amiodarone include serious hemodynamic side effects (principally hypotension and bradycardia), major problems with administration of the drug as currently formulated and packaged, and high cost. Unless premixed, amiodarone must be reconstituted from a concentrate of the drug suspended in a soaplike vehicle; storage in glass ampules adds to the delay and inconvenience. Over time amiodarone is adsorbed onto plastic surfaces, precluding the use of premixed and preloaded syringes. Several critical drug interactions occur. For example, precipitation occurs when amiodarone is mixed with heparin and sodium bicarbonate.

Relevant Research: The ARREST Trial (Amiodarone in Out-of-Hospital Resuscitation of Refractory Sustained Ventricular Tachyarrhythmias)

Methods: Investigators conducted a randomized, double-blind, placebo-controlled study of IV amiodarone in patients with VF cardiac arrest (or pulseless VT) who were not resuscitated after 3 or more precordial shocks. These patients were randomly assigned to receive 300 mg of IV amiodarone (246 patients) or placebo (258 patients).

Results: The 2 groups had similar clinical profiles with no significant difference in duration of resuscitation attempt (42 ± 16.4 and 43 ± 16.3 minutes, respectively), number of shocks delivered (4 ± 3 and 6 ± 5), or proportion of patients who required more antiarrhythmic drugs after receiving the study drug (66% and 73%). More patients in the amiodarone group than in the placebo group had hypotension (59% vs 48%, $P = .04$) or bradycardia (41% vs 25%, $P = .004$) after receiving the study drug. Recipients of amiodarone were more likely to survive to be admitted to the hospital (44%) than were placebo recipients (34%, $P = .03$). The benefit of amiodarone was consistent among all subgroups and at all times of drug administration. The adjusted odds ratio for survival to hospital admission in the amiodarone group versus the placebo group was 1.6 (95% confidence interval, 1.1 to 2.4; $P = .02$). The trial lacked sufficient statistical power to detect differences in survival to hospital discharge, which differed only slightly between the 2 groups.

Conclusions: In patients with out-of-hospital cardiac arrest due to refractory ventricular arrhythmias, treatment with amiodarone resulted in a higher rate of survival to hospital admission. Whether this benefit extends to survival to discharge from the hospital merits further investigation.

—*Condensed from Kudenchuk et al.*[33]

Foundation Facts

Intravenous amiodarone is the preferred treatment for shock-refractory VF when an antiarrhythmic agent is thought to be indicated.

- Lidocaine is an acceptable alternative when amiodarone is unavailable.

Critical Concept

Pharmacology of Amiodarone

Indications Approved by the FDA

- Frequently recurring VF and hemodynamically unstable VT refractory to other therapy
- Hemodynamically unstable VT

Intravenous Dose for VF/VT Cardiac Arrest (300-mg dose not FDA approved—eg, "off label")

- 300-mg rapid infusion diluted in 20 to 30 mL D_5W
- May repeat ONCE 150-mg infusion in 3 to 5 minutes for refractory VF/VT

In the ARREST trial amiodarone was drawn up in a 30-mL syringe and diluted with 20 mL D_5W or NS in the syringe. This mixture was then pushed into a line through which wide open fluid was also running. Some EMS agencies administer amiodarone IV push and then flush with a 20- to 30-mL bolus of fluid and a wide open line. The rationale for the 30-mL mixture in the ARREST trial was to dilute the drug initially, avoiding an adverse effect on a peripheral vein.

Intravenous Dosage for Recurrent VT or Prophylaxis After Cardiac Arrest

- 150 mg over 10 minutes (15 mg/min); repeat as needed for recurrent or refractory arrhythmias, *then*
- 1 mg/min for 6 hours, *then*
- 0.5 mg/min for remaining 18 hours
- Maximum total dose: 2.2 g per 24 hours

Contraindications and Precautions

- Sinus node dysfunction
- Sinus bradycardia
- Second-degree and third-degree heart block
- Known hypersensitivity from past exposure
- Careful rhythm and blood pressure monitoring are required

Special Resuscitation Considerations: Possible Delays in Achieving Full Electrophysiologic Effects

- Reconstitution is complicated and time-consuming, requiring aspiration from 2 separate glass vials (for the 300-mg cardiac arrest dose) with a large-bore needle and then mixing with 20 to 30 mL of D_5W
- The diluent, *polysorbate-80,* has soaplike properties, leading to foaming when the mixture is shaken vigorously
- Foaming can cause delays during drug aspiration from the 150 mg/3 mL glass vial
- Foaming can cause underdosing (manufacturer states that volume adjusts for this problem)
- Drug is adsorbed onto plastic after prolonged contact (10% after 2 hours)
- Drug precipitates with sodium bicarbonate and heparin
- Positive benefit for longer-term outcomes (eg, discharge alive from the hospital) has not been demonstrated

FAQ

Can amiodarone be repeated during cardiac arrest?

Amiodarone may be administered for VF or pulseless VT unresponsive to CPR, shock, and a vasopressor.

- An initial dose of 300 mg IV/IO can be followed by 1 dose of 150 mg IV/IO.
- Due to uncertain efficacy and unknown drug-drug interactions, amiodarone and lidocaine are not used concomitantly.

Relevant Research: The ALIVE Trial (*Amiodarone* vs *Lidocaine In* Prehospital Refractory *Ventricular* Fibrillation *Evaluation*)

Background: Although *lidocaine* has been the recommended treatment in cardiac arrest due to unresponsive VF, there have been no large-scale, controlled clinical trials to show that lidocaine is superior to placebo or other antiarrhythmic agents. The 2000 American Heart Association/International Liaison Committee on Resuscitation guidelines classify intravenous lidocaine as "Indeterminate," meaning "to be considered," and intravenous amiodarone as Class IIb, or "possibly effective." The ALIVE trial hypothesis was that amiodarone would produce better outcomes than lidocaine in these patients and would eliminate some uncertainty surrounding the most effective treatment.

Methods: ALIVE was a blinded, randomized trial of 5 mg/kg IV amiodarone or placebo versus 1.5 mg/kg lidocaine or placebo in patients with out-of-hospital VF resistant to 3 shocks and intravenous epinephrine followed by a fourth shock, or in those experiencing recurrent VF after successful defibrillation. VF persisting after the first drug dose was treated with an additional 2.5 mg/kg amiodarone or placebo or an additional 1.5 mg/kg lidocaine or placebo. The drugs were administered by the Toronto EMS system. The primary end point was survival to hospital admission. The secondary end point was discharge alive from the hospital.

Group Characteristics: A total of 347 patients were randomized, 180 to amiodarone and 167 to lidocaine. The following overall characteristics were observed: mean age, 67 years; witnessed cardiac arrest, 78%; CPR by bystanders, 27%; mean interval from dispatch to paramedic arrival, 7.4 minutes; mean interval to first defibrillation, 8.4 minutes in amiodarone group, 8.7 minutes in lidocaine group; and mean interval from dispatch to first drug administration, 25 minutes in the 2 drug groups. Initial rhythms and last recorded rhythm before administration of the study drug were the same. The amiodarone and lidocaine groups were similar in number of shocks before study drug and bradycardia treatment and pressor treatment before and after the study drug. Transient spontaneous circulation, however, occurred significantly more often in the amiodarone group *before* administration of the study drug.

Results: Of 180 patients in the amiodarone group, 41 (22%) survived to hospital admission, compared with 20 (12%) of 167 patients in the lidocaine group. This represents a 53% risk reduction with amiodarone treatment of resistant VF ($P = .0083$, odds ratio = 2.17). There was no significant difference between the 2 groups in the secondary end point of discharge alive from the hospital: 9 (5%) amiodarone patients versus 5 (3%) lidocaine patients ($P = .3427$). When adjusted for factors that may influence outcome, treatment with amiodarone, time to drug administration, and spontaneous transient return of circulation before drug administration were positive predictors of survival to hospital admission.

Conclusion: In patients with out-of-hospital, shock-resistant VF, intravenous amiodarone is substantially more effective than lidocaine as an adjunct to ACLS with respect to survival to hospital admission. Based on Dorian et al.[34][35]

Other Antiarrhythmics to Consider: Lidocaine

Intravenous lidocaine is an acceptable drug to consider as an alternative to amiodarone for use in treating *persistent* or *recurrent* VF/pulseless VT when amiodarone is not available. But there is no evidence that lidocaine improves ROSC or survival to hospital admission when compared with amiodarone. Although use of lidocaine is acceptable, it has a Class Indeterminate recommendation for these indications because of the lack of studies with a high level of evidence demonstrating an association between lidocaine use and improved survival from VF arrest, including ROSC. To treat *refractory* or *recurrent* VF, lidocaine is administered only after a treatment sequence of high-quality CPR, shocks, an adrenergic agent (either IV epinephrine or vasopressin), and 1 or more additional shocks.

The Evidence

The use of lidocaine for ventricular arrhythmias was initially supported by evidence from animal studies and by extrapolation from the historical use of lidocaine to suppress premature ventricular contractions and to prevent VF after acute myocardial infarction. Administration of lidocaine improved rates of resuscitation and admission alive to the hospital in one retrospective prehospital study (see "Relevant Research: Lidocaine in Out-of-Hospital Ventricular Fibrillation: Does It Improve Survival?"). But other trials of lidocaine and comparisons of lidocaine and bretylium (no longer available or recommended) found no statistically significant differences in outcomes. One small randomized comparison of amiodarone and lidocaine found a greater likelihood of successful resuscitation with amiodarone. A randomized comparison of lidocaine and epinephrine demonstrated a higher incidence of asystole with lidocaine use and no difference in ROSC. In an in-hospital, retrospective, uncontrolled Canadian study, investigators observed an association between the use of lidocaine and a lower rate of short-term resuscitation success. But this study, a retrospective, uncontrolled study, was flawed by the phenomenon that patients destined not to be resuscitated during a resuscitation attempt are treated for much longer periods; the longer patients are treated, the more medications they receive. As a result, researchers can observe an association between the use of pharmacologic agents and a negative outcome. This association must not be misinterpreted as a cause-and-effect relationship.

Lidocaine has practical advantages for use in persistent VF/pulseless VT. These advantages include no serious side effects when administered rapidly, much lower cost, availability in rapid-administration syringes that are premixed and prefilled, and wide familiarity with the drug from decades of use.

Pharmacology of Lidocaine

Indications

- Hemodynamically significant ventricular ectopy
- Persistent VF/pulseless VT (alternative to amiodarone)
- Stable VT (alternative to procainamide or amiodarone)

Dose for VF/VT Cardiac Arrest

- Initial bolus: 1 to 1.5 mg/kg IV push
- Repeat dose: 0.5 to 0.75 mg/kg IV in 3 to 5 minutes
- Maximum total dose: 3 mg/kg
- Endotracheal administration: 2 to 4 mg/kg

Dose for Perfusing VT

- Initial bolus: 1 to 1.5 mg/kg IV push
- Repeat dose: 0.5 mg to 0.75 mg/kg every 5 to 10 minutes
- Maximum total dose: 3 mg/kg
- Maintenance infusion: 1 to 4 mg/min (30 to 50 µg/kg per minute)

Contraindications and Precautions

- Not recommended for prophylactic use in acute myocardial infarction
- Reduce dose in hepatic failure or congestive heart failure
- Stop infusion if neurologic abnormalities develop

Relevant Research: "Lidocaine in Out-of-Hospital Ventricular Fibrillation: Does It Improve Survival?"

Background: This study was designed to describe the role of lidocaine in patients with out-of-hospital cardiac arrest caused by VF. Subjects comprised all patients with out-of-hospital cardiac arrest found in VF in Goteborg, Sweden, between 1980 and 1992, for whom EMS personnel started CPR.

Results: Detailed records were available for 1212 patients. Lidocaine was given in 405 of these cases (33%). Among patients with sustained VF, those who received lidocaine had ROSC more frequently (P <.001) and were hospitalized alive more frequently (38% vs 18%, P <.01) than patients who did not receive lidocaine. But the rate of survival to hospital discharge did not significantly differ between the 2 groups. Among patients who were converted to a pulse-generating rhythm, those who then received prophylactic lidocaine were more frequently admitted to the hospital than those who did not receive lidocaine (94% vs 84%, P <.05). Nonetheless, the rate of discharge did not differ significantly between the 2 groups.

Conclusions: This retrospective analysis compared outcomes of patients given lidocaine during sustained VF or after conversion to a pulse-generating rhythm with outcomes of patients not given lidocaine. Lidocaine treatment was associated with a higher rate of ROSC and a higher rate of hospital admission but not with an increased rate of survival to hospital discharge.

—*Condensed from Herlitz et al.*[36]

Magnesium

Magnesium is recommended for use in patients with persistent VF/VT arrest who are known or *suspected* to be in a hypomagnesemic state. Clinicians probably administer magnesium less frequently than indicated because of failure to suspect hypomagnesemia in patient groups known to be at high risk for the condition (ie, the elderly, alcohol abusers, and those with chronic malnutrition). Risk factors for hypomagnesemia may be noted in the medical record, which can be reviewed during the course of resuscitation, or elicited from family members (ie, patient history). Hypomagnesemia may also be evident on the ECG (prior prolongation of the QT_c interval).

IV magnesium can terminate torsades de pointes (irregular/polymorphic VT associated with prolonged QT interval).

Magnesium is unlikely to be effective in terminating irregular/polymorphic VT in patients with a normal QT interval.

Dose

- Cardiac arrest: 1 to 2 g diluted in 10 mL D$_5$W IV/IO push, typically over 5 to 20 minutes
- After resuscitation: 1 to 2 g mixed in 50 to 100 mL D$_5$W, given over 5 to 60 minutes

Relevant Research: "Randomized Trial of Magnesium in In-Hospital Cardiac Arrest"

Background: The apparent benefit of magnesium in acute myocardial infarction and the persistently poor outcome after cardiac arrest have led to use of magnesium in CPR. Because few data on the use of magnesium in cardiac arrest were available, we undertook a randomized placebo-controlled trial (MAGIC trial).

Methods: Patients treated for cardiac arrest by the Duke Hospital code team were randomly assigned to receive intravenous magnesium (2 g bolus followed by 8 g over 24 hours, 76 patients) or placebo (80 patients). Only patients in intensive care or general wards were eligible; those whose cardiac arrest occurred in the emergency, operating, or recovery rooms were excluded. The primary end point was ROSC, defined as attainment of any measurable blood pressure or palpable pulse for at least 1 hour after cardiac arrest. The secondary end points were survival to 24 hours, survival to hospital discharge, and neurologic outcome. Analysis was by intention to treat.

Findings: There were no significant differences between the magnesium and placebo groups in the proportion with ROSC (41 [54%] vs 48 [60%], $P = .44$), survival to 24 hours (33 [43%] vs 40 [50%], $P = .41$), survival to hospital discharge (16 [21%] vs 17 [21%], $P = .98$), or Glasgow coma scale score (median, 15 in both groups).

Interpretation: Empirical magnesium supplementation did not improve the rate of successful resuscitation, survival to 24 hours, or survival to hospital discharge overall or in any subpopulation of patients with in-hospital cardiac arrest.

—Condensed from Thel et al.[37]

The Evidence

Evidence on the value of magnesium in cardiac arrest has been gathered, but the study investigators concluded that magnesium has no particular positive effects[37] (see "Relevant Research: Randomized Trial of Magnesium in In-Hospital Cardiac Arrest"). In the presence of torsades de pointes or suspected hypomagnesemia, however, magnesium does improve outcomes. Magnesium administration in resuscitation may be associated with a higher incidence of hypotension despite a potential for improved neurologic outcome in survivors.

Interventions Not Supported by Outcome Evidence

Procainamide in VF and Pulseless VT

Use of procainamide in cardiac arrest is supported by one retrospective comparison study of only 20 patients. Administration of procainamide in cardiac arrest is limited by the need for slow infusion and by uncertain efficacy in emergent circumstances. Procainamide is no longer recommended for refractory VF or recurrent VF/VT during cardiac arrest and is not included in the ACLS Pulseless Arrest Algorithm.

Antiarrhythmic Cocktails and Combinations

Amiodarone is the only agent administered during cardiac arrest shown to increase short-term outcome (admission to the hospital alive). If amiodarone is unavailable, lidocaine is an acceptable alternative to amiodarone, but data supporting short-term and long-term efficacy is lacking. Similar to administration of antiarrhythmic agents following resuscitation from cardiac arrest (see below), a single agent should be used during resuscitation. There is no evidence supporting combination therapy, such as amiodarone alternating with lidocaine. Combination therapy has no proven benefit and could be harmful because of the proarrhythmic effects that can occur when agents are administered in combination. Most important, interruption of CPR to assess rhythm and administer antiarrhythmic agents is discouraged.

Prophylactic Use of Antiarrhythmic Medications After Cardiac Arrest

Because of methodological challenges and sample size barriers, researchers have been unable to complete studies that address the value of prophylactic antiarrhythmic drugs after shock-terminated VF/VT. Both experts and clinicians have argued that if VF/VT is successfully terminated after antiarrhythmic agents have been administered, then the

FYI **Guidelines 2005** **Procainamide**	Administration of procainamide in cardiac arrest is limited by the need for slow infusion and by uncertain efficacy in emergent circumstances. • Procainamide is no longer recommended during cardiac arrest.
FAQ **Can amiodarone and lidocaine be alternated?**	Combination therapy has no proven benefit and could be harmful because of the proarrhythmic effects that can occur when agents are given in combination. • Most important, interruption of CPR to assess rhythm and administer antiarrhythmic agents is discouraged.
FYI **Antiarrhythmics After Resuscitation**	If VF/VT is successfully terminated after administration of an antiarrhythmic, the same agent may be continued for 6 to 24 hours. Many experts and clinicians contend that this therapy reduces the probability of recurrent arrhythmias. Based more on tradition than science, this practice remains acceptable as long as there remains no evidence of harm. • If VF, VT, or frequent ventricular premature beats occur, consider causes such as ischemia, electrolyte imbalance, and hypoxia

same antiarrhythmic agents should be continued for the next 6 to 24 hours. The rationale contends that this therapy reduces the probability of recurrent arrhythmias. Based more on tradition than science, this practice remains acceptable as long as there remains no evidence of harm.

Identify and Treat or Eliminate the Arrhythmia Trigger?

One important question after resuscitation from cardiac arrest involves the etiology, or trigger, of the arrest rhythm. In adults an acute coronary syndrome is a leading cause and precipitates cardiac arrest by ischemia. Frequent causes of malignant arrhythmias in addition to ischemia include electrolyte abnormalities, hypoxemia, hypotension, and drug-induced arrhythmias (including proarrhythmic effects of drugs). In patients with STEMI treatment involves consideration of reperfusion therapy. The risk-benefit ratio for fibrinolytics and logistical considerations for percutaneous coronary intervention are complicated. Alternatively, in the absence of ischemia, a "substrate" of electrical instability can cause cardiac arrest, impacting both short-term and long-term management. For these reasons cardiology and electrophysiology subspecialty consultations are important early after resuscitation.

Fibrinolytic Therapy During *Cardiac Arrest*

Adults have been successfully resuscitated following administration of fibrinolytics (tissue plasminogen activator, or tPA) after initial failure of standard CPR techniques, particularly when the condition leading to the arrest was acute pulmonary embolism or other presumed cardiac cause. Evidence from one large clinical trial, however, failed

to show any significant treatment effect when tPA was given to out-of-hospital patients with undifferentiated PEA cardiac arrest unresponsive to initial interventions. There is insufficient evidence to recommend the routine use of fibrinolysis for cardiac arrest. It may be considered on a case-by-case basis when pulmonary embolus is suspected. Ongoing CPR is not a contraindication to fibrinolysis.

References

1. Wik L. Rediscovering the importance of chest compressions to improve outcome form cardiac arrest. *Resuscitation*. 2003;58:267-269.

2. Larsen MP, Eisenberg MS, Cummins RO, Hallstrom AP. Predicting survival from out-of-hospital cardiac arrest: a graphic model. *Ann Emerg Med*. 1993;22:1652-1658.

3. Holmberg M, Holmberg S, Herlitz J. Incidence, duration and survival of ventricular fibrillation in out-of-hospital cardiac arrest patients in Sweden. *Resuscitation*. 2000;44:7-17.

4. Valenzuela TD, Roe DJ, Cretin S, Spaite DW, Larsen MP. Estimating effectiveness of cardiac arrest interventions: a logistic regression survival model. *Circulation*. 1997;96:3308-3313.

5. Wik L, Hansen TB, Fylling F, Steen T, Vaagenes P, Auestad BH, Steen PA. Delaying defibrillation to give basic cardiopulmonary resuscitation to patients with out-of-hospital ventricular fibrillation: a randomized trial. *JAMA*. 2003;289:1389-1395.

6. Weaver WD, Copass MK, Bufi D, Ray R, Hallstrom AP, Cobb LA. Improved neurologic recovery and survival after early defibrillation. *Circulation*. 1984;69:943-948.

7. Cummins RO, Eisenberg MS, Hallstrom AP, Litwin PE. Survival of out-of-hospital cardiac arrest with early initiation of cardiopulmonary resuscitation. *Am J Emerg Med*. 1985;3:114-119.

8. Waalewijn RA, Nijpels MA, Tijssen JG, Koster RW. Prevention of deterioration of ventricular fibrillation by basic life support during out-of-hospital cardiac arrest. *Resuscitation*. 2002;54:31-36.

9. Cobb LA, Fahrenbruch CE, Walsh TR, Copass MK, Olsufka M, Breskin M, Hallstrom AP. Influence of cardiopulmonary resuscitation prior to defibrillation in patients with out-of-hospital ventricular fibrillation. *JAMA*. 1999;281:1182-1188.

10. Berg RA, Sanders AB, Kern KB, Hilwig RW, Heidenreich JW, Porter ME, Ewy GA. Adverse hemodynamic effects of interrupting chest compressions for rescue breathing during cardiopulmonary resuscitation for ventricular fibrillation cardiac arrest. *Circulation*. 2001;104:2465-2470.

11. Kern KB, Hilwig RW, Berg RA, Sanders AB, Ewy GA. Importance of continuous chest compressions during cardiopulmonary resuscitation: improved outcome during a simulated single lay-rescuer scenario. *Circulation*. 2002;105:645-649.

12. Abella BS, Alvarado JP, Myklebust H, Edelson DP, Barry A, O'Hearn N, Vanden Hoek TL, Becker LB. Quality of cardiopulmonary resuscitation during in-hospital cardiac arrest. *JAMA*. 2005;293:305-310.

13. Hess EP, White RD. Ventricular fibrillation is not provoked by chest compression during post-shock organized rhythms in out-of-hospital cardiac arrest. *Resuscitation*. 2005;66:7-11.

14. Stiell IG, Walker RG, Nesbitt LP, Chapman FW, Cousineau D, Christenson J, Bradford P, Sookram S, Berringer R, Lank P, Wells GA. BIPHASIC Trial: a randomized comparison of fixed lower versus escalating higher energy levels for defibrillation in out-of-hospital cardiac arrest. *Circulation*. 2007;115:1517.

15. Yakaitis RW, Otto CW, Blitt CD. Relative importance of alpha and beta adrenergic receptors during resuscitation. *Crit Care Med*. 1979;7:293-296.

16. Michael JR, Guerci AD, Koehler RC, Shi AY, Tsitlik J, Chandra N, Niedermeyer E, Rogers MC, Traystman RJ, Weisfeldt ML. Mechanisms by which epinephrine augments cerebral and myocardial perfusion during cardiopulmonary resuscitation in dogs. *Circulation*. 1984;69:822-835.

17. Ditchey RV, Lindenfeld J. Failure of epinephrine to improve the balance between myocardial oxygen supply and demand during closed-chest resuscitation in dogs. *Circulation*. 1988;78:382-389.

18. Oyama H, Suzuki Y, Satoh S, Kajita Y, Takayasu M, Shibuya M, Sugita K. Role of nitric oxide in the cerebral vasodilatory responses to vasopressin and oxytocin in dogs. *J Cereb Blood Flow Metab*. 1993;13:285-290.

19. Lindner KH, Strohmenger HU, Ensinger H, Hetzel WD, Ahnefeld FW, Georgieff M. Stress hormone response during and after cardiopulmonary resuscitation. *Anesthesiology*. 1992;77:662-668.

20. Kern KB, Ewy GA, Voorhees WD, Babbs CF, Tacker WA. Myocardial perfusion pressure: a predictor of 24-hour survival during prolonged cardiac arrest in dogs. *Resuscitation*. 1988;16:241-250.

21. Shaffner DH, Eleff SM, Brambrink AM, Sugimoto H, Izuta M, Koehler RC, Traystman RJ. Effect of arrest time and cerebral perfusion pressure during cardiopulmonary resuscitation on cerebral blood flow, metabolism, adenosine triphosphate recovery, and pH in dogs. *Crit Care Med*. 1999;27:1335-1342.

22. Ahlquist RP. Development of the concept of alpha and beta adrenotropic receptors. *Ann N Y Acad Sci*. 1967;139:549-552.

23. Zaritsky AL. Catecholamines, inotropic medications, and vasopressor agents. In: Chernow B, ed. *The Pharmacologic Approach to the Critically Ill Patient*. 3rd ed. Baltimore, Md: Williams & Wilkins; 1994:387-404.

24. Hornchen U, Lussi C, Schuttler J. Potential risks of high-dose epinephrine for resuscitation from ventricular fibrillation in a porcine model. *J Cardiothorac Vasc Anesth*. 1993;7:184-187.

25. Tang W, Weil MH, Sun S, Noc M, Yang L, Gazmuri RJ. Epinephrine increases the severity of postresuscitation myocardial dysfunction. *Circulation*. 1995;92:3089-3093.

26. Rivers EP, Wortsman J, Rady MY, Blake HC, McGeorge FT, Buderer NM. The effect of the total cumulative epinephrine dose administered during human CPR on hemodynamic, oxygen transport, and utilization variables in the postresuscitation period. *Chest*. 1994;106:1499-1507.

27. Gueugniaud PY, Mols P, Goldstein P, Pham E, Dubien PY, Deweerdt C, Vergnion M, Petit P, Carli P. A comparison of repeated high doses and repeated standard doses of epinephrine for cardiac arrest outside the hospital. European Epinephrine Study Group. *N Engl J Med*. 1998;339:1595-1601.

28. Vandycke C, Martens P. High dose versus standard dose epinephrine in cardiac arrest - a meta-analysis. *Resuscitation*. 2000;45:161-166.

29. Lindner KH, Prengel AW, Pfenninger EG, Lindner IM, Strohmenger HU, Georgieff M, Lurie KG. Vasopressin improves vital organ blood flow during closed-chest cardiopulmonary resuscitation in pigs. *Circulation*. 1995;91:215-221.

30. Stiell IG, Hebert PC, Wells GA, Vandemheen KL, Tang AS, Higginson LA, Dreyer JF, Clement C, Battram E, Watpool I, Mason S, Klassen T, Weitzman BN. Vasopressin versus epinephrine for inhospital cardiac arrest: a randomised controlled trial. *Lancet*. 2001;358:105-109.

31. Wenzel V, Krismer AC, Arntz HR, Sitter H, Stadlbauer KH, Lindner KH. A comparison of vasopressin and epinephrine for out-of-hospital cardiopulmonary resuscitation. *N Engl J Med*. 2004;350:105-113.

32. American Heart Association in collaboration with International Liaison Committee on Resuscitation. Guidelines for Cardiopulmonary Resuscitation and Emergency Cardiovascular Care—an International Consensus on Science. *Resuscitation*. 2000;46:3-430.

33. Kudenchuk PJ, Cobb LA, Copass MK, Cummins RO, Doherty AM, Fahrenbruch CE, Hallstrom AP, Murray WA, Olsufka M, Walsh T. Amiodarone for resuscitation after out-of-hospital cardiac arrest due to ventricular fibrillation. *N Engl J Med*. 1999;341:871-878.

34. Dorian P, Cass D, Gelaznikas R, Cooper R, Schwartz B. ALIVE: a randomized, blinded trial of intravenous amiodarone versus lidocaine in shock resistant ventricular fibrillation. *Circulation*. 2001;104:II-765.

35. Dorian P, Cass D, Schwartz B, Cooper R, Gelaznikas R, Barr A. Amiodarone as compared with lidocaine for shock-resistant ventricular fibrillation. *N Engl J Med*. 2002;346:884-890.

36. Herlitz J, Ekstrom L, Wennerblom B, Axelsson A, Bang A, Lindkvist J, Persson NG, Holmberg S. Lidocaine in out-of-hospital ventricular fibrillation. Does it improve survival? *Resuscitation*. 1997;33:199-205.

37. Thel MC, Armstrong AL, McNulty SE, Califf RM, O'Connor CM. Randomised trial of magnesium in in-hospital cardiac arrest. Duke Internal Medicine Housestaff. *Lancet*. 1997;350:1272-1276.

Chapter 6

Pulseless Arrest: Asystole/PEA

This Chapter

- **Cardiac arrhythmias associated with pulseless arrest**
- **No shocks or pacing for asystole**
- **Atropine without proven benefit**
- **When to stop resuscitation**

Overview

Asystole, or more appropriately ventricular asystole, is often a terminal or end-stage rhythm with a poor prognosis and outcome. Pulseless electrical activity (PEA) is not a single rhythm but any organized rhythm having lack of pulse as a feature. Any measurable blood pressure is also absent, although this should never be measured in an unresponsive patient without a pulse. This heterogeneous group of pulseless rhythms includes pseudo-electromechanical dissociation (pseudo-EMD), idioventricular rhythms, ventricular escape rhythms, postdefibrillation idioventricular rhythms, and bradyasystolic rhythms. Asystole and PEA are discussed together because they often occur during cardiac arrest and their treatments are similar. During a resuscitation attempt, brief periods of an organized complex may appear

on the monitor screen, but spontaneous circulation rarely emerges. These rhythms and their management appear on the right side of the ACLS Pulseless Arrest Algorithm (Figure 1).

The survival rate from cardiac arrest with asystole or PEA is dismal. Often asystole represents "end-stage" ventricular fibrillation (VF) as the final rhythm, following fine VF (Figure 2A). When cardiopulmonary resuscitation (CPR) or defibrillation has been delayed, asystole and agonal rhythms often follow defibrillation (Figure 2B). This pattern is part of the rationale for a brief period of CPR before defibrillation in cases of delayed CPR and defibrillation and for immediate resumption of CPR after defibrillation. In other cases an end-stage or critical comorbidity triggered cardiac arrest. In these situations any hope for resuscitation is the rapid identification and treatment of an immediately reversible cause.

Research with cardiac ultrasonography and indwelling pressure catheters has confirmed that pulseless patients with electrical activity have associated mechanical contractions, but these contractions are too weak to produce a blood pressure detectable by palpation or noninvasive blood pressure monitoring. PEA is often caused by reversible conditions and can be treated if those conditions are identified and corrected.

Foundation Facts **Pulseless Electrical Rhythm**	PEA is not a single rhythm but any organized rhythm without a detectable pulse or blood pressure. Some examples of this heterogeneous group of pulseless rhythms are • Bradyasystolic rhythms • Idioventricular rhythms • Ventricular escape rhythms • Supraventricular rhythms without a pulse

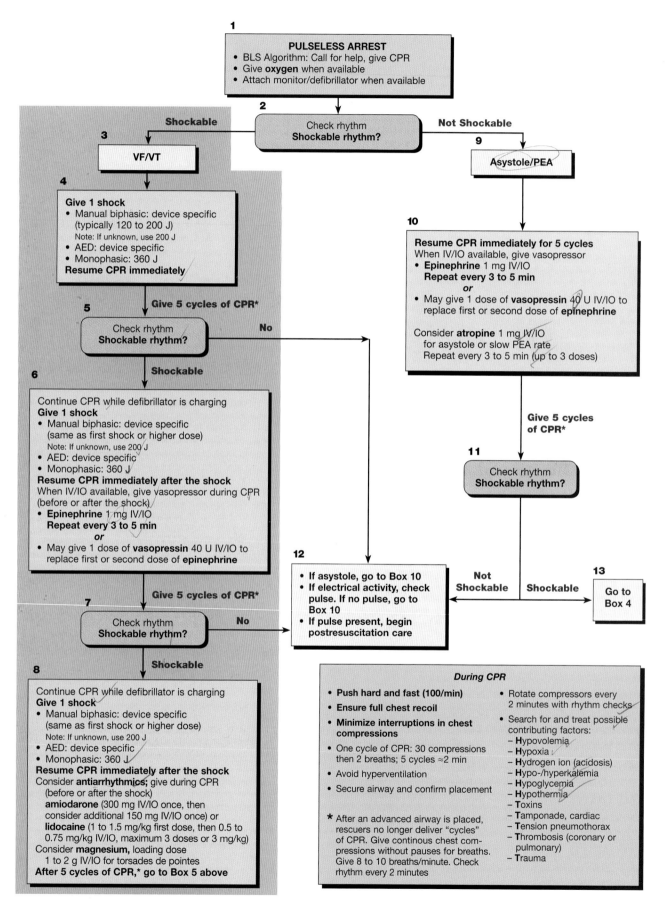

1

PULSELESS ARREST
- BLS Algorithm: Call for help, give CPR
- Give **oxygen** when available
- Attach monitor/defibrillator when available

2

Check rhythm
Shockable rhythm?

Shockable | Not Shockable

3

VF/VT

9

Asystole/PEA

4

Give 1 shock
- Manual biphasic: device specific (typically 120 to 200 J)
  Note: If unknown, use 200 J
- AED: device specific
- Monophasic: 360 J
Resume CPR immediately

5

Give 5 cycles of CPR*

Check rhythm
Shockable rhythm?

No

Shockable

6

Continue CPR while defibrillator is charging
Give 1 shock
- Manual biphasic: device specific (same as first shock or higher dose)
  Note: If unknown, use 200 J
- AED: device specific
- Monophasic: 360 J
Resume CPR immediately after the shock
When IV/IO available, give vasopressor during CPR (before or after the shock)
- **Epinephrine** 1 mg IV/IO
  Repeat every 3 to 5 min
      or
- May give 1 dose of **vasopressin** 40 U IV/IO to replace first or second dose of **epinephrine**

10

Resume CPR immediately for 5 cycles
When IV/IO available, give vasopressor
- **Epinephrine** 1 mg IV/IO
  Repeat every 3 to 5 min
      or
- May give 1 dose of **vasopressin** 40 U IV/IO to replace first or second dose of **epinephrine**

Consider **atropine** 1 mg IV/IO
  for asystole or slow PEA rate
  Repeat every 3 to 5 min (up to 3 doses)

Give 5 cycles of CPR*

11

Check rhythm
Shockable rhythm?

Not Shockable | Shockable

7

Give 5 cycles of CPR*

Check rhythm
Shockable rhythm?

No

Shockable

12

- If asystole, go to Box 10
- If electrical activity, check pulse. If no pulse, go to Box 10
- If pulse present, begin postresuscitation care

13

Go to Box 4

8

Continue CPR while defibrillator is charging
Give 1 shock
- Manual biphasic: device specific (same as first shock or higher dose)
  Note: If unknown, use 200 J
- AED: device specific
- Monophasic: 360 J
Resume CPR immediately after the shock
Consider **antiarrhythmics;** give during CPR (before or after the shock)
  amiodarone (300 mg IV/IO once, then consider additional 150 mg IV/IO once) or **lidocaine** (1 to 1.5 mg/kg first dose, then 0.5 to 0.75 mg/kg IV/IO, maximum 3 doses or 3 mg/kg)
Consider **magnesium**, loading dose 1 to 2 g IV/IO for torsades de pointes
After 5 cycles of CPR,* go to Box 5 above

During CPR
- **Push hard and fast (100/min)**
- **Ensure full chest recoil**
- **Minimize interruptions in chest compressions**
- One cycle of CPR: 30 compressions then 2 breaths; 5 cycles ≈2 min
- Avoid hyperventilation
- Secure airway and confirm placement

- Rotate compressors every 2 minutes with rhythm checks
- Search for and treat possible contributing factors:
  – **H**ypovolemia
  – **H**ypoxia
  – **H**ydrogen ion (acidosis)
  – **H**ypo-/hyperkalemia
  – **H**ypoglycemia
  – **H**ypothermia
  – **T**oxins
  – **T**amponade, cardiac
  – **T**ension pneumothorax
  – **T**hrombosis (coronary or pulmonary)
  – **T**rauma

* After an advanced airway is placed, rescuers no longer deliver "cycles" of CPR. Give continous chest compressions without pauses for breaths. Give 8 to 10 breaths/minute. Check rhythm every 2 minutes

Figure 1. ACLS Pulseless Arrest Algorithm. Right Side of Algorithm PEA/Asystole

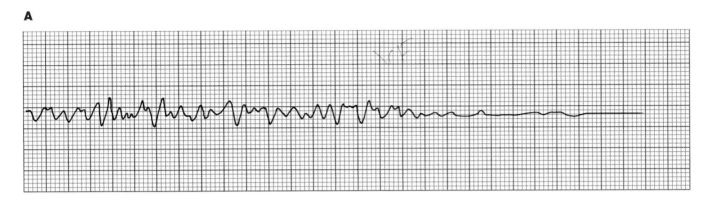

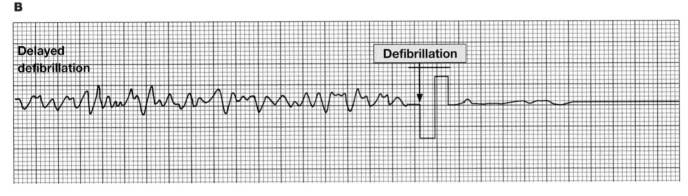

Figure 2. A, Ventricular fibrillation deteriorating to asystole over time. Effective chest compressions may delay the "decay" of VF into asystole until an AED or manual defibrillator arrives. **B,** Ventricular fibrillation resulting in asystole after delayed defibrillation. Prognosis is poor when this rhythm follows a shock.

Rapid Identification of a Reversible Cause

In every cardiac arrest the potential cause of the arrest is an important consideration. In many patients who have return of spontaneous circulation (ROSC), this etiology will become most important during the postarrest period. For example, the leading cause of adult cardiac arrest is one of the acute coronary syndromes. In other cases an extracardiac cause may need to be treated during the arrest for optimal outcome.

The ACLS Provider Course teaches ACLS providers to perform the BLS Primary ABCD Survey and the ACLS Secondary ABCD Survey in a thoughtful and expeditious manner. A major component of the "thoughtful approach" is constantly to consider the secondary *D, Differential Diagnoses,* and to think carefully about what could be causing the arrest. Table 1 lists an *aide mémoire* called the *H's and the T's.* The H's and the T's is an easy way to recall possible reversible causes of arrest, allowing a rapid review of the differential diagnoses. ACLS instructors will note that a list of the more common triggers or comorbidities complicating resuscitation is included in the *ACLS Provider Manual* and Table 2. The team leader should concurrently review and identify, if possible, any precipitating cause of cardiac arrest as part of the resuscitation protocol. Part 2 of this text,

for the experienced provider, deals in more detail with these special resuscitation situations. Examples include electrolyte abnormalities, toxic drug effects and overdoses, hypothermia, and pulmonary embolism.

The mechanisms by which these conditions can produce PEA are usually understandable from the simple application of mechanics and physiology. For example, PEA can develop from hypovolemia due to blood loss. This mechanism would be clinically apparent with a history of trauma but clinically occult with an aortic dissection. The postoperative patient may suffer major pulmonary emboli due to obstruction of pulmonary vessels. Blood flow from the right ventricle to the

Table 1. Most Common Causes of PEA

H's	T's
Hypovolemia	Toxins
Hypoxia	Tamponade (cardiac)
Hydrogen ion (acidosis)	Tension pneumothorax
Hyper-/hypokalemia	Thrombosis (coronary and pulmonary)
Hypoglycemia	Trauma
Hypothermia	

Table 2. Frequent Causes of PEA (H's and T's)

Condition	Clues From ECG and Monitor	Clues From History and Physical Exam	Recommended Treatment
Hypovolemia	Narrow complex Rapid rate	Trauma, bleeding, flat neck veins	Volume infusion
Hypoxia	Slow rate (hypoxia)	Cyanosis, blood gases, airway problems	Oxygenation, ventilation
Hydrogen ion (acidosis)	Smaller-amplitude QRS complexes	History of diabetes, bicarbonate-responsive preexisting acidosis, renal failure	Sodium bicarbonate, hyperventilation
Hyperkalemia or	Both hyperkalemia and hypokalemia cause wide-complex QRS *"High potassium" ECG:* • T waves taller and peaked • P waves get smaller • QRS widens • Sine-wave PEA	History of renal failure, diabetes, recent dialysis, dialysis fistulas, medications	*Hyperkalemia:* • Sodium bicarbonate • Glucose plus insulin • Calcium chloride • Kayexalate/sorbitol • Dialysis (long term) • Possibly albuterol
Hypokalemia	*"Low potassium" ECG:* • T waves flatten • Prominent U waves • QRS widens • QT prolongs • Wide-complex tachycardia	Abnormal loss of potassium, diuretic use	*Hypokalemia:* • Rapid but controlled infusion of potassium • Add magnesium if cardiac arrest
Hypothermia	J or Osborne waves	History of exposure to cold, central body temperature	See Hypothermia Algorithm *(ECC Handbook)*
Toxins (drug overdose): tricyclics, digoxin, β-blockers, calcium channel blockers	Various effects on ECG, predominantly prolongation of QT interval	Bradycardia, empty bottles at the scene, pupils, neurologic exam	Drug screens, intubation, lavage, activated charcoal, lactulose per local protocols, specific antidotes and agents per toxidrome
Tamponade, cardiac	Narrow complex Rapid rate	History of pericardial effusion, no pulse felt with CPR, vein distention, chest trauma	Pericardiocentesis
Tension pneumothorax	Narrow complex Slow rate (hypoxia)	History, no pulse felt with CPR, neck vein distention, tracheal deviation, unequal breath sounds, difficult to ventilate patient	Needle decompression
Thrombosis, heart: acute, extensive MI	Abnormal 12-lead ECG: • Q waves • ST-segment changes • T waves, inversions	Chest discomfort, angina, associated ACS symptoms, cardiac markers	See ACS STEMI Reperfusion Therapy
Thrombosis, lungs: massive pulmonary embolism	Narrow complex Rapid rate	History of prior pulmonary embolism, no pulse felt with CPR, distended neck veins, prior positive test for DVT or PE	Surgical embolectomy, fibrinolytics

DVT indicates deep vein thrombosis; and PE, pulmonary embolus.

left ventricle is significantly reduced because of impaired flow through the lungs, complicated by profound hypoxemia. The elderly and diabetic patients may have cardiogenic shock due to acute myocardial infarction (AMI) with painless infarcts. They present with a history of weakness and possibly dyspnea, leading to prostration before secondary VF occurs. Pericardial tamponade restricts filling of the left ventricle, primarily by pushing the interventricular septum against the left ventricular wall and outflow tract to the aorta. Sudden acute dyspnea and immediate collapse with PEA is most often due to major pulmonary emboli. Other pulmonary causes should be considered as well, including near-fatal asthma and tension pneumothorax.

QRS Rate and Width: Clues to the Cause of PEA

The rate and QRS width of the pulseless *electrical activity* can sometimes offer a clue to an underlying reversible cause of arrest. Consider whether the electrical activity (QRS complex) is wide versus narrow and fast versus slow. Most clinical studies have observed poor survival rates from PEA that presents with a wide complex QRS and a slow rate. These rhythms often indicate dysfunction of the myocardium or the cardiac conduction system, such as

occurs with massive STEMI. These rhythms can represent the last electrical activity of a dying myocardium, or they may indicate specific critical rhythm disturbances. For example, severe hyperkalemia, hypothermia, hypoxia, preexisting acidosis, and a large variety of drug overdoses can produce wide-complex PEA.

Overdoses of tricyclic antidepressants, β-blockers, calcium channel blockers, and digitalis will produce a slow, wide-complex PEA. In contrast, a fast, narrow-complex PEA indicates a relatively normal heart responding exactly as it should to severe hypovolemia, febrile infections, pulmonary emboli, or cardiac tamponade. Table 3 summarizes some of the former nomenclature used for PEA and lists several causes of PEA that is fast or slow and wide or narrow.

Asystole

Definition

The word *asystole* (from the Greek word *systole*, "contraction") means the total absence of ventricular contractile activity. Without contractions the surface ECG monitor, properly attached and calibrated, displays predominantly a "flat line"; agonal deflections may occasionally appear.

Table 3. Using QRS Rate and Width as Clues to the Cause of PEA

Rate of Complexes	Width of Complexes	
	Narrow More likely to have noncardiac cause; low volume, low vascular tone	**Wide** More often due to cardiac cause; also drug and electrolyte toxicities
Fast (>60 bpm)	Former nomenclature: • Sinus (P wave) EMD • Pseudo-EMD • PSVT Possible causes: • Hypovolemia • Shock • Cardiac tamponade • Massive pulmonary embolus	Former nomenclature: • VF • VT Possible causes: • Unstable VT • Unstable wide-complex tachycardia • Electrolyte abnormalities (potassium, calcium) • Acute coronary syndromes
Slow (<60 bpm)	Former nomenclature: • EMD • Pseudo-EMD • Postdefibrillation rhythms • Idioventricular rhythms Possible causes: • Hypoxia • Acidosis	Former nomenclature: • Bradyasystolic rhythms • Idioventricular rhythms • Ventricular escape rhythms Possible causes: • Drug overdose, toxicities • Electrolyte abnormalities (potassium, calcium) • Acute coronary syndromes

PSVT indicates paroxysmal supraventricular tachycardia.

Clinicians have come to use the term *ventricular asystole* (Figure 3) when they see a total absence of electrical activity on the monitor. The depolarization implied by a QRS complex does not occur, no ventricular contraction occurs, no blood is pumped, no arteries fill, and no peripheral pulse is felt. Attempts to distinguish among "slow PEA," "asystole," "fine ventricular fibrillation," "coarse asystole," and "VF with an isoelectric vector that masquerades as asystole" are of little clinical use.

Causes and Triggers of Asystole

In about 1 of every 8 patients who develop cardiac arrest, a progressively profound bradycardia that ends in asystole is observed after several minutes.[1] This is called a *bradyasystolic arrest.* Direct transition over several seconds from a rhythm that produces spontaneous circulation to asystolic cardiac arrest is uncommon. Typically the patient "passes through" other cardiac arrest rhythms, most commonly progressively slowing bradycardia, various types of heart block, PEA, "cardiac arrest," and then asystole. Case reports and case series of unexpected, sudden cardiac arrest due to asystole frequently identify some profound vasovagal stimulus as the precipitating cause.

Who Survives Asystole?

Patients in cardiac arrest whose first monitor display reveals "asystole" have a dismal rate of survival to hospital discharge. Studies reporting survival from out-of-hospital cardiac arrest seldom list survival greater than 1% for patients found to be in asystole on initial rhythm assessment. In fact, many experts think survival rates in the range of 1% for asystole represent misclassification caused by unconnected monitor/defibrillator electrodes or reduced gain control levels. But investigators from Göteborg, Sweden, in an excellent review of 16 years of data, observed an admission rate of 10% and a survival to discharge rate of 2% for all cardiac arrest victims with asystole as the first recorded rhythm[2] (see "Relevant Research"). So when positive factors (eg, witnessed arrest, younger age, noncardiac cause, and short intervals from collapse to basic and advanced life support) are present, the survival rate can be much higher.

Confirmation of Asystole

ACLS providers and students should recognize that *asystole* is a specific diagnosis. A flat line is not. The term *flat line* is nonspecific; it could apply to several conditions, of which true asystole is only one.

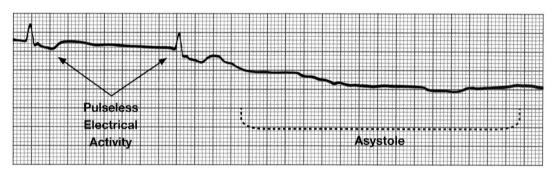

Figure 3. The "rhythm" of pulseless electrical activity and ventricular asystole. This patient is pulseless and unresponsive. Note the 2 QRS-like complexes at the start of this rhythm display. These complexes represent a minimum of electrical activity, probably ventricular escape beats. Ventricular electrical activity ceases after 2 beats, and asystole is present.

FAQ **Who has the best (but small) chance of survival from asystole?**	Patients with a rapidly identified and correctable cause of arrest have the best chance of survival (2% to 10%) from asystole. Other factors associated with a better chance of ROSC include • Witnessed arrest with short intervals from collapse to basic and advanced life support • Younger age • Noncardiac cause
Critical Concept **High-Quality CPR First**	When considering patient and technical problems and causes of asystole, it is mandatory that there is minimal interruption in CPR. • Remember, pulse checks are performed only if an organized rhythm is identified. • Assessment of technical problems should rarely, if ever, interrupt CPR.

Relevant Research: "Can We Define Patients With No Chance and Those With Some Chance of Survival When Found in Asystole Out of Hospital?"

Investigators analyzed 16 years of data on out-of-hospital cardiac arrest in which asystole was the first arrhythmia recorded by emergency medical services (EMS) personnel. All arrests were included regardless of the age of victim or origin of arrest. Between 1981 and 1997 EMS personnel in Göteborg, Sweden, attended 4662 cardiac arrests. Asystole was the first-recorded arrhythmia for 1635 patients (35%). Of these patients, 10% (156) were admitted alive to the hospital and 2% (32) were discharged alive.

The following characteristics were associated with survival: younger age (median age 58 vs 68 years), witnessed arrest (78% vs 50%), shorter intervals from collapse to arrival of ambulance (3.5 vs 6 minutes) and mobile coronary care unit (5 vs 10 minutes), atropine given less often, noncardiac cause of arrest (48% vs 27%), and higher level of consciousness on arrival at the emergency department.

Multivariate analysis of all patients with asystole indicated lower age ($P = .01$) and witnessed arrest ($P = .03$) as independent predictors of increased survival. Multivariate analysis of witnessed arrests indicated short time to arrival of the mobile coronary care unit ($P < .001$) and no atropine ($P = .05$) as independent predictors of survival. Fifty-five percent of patients discharged alive had no or small neurologic deficits (cerebral performance category 1 or 2). No patients older than 70 years with unwitnessed arrest (n = 211) survived to discharge.

—Condensed from Engdahl et al.[2]

Differential Diagnoses for a Flat Line

The other "diagnoses" are mainly technical and operational problems that must be identified and eliminated if present. These may include

- Power "OFF" to monitor or defibrillator
- Batteries dead
- Monitor gain too low
- Monitor cable not connected to patient, lead connector, or monitor

Some of these problems do not apply to all defibrillators.

An Unplugged Defibrillator With a Dead Battery

A totally blank monitor screen means NO POWER. Surprisingly common errors are failure to plug the unit back into line power when it has been operating on batteries or inadvertently disconnecting the power cord. If the defibrillator/monitor is used for routine monitoring, the batteries will support display of the rhythm on the monitor while steadily discharging. A point can be reached where the rhythm displays normally but the batteries are too low to support multiple rapid charges and discharges of the defibrillator. Performing a routine checklist at appropriate intervals avoids this difficulty.

False or Occult Asystole

One cause of a flat line comes from the so-called "VF-has-a-vector" theory.[3] This frequently repeated theory remains viable despite the virtually total absence of confirmation in human studies. If VF moves through the myocardium with a sustained *direction* (or *vector*), then the monitor may display a flat line in any lead that records at 90 degrees to the direction of VF. This fact led to the practice of shocking asystole in case VF was masquerading as "occult" or "false" asystole. In studies addressing this concept, there was no benefit from shock delivery for asystole. In fact, in all outcomes studied, including ROSC and survival, the group that received shocks showed a trend toward a *worse* outcome than the group that did not receive shocks. With recent recognition of the importance of minimizing interruptions in chest compressions, it is difficult to justify any interruption in chest compressions to attempt shock delivery for asystole.

FAQ **Should we teach to shock asystole in case fine VF or "occult" VF is present?**	<ul><li>In studies addressing this question, there was no benefit from shock delivery for asystole.</li><li>In fact, in all outcomes studied, including ROSC and survival, the group that received shocks showed a trend toward a *worse* outcome than the group that did not receive shocks.</li></ul>

Shock for Asystole—Lack of Evidence

In 1984 Thompson et al from Milwaukee were the first to study Ewy's theory[3] that empiric shocks to asystole might "discover" people in occult VF and increase the dismal save rate for asystole. They entered 119 patients in initial asystole into the prospective study and observed that 10 patients showed a change in rhythm after a shock, and 6 of these people reached the hospital. None of the 6 survived to admission. Although the authors concluded that the result "justifies continuation of the study," no follow-up publication has ever appeared.

In 1985 Ornato and Gonzales published their data about whether electrical shock for asystole had any value. In a study of 24 patients they observed, without presenting specific figures, that "shock was more effective than epinephrine, atropine or calcium chloride in altering the rhythm from asystole." They concluded that "the rhythm diagnosed as asystole may actually be VF in many cases."

In 1989 Losek et al[4] published a retrospective review of initial shock of 49 children in asystole compared with 41 asystolic children who were not shocked. A change in rhythm occurred in 10 of the 49 (20%) children who received shocks; 3 of the 10 had ROSC, but none survived to hospital discharge. A change in rhythm occurred in 9 of the 41 (22%) children not shocked; 6 of the 9 had ROSC, and 1 survived. The authors concluded that immediate shock of asystole in children had no value and should not be recommended.

In 1993 the Nine City High-Dose Epinephrine Study Group published an analysis of 77 asystolic patients who received initial shock compared with 117 who received standard therapy. In all outcomes studied, the shock group had a *worse* outcome than the no-shock group: ROSC occurred in 16% of the shock group and 23% of the no-shock group; survival to hospital discharge was 0% in the shock group and 2% in the no-shock group. Although no statistical significance was associated with these differences, the authors concluded that the no-shock group displayed a "tendency" to do better. The authors saw no justification for a study with a much larger sample size; they saw little reason to continue studying this question.

In the past decade the only published advocacy for empiric shocks for asystole have been in letters to the editor and an occasional editorial expressing rational conjecture rather than empiric evidence. Based on the 4 studies noted above and the absence of any significant data subsequently, the American Heart Association ACLS Subcommittee and topic experts at the guidelines consensus conference do not recommend empiric shocks to asystole. Extrapolation of data from studies of the possible harm of electric shock supports a Class III recommendation (no benefit, possible harm) for this approach.

The Flat Line Protocol

The differential diagnoses for a flat line seen on an in-hospital or out-of-hospital monitor can be narrowed by following a *flat line protocol* such as the one outlined in Table 4.

Pacing for Asystole?

Previous reports of success with transcutaneous pacing (TCP) in the treatment of asystole are rare and in effect only anecdotes. It was thought that if TCP was to be effective at all, it needed to be performed early, as soon after asystole began as possible. Clinical experience and 1 prospective, randomized, clinical trial showed that prehospital pacing is ineffective, and the AHA did not recommend routine pacing for out-of-hospital asystolic cardiac arrest in the *ECC Guidelines 2000.* Because of the emphasis on continued and uninterrupted high-quality CPR in the *2005 AHA Guidelines for CPR and ECC,* and a lack of evidence and potential for harm when chest compressions are interrupted, pacing is no longer recommended.

The Evidence

Advocates of TCP for asystole in the past argued that patients in cardiac arrest for no more than 5 minutes should be able to respond to a pacing stimulus. In theory there should exist large cohorts of asystolic patients who are responsive to pacing. Patients with a normally functioning myocardium but a temporarily disturbed cardiac conduction system fall into this category. These patients would include people who suddenly develop a bradyasystolic arrest in an emergency or critical care setting, people with myocardial "stunning" after a defibrillation shock, overdose victims who have ingested cardiotoxic drugs, and that heterogeneous group of people referred to previously who respond with asystole to a massive stimulation of the vagal nerve.[5]

Table 4. The Flat Line Protocol: Recommended Steps to Follow When a Flat Line Appears on the Monitor/ Defibrillator Screen

- Check power to both defibrillator and monitor (some devices have separate POWER ON controls for the defibrillator and monitor).
- When using 3-lead monitor cables, check all connections:
  - Defibrillator → monitor cables
  - Monitor cables → monitor leads
  - Monitor leads → patient's chest
- When using "quick-look" paddles to assess the rhythm, check the following connections:
  - Defibrillator → paddle cables
  - Paddle cables → paddles
  - Paddles → conductive interface (adhesive pads on chest or conductive gel or paste)
  - Conductive interface → patient's skin (dry, not wet; clean, not dirty; close contact, not blocked by chest hair)
- Check GAIN or SENSITIVITY setting on the defibrillator/monitor (if turned LOW or OFF, any rhythm, even normal sinus, will appear as a flat line).
- Check the setting for LEAD SELECT control: set for paddles? lead I? lead II? lead III?
- When set on LEAD SELECT, do a quick check in each of the 3 leads to see what rhythm is displayed (vector of VF concept).
- When set on PADDLES and the quick look shows a flat line, check for VF with a vector by moving the lead axis between the 2 paddles 90 degrees (ie, move paddle at upper right sternal border to upper left sternal border; move paddle at left apex to right lower sternal border).
- If using adhesive pads, do *not* unstick the pads and rotate them 90 degrees. Instead connect 3-lead limb leads.

Early pacing, with direct stimulation of the myocardium rather than pharmacologic stimulation of the conduction system, may produce life-sustaining heart contractions for a limited time.[6] It was further hypothesized that TCP bought time while awaiting correction of drug-induced rhythm disturbances, electrolyte abnormalities, acidosis, or hypoxia.

Patients in out-of-hospital cardiac arrest due to either primary asystole or postshock asystole who are treated early by first-responding emergency medical technicians were thought to be better theoretical candidates for pacing because of a short arrest-to-pacing interval. But a randomized, controlled trial of out-of-hospital TCP from King County, Washington, found no case of a pacing-dependent return of circulation in more than 120 cases of early TCP for primary or postshock asystole.[7]

Drugs for Asystole and PEA

No drug administered for asystole or PEA has been shown to improve survival in randomized, controlled trials. Hence, the emphasis on treatment of asystole and PEA is high-quality CPR, primarily chest compressions, and the search for an immediately reversible cause.

Vasopressors

Epinephrine for Asystole and PEA

The Recommendation: Class Indeterminate

Continued use of epinephrine for persistent asystole and PEA is a Class Indeterminate recommendation without evidence of improvement in survival. Providers should continue to search actively for reversible causes.

Why, Then, Does Everyone Get Epinephrine?

Epinephrine, or adrenaline, has been present in every resuscitation protocol, even predating defibrillation. The original protocols were assembled by reasonable clinicians who were extrapolating drugs and doses from decades of animal and laboratory research. The widely accepted principle was that by producing marked vasoconstriction, epinephrine would increase diastolic blood pressure, thereby increasing blood flow to the brain and heart.

Whether this practice contributed significantly to cardiac resuscitation in humans was never submitted to rigorous

FAQ

Is pacing no longer recommended for asystole?

Is this a change?

- Previously pacing was a Class IIb recommendation, but the *ECC Guidelines 2000* did not recommend routine pacing for out-of-hospital asystolic cardiac arrest.
- Because of the emphasis on continued and uninterrupted high-quality CPR in the *2005 AHA Guidelines for CPR and ECC*, and a lack of evidence and potential for harm when chest compressions are interrupted, pacing is no longer recommended.

scientific review. It was not until the last 2 decades of the 20th century, during an upsurge of interest in high-dose epinephrine, that the level of evidence supporting the value of epinephrine in human resuscitation came under question.

What Happened to High-Dose Epinephrine?

The *1992 ECC Guidelines* accepted the use of higher doses of epinephrine in either escalating doses (1, 3, 5 mg), intermediate doses (5 mg per dose rather than 1 mg), or high doses based on body weight (up to 0.2 mg/kg). These doses were based on results of a series of randomized, controlled trials of high-dose epinephrine that demonstrated positive, but not definitive, effects. By 2000 a growing body of indirect evidence suggested that high-dose epinephrine therapy might be harmful. In successfully resuscitated patients clinicians observed that the more epinephrine administered during the resuscitation, the worse the cerebral function in the postresuscitation period.[8] Although high-dose epinephrine appeared to be better at "restarting the heart," this effect was not equivalent to "restarting the head." The *ECC Guidelines 2000* considered higher doses of epinephrine as Class Indeterminate, acceptable but not recommended.

Vasopressin for Asystole and PEA

Studies have compared epinephrine and vasopressin in patients with PEA and asystole. These studies failed to show that either vasopressin or epinephrine is superior for treatment of PEA regardless of the order of administration. In the case of asystole, a single post hoc analysis of a larger study found a survival benefit of vasopressin over epinephrine but did not find an increase in intact neurologic survival. On the basis of these findings, providers may consider vasopressin for treatment of asystole, but there is insufficient evidence to recommend for or against its use in PEA. Further studies are required.

Atropine for Asystole and PEA

Asystole can be precipitated or exacerbated by excessive vagal tone, and administration of a vagolytic medication is consistent with a physiologic approach. However, no prospective, controlled studies support the use of atropine in asystole or slow PEA arrest. Administration of atropine for asystole is supported by a retrospective review of intubated patients with refractory asystole who showed improved survival to hospital admission with atropine and a case series that documented conversion from asystole to sinus rhythm in 7 of 8 patients.

The Recommendation and the Evidence: Class Indeterminate

The recommendation for atropine in asystolic cardiac arrest is based on the assumption that some patients experience asystolic cardiac arrest due to excessive vagal or parasympathetic tone. The many unusual causes of asystolic arrest presented above all fall in the category of profound vagal discharge. As a powerful antagonist to vagal activity, atropine would be expected to have a positive effect in such patients, and case reports and 1 retrospective case-control series support this concept.

Other published studies observe no benefit. These studies include a simple case series of 8 patients; an observational series of 33 asystolic or bradycardic patients treated aggressively with atropine, epinephrine, and isoproterenol; a prospective, controlled study of 11 patients getting atropine and 11 control subjects; and well-designed animal studies. A prospective, randomized trial to establish the true benefit, if any, of atropine for asystolic cardiac arrest has never been published. The most active research on atropine has been in animal models, but even in those studies investigators have observed a negative effect from higher doses of atropine.

Atropine should not be used when the lack of cardiac activity has a clear explanation, such as in hypothermic arrest. The dosage of atropine can vary by dose (0.03 to 0.04 mg/kg) and by interval (every 3 to 5 minutes). In practice most clinicians use the more aggressive approach of atropine 1 mg every 3 minutes until 0.04 mg/kg has been infused. The only evidence that supports the effectiveness of this approach comes from rational conjecture and extrapolation from studies done for other purposes.

Epinephrine, Atropine and Empiric Fluids, and Calcium Chloride

Clinicians and some resuscitation experts have proposed—usually in letters to the editor—a number of nonspecific temporizing and therapeutic interventions. No evidence higher than level 8 (common sense) supports these actions, so all are considered Class Indeterminate. For example, if the lungs are clear and you suspect hypovolemia, you can infuse an empiric 500 mL bolus of normal saline while giving additional consideration to the true intravascular volume status. In settings where patients with renal failure are common (eg, near dialysis facilities), PEA protocols can include empiric administration of 10 mL of a 10% solution of calcium chloride. Life-threatening hyperkalemia is well known to produce a wide, bizarre cardiac rhythm that is classic PEA.

Epinephrine is recommended and atropine should be considered (slow rate) for PEA in the ACLS Pulseless Arrest Algorithm, although the level of evidence supporting their use is insufficient to merit anything more than a Class Indeterminate recommendation. The International Guidelines Committees had no evidence to review on the use of vasopressin in PEA.

Other Drugs/Interventions Not Supported by Outcome

Sodium Bicarbonate: The Recommendations

Sodium bicarbonate 1 mEq/kg is definitely helpful in the asystolic patient known to have preexisting hyperkalemia, in known overdose with tricyclic antidepressants, and to alkalinize the urine in drug overdose. It may be helpful to give sodium bicarbonate immediately after intubation in patients who experienced a long arrest interval before intubation. Sodium bicarbonate is ineffective and may be harmful in nonintubated patients likely to have hypercarbic acidosis.

Aminophylline for Asystole?

Aminophylline is a nonspecific adenosine receptor antagonist that in theory might have had some benefit in asystole. Case reports and 1 very optimistic case series led to at least 2 prospective, randomized trials of aminophylline in out-of-hospital asystolic cardiac arrest. The more sophisticated the study, however, the fewer benefits observed with aminophylline. Since publication of the negative findings by Mader et al in 1999, little research has been published, and this drug is of historical interest.

Pulseless Electrical Activity (PEA)

As defined above, any organized rhythm without a pulse is called *pulseless electrical activity.* **There is also no measurable blood pressure, but taking a blood pressure measurement is never indicated in an unresponsive and pulseless patient.** PEA is a heterogeneous group of rhythms that includes supraventricular rhythms without a detectable pulse or blood pressure. It should be noted that maintenance of an organized supraventricular rhythm without a pulse or blood pressure, such as sinus tachycardia, is usually short lived, and deterioration to other, more sinister rhythms usually develops in minutes.

Issues of Definition
Whatever Became of Electromechanical Dissociation?

When electrical activity appears regular and organized on the monitor but the palpating finger feels no pulse, clinicians had traditionally used the term *electromechanical dissociation.* In the early 1990s the international resuscitation community adopted the expression *pulseless electrical activity.* This term is a more suitable phrase that embraces a heterogeneous collection of pseudo-EMD, idioventricular rhythms, ventricular escape rhythms, post-defibrillation idioventricular rhythms, and bradyasystolic rhythms. PEA more precisely describes the phenomenon without the implication of anatomy or etiology contained in the other terms.

PEA by definition is a rhythmic display of some type of organized electrical activity other than VF or ventricular tachycardia (VT) but without an accompanying pulse that can be detected by palpation of any artery. The former term *electromechanical dissociation* was too specific and narrow. Strictly speaking, EMD means that organized electrical depolarization occurs throughout the myocardium; no synchronous shortening of the myocardial fiber occurs, and mechanical contractions are absent. The absence of a pulse and the presence of electrical activity defines this group of arrhythmias.

Electrical Activity Without a Pulse: Any Mechanical Activity

Although electrical activity without a palpable pulse implies the absence of cardiac output, this characterization may not reflect the true cardiac condition. Research with cardiac ultrasonography and indwelling pressure catheters has confirmed that a pulseless patient with electrical activity may possess associated mechanical contractions at the onset of PEA. These contractions are too weak to produce the 45 to 60 mm Hg of pressure required for detection by manual palpation or sphygmomanometry.

The critical point is for resuscitation providers to understand that PEA may be associated with clinical states that are reversible if identified early and treated appropriately because there may be some small but appreciable cardiac output. Unless a specific cause can be identified and an intervention performed to improve the condition, rhythm degeneration usually follows quickly. Degeneration of PEA into an agonal ventricular rhythm or asystole is most common.

Pseudo-PEA?

Immediate assessment of blood flow by Doppler ultrasound may reveal an actively contracting heart and significant blood flow. But the blood pressure and flow may fall below the threshold of detection of simple arterial palpation, a condition originally termed *pseudo-EMD*.[9] Patients with PEA and a Doppler-detectable blood flow are treated aggressively. Depending on the assessment of the probable cause, these patients may need volume expansion,

Table 5. Frequency of PEA and Survival to Hospital Discharge in 9 Studies*

Location and Period of Study	Index Population	Number of Arrests	PEA Arrests	Survival to Hospital Admission	Survival to Hospital Discharge	Comment
Adults Only, Nontrauma Only						
Scotland; 1994	Adults only, nontrauma	258	4% (10/258) EMD 28% (72/258) bradycardia	—	10% (1/10)	Only arrests witnessed by EMS personnel
Houston, TX; 2 years	Adults only, nontrauma	2404	7% (168/2404) EMD 5% (120/2404) IVR 12% (288/2404) PEA	—	7% (12/168) EMD 5% (6/120) IVR 6% (18/288) PEA	2 tiers: EMT-Ds + paramedics
Helsinki, Finland; 1990	Adults only, nontrauma	489	21% (103/489)	26% (27/103)	6% (6/103)	2nd tier: doctors on ambulances
Seattle, WA; 1980-1986	Adults only, nontrauma	5145	4% (206/5145)	—	6% (12/206)	2 tiers: EMT-Ds + paramedics
Milwaukee, WI; 1980-1985	Adults only, nontrauma	503	503	19% (96/503)	4% (20/503)	50% of PEA arrests respiratory in origin
Tucson, AZ; 16 months	Adults only, nontrauma	298	27% (80/298)	20% (16/80)	4% (3/80)	2 tiers: EMT-Ds + paramedics
Adults Only, Trauma + Nontrauma						
Helsinki, Finland; 1996	Adults + trauma	344	21% (72/344)	28% (20/72)	3% (2/72)	2nd tier: doctors on ambulances
Adults + Children, Nontrauma + Trauma						
Göteborg, Sweden; 1980-1997	Adults + children + trauma	4662	23% (1069/4662)	15% (158/1069)	2% (26/1069)	1st tier: standard ambulance; 2nd tier: mobile CCU
Glamorgan, Scotland; 2.7 years	Adults + children + trauma	954	9% (86/954)	6% (5/86)	2% (2/86)	1st tier: standard ambulance; 2nd tier: MD response

IVR indicates idioventricular rhythm; EMT-D, emergency medical technician-defibrillation; and CCU, coronary care unit.
*Studies listed in order of decreasing magnitude of survival to hospital discharge.

norepinephrine, dopamine, or some combination of the three. They might benefit from early TCP because the myocardium is healthy and only a temporarily disturbed cardiac conduction system stands between survival and death. Although in general PEA leads to poor outcomes, reversible causes should always be targeted and never missed when present. Look for the H's and T's listed earlier.

Frequency of, and Survival From, PEA

Because of imprecise and variable nomenclature, researchers have encountered difficulties obtaining definitive information about the frequency of PEA in out-of-hospital cardiac arrest. Published rates of survival to hospital discharge vary considerably, from 1% to more than 10% (Table 5). Given the wide range of causes of PEA arrest, such variation in frequency and survival would be expected.

Research and Reporting

Another source of imprecision in our understanding of PEA stems from researchers' use of inconsistent denominators. Table 5 demonstrates this problem. Table 5 lists frequency and survival data from 9 studies. Notice that the authors of different studies used 3 markedly different denominators in calculating the frequency and survival rates: adult cardiac arrest due to nontraumatic causes (6 studies); adult cardiac arrest only, both traumatic and nontraumatic causes (1 study); and both adult and pediatric cardiac arrests due to both nontraumatic and traumatic causes (2 studies).

Note that with broader, less precise denominators in the studies, the frequency of PEA increases somewhat but the survival rate decreases. This result would be expected because both traumatic cardiac arrests and pediatric cardiac arrests are more likely to be associated with non-VF arrest rhythms, primarily PEA. The rate of survival from non-VF arrest is much lower than the rate of survival from VF/pulseless VT arrest. Almost no one with blunt traumatic cardiac arrest and with very penetrating injuries as a cause survives. So when survival data from these 2 types of arrest are analyzed together, the overall survival rate will be lower.

Standard reporting recommendations known as the *Utstein style* have been developed, and one of the major purposes of these guidelines is to help establish standardized nomenclature for reporting outcomes from cardiac arrest.[10,11] But for most of these published studies, researchers initiated data collection before publication and dissemination of the Utstein style guidelines. Subsequent research is helping to clarify the epidemiology of PEA.[2,12-14]

Special Considerations When Treating Asystole and PEA

Rapid Scene Survey Evidence for DNAR?

A common scenario, both in and out of hospital, occurs when providers respond to an emergency alarm and observe a person who appears far removed from life. A flat line on the monitor screen is often a confirmation of death. A rapid scene survey should be performed to determine if any reason exists not to initiate CPR.

The Person Is Obviously Dead

Providers should observe and note any *clinical* indicators that a resuscitation attempt is not indicated. For example, are there signs of death? If yes, do not start or attempt resuscitation. In general the most common reasons for healthcare professionals not to start a resuscitation attempt for a person in cardiac arrest are

- The patient has a valid Do Not Attempt Resuscitation (DNAR) order
- The patient has signs of *irreversible death,* such as rigor mortis, decapitation, or dependent lividity
- The vital functions have deteriorated despite maximal therapy for such conditions as overwhelming septic or cardiogenic shock such that *no physiologic* benefit can be expected

Patient Self-Determination?

The concept of *patient self-determination, that a person has the right to make decisions about healthcare treatment at the end of life,* is now widely accepted internationally. In the United States it is a matter of both ethics and law.[15] EMS and hospital providers should be familiar with local policies, procedures, and practice. A few questions during the initial scene survey could provide guidance:

- Could DNAR be an appropriate approach for this patient?
- Are there any *objective* indicators of DNAR status, such as an alert bracelet or anklet? written documents? family statements? If yes, do not start or attempt resuscitation.

Family and Patient Wishes?

People call for emergency help for many reasons. Many families call 911 not to request resuscitation but to request help in coping with the dead. Physicians caring for terminally ill patients are now more aware that hospice programs frequently can address these issues; we encourage physicians to support the patient and family by referring them to these excellent programs. Making a terminally ill patient comfortable is more important than sustaining a few more moments of agonizing life for the patient and family. Legal barriers are often cited as reasons to withhold comfort measures and initiate resuscitation. Public knowledge and EMS planning are beginning to remove many of these concerns. People should be able to call for and receive emergency comfort and care, but they should not receive an unwanted attempt at resuscitation.

Calling the Code: When to Stop Resuscitative Efforts

In most resuscitation attempts this question seems to "sneak up" on the team. The question of whether the resuscitation attempt has reached the point where efforts should cease is best answered after consideration of the quality of the resuscitation attempt, the presence of atypical clinical events or features, and whether *cease-efforts protocols* are in place in the setting of the resuscitation.

The resuscitation team must make a conscientious and competent effort to give patients a trial of CPR and ACLS, provided that the patient has not expressed a decision to forego resuscitative efforts. The final decision to stop efforts can never be as simple as an isolated time interval, but clinical judgment and respect for human dignity must enter into decision making. There is little data to guide this decision, but the following considerations are important and can guide ACLS team leaders.

Consider Quality of Resuscitation

The resuscitation team leader should quickly review, in almost a checklist fashion, a series of questions similar to the following:

- Was there an adequate trial of BLS? of ACLS?
- Has the team achieved endotracheal intubation?
- Performed effective ventilation?
- Shocked VF if present?
- Obtained intravenous (IV) access?
- Given epinephrine IV? atropine IV?
- Ruled out or corrected reversible causes?
- Documented continuous asystole for more than 5 to 10 minutes after all of the above have been accomplished?

Atypical Features Present?

Even within the context of persistent asystole, exceptions and unusual circumstances can come into play. These exceptions are clinical features that in general would justify prolonging the resuscitation attempt beyond what would be appropriate for prolonged asystole:

- Young age?
- Asystole persists because of toxins or electrolyte abnormalities?
- Profound hypothermia?

- Therapeutic or illicit drug overdose?
- Suicide attempt?
- Nearby family or loved ones expressing opposition to stopping efforts?
- Victim of cold-water submersion?

A particularly challenging situation can arise when the person in cardiac arrest experiences effective circulation from the chest compressions of CPR. The blood flow can be sufficient to maintain higher brainstem functions such as gasping respirations, avoidance or protective movements, and even near consciousness. Although a rarely observed phenomenon, there are case reports, most often of young adults with drug overdoses, of CPR maintaining near consciousness for up to 6 hours.[16,17]

Cease-Efforts Protocols in Place?

The final decision to stop efforts is never as simple as an isolated time interval. Clinical judgment and a respect for human dignity must enter the decision making. Many knowledgeable observers believe that the resuscitation community has erred greatly in the tendency to try prolonged, excessive resuscitative efforts.

Physician orders to "discontinue resuscitative efforts"* are both clinically and ethically appropriate when the recommendations noted above are followed. Healthcare professionals in settings where resuscitation attempts are regular events should conduct advance planning for how to handle the emotional, social, and legal aspects of unsuccessful resuscitation attempts. Such *cease-efforts protocols* receive uniform approbation in virtually every setting when initiated. These protocols should include suggestions for how to encourage and support family presence at resuscitation attempts.

Transport of Patients in Cardiac Arrest

Unless special situations are present (as partially listed above), evidence for nontraumatic and blunt traumatic out-of-hospital cardiac arrest confirms that ACLS care in the emergency department (ED) offers no advantage over ACLS care in the field. Stated succinctly, if ACLS care in the field cannot resuscitate the patient, ED care will not resuscitate the patient. Civil rules, administrative concerns, medical insurance requirements, and even reimbursement enhancement have frequently led to requirements to transport all cardiac arrest victims to a hospital or ED. If these requirements are nonselective, they are inappropriate, futile, and ethically unacceptable. Cessation of efforts in the out-of-hospital setting, following system-specific criteria

---

*A persistent puzzle in American hospitals is how the phrase "call the code" became a ubiquitous substitute for more formal expressions to stop the attempt to resuscitate.

and under direct medical control, should be standard practice in all EMS systems.

Here is a short list of some of the most important AHA recommendations for cease-efforts protocols:

- Field protocols to cease resuscitative efforts or to pronounce death outside the hospital have been recommended for more than a decade. States should take all administrative, legislative, and regulatory steps necessary to allow rescuers to cease resuscitative efforts in the field.
- EMS systems directors should provide clear instructions to EMS personnel about leaving the body at the scene, what to do about death certification, and what to tell the family about arranging for the funeral home to pick up the deceased relative.
- EMS system directors should consider on-scene EMS-employed family advocates and a program involving local clergy members willing to assume on-call responsibility for 24/7 religious or nondenominational counseling.
- Larger EMS systems should consider having special-duty field officers respond to the site of an out-of-hospital death pronouncement to replace the departing field personnel and to provide more support and information to the family and loved ones. EMS personnel must be trained to deal sensitively with family members and others at the scene.
- Terminally ill patients in private homes, hospice programs, or nursing homes have the ethical and legal right to decline resuscitative attempts while maintaining access to emergency treatment for acute medical illness or traumatic injuries, comfort measures to relieve suffering, and transport by ambulance to a medical facility.
- Personal physicians are responsible for helping patients who are entering the terminal stages of an illness plan for death. Physicians must be familiar with local laws related to certification and pronouncement of death, the role of the coroner and police, and disposition of the body.
- Physicians have a responsibility to initiate frank discussions with patients and family members about comfort measures and hygiene, pain control and end-of-life support, when (and when not) to call the EMS system, use of a local hospice, when and how to contact the personal physician, funeral plans, disposition of the body, psychological concerns surrounding death and dying, and bereavement counseling and ministerial support.
- Most in-hospital DNAR orders are not transferable outside the hospital. An additional out-of-hospital DNAR form must be completed. Failure to address these issues may result in unnecessary confusion and inappropriate care.
- Many patients prefer to die at home surrounded by loved ones. The hospice movement and many societies for specific diseases provide excellent guidelines for planning an expected death at home.

References

1. Bayes de Luna A, Coumel P, Leclercq JF. Ambulatory sudden cardiac death: mechanisms of production of fatal arrhythmia on the basis of data from 157 cases. *Am Heart J*. 1989;117:151-159.

2. Engdahl J, Bang A, Lindqvist J, Herlitz J. Can we define patients with no and those with some chance of survival when found in asystole out of hospital? *Am J Cardiol*. 2000;86: 610-614.

3. Ewy GA. Ventricular fibrillation masquerading as asystole. *Ann Emerg Med*. 1984;13:811-812.

4. Losek JD, Hennes H, Glaeser PW, Smith DS, Hendley G. Prehospital countershock treatment of pediatric asystole. *Am J Emerg Med*. 1989;7:571-575.

5. Lipton JD, Forstater AT. Recurrent asystole associated with vasovagal reaction during venipuncture. *J Emerg Med*. 1993;11:723-727.

6. Hedges JR, Syverud SA, Dalsey WC, Feero S, Easter R, Shultz B. Prehospital trial of emergency transcutaneous cardiac pacing. *Circulation*. 1987;76:1337-1343.

7. Cummins RO, Graves JR, Larsen MP, Hallstrom AP, Hearne TR, Ciliberti J, Nicola RM, Horan S. Out-of-hospital transcutaneous pacing by emergency medical technicians in patients with asystolic cardiac arrest. *N Engl J Med*. 1993;328: 1377-1382.

8. Cummins RO, Hazinski MF. The next chapter in the high-dose epinephrine story: unfavorable neurologic outcomes? [editorial] *Ann Intern Med*. 1998;129:501-502.

9. Paradis NA, Martin GB, Goetting MG, Rivers EP, Feingold M, Nowak RM. Aortic pressure during human cardiac arrest. Identification of pseudo-electromechanical dissociation. *Chest*. 1992;101:123-128.

10. Cummins RO, Chamberlain DA, Abramson NS, Allen M, Baskett P, Becker L, Bossaert L, Delooz H, Dick W, Eisenberg M, et al Recommended guidelines for uniform reporting of data from out-of-hospital cardiac arrest: the Utstein Style. Task Force of the American Heart Association, the European Resuscitation Council, the Heart and Stroke Foundation of Canada, and the Australian Resuscitation Council. *Ann Emerg Med*. 1991;20:861-874.

11. Cummins RO, Chamberlain D, Hazinski MF, Nadkarni V, Kloeck W, Kramer E, Becker L, Robertson C, Koster R, Zaritsky A, Bossaert L, Ornato JP, Callanan V, Allen M, Steen P, Connolly B, Sanders A, Idris A, Cobbe S. Recommended guidelines for reviewing, reporting, and conducting research on in-hospital resuscitation: the in-hospital 'Utstein style.' American Heart Association. *Circulation*. 1997;95:2213-2239.

12. Engdahl J, Bang A, Lindqvist J, Herlitz J. Factors affecting short- and long-term prognosis among 1069 patients with out-of-hospital cardiac arrest and pulseless electrical activity. *Resuscitation*. 2001;51:17-25.

13. Herlitz J, Bang A, Gunnarsson J, Engdahl J, Karlson BW, Lindqvist J, Waagstein L. Factors associated with survival to hospital discharge among patients hospitalised alive after out of hospital cardiac arrest: Change in outcome over 20 years in the community of Goteborg, Sweden. *Heart*. 2003;89:25-30.

14. Herlitz J, Engdahl J, Svensson L, Young M, Angquist KA, Holmberg S. Characteristics and outcome among children suffering from out of hospital cardiac arrest in Sweden. *Resuscitation*. 2005;64:37-40.

15. Wolf SM, Boyle P, Callahan D, Fins JJ, Jennings B, Nelson JL, Barondess JA, Brock DW, Dresser R, Emanuel L, et al. Sources of concern about the Patient Self-Determination Act. *N Engl J Med*. 1991;325:1666-1671.

16. Orzel JA. Tricyclic antidepressant poisoning and prolonged external cardiac massage during asystole. *Br Med J (Clin Res Ed)*. 1981;283:1399.

17. Orr DA, Bramble MG. Tricyclic antidepressant poisoning and prolonged external cardiac massage during asystole. *Br Med J (Clin Res Ed)*. 1981;283:1107-1108.

Chapter 7

Bradycardia

Key Points

- If bradycardia produces signs and symptoms (eg, acute altered mental status, ongoing severe ischemic chest pain, congestive heart failure, hypotension or other signs of shock) that persist despite adequate airway and breathing, immediately prepare to provide pacing.
- Transcutaneous pacing (TCP) is indicated for symptomatic bradycardia refractory to atropine (when atropine is indicated). Unless patients are unstable and deteriorating, sedation is recommended before TCP. Preparation for TCP should be made early. For symptomatic high-degree (second-degree or third-degree atrioventricular [AV] block), provide TCP without delay.
- Atropine is useful in treating symptomatic sinus bradycardia and may be beneficial in the presence of AV block at the nodal level or for ventricular asystole.
- In second-degree type I AV block (Wenckebach), where vagal activity is an etiologic factor, atropine administration may lessen the degree of block. Atropine is not indicated in the treatment of bradycardia from AV block at the His-Purkinje level (type II AV block and third-degree block with new wide QRS complexes). In such instances without significant vagal effect atropine rarely accelerates sinus rate and AV node conduction, but it may be difficult in an emergency to accurately make this clinical distinction.
- Atropine should be used cautiously in the presence of an acute coronary syndrome (ACS) or infarction because increases in heart rate may worsen ischemia or increase the zone of infarction. Ventricular fibrillation (VF) or ventricular tachycardia (VT) is a potential but uncommon complication of atropine administration.

Introduction

A *bradyarrhythmia* is a rhythm disorder with a heart rate less than 60 per minute. This term is commonly used interchangeably with the term *bradycardia* to define a sinus bradycardia when a rate limit of 60 is used since this is the lower limit of normal sinus rhythm. But a bradyarrhythmia also includes any rhythm disorder with a rate less than 60 per minute. Although cardiologists typically define bradycardia as a heart rate <60 per minute, this heart rate may be physiologically normal and appropriate and may produce effective systemic perfusion for many people, including trained athletes.

Absolute and Relative Bradycardia

Clinicians must be able to recognize both *absolute bradycardia* (heart rate <60 per minute) and *relative bradycardia*. A slow heart rate may be physiologically normal for some patients and inadequate for others. A relative bradycardia is a heart rate that is less than expected relative to the patient's condition. For example, a heart rate of 70 per minute in a hypotensive and septic patient represents a relative bradycardia. Under these clinical circumstances a much higher rate, usually sinus tachycardia, would be present as a compensatory response. It is important to note, however, that attempts to increase the heart rate using chronotropic agents and pacing are not indicated unless drug toxicity or high-degree AV block is complicating the clinical situation.

Definition

For purposes of the ACLS Experienced Provider Course and instructor teaching, the term *bradycardia* is used for bradyarrhythmia. In this context a bradycardia can be sinus bradycardia or third-degree AV block. In fact, the Bradycardia Algorithm (Figure 1) can be implemented without the delay that would be needed to initially identify the underlying rhythm disorder: Just the fact that the patient has a symptomatic bradycardia is enough to start. There are only 2 initial considerations:

1. A bradycardia is present
2. Signs or symptoms are due to the bradycardia

The next consideration is identification of the rhythm disorder and then "tailoring" and "titrating" therapy to the arrhythmia and patient.

Bradycardia and *Symptoms*

In managing patients with a bradycardia, the responsible clinician must first evaluate whether the slow heart rate is hemodynamically significant and produces related symptoms. Recall that heart rate is a major determinant of cardiac output: Cardiac Output = Heart Rate × Stroke Volume. When cardiac function is depressed or limited and stroke volume cannot compensate, cardiac output will fall and patients will eventually become symptomatic.

The clinical sign hypotension, for example, may be due to myocardial dysfunction or hypovolemia rather than to a slowly beating heart even when it is associated with bradycardia (↓ Cardiac Output = Heart Rate × ↓ Stroke Volume). Clinicians are required to treat bradycardia only when the bradycardia itself causes serious signs

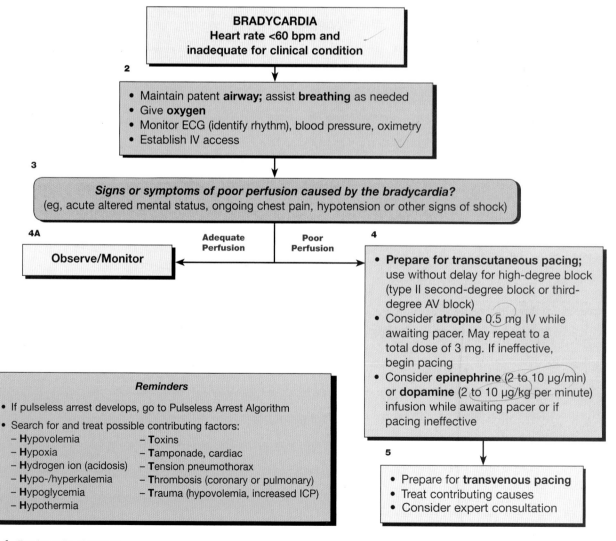

Figure 1. Bradycardia Algorithm.

Foundation Facts **Determinants of Cardiac Output**	Cardiac output per minute is determined by the heart rate per minute and the heart's stroke volume with each mechanical contraction. **Cardiac Output = Heart Rate × Stroke Volume**

and symptoms. Clinical *symptoms* that may be caused by bradycardia include angina or angina with exertion; shortness of breath or dyspnea on exertion; weakness; fatigue; exercise intolerance; lightheadedness, dizziness, or syncope; and decreased level of consciousness. Clinical *signs* include the following:

- Hypotension, postural hypotension, or shock
- Pulmonary congestion (on physical exam or chest x-ray), congestive heart failure, or acute pulmonary edema
- Rate-related ischemic ventricular arrhythmias or ischemic ECG changes

Intervention Sequence for Hemodynamically Significant Bradycardia at Rest

The Bradycardia Algorithm (Figure 1) lists interventions in a sequence assuming worsening clinical condition. When patients have signs and symptoms so severe as to be considered "pre–cardiac arrest," perform multiple interventions in rapid sequence. In such situations near-simultaneous provision of atropine, preparation for pacing, and IV catecholamine infusion (epinephrine or dopamine) if required are appropriate.

Atropine 0.5 mg

The sinus and AV nodes are innervated by the vagus nerve. Atropine works by blocking the effects of vagal nerve discharges on the sinus and AV nodes. Areas of the heart not served by the vagus nerve will not respond to

atropine. Atropine is useful in treating symptomatic sinus bradycardia and may be beneficial in the presence of AV block at the nodal level. In the absence of reversible causes, atropine remains the first-line drug for acute symptomatic bradycardia. Atropine improves heart rate and signs and symptoms associated with bradycardia. In clinical studies an initial dose of 0.5 mg, repeated as needed to a total dose of 1.5 mg, was effective in both in-hospital and out-of-hospital treatment of symptomatic bradycardia.[1-3] Current ACLS Guidelines limit the total dose of atropine to a total maximal dose of 3 mg.

Atropine is not indicated in the treatment of bradycardia from AV block at the His-Purkinje level (type II AV block and third-degree block with new wide QRS complexes). Paradoxical responses to atropine have been reported with anesthesia after heart transplantation.[4-7] Theoretically atropine may increase the rate of sinus node discharge and accelerate AV conduction, worsening the degree of AV block.

Atropine should be used cautiously in the presence of ACS or infarction because excessive increases in heart rate may worsen ischemia or increase the zone of infarction. In rare cases VF and VT have followed IV administration of atropine. A transplanted heart, lacking vagal innervation, typically does not respond to atropine and has only a blunted response to sympathetic stimulation.[10]

FAQ **Will atropine increase the degree of high-degree AV block?** **Can atropine be used if the level of block is uncertain or pacing is not immediately available?**	Theoretically, atropine may paradoxically increase the rate of sinus node discharge and accelerate AV conduction, worsening the degree of block or decreasing the ventricular rate. But the paucity of clinical reports of this complication in the literature since this caution was initially included in the *1992 ECC Guidelines* suggests that it is uncommon. Atropine should not be used if the block is definitely infranodal. If uncertain, preparation for and provision of transcutaneous pacing is always appropriate and is recommended when clinicians are concerned about the use of atropine in patients with higher-level blocks. In certain clinical situations, atropine may be useful while sedation of the patient is achieved or when TCP is not immediately available for a rapidly deteriorating patient.

Atropine Dosing

The *2005 American Heart Association Guidelines for Cardiopulmonary Resuscitation and Emergency Cardiovascular Care* recommend only 2 dosing regimens for atropine, except in special circumstances.

- Atropine 0.5 mg for symptomatic bradycardia. This dose can be repeated every 3 to 5 minutes up to a maximal total dose of 3 mg.
- Atropine 1 mg, as noted in the ACLS Pulseless Arrest Algorithm.

Atropine Cautions

- Atropine may produce a paradoxical decrease in heart rate at lower doses (<0.5 mg).[8,9]
- Carefully assess the need for further doses and correctable comorbidities (eg, volume, ischemia) in patients with an ACS.

Transcutaneous Pacing

Transcutaneous pacing is initiated quickly in patients who do not respond to atropine or who are severely symptomatic and clinically deteriorating, especially when the QRS complex is wide. Verify patient tolerance, electrical capture, and effective mechanical function. Pacing may fail to produce effective cardiac contractions, so the patient's pulse and systemic perfusion need close monitoring. Transcutaneous pacing can be painful, so use analgesia and sedation as needed and tolerated. Note that some sedatives may adversely affect the underlying rhythm.

Most recent-model defibrillator/monitors can perform TCP, making this intervention widely available. Unlike the skill required for insertion of *transvenous* pacemakers, transcutaneous pacing requires no invasive skills and can easily be mastered by most ECC providers. As a bedside intervention TCP has the advantages of speed and simplicity over transvenous pacing. Details and specifics of TCP are reviewed at the end of this chapter.

Alternative Chronotropic Drugs to Consider

After the maximum dose of atropine is administered, consider administration of chronotropic infusion of epinephrine or dopamine if TCP is still not available.

Epinephrine 2 to 10 µg/min

If the patient has severe symptoms (eg, severe bradycardia with hypotension), the drug of choice is a catecholamine infusion (either epinephrine or dopamine). An epinephrine infusion of 2 to 10 µg/min is titrated on the basis of heart rate, blood pressure, and systemic perfusion. Epinephrine infusion is also appropriate if the patient has symptomatic bradycardia unresponsive to dopamine.

Dopamine 2 to 10 µg/kg per minute

After the maximum dose of atropine is administered, add a chronotropic infusion. Dopamine in doses of 2 to 10 µg/kg per minute can be titrated. Dopamine can be added to epinephrine or administered alone. This agent may cause splanchnic vasodilation and hypovolemia when given in low doses, complicating the clinical picture. For this reason it is necessary to assess intravascular volume whenever you give dopamine in low doses.

Isoproterenol No Longer Recommended

Isoproterenol can increase infarct size and cause life-threatening ventricular arrhythmias, so it requires careful titration. It is no longer included or recommended in the Bradycardia Algorithm. Isoproterenol is contraindicated in acetylcholinesterase-induced bradycardias, although it may be useful at high doses in refractory bradycardia induced by β-antagonist receptor blockade.

Glucagon in Special Situations

A case series of patients documented improvement in heart rate, symptoms, and signs associated with bradycardia when IV glucagon (3 mg initially, followed by infusion at 3 mg/h if necessary) was given to in-hospital patients with drug-induced (eg, β-blocker or calcium channel blocker overdose) symptomatic bradycardia not responding to atropine.[11]

Bradycardias—Refining the Diagnosis and Treatment

Sinus Bradycardia

Sinus bradycardia (Figure 2) is a slow heart rate with regular P waves followed at a consistent and normal interval by QRS complexes that are normal in configuration and width. The sinus node is the pacemaker for this rhythm, and the heart rate is less than 60 per minute. Sinus bradycardia is often a symptom of other conditions (eg, good physical conditioning, vagal impulses, or drug effects) rather than a primary arrhythmia that requires treatment. In ACS it commonly is seen in inferior myocardial infarction (MI).

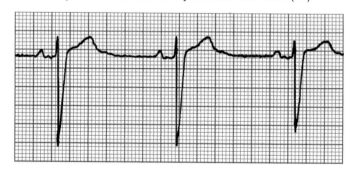

Figure 2. Sinus bradycardia. Sinus rate is 46 per minute and rhythm is regular.

Pathophysiology

- Sinus bradycardia is caused by a slow rate of spontaneous impulses originating at the sinoatrial node.
- Sinus bradycardia is typically a physical sign of other problems rather than a primary arrhythmia.

Defining ECG Criteria (Figure 2)

The key defining criteria of sinus bradycardia on the ECG are regular P waves followed by regular QRS complexes at a rate less than 60 per minute.

- **Rate:** Less than 60 per minute.
- **Rhythm:** Regular sinus.
- **PR interval:** Regular; 0.12-0.20 second.
- **P waves:** Size and shape normal; every P wave is followed by a QRS complex; every QRS complex is preceded by a P wave.
- **QRS complex:** Narrow; <0.12 second (often <0.11 second) in the absence of intraventricular conduction defects.

Clinical Manifestations

- Most people with sinus bradycardia are asymptomatic at rest.
- With increased activity if the heart rate remains slow or does not rise sufficiently with exertion, a patient may become symptomatic.
- Common symptoms include fatigue, shortness of breath, dizziness or lightheadedness, and frank syncope. Common physical signs include hypotension, diaphoresis, pulmonary congestion, and frank pulmonary edema.
- The ECG can independently display acute ST-segment or T-wave deviations or ventricular arrhythmias. The QT interval normally lengthens as heart rate decreases.

Common Etiologies

- Sinus bradycardia is often appropriate ("normal") for well-conditioned people. With age resting heart rate also declines. It is not uncommon to observe significant sinus bradycardia during nighttime telemetry monitoring of patients.
- Sinus bradycardia can occur after an event that stimulates the vasovagal reflex or increases vagal tone, such as vomiting, a Valsalva maneuver, rectal stimuli, or inadvertent pressure on the carotid sinus in the elderly ("shaver's syncope").
- In most patients the blood supply of the sinoatrial node comes from the right coronary artery. For this reason ACS related to the right coronary artery can produce sinus node ischemia and sinus bradycardia.

- Sinus bradycardia can occur as a pharmacological or adverse clinical drug effect of a number of agents, including β-blockers, calcium channel blockers, digoxin, quinidine, amiodarone, and other agents that prolong the refractory period of the sinus node.

Recommended Therapy

- Sinus bradycardia rarely produces rate-related, serious signs and symptoms that merit emergent treatment unless associated with significant comorbidity (eg, inferior ST-elevation myocardial infarction [STEMI]) or ischemia.
- When hemodynamically significant sinus bradycardia does occur, follow the intervention sequence listed in the Bradycardia Algorithm.
- Try to determine the cause and treat it. Also treat any significant complicating factors (eg, hypoxia)

Atrioventricular Block

Atrioventricular block is a delay or interruption in conduction between the atria and ventricles. The delay can occur at many levels in the conduction system and may occur insidiously or abruptly. To effectively anticipate progression in AV block, providers need to understand the conduction system, external influences on conduction tissue, and comorbidities that may precipitate high-degree AV block.

Common Etiologies

AV block may be caused by

- Pathological lesions along the conduction pathway (eg, calcium, fibrosis, necrosis).
- Enhanced vagal stimulation (inferior MI, carotid sinus sensitivity or massage).
- Increases in the refractory period of the conduction pathway (drugs).
- Physiologic block due to shortening of the length of the supraventricular cycle. As the length of the supraventricular cycle becomes shorter (as with rapid atrial flutter), it eventually becomes shorter than the normal refractory period of the AV node. At this point of encroachment on the refractory period of the AV node, conduction will not occur. Electrical impulses are "blocked" from progressing to the ventricle. The AV node may, for example, allow conduction at 150 per minute but not at 300 per minute. This conduction pattern becomes a 2:1 AV block. This "protects" the ventricle from excessive rates.

Summary—Sinus Bradycardia

Sinus Bradycardia	
Pathophysiology	• Impulses originate at SA node at a slow rate • Not pathological; not an abnormal arrhythmia • More a physical sign
Defining Criteria per ECG **Key:** Regular P waves followed by regular QRS complexes at rate <60 beats/min **Note:** Often a physical sign rather than an abnormal rhythm	• **Rate:** <60 beats/min • **Rhythm:** regular sinus • **PR:** regular; <0.20 sec • **P waves:** size and shape normal; every P wave is followed by a QRS complex; every QRS complex is preceded by a P wave • **QRS complex:** narrow; <0.12 sec in absence of intraventricular conduction defect
Clinical Manifestations	• At rest, usually asymptomatic • With increased activity, persistent slow rate will lead to symptoms of easy fatigue, SOB, dizziness or lightheadedness, syncope, hypotension
Common Etiologies	• Normal for well-conditioned people • A vasovagal event such as vomiting, valsalva, rectal stimuli, inadvertent pressure on carotid sinus ("shaver's syncope") • Acute MIs that affect circulation to SA node (right coronary artery); most often inferior AMIs • Adverse drug effects, eg, blocking agents (β or calcium channel), digoxin, quinidine
Recommended Therapy	• Treatment rarely indicated • Treat only if patient has significant signs or symptoms due to the bradycardia • Oxygen is always appropriate **Intervention sequence for bradycardia** • *Atropine* 0.5 mg IV if vagal mechanism • *Transcutaneous pacing* if available **If signs and symptoms are severe, consider catecholamine infusion if atropine and pacing fail:** • *Dopamine* 2 to 10 µg/kg per min • *Epinephrine* 2 to 10 µg/min

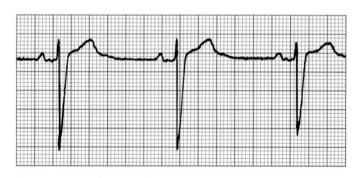

Sinus bradycardia: rate of 45 bpm; with borderline first-degree AV block (PR ≈ 0.20 sec)

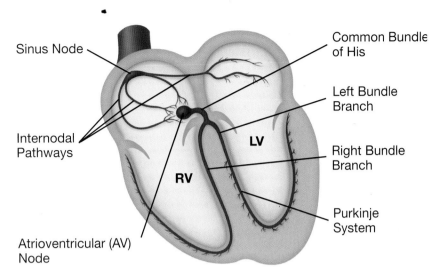

Figure 3. Relationship of the AV node to the anatomy of the conduction system. Although often portrayed as a "discrete structure," the AV node is a complicated network of fibers with different electrophysiologic properties.

Classification of AV Block

Atrioventricular block may be classified according to the *site* or *degree* of block. The AV node is anatomically a complicated network of fibers—not a discrete structure—and located inferiorly in the right atrium, anterior to the ostium of the coronary sinus and above the tricuspid valve. The speed of conduction is normally slowed through the AV node, and the upper limit of normal of the PR interval is 0.20 second. These fibers converge at their lower margin to form a discrete bundle of fibers, the *bundle of His* (or *AV*

bundle). This structure penetrates the annulus fibrosis and arrives at the upper margin of the muscular intraventricular septum. Here the infranodal structure of the conduction system gives origin to the bundle branches (Figure 3).

Site of Block

- Junction of AV node with atria or within AV nodal tissue
- Infranodal, occurring anatomically at either the bundle of His or the bundle branches

Table 1. Major ECG Features of First-Degree, Second-Degree, and Third-Degree Heart Block

ECG Feature	First-Degree	Second-Degree	Third-Degree
Rate **Atrial** **Ventricular**	Unaffected Same as atrial rate	Unaffected Slower than atrial rate	Unaffected Slower than atrial rate
Ventricular rhythm	Same as atrial rhythm or regular	**Type I:** Irregular (may be regularly irregular in a repetitive pattern) **Type II:** Regular or irregular	Ventricular escape beats are usually regular
P-QRS relationship	Consistent: 1:1	**Type I:** Variable PR intervals before the dropped QRS complex **Type II:** Fixed PR intervals before the dropped QRS complex	Absent (AV dissociation)
QRS duration	Unaffected	**Type I:** Narrow **Type II:** Most often wide; rarely narrow	Usually wide but can be narrow, depending on site of escape rhythm
Site of block	Anywhere from AV node to bundle branches, though typically in AV node	**Type I:** AV node **Type II:** Typically in or below the bundle of His	Anywhere from AV node to bundle branches

Degree of Block

- First-degree AV block.
- Second-degree AV block (either type I or type II). In second-degree block there are more atrial than ventricular complexes, and it is further described by the number of atrial to ventricular beats, for example, 2:1 or 4:1 (expressed as "two-to-one" or "four-to-one") or greater.
- Third-degree or complete AV block.

The 3 degrees of block can generally be used to infer the sites of block: junction of atria and AV node (supranodal), within the AV node, or below the AV node (infranodal). The site of block is important because the pathogenesis, treatment, and prognosis vary with each site. There are exceptions to this classification, but the details involve complicated electrophysiology. Table 1 presents the major general ECG features of first-degree, second-degree, and third-degree heart block.

First-Degree AV Block

First-degree AV block (Figure 4) is a *delay* in passage of the depolarization impulse from atria to ventricles. This delay manifests as prolongation of the PR interval. The specific site of block can be anywhere from the AV node to the bundle branches, although typically it occurs in the AV node.

Pathophysiology

- In first-degree AV block conduction of the sinus impulse is slowed (partially blocked) at the AV node for a fixed amount of time.
- First-degree AV block can be a normal physiologic variant without a specific pathophysiology.
- In some clinical circumstances first-degree AV block is caused by an extracardiac condition (eg, excess vagal tone, drug toxicity).

Defining ECG Criteria (Figure 4)

The key defining criterion on the ECG is a PR interval greater than 0.20 second.

- **Rate:** First-degree heart block can be seen with both sinus bradycardia and sinus tachycardia.
- **Rhythm:** Sinus, regular; both atria and ventricles.
- **PR interval:** Prolonged (>0.20 second) but does not vary *(fixed)*.
- **P waves:** Size and shape normal; every P wave is followed by a QRS complex; every QRS complex is preceded by a P wave.
- **QRS complex:** Less than 0.12 second in the absence of intraventricular conduction defects.

Clinical Manifestations

- The patient with first-degree AV block is usually asymptomatic.

Common Etiologies

- Many first-degree AV blocks are due to the adverse effects of drugs, most commonly drugs known to block conduction through the AV node: β-blockers, calcium channel blockers, and digoxin. It can also be a manifestation of pathology in the conduction system associated with aging and other disease states.
- First-degree AV block can occur after an event that stimulates vagal activity, such as vomiting, a Valsalva maneuver, rectal stimuli, or inadvertent pressure on the carotid sinus (shaver's syncope).
- Acute coronary syndromes involving the right coronary artery will often affect circulation to the AV node, creating AV nodal ischemia and slowing AV nodal conduction.

Recommended Therapy

- Treatment of first-degree AV block is almost never necessary or indicated because few patients have significant signs or symptoms related to the first-degree AV block. If symptoms or signs are present, always search for and consider an alternate cause.
- When a patient develops new-onset first-degree AV block, be alert for progression of the block to second-degree AV block, either type I or type II, and consider a cause.

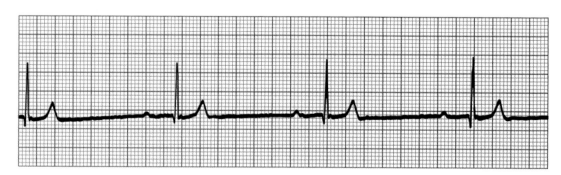

Figure 4. First-degree AV block. The PR interval is prolonged to about 0.34 second. Also present is sinus bradycardia.

First-Degree AV Block	
Pathophysiology	• Impulse conduction is slowed *(partial block)* at the AV node by a fixed amount • Closer to being a physical sign than an abnormal arrhythmia
Defining Criteria per ECG **Key:** PR interval >0.20 sec	• **Rate:** First-degree AV block can be seen with both sinus bradycardia and sinus tachycardia • **Rhythm:** sinus, regular, both atria and ventricles • **PR:** prolonged, >0.20 sec, but does not vary *(fixed)* • **P waves:** size and shape normal; every P wave is followed by a QRS complex; every QRS complex is preceded by a P wave • **QRS complex:** narrow; <0.12 sec in absence of intraventricular conduction defect
Clinical Manifestations	• Usually asymptomatic at rest • Rarely, if bradycardia worsens, person may become symptomatic from the slow rate
Common Etiologies	• Large majority of first-degree AV blocks are due to drugs, usually the AV nodal blockers: β-blockers, calcium channel blockers, and digoxin • Any condition that stimulates the parasympathetic nervous system (eg, vasovagal reflex) • Acute MIs that affect circulation to AV node (right coronary artery); most often inferior AMIs
Recommended Therapy	• Treat only when patient has significant signs or symptoms that are due to the bradycardia • Be alert to block deteriorating to second-degree, type I or type II block • Oxygen is always appropriate **Intervention sequence for symptomatic bradycardia** • *Atropine* 0.5 mg IV if vagal mechanism • *Transcutaneous pacing* if available **If signs and symptoms are severe, consider catecholamine infusions:** • *Dopamine* 2 to 10 µg/kg per min • *Epinephrine* 2 to 10 µg/min

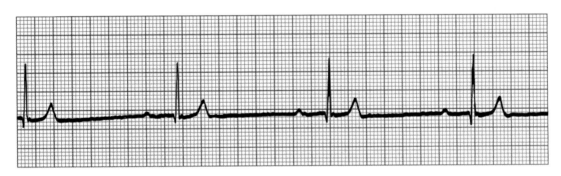

First-degree AV block at rate of 37 bpm; PR interval 0.28 sec

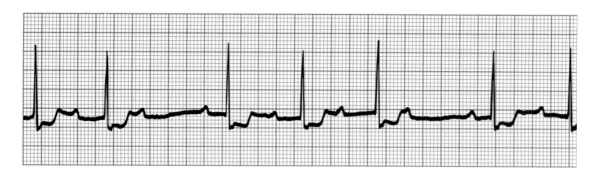

Figure 5. Type I second-degree AV block. Atrial rhythm is nearly regular. But there are pauses in ventricular rhythm because the depolarization impulse associated with every fourth P wave does not conduct into the ventricles. Note progressive prolongation of the PR interval, indicating increasing conduction delay in the AV node before the nonconducted impulse ("blocked atrial to ventricular conduction"). In the center of the strip there are 4 P waves and 3 QRS complexes, representing a 4:3 cycle. The QRS complexes are normal.

Second-Degree AV Block (Mobitz I or Wenckebach)

In second-degree AV block some atrial impulses are conducted through the AV node and others are blocked—that is, "not every P wave is followed by a QRS complex."[12-14] Second-degree AV block is divided into 2 types:

- *Type I second-degree AV block* (also referred to as *Mobitz I or Wenckebach*)
- *Type II second-degree AV block* (also referred to as *Mobitz II*)

Type I second-degree AV block almost always occurs at the level of the AV node and is characterized by a progressive prolongation of the PR interval. Conduction velocity slows through the AV node until an impulse is completely blocked. Usually only a single impulse is blocked, and the pattern is then repeated. The sequence of the block can be described by the ratio of the P waves to the QRS complexes (eg, 2:1 means every other P wave is not followed by a QRS complex; 3:2 means that every third P wave is not followed by a QRS complex).

Pathophysiology

- Type I second-degree AV block (Mobitz I or Wenckebach) almost always occurs at the level of the AV node (rather than at an *infranodal* level, ie, at the bundle of His or bundle branches). The AV node cells can demonstrate a gradual and progressive conduction delay in response to a depolarization stimulus.
- Type I second-degree block is more often caused by increased parasympathetic tone than by ischemia. Because type I block seldom indicates AV node ischemia, except in the presence of ACS, this form of second-degree block is not as ominous clinically as type II second-degree block (see below). In addition, it uncommonly progresses to a high-degree AV block with slow escape rhythm.

- An increase in parasympathetic tone can cause impulse conduction through the AV node to become slower and slower. This slowed conduction causes the PR interval to increase until one depolarization impulse from the atria is completely blocked before it depolarizes the ventricle ("dropped" QRS complex or "dropped beat").
  - This pattern is repeated, resulting in "group beating" (eg, 3 conducted sinus depolarizations with progressive lengthening in PR intervals and a fourth sinus depolarization that is not followed by a QRS complex). Such a "group" is referred to as 4:3 *conduction*.
  - The conduction ratio can change (eg, 4:3, 3:2, 2:1), although it may remain constant.
  - Type I second-degree AV block is usually transient. The prognosis is generally good.

Defining ECG Criteria (Figure 5)

The key defining criterion on the ECG is progressive lengthening of the PR interval until one P wave is not followed by a QRS complex. This represents the nonconducted or "dropped" depolarization impulse or "dropped beat (QRS complex)."

- **Rate:** The atrial rate is unaffected. But the overall atrial rate is usually slightly faster than the overall ventricular rate because some atrial depolarization impulses are not conducted to the ventricles ("blocked complexes" or "dropped beats [QRS complex]").
- **Rhythm:** The atrial rhythm is usually regular. The ventricular rhythm is usually regularly irregular except in the presence of 2:1 AV block or a changing conduction sequence.
- **PR interval:** The PR interval progressively lengthens from cycle to cycle; then one P wave is not followed by a QRS complex (the nonconducted impulse or "dropped" QRS complex). There is

progressive shortening of the RR interval before the blocked impulse. The RR interval that brackets the nonconducted P wave is less than twice the normal cycle length.

- **P waves:** The size and shape remain normal; occasionally a P wave is not followed by a QRS complex (the blocked impulse or "dropped" QRS complex).
- **QRS complex:** The QRS complex is usually *narrow* (often <0.12 sec), but a QRS "drops out" periodically (ie, a QRS complex does not follow every P wave).

Clinical Manifestations

In type I second-degree AV block the symptoms and signs are related to the severity of the bradycardia.

- **Symptoms:** With minimal exertion patients may experience chest discomfort, shortness of breath, and decreased level of consciousness.
- **Signs:** Occasionally the bradycardia is slow enough to produce hypotension, shock, pulmonary congestion, congestive heart failure, and angina.

Common Etiologies

- The most frequent causes of type I second-degree AV block are drugs that slow conduction through the AV node: β-blockers, calcium channel blockers, and digoxin.
- The second most common cause of type I second-degree AV block is any condition that stimulates the parasympathetic system, increasing parasympathetic tone. Such conditions include any event that stimulates the vasovagal reflex, such as vomiting, a Valsalva maneuver, or rectal stimuli.

- Circulation to the AV node comes from the right coronary artery in most patients. For this reason acute coronary syndromes that affect the *right* coronary artery (or a dominant left circumflex coronary artery) can produce type I second-degree AV nodal block.

Recommended Therapy

Specific treatment is rarely needed unless severe signs and symptoms are present. Clinicians should remain comfortable with *watchful waiting* and avoid unnecessary administration of atropine simply to treat the observed block.

- Place a high priority on identifying the underlying cause.
- If the bradycardia resulting from the nonconducted P wave leads to serious signs and symptoms, initiate the bradycardia algorithm intervention sequence.
- If a vagal mechanism appears to be the cause of the type I block, administer atropine 0.5 mg IV. Further treatment is rarely necessary (see the Bradycardia Algorithm for additional therapies).

Second-Degree AV Block (Mobitz II or Infranodal)

Type II second-degree AV block (Figure 6) occurs below the level of the AV node (infranodal) at either the bundle of His or the bundle branches. A hallmark of this type of second-degree AV block is that the PR interval does not lengthen before a blocked impulse; the blocking of the impulse is an abrupt event. More than 1 nonconducted impulse may occur in succession.

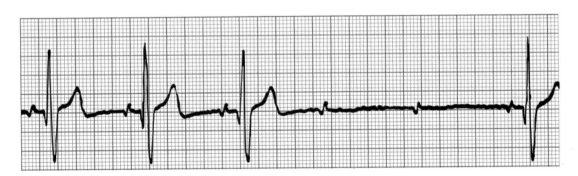

Figure 6. Type II second-degree AV block. In this example 3 conducted sinus impulses are followed by 2 nonconducted P waves. The PR interval of the conducted P waves remains constant, and the QRS complex is wide.

Second-Degree AV Block Type I (Mobitz I or Wenckebach)	
Pathophysiology	• Site of pathology: AV node • AV node blood supply comes from branches of the right coronary artery • Impulse conduction is increasingly slowed at the AV node (causing increasing PR interval) • Until one sinus impulse is completely blocked and a QRS complex fails to follow
Defining Criteria per ECG **Key:** There is progressive lengthening of the PR interval until one P wave is not followed by a QRS complex (the dropped beat)	• **Rate:** atrial rate just slightly faster than ventricular (because of dropped beats); usually normal range • **Rhythm:** regular for atrial beats; irregular for ventricular (because of dropped beats); can show regular P waves marching through irregular QRS • **PR:** progressive lengthening of the PR interval occurs from cycle to cycle; then one P wave is not followed by a QRS complex (the "dropped beat") • **P waves:** size and shape remain normal; occasional P wave not followed by a QRS complex (the "dropped beat") • **QRS complex:** <0.12 sec most often, but a QRS "drops out" periodically
Clinical Manifestations—Rate-Related	**Due to bradycardia:** • **Symptoms:** chest pain, shortness of breath, decreased level of consciousness • **Signs:** hypotension, shock, pulmonary congestion, CHF, angina
Common Etiologies	• AV nodal blocking agents: β-blockers, calcium channel blockers, digoxin • Conditions that stimulate the parasympathetic system • An acute coronary syndrome that involves the *right* coronary artery
Recommended Therapy **Key:** Treat only when patient has significant signs or symptoms that are due to the bradycardia	**Intervention sequence for symptomatic bradycardia:** • *Atropine* 0.5 mg IV if vagal mechanism • *Transcutaneous pacing* if available **If signs and symptoms are severe, consider catecholamine infusions:** • *Dopamine* 2 to 10 µg/kg per min • *Epinephrine* 2 to 10 µg/min

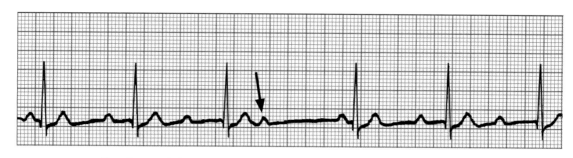

Type I second-degree AV block. Note progressive lengthening of PR interval

until one P wave (arrow) is not followed by a QRS.

Pathophysiology

- In the type II form of second-degree AV block the conduction pathology occurs *below* the level of the AV node (infranodal) at either the bundle of His (uncommon) or the bundle branches (more common).
- Conduction of impulses through the AV node is normal with type II second-degree AV block. For this reason no conduction delays occur (ie, no first-degree block), and the PR interval does not lengthen before the nonconducted impulse (ie, no type I second-degree AV block).
- The bundle of His and Purkinje fibers are fast-response cells that tend to be depolarized as an "all or none" phenomenon. This explains why there is no progressive lengthening of the PR interval but instead either a conduction or nonconduction of the impulse from the atria to the ventricles.
- Type II second-degree AV block is associated with a poorer prognosis. Often it progresses to complete heart block.

Defining ECG Criteria (Figure 6)

- The hallmark of type II second-degree AV block is that the PR interval remains constant before an atrial impulse is blocked (not conducted to the ventricles), resulting in "a P wave not followed by a QRS complex." Unlike type I block, in type II block the PR interval does not lengthen before a nonconducted impulse ("dropped beat" [QRS complex] or "blocked impulse").
- **Atrial rate:** The atrial rate is usually between 60 and 100 per minute.
- **Ventricular rate:** By definition the ventricular rate is slower than the atrial rate because some impulses are blocked between the atria and the ventricles so that ventricular depolarization does not follow some P waves.
- **Rhythm:** The atrial rhythm is regular; the nonconducted impulses render the ventricular rhythm irregular.
- **PR interval:** The PR interval may be normal or prolonged, but it will remain constant. There is no progressive prolongation of the PR interval as is observed with type I second-degree block.
- **P waves:** The P waves are typical in size and shape; by definition the P-wave impulses that are blocked will not be followed by a QRS complex.
- **QRS complex:** The QRS complexes can be either narrow (<0.12 second) or wide (≥0.12 second).
  - If the block is high (near the AV node), the QRS complex is narrow (<0.12 second) and the ventricular rate is faster.
    - When the block occurs at the His bundle, the QRS complex is narrow because normal conduction occurs through the ventricles (unless concurrent bundle branch block is present).
  - If the block is low (in relation to the AV node), the QRS complex is wide (≥0.12 second) and the ventricular rate is slower.
    - When the block is below the His bundle, the QRS complex is wide because of less effective conduction through the ventricles.
  - The rhythm may be irregular when block is intermittent or when the conduction ratio is variable. With a constant conduction ratio (eg, 2:1), the ventricular rhythm is regular.

Clinical Manifestations

In type II second-degree AV block the following symptoms can result from the bradycardia:

- **Symptoms:** Chest discomfort, shortness of breath, and decreased level of consciousness
- **Signs:** Hypotension, shock, pulmonary congestion, congestive heart failure, angina, or acute ST deviation

Common Etiologies

- Type II second-degree AV block is usually associated with a pathologic lesion in the conduction pathway.
- Unlike type I second-degree AV block, type II second-degree AV block is rarely the result of increased parasympathetic tone or a drug effect.
- New-onset type II second-degree block is most frequently caused by an ACS that involves the *left* coronary artery. More specifically type II block develops with occlusion of one of the septal branches of the left anterior descending coronary artery. This occlusion also produces bundle branch blocks.

Recommended Therapy

Note: New-onset type II second-degree heart block in the clinical context of an ACS is an indication for consideration for insertion of a transvenous pacemaker. The Bradycardia Algorithm provides specific instructions for the management of symptomatic bradycardia associated with type II second-degree AV block or new third-degree AV block:

- Prepare for a transvenous pacer.
- If symptoms develop, use a transcutaneous pacemaker until a transvenous pacer is placed.

The intervention sequence for new-onset type II second-degree AV block with serious signs and symptoms is as follows:

- Consider atropine 0.5 mg (this is seldom effective for infranodal block) while awaiting pacer.
- Use TCP if available as a bridge to transvenous pacing. Verify patient tolerance and electrical capture

Second-Degree Heart Block Type II (Infranodal) (Mobitz II or Non-Wenckebach)	
Pathophysiology	• The pathology, ie, the site of the block, is most often *below* the AV node (infranodal); at the bundle of His (infrequent) or at the bundle branches • Impulse conduction is normal through the node, thus no first-degree block and no prior PR prolongation
Defining Criteria per ECG	• **Atrial Rate:** usually 60-100 beats/min • **Ventricular rate:** by definition (due to the blocked impulses) slower than atrial rate • **Rhythm:** atrial = regular; ventricular = irregular (because of blocked impulses) • **PR:** constant and set; no progressive prolongation as with type I—a distinguishing characteristic. • **P waves:** typical in size and shape; by definition some P waves will not be followed by a QRS complex • **QRS complex:** narrow (<0.12 sec) implies high block relative to the AV node; wide (≥0.12 sec) implies low block relative to the AV node
Clinical Manifestations— Rate-Related	**Due to bradycardia:** • **Symptoms:** chest pain, shortness of breath, decreased level of consciousness • **Signs:** hypotension, shock, pulmonary congestions, CHF, acute MI
Common Etiologies	• An acute coronary syndrome that involves branches of the *left* coronary artery
Recommended Therapy **Pearl:** New onset type II second-degree AV block in clinical context of acute coronary syndrome is indication for transvenous pacemaker insertion	**Intervention sequence for bradycardia due to type II second-degree *or* third-degree AV block:** • Use *transcutaneous pacing* if available as a bridge to transvenous pacing (verify patient tolerance and mechanical capture. Use sedation and analgesia as needed.) • Atropine is seldom effective for infranodal block • Prepare for *transvenous* pacer **If signs/symptoms are severe and unresponsive to TCP, and transvenous pacing is delayed, consider catecholamine infusions:** • *Dopamine* 2 to 10 µg/kg per min • *Epinephrine* 2 to 10 µg/min

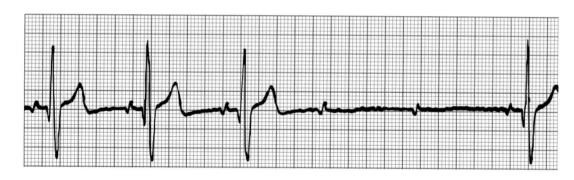

Type II (high block): regular PR-QRS intervals until 2 dropped beats occur; borderline normal QRS complexes indicate high nodal or nodal block

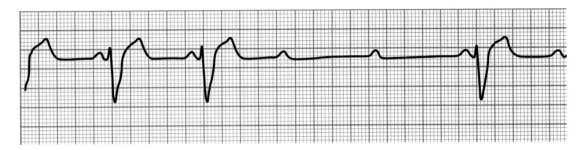

Type II (infranodal block): regular PR-QRS intervals until dropped beats; wide QRS complexes indicate infranodal block

with effective systemic perfusion; use sedation and analgesia as needed and tolerated.

- If severe signs and symptoms are unresponsive to atropine (if used) and TCP and there are delays to placement of a transvenous pacer, then initiate a catecholamine infusion:
  - Epinephrine 2 to 10 μg/min
  - Dopamine 2 to 10 μg/kg per minute
- Immediately consult cardiology and begin preparations for a transvenous pacemaker.

Third-Degree AV Block

Third-degree AV block (Figure 7) results from injury or damage to the cardiac conduction system so that no impulses are conducted from the atria to the ventricles. The atrial rate is typically faster than the ventricular rate when third-degree AV block is present. In third-degree AV block, there is no relationship between the atrial and ventricular complexes—by definition AV dissociation. *AV dissociation* is a broader term that describes rhythms in which there is no link between the atrial and ventricular conduction. There

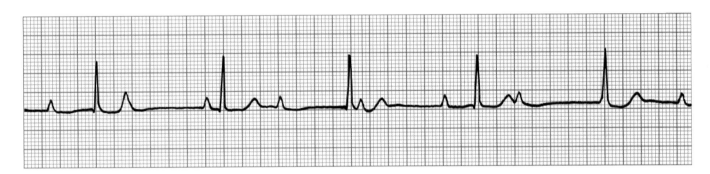

A

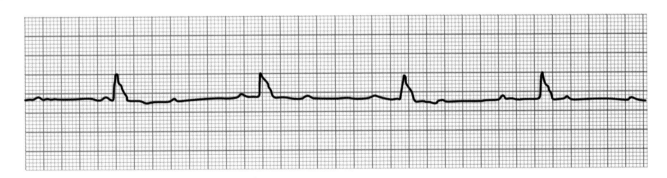

B

Figure 7. A, Third-degree AV block occurring just below the level of the AV node (above bifurcation of the His bundle). Atrial rhythm is slightly irregular owing to the presence of sinus arrhythmia. Ventricular rhythm is regular at a slower rate (44 per minute). There is no constant PR interval. QRS complexes are narrow, indicating that they originate above the bifurcation of the His bundle. **B,** Third-degree AV block occurring at the ventricular level. There is no relation between the atrial and ventricular depolarizations (complexes) indicating AV dissociation. Ventricular rhythm is regular at a very slow rate (38 per minute). The QRS is wide because the block is in the bundle branches and the ventricular escape rhythm originates distal to that level.

is independent contraction of the atria and ventricles. AV dissociation in never a primary rhythm disturbance but always has an underlying cause. Ventricular tachycardia is another form of AV dissociation.

Pathophysiology

- Third-degree AV block (complete heart block) is caused by injury or damage to the cardiac conduction system such that no impulses (*complete*) can pass (*blocked*) between atria and ventricles by either forward (antegrade) or backward (retrograde) conduction. Atrial impulses are not conducted to the ventricles and ventricular and atrial complexes have no relationship.
- This complete block can occur at several different anatomic areas, and each anatomic level of block may be associated with a different pathogenesis, treatment, and prognosis:
  — AV node ("high" or "supra" or "junctional" nodal block)
    ▪ At this anatomic site a junctional escape pacemaker frequently will initiate ventricular depolarization. This is usually a stable subsidiary pacemaker with a rate of 40 to 60 per minute.
    ▪ Because this anatomic site is located above the bifurcation of the bundle of His, the sequence of ventricular depolarization usually is normal, resulting in a normal QRS complex (<0.12 second). (Figure 7A).
    ▪ This type of third-degree AV block can result from increased parasympathetic tone associated with inferior infarction, from toxic drug effects (eg, digitalis, propranolol), or from damage to the AV node.
    ▪ Third-degree AV block with a junctional escape rhythm may be transient and associated with a favorable prognosis.
  — Bundle of His block (rare)
  — Bundle branch block ("low" or "infra" nodal block)
    ▪ Third-degree block at the bundle branches indicates the presence of extensive infranodal conduction system disease.
    ▪ When this type of third-degree block is new in onset, it is usually associated with extensive anterior MI.
    ▪ The only escape mechanism available is in the ventricle distal to the site of block. Such a ventricular escape pacemaker has an intrinsic rate that is slow (<40 per minute). Like any depolarization originating in a ventricle, the QRS complex will be wide (≥0.12 second) (Figure 7B). It is not a stable pacemaker, and episodes of ventricular asystole are common.

Defining ECG Criteria (Figure 7)

The key defining criterion for third-degree block is that the atria and ventricles depolarize independently with no relationship to one another: there is *dissociation*.

- **Atrial rate:** The atrial rate is usually 60 to 100 per minute. The atrial impulses are completely independent of (*dissociated* from) the ventricular impulses.
- **Ventricular rate:** The ventricular rate is determined by the rate of the ventricular escape pacemaker.
  – With complete heart block the ventricular escape rate is slower than the atrial rate; the ventricular rate is typically 20 to 40 per minute.
  – With AV dissociation the ventricular escape rate is faster than the atrial rate; the ventricular rate is typically 40 to 55 per minute.
- **Rhythm:** Both the atrial rhythm and the ventricular rhythm are regular, but each is independent of (*dissociated* from) the other.
- **PR interval:** By definition there is no relationship between the P wave and QRS complex.
- **P waves:** The P waves are normal in size and shape.
- **QRS complex:** A narrow (<0.12 second) QRS complex implies a high block (near the AV node, within the His bundle, above the level of the bifurcation of the His bundle into the right and left bundle branches) without bundle branch block; a wide (≥0.12 second) QRS complex implies low block within the bundle branches.

Clinical Manifestations

- **Symptoms:** Chest pain, shortness of breath, decreased level of consciousness, and syncope
- **Signs:** Hypotension, shock, pulmonary congestion, signs of congestive heart failure, angina, or AMI

Common Etiologies

- Third-degree AV block is most often due to an ACS that involves the *left* coronary artery. In particular the involvement is with the left anterior descending artery, the branches to the interventricular septum, and the corresponding bundle branches.
- Third-degree AV block can occur just below the AV node, with a resultant junctional escape rhythm. This type of AV block can result from increased parasympathetic tone associated with inferior infarction or toxic drug effects (eg, digitalis, propranolol) or from injury to the AV node and surrounding tissue.

Recommended Therapy

Note: New-onset third-degree AV block in the clinical context of an ACS is an indication for insertion of a transvenous pacemaker. The Bradycardia Algorithm indicates the following treatment for symptomatic type II second-degree AV block or symptomatic third-degree AV block:

- Prepare for a transvenous pacer.
- If symptoms develop, use a transcutaneous pacemaker until a transvenous pacer is placed.

The intervention sequence for new-onset third-degree AV block with serious signs and symptoms is as follows (some may be initiated concurrently):

- Begin TCP immediately when available if the patient is unstable due to AV block. Use sedation and analgesia as needed.
- If TCP is not immediately available, consider atropine 0.5 mg; use atropine only if the QRS complex is narrow; atropine is not effective in infranodal (wide QRS) block.
- If severe signs and symptoms are unresponsive to atropine (if used) and TCP and there are delays to placement of a transvenous pacer, then initiate a catecholamine infusion:
  - Epinephrine 2 to 10 µg/min
  - Dopamine 2 to 10 µg/kg per minute
- Consult cardiology and begin preparations for a transvenous pacer. Use TCP if available as a bridge to transvenous pacing. Verify patient tolerance and mechanical capture.

Note: If the patient has third-degree AV block and a ventricular escape rhythm, the ventricular escape rhythm is the only source of ventricular depolarization. ***Do not administer lidocaine or amiodarone to these patients.*** Lidocaine may suppress the ventricular escape rhythm and cause cardiac standstill.

Other Terminology

The classification of AV blocks is simplified to allow providers to initiate emergency therapy for a large number of patients in circumstances where detailed consideration and differential rhythm diagnosis may not be possible. In some instances questions of a more advanced context may arise. Although such questions are beyond the scope of this chapter, a brief summary of the more common terminology is provided here to facilitate understanding.

2:1 AV Block

A 2:1 AV conduction ratio is often mistakenly classified as type II AV block when it can be either type I or type II second-degree AV block. Because 2 consecutive PR intervals are not recorded, an assessment of the PR interval for progressive prolongation or a fixed interval cannot aid in the differential diagnosis. But certain "clues" can be used. For example, if the PR interval of the conducted beat is prolonged and the QRS complex is narrow, the block is more likely type I second-degree AV block. If there is a preexisting bundle branch block or if the QRS complexes are wide, it may not be possible to differentiate between type I and type II second-degree AV block. If the patient has responded to atropine—given for an indicated reason—the block is likely in the AV nodal portion under vagal influence. But the opposite may not be true. If atropine increases sinus node discharge but minimally increases AV conduction, AV block may paradoxically increase. So neither atropine nor response to autonomic drugs and maneuvers (eg, carotid sinus massage) should be used for diagnostic purposes.

Third-Degree AV Block and AV Dissociation

Pathophysiology **Pearl:** *AV dissociation* is the defining class; *third-degree* or *complete AV block* is one type of AV dissociation. By convention (outdated): if ventricular escape depolarization is faster than atrial rate = *"AV dissociation"*; if slower = "third-degree AV block"	Injury or damage to the cardiac conduction system so that no impulses *(complete block)* pass between atria and ventricles (neither antegrade nor retrograde) This complete block can occur at several different anatomic areas: • AV node ("high" or "supra" or "junctional" *nodal block*) • Bundle of His • Bundle branches ("low-nodal" or "infranodal" block)

Defining Criteria per ECG
Key: The third-degree block (see pathophysiology) causes the atria and ventricles to depolarize independently, with no relationship between the two (AV dissociation)
	• **Atrial rate:** usually 60-100 beats/min; impulses completely independent ("dissociated") from ventricular rate
	• **Ventricular rate:** depends on rate of the ventricular escape beats that arise:
	  — Ventricular escape beat rate slower than atrial rate = third-degree AV block (20-40 bpm)
	  — Ventricular escape beat rate faster than atrial rate = AV dissociation (40-55 bpm)
	• **Rhythm:** both atrial rhythm and ventricular rhythm are regular but independent ("dissociated")
	• **PR:** by definition there is no relationship between P wave and R wave
	• **P waves:** typical in size and shape
	• **QRS complex:** narrow (<0.12 sec) implies high block relative to the AV node; wide (≥0.12 sec) implies low block relative to the AV node

Clinical Manifestations— Rate-Related	**Due to bradycardia:** • **Symptoms:** chest pain, shortness of breath, decreased level of consciousness • **Signs:** hypotension, shock, pulmonary congestions, CHF, acute MI
Common Etiologies	• An acute coronary syndrome that involves branches of the *left* coronary artery • In particular, the LAD (left anterior descending) and branches to the interventricular septum (supply bundle branches)
Recommended Therapy **Pearl:** New onset third-degree AV block in clinical context of acute coronary syndrome is indication for transvenous pacemaker insertion **Pearl:** *Never treat third-degree AV block plus ventricular escape beats with lidocaine or amiodarone*	**Intervention sequence for bradycardia due to type II second-degree *or* third-degree AV block:** • Prepare for *transvenous* pacer • Use *transcutaneous pacing* if available as a bridge to transvenous pacing (verify patient tolerance and mechanical capture; use sedation and analgesia as needed) **If signs/symptoms are severe and unresponsive to TCP, and transvenous pacing is delayed, consider catecholamine infusions:** • *Dopamine* 2 to 10 µg/kg per min • *Epinephrine* 2 to 10 µg/min

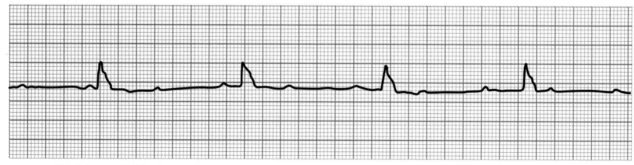

Third-degree AV block: regular P waves at 50 to 55 bpm; regular ventricular "escape beats" at 35 to 40 bpm; no relationship between P waves and escape beats

AV Dissociation

AV dissociation denotes independent contractions of the atria and ventricles. AV dissociation is not a primary rhythm disorder per se, but the result of an underlying rhythm abnormality. Treatment is directed by the presence or absence of symptoms and the nature of the underlying rhythm disorder.

- Normal sinus rhythm may slow (or a bradycardia may be present), and a subsidiary pacemaker can emerge. For example, a junctional escape rhythm may emerge in patients with significant sinus bradycardia or sinus node dysfunction. In MI and sinus bradycardia an idioventricular rhythm can emerge. When the rate of this rhythm is increased but less than 100 per minute, it is sometimes referred to as an accelerated idioventricular rhythm, or AIVR.
- A latent and irritable focus can itself accelerate and "take over" control of the ventricles. This occurs with VT. If the VT is not conducted retrograde into the atria, independent atrial activity may be seen "marching through" the VT. This is one of the "footprints" of VT, denoting independent atrial and ventricular activity.
- When AV block prevents impulses from reaching the ventricles, a subsidiary ventricular pacemaker can take over. If the AV block is complete, patients have complete AV dissociation.

High-Degree and Advanced AV Block

In high-degree AV block the AV conduction ratio is by definition 3:1 or greater and may be variable. This variability can result in an irregularity in both the PR intervals and ventricular rate, making classification difficult. Multiple levels of block may be present, and the electrophysiologic events can be complex. The term *advanced AV block* is often used interchangeably, but it most often refers to high-degree AV block occurring below the AV node and distal in the conduction system. The variability and difficulty in classification can lead to delay in initiating therapy (see below).

Management of Symptomatic High-Degree AV Block of Uncertain Classification (Site of Block)

Recommended Therapy

Fortunately most high-degree AV block is transient and asymptomatic or mildly symptomatic. The occurrence of high-degree AV block is largely prognostic and does not require immediate intervention with either pacing or drug therapy. Definitive therapy for significantly symptomatic high-degree AV block is *immediate transcutaneous pacing*. Transcutaneous pacing is started as soon as possible and is not delayed for drug therapy, including assessment of response to atropine or before sedation for patient comfort. Cardiology consultation is indicated for transvenous pacing pending evaluation for permanent pacing.

The intervention sequence for new-onset high-degree AV block of uncertain origin with serious signs and symptoms is similar to second or third-degree AV block with serious or significant signs and symptoms:

- **Do not delay. If you are uncertain of the diagnosis or type of AV block, follow the Bradycardia Algorithm.**
- Consider atropine 0.5 mg if TCP is not immediately available.

Foundation Facts AV Dissociation and AV Block	Patients with complete AV block have complete AV dissociation, but • *Not all patients with complete AV dissociation have AV block. The terms are not synonymous.*

FAQ Atropine and High-Degree AV Block	Can atropine be used for second-degree and third-degree AV block of uncertain level (AV nodal vs infranodal) while pacing is initiated? • For a hemodynamically stable and symptomatic patient, atropine and preparation for pacing with presedation may be an initial strategy. In critical or very unstable patients, immediate pacing is indicated, and atropine may be given while pacing is initiated. Drug therapy (atropine or chronotropic therapy) should not delay pacing in these patients. Will any type of high-degree AV block respond to atropine? • It may be difficult to identify the site of block in some higher degrees of AV block, eg, AV nodal or infranodal (see below). If AV block occurs in the portion of the AV node under vagal innervation, atropine may be effective.

Use TCP without delay for symptomatic high-degree (second-degree or third-degree) AV block. *Atropine sulfate reverses cholinergic-mediated decreases in heart rate and is a temporizing measure that can be used while preparing a transcutaneous pacemaker for these patients.* Atropine is useful for treating symptomatic sinus bradycardia and may be beneficial for any type of AV block at the nodal level.

- Use TCP when available as a bridge to transvenous pacing. Verify patient tolerance and electrical capture with effective systemic perfusion; use sedation and analgesia as needed and tolerated.
- If severe signs and symptoms are unresponsive to atropine (if used) and TCP and there are delays to placement of a transvenous pacer, then initiate a catecholamine infusion:
  - Epinephrine 2 to 10 µg/min (chronotropic infusion, titrated)
  - Dopamine 2 to 10 µg/kg per minute (chronotropic infusion, titrated)
- Consult Cardiology for a transvenous pacemaker and evaluation.

Critical Concepts: Management of AV Block in ACS

Sinus Bradycardia

Approximately 30% of patients with AMI will develop sinus bradycardia. Patients with inferior wall infarcts secondary to occlusion of the right coronary artery often present with sinus bradycardia caused by ischemia of the sinus and/or AV node. Sinus bradycardia may also occur with reperfusion of the right coronary artery. Atropine-resistant bradycardia and AV block may occur, possibly from accumulation of adenosine in ischemic nodal tissue. Initial treatment with atropine is indicated only when serious signs and symptoms are related to the decreased rate.

Second-Degree or Third-Degree AV Block

Approximately 20% of patients with AMI will develop second-degree or third-degree AV block. Of those who develop AV block, 42% demonstrate the block on admission, and 66% demonstrate the block within the first 24 hours of

presentation. In the majority of cases these abnormalities are the result of myocardial ischemia or infarction with necrosis of the cardiac pacemaker sites or the conduction system. Other factors responsible for the development of AV block include altered autonomic influence, systemic hypoxia, electrolyte disturbances, acid-base disorders, and complications of various medical therapies.

AV block per se is rarely fatal; if death occurs, it is usually caused by an extensive MI with cardiac dysfunction. AV block is not an independent predictor of mortality, and it is a poor predictor of mortality in patients who survive to discharge.

The prognosis for patients with AV block is related most consistently to the size and site of infarction (anterior or inferior). Treatment is influenced by the level of block in the conduction system, the presence and rate of escape rhythms, and the degree of hemodynamic compromise.

Use of Atropine

There are several caveats about the use of atropine for bradyarrhythmias associated with ACS:

- In general atropine treatment of AV block is not required unless serious rate-related signs and symptoms develop.
- In prehospital settings and emergency departments, use of atropine for hemodynamically significant bradyarrhythmias produces the same effects in patients with and without AMI.
- Atropine is inappropriate for bradycardia in patients who have had a heart transplant because denervated hearts will not respond to atropine.
- In general atropine should not be used to treat type II second-degree AV block with wide QRS because it will have no effect on infranodal AV block. Theoretically, an

Be prepared for TCP in the presence of high-degree AV block. Atropine can be considered for high-degree AV block, but the presence of a wide QRS complex indicates that the origin of the block is below the AV node and will not respond to atropine.

- Do not delay pacing for drug therapy (including presedation) in the highly symptomatic or hemodynamically unstable patient. If high-degree AV block fails to respond to pacing, begin an infusion of dopamine or epinephrine.
- Titrate these drugs and use caution: watch for ventricular ectopy, especially in the setting of ischemia.

atropine-induced increase in sinus rate may actually enhance AV block or precipitate third-degree AV block.

- Atropine treatment of third-degree AV block:
  - **Do not use atropine** for treatment of third-degree AV block with a new wide QRS complex presumed to be due to AMI. **Also do not administer lidocaine or amiodarone to these patients.** Lidocaine or amiodarone may suppress a slow ventricular escape rhythm and result in ventricular standstill.

Use of Pacing

Transcutaneous pacing has dramatically changed the approach to pacing for patients with AMI in recent years.[8] This noninvasive technique alleviates the risks of bleeding from venipuncture sites required for transvenous pacing. Bleeding from noncompressible vascular puncture sites may be difficult to control, a particularly important consideration in patients who may be candidates for fibrinolytic therapy. Transcutaneous pacing provides an emergency bridge to transvenous pacing for patients with appropriate indications. In the setting of an ACS, any of the following abnormalities place the patient at risk for complete AV block or another hemodynamically significant deterioration:

- Hemodynamically unstable bradycardia (rate <50 per minute) unresponsive to atropine
- Type II second-degree AV block
- Third-degree AV block
- Newly acquired left, right, or alternating bundle branch block (BBB) or bifascicular block
- Left anterior fascicular block
- Newly acquired or age-indeterminate left BBB
- Right or left BBB plus first-degree AV block

When these abnormalities occur, consider standby placement of a transcutaneous pacing device. For more details see "Emergency Cardiac Pacing," below.

Emergency Cardiac Pacing

Since the first successful cardiac pacing during the 19th century, a variety of devices for pacing the heart have been developed. All cardiac pacemakers deliver an electrical stimulus through electrodes to the heart, causing myocardial depolarization and subsequent cardiac contraction. A transcutaneous pacing system delivers pacing impulses to the heart through the skin using cutaneous electrodes. Transvenous pacemakers use electrodes that have been passed through large central veins to the right chambers of the heart.

Every pacing system requires a pulse generator. The pulse generator can be located outside the patient's body (external pacemakers) or surgically implanted inside the body (internal or permanent pacemakers).

Table 2 summarizes the types of pacemakers now available. The introduction of new TCP systems during the 1980s led to more widespread use of pacing in emergency cardiac care, and these systems are summarized here.[16] ACLS providers require knowledge about implantable pacemakers because these devices may produce a pacing artifact that can be confused with arrhythmias.

Indications for Emergency and "Standby" Pacing

Emergency Pacing

Transcutaneous pacing is an indicated intervention for symptomatic bradycardias. It should be started immediately for patients who are unstable, particularly those with high-degree (Mobitz type II second-degree or third-degree) block. Transcutaneous pacing can be painful, and some limitations apply. Pacing spikes may be present, but electrical stimulation may fail to produce effective mechanical capture. After starting pacing, carefully assess the patient for clinical response. Because heart rate is a major determinant of myocardial oxygen consumption, set the pacing rate to the lowest effective rate based on clinical assessment and symptom resolution. If cardiovascular symptoms are not caused by the bradycardia, the patient may not improve despite effective pacing.

Standby Pacing

The indications for *standby pacing* are multiple and most often occur in the setting of an ACS. These patients typically are clinically stable yet at risk for decompensation in the near future. Often it is the location and size of MI that is ominous in these patients. The development of the rhythm disorder is a secondary event, and pacing has not altered outcome in the past. Priority is given to reperfusion of patients with STEMI, and treatment of symptomatic AV block is supportive in the vast majority of patients.

FYI **AV Block in AMI**	Management of transient and persistent conduction abnormalities in AMI is complicated and requires expert consultation. For more on this topic see the American College of Cardiology/American Heart Association Guidelines for the Management of ST-Elevation Myocardial Infarction,[15] available at http://www.acc.org/qualityandscience/clinical/guidelines/stemi/Guideline1/index.htm.

Table 2. Types of Cardiac Pacers

Type of Pacemaker	Electrode Location	Pulse Generator Location	Synonyms
Transcutaneous	Skin (anterior chest wall and back)	External	External Noninvasive
Transvenous	Venous (catheter with tip in right ventricle, right atrium, or both)	External	Temporary transvenous Permanent transvenous
Transthoracic	Through anterior chest wall into heart	External	Transmyocardial (no longer used)
Transesophageal	Esophagus	External	Esophageal
Epicardial	Epicardium (electrodes placed on heart surface during surgery)	External or internal External generator may be used postoperatively with temporary wires. Permanent wires may also be placed at the time of surgery with later implantation of permanent generator (if needed)	Temporary or permanent epicardial
"Permanent"	Venous or epicardial	Internal	Implanted Internal

But TCP is widely available and inexpensive. When ACLS providers are concerned about the possibility of the development of high-degree symptomatic AV block, preparations for TCP should be initiated. Standby TCP has also been used successfully during surgery for high-risk patients who have bifascicular or left bundle branch block with additional first-degree block.[17,18] A transcutaneous pacemaker can be placed in standby mode for these and other at-risk patients. If then needed to treat hemodynamically significant bradycardia, the device provides a therapeutic bridge until a transvenous pacemaker can be placed under more controlled circumstances.

Pacing for Pulseless Bradyasystolic Cardiac Arrest

Pacing has been studied extensively in the treatment of pulseless patients with bradycardia or asystole. Some studies had shown encouraging results in such patients when pacing was initiated within 10 minutes of cardiac arrest, but recent studies have documented no improvement in either short-term outcomes (admission to hospital) or long-term outcomes (survival to hospital discharge).[19-21]

Prehospital studies of TCP for asystolic arrest or postshock asystole have also shown no benefit of pacing.[22] In a level 1, prospective, controlled trial of TCP for cardiac arrest, investigators observed no benefit even when CPR was combined with pacing, nor did they observe any benefit when the asystole was of only brief duration after a defibrillatory shock.[21]

Pacing for Drug-Induced Cardiac Arrest

An exception to the negative results of pacing for cardiac arrest is patients in overdose-induced cardiac arrest. Pacing may be successful for the treatment of profound bradycardia or pulseless electrical activity.[23-27] Emergency pacing may also benefit patients with pulseless electrical activity due to acidosis or electrolyte abnormalities. Such patients often possess a normal myocardium with only temporary impairment of the conduction system.

Foundation Facts **Pacemaker Pacing and "Standby" Rate**	Because heart rate is a major determinant of myocardial oxygen consumption, set the pacing rate to the lowest effective rate based on clinical assessment and symptom resolution. • Increasing the pacing rate may have a variable effect on cardiac output because factors beyond heart rate (eg, stroke volume, left ventricular function, clinical condition) may be operative.

While attempts are made to correct electrolyte abnormalities or profound acidosis, pacing can stimulate effective myocardial contractions. Similarly pacing can be life sustaining as the conduction system recovers from the cardiotoxic effects of a drug overdose or poisoning with other substances.[26]

Contraindications to Cardiac Pacing

Severe hypothermia is one of the few relative contraindications to cardiac pacing in patients with bradycardia. Bradycardia may be physiologic in these patients; the bradycardia is an appropriate response to a decreased metabolic rate associated with hypothermia. More important, the hypothermic ventricle is more prone to fibrillation with any sort of irritation, such as that of ventricular pacing. If the hypothermic ventricle begins to fibrillate, it is more resistant to defibrillation.

Transcutaneous pacing is not effective in the treatment of bradycardia caused by hypoxia or ischemia. Transcutaneous pacing has not been effective in improving the survival rate of children with out-of-hospital unwitnessed cardiac arrest. But emergency TCP may be lifesaving in selected cases of bradycardia caused by congenital heart defects, complete heart block, abnormal sinus node function, complications following cardiovascular surgery, drug overdose, or a failing implanted pacemaker.[28]

Principles and Technique of Transcutaneous Pacing

In TCP the heart is stimulated with externally applied cutaneous electrodes that deliver an electrical impulse. This impulse is conducted through the intact chest wall to activate the myocardium.[29-31] This technique has been referred to as *external pacing, noninvasive pacing, external transthoracic pacing,* and *trans-chest pacing. Transcutaneous pacing* is the preferred term because it best conveys the concept of pacing the heart through electrodes attached to the skin surface.

Transcutaneous pacing should not be termed "noninvasive" because electrical current is introduced into the body and has the potential to cause cardiac and tissue damage.[32-34] The term *external* also is used in pacemaker terminology to refer to pacing with any pulse generator that is not implanted in the body. So *external pacing* may refer to transvenous, transthoracic, transesophageal, or transcutaneous pacing.

Transcutaneous pacing is the initial pacing method of choice in emergency cardiac care because it can be instituted rapidly and because it is the least invasive pacing technique available. Because no vascular puncture is required for electrode placement, this technique is preferred in patients who have received or who may require fibrinolytic therapy.

Most manufacturers now produce defibrillators with a built-in transcutaneous pacemaker, offering the rapid availability of pacing. Multifunction electrodes allow hands-off defibrillation, pacing, and ECG monitoring through a single pair of anterior-posterior or sternal-apex adhesive chest wall electrodes.

Limited experience suggests that TCP also may be useful in treating refractory tachyarrhythmias by overdrive pacing.[35-37] But overdrive pacing may also accelerate the tachycardia.

History of Cardiac Pacing

Origins

The modern age of cardiac pacing in humans began in 1952 with the first successful resuscitation using the transcutaneous technique, later reported by Paul Zoll and colleagues.[29] This technique was largely abandoned by the 1960s because it was extremely painful and produced marked muscle contraction and cutaneous burns, especially with prolonged use. In addition, work by Lillehei, Bakken, and Furman led to successful transvenous pacing in the late 1950s and early 1960s.[30,38,39]

Modern Refinements

Refinements in electrode size and pulse characteristics led to the reintroduction of transcutaneous pacing into clinical practice in the 1980s.[31,40] Increasing the pulse duration from 2 to 20 milliseconds or longer was found to decrease the current output required for cardiac capture.[41] Longer impulse durations also make induction of VF less likely than when shorter impulse durations are used. The pacing stimulus is safe. In animal studies[42] the "safety factor" for VF induction (ratio of fibrillation current to pacing current) of transcutaneous pacing is 12 to 15. This means that 12 to 15 times the pacing current would be required to fibrillate the heart. Electrodes with a larger surface area (8 cm in diameter) decrease the current density at the skin, thereby decreasing pain and tissue burns.

Trials of transcutaneous pacemakers using the newer impulse and electrode characteristics have demonstrated the success of these modifications in overcoming the limitations of earlier transcutaneous pacemakers.[43] The mean current required for electrical capture is usually 50 to 100 mA. Although some patients can tolerate pacing at their capture threshold, IV analgesia and sedation should generally be provided when pacing with currents of approximately 50 mA or more.

Equipment for Transcutaneous Pacing

Transcutaneous pacemakers should be available in all emergency departments and in many in-hospital and out-of-hospital care settings. The pacemakers introduced in the early 1980s were largely asynchronous devices with a limited selection of rate and output options. More recent units have demand-mode pacing with more output options. In newer units pacing is often combined with a defibrillator in a single unit.

Most transcutaneous pacemakers have similar basic features:

- **Operation mode:** Both a fixed-rate (nondemand or asynchronous) mode and a demand mode.

- **Rate selection:** A range from 30 to 180 per minute.

- **Current output:** Adjustable from 0 to 200 mA.

- **Pulse duration:** Varies from 20 to 40 ms but is not operator adjustable. (Rectangular pacing-pulse markers of 20 to 40 ms are visible on the recorder.)

- **Monitor blanking:** A feature that prevents the large electrical spike from the pacemaker impulse from obscuring interpretation of the much smaller ECG complex. The majority of commercially available TCP units are integrated monitor/defibrillator/pacing devices that automatically blank the pacing complex. Without this feature large pacing artifacts can mask treatable VF or otherwise make rhythm interpretation difficult.

A preliminary trial of TCP should be undertaken to ensure that capture can be achieved and pacing is tolerated by the patient. If the patient is having difficulty tolerating the discomfort caused by TCP, administer medications such as diazepam (for treatment of anxiety and muscle contractions) and morphine (for analgesia).

Transcutaneous Pacing: Step-by-Step Technique (Figure 8)

- Attach the 2 pacing electrodes to the patient's chest.
  - Place the anterior electrode to the left of the sternum, centered as close as possible to the point of maximal cardiac impulse.
  - Place the posterior electrode on the back, between the shoulder blades, to the left of the thoracic spinal column.
  - Shaving may be required to ensure good contact on patients with excessive body hair; alternative pacing electrode positions may be needed.
- Set the *pacing rate* (usually 60 to 80 per minute—see discussion above).
- Set the *pacing current.* Start with the minimal setting and slowly increase the output until the *pacing spike* of the pacemaker appears on the monitor screen

(Figure 8B). Continue increasing the output until *pacing capture* is achieved (see next bullet).

- Monitor the ECG to assess *electrical* pacing capture. Pacing capture is present when each pacer spike is followed by a ventricular depolarization with a visible QRS complex and repolarization with a T wave (Figure 8C).
- Each pacer spike that "captures" the ventricle will produce a wide QRS complex, a consistent ST segment, and a broad, slurred T wave that is opposite in polarity (direction) from the QRS complex (Figure 8C).
- Do not mistake the wide, slurred afterpotential following an external pacing spike for evidence of ventricular depolarization associated with electrical capture.
- Assess ventricular *function* and *cardiac output* (so-called *hemodynamic* or *mechanical capture)* during pacing by the patient's pulse and blood pressure. Attempt to palpate the patient's pulse at the right carotid or right femoral artery to avoid confusing a pulse with the muscle contractions caused by the pacer.
- Continue pacing at a pacemaker output level slightly higher (10%) than the threshold of initial electrical capture (the threshold is the minimal pacemaker output associated with consistent pacing capture).

Transcutaneous Pacing: Complications and Corrections

Following are the major complications or problems encountered during TCP and corrective measures to address them.

- **Failure to recognize the presence of underlying treatable VF.** Critically ill patients in need of emergency pacing are at risk for the development of sudden unstable VT or VF. The presence of VF/pulseless VT can be obscured by a large pacing artifact on an ECG monitor. The development of VF/pulseless VT is more likely to be obscured if the monitor lacks the feature of pacing stimulus dampening or blanking. In some clinical situations a patient may be attached to a bedside or transport monitor when pacing is needed. If pacing is initiated without switching to a dampened monitor, the rhythm may be uninterpretable and the development of VF may be undetected.
  - **Correction.** Perform TCP with an integrated monitor constructed to display an interpretable rhythm during pacing stimuli.
- **Failure to capture.** Failure to achieve effective cardiac contractions with pacing is most often caused by misplacement of pacing pads relative to patient size and shape or from inadequate pacemaker output. In

adults capture thresholds do not appear to be related to body weight or surface area. Current is poorly conducted through barrel-shaped chests (eg, severe emphysema) or through large amounts of intrathoracic air (eg, bullous emphysema, pneumothorax). The hearts of some patients may be refractory to pacing. A large pericardial effusion, tamponade, and recent thoracic surgery also will increase the output required for capture.

- **Correction.** Often patients are semiconscious or so symptomatic that moving them to gain access to the back for pad placement is difficult. Although it is acceptable to use the same sternal-to-apex pacing route used for defibrillation, pad-to-pad impedance is lower and current flow is higher with the anterior-posterior placement described above. Make sure an anterior-posterior pacing route is used. The left scapula and the thoracic column may also reduce current flow between the pacing pads. The optimal pad position often has to be located by trial and error.

- **Failure to recognize failure to capture.** This complication is primarily due to the size of the pacing artifact on the ECG screen, a technical problem inherent in systems without dampening circuitry. The rhythmic skeletal muscle contractions that occur during external pacing also can make it difficult to determine if capture occurs.

  - **Correction.** Bedside ultrasound has been used to assess the effectiveness of TCP capture. Newer devices that integrate monitoring, defibrillation, and pacing in a single instrument eliminate this problem by their intrinsic dampening circuitry.

- **Failure to recognize "electrical" capture without effective myocardial function.** The ultimate objective of TCP is to produce hemodynamically effective cardiac contractions through effective depolarization of the ventricles. This requires effective excitation-mechanical coupling (see "FYI: Electrical Capture and Effective Myocardial Function: Excitation-Contraction Coupling"). Electrical capture with ventricular depolarization (wide QRS complexes with broad T waves of opposite polarity) may occur without effective cardiac output, an example of true "electromechanical dissociation." This complication often occurs during the first minute or two of TCP.

  - **Correction.** Increasing the pacing output beyond that required for electrical capture may result in hemodynamically effective mechanical capture. Provide chest compressions whenever pacing with electrical capture fails to sustain a palpable pulse. Several minutes of simultaneous pacing and chest compressions have been reported to reestablish "electromechanical association" in some patients.

- **Pacing-induced arrhythmias or VF.** Pacing-induced arrhythmias are more of a theoretical than a documented complication of pacing. Most observers consider VF associated with pacing to be coincidental and not cause-and-effect in critically ill patients. The current output required for TCP is several factors lower than the current output required to induce fibrillation.

- **Pain and discomfort.** Some conscious patients, paced for symptomatic bradycardias, will experience discomfort from the muscle contractions stimulated by pacing. Others find the pacing stimulus itself painful and intolerable. Pain from electrical skin and muscle stimulation was a significant complication of early devices.[37] The units now used for conscious patients are well tolerated, with most patients rating the discomfort as "mild or moderate" and "easily tolerable." In other studies up to 1 of 3 patients rates the pain as severe or intolerable.

  - **Correction.** If not contraindicated, analgesia with incremental doses of a narcotic, sedation with a benzodiazepine, or both can reduce the pain of TCP to an acceptable level. Some clinicians use procedural sedation protocols for patients needing emergency TCP. Often all that is needed is a brief period of TCP while preparing for transvenous pacemaker insertion.

  - **Prevention.** When standby TCP is indicated, clinicians should always provide a brief period of "trial pacing" to document that capture is possible, to familiarize the patient with the sensations of pacing, and to determine if parenteral analgesia and sedation will be necessary if pacing is required. Set the pacer at a rate slightly faster than the patient's intrinsic rate to achieve capture and then return the device to standby mode.

Figure 8. Transcutaneous pacing (TCP). **A**, Bradycardia (third-degree heart block), no pacing. (*Note:* Rates and intervals are slightly altered because of monitor compensation for pacing stimulus.) QRS rate = 41 per minute; observed P waves = 187 per minute; QRS is very wide (0.24 second); ventricular escape beats are present; polarity of QRS and T wave is positive. Patient had shortness of breath (SOB) at rest, severe SOB with walking, and near syncope. **B**, TCP initiated at low current (35 mA) and slow rate (50 per minute). The current is below the threshold needed to capture the myocardium. With TCP, monitor electrodes are attached in a modified lead II position. As current (in mA) is gradually increased, the monitor leads detect the pacing stimuli as squared-off, negative markers. Transcutaneous pacemakers incorporate standard ECG monitoring circuitry, but they also have filters to dampen the pacing stimuli. A monitor without these filters records "border-to-border" tracings (off the edge of the screen or paper at the top and bottom borders) that cannot be interpreted. **C**, Pacing current is turned up above threshold (60 mA at 71 per minute), "capturing" the myocardium. TCP stimulation does not work through the normal cardiac conduction system but by direct electrical stimulation of the myocardium. For this reason a successful capture, where TCP stimulation results in a myocardial contraction, resembles a premature ventricular contraction with a wide QRS complex with the initial deflection and the terminal deflection *always* in opposite directions. So-called "mechanical capture" implies effective myocardial contractions with production of blood flow (usually assessed by a palpable carotid pulse), and cannot be determined by the rhythm display. These terms are discussed further in the text.

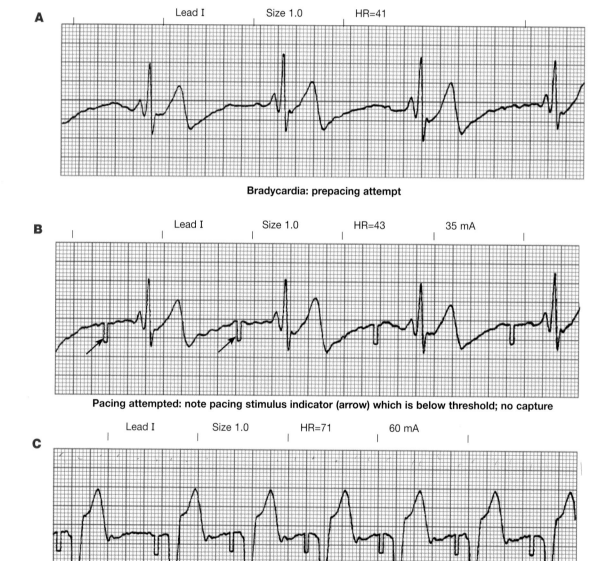

A   Lead I   Size 1.0   HR=41

Bradycardia: prepacing attempt

B   Lead I   Size 1.0   HR=43   35 mA

Pacing attempted: note pacing stimulus indicator (arrow) which is below threshold; no capture

C   Lead I   Size 1.0   HR=71   60 mA

Pacing above threshold (60 mA): with capture (QRS complex broad and ventricular; T wave opposite QRS)

Transcutaneous Pacing
A. Bradycardia: no pacing
B. Pacing stimulus below threshold: no capture
C. Pacing stimulus above threshold: capture occurs

Rhythm Strip (Figure 8)	Comments
A. Bradycardia (third-degree AV block): no pacing (**Note:** Rates and intervals slightly altered due to monitor compensation for pacing stimulus)	• QRS rate = 41 beats/min • P waves = 187 beats/min • QRS = very wide, 0.24 sec; ventricular escape beats • QRS and T wave polarity = both positive • Patient: SOB at rest; severe SOB with walking; near syncope
B. Transcutaneous pacing initiated at low current (35 mA) and slow rate (50 beats/min). Below the threshold current needed to stimulate the myocardium	• With TCP, monitor electrodes are attached in modified lead II position • As current (in milliamperes) is gradually increased, the monitor leads detect the pacing stimuli as a squared off, negative marker • TC pacemakers incorporate standard ECG monitoring circuitry but incorporate filters to dampen the pacing stimuli • A monitor without these filters records "border-to-border" tracings (off the edge of the screen or paper at the top and bottom borders) that cannot be interpreted
C. Pacing current turned up above threshold (60 mA at 71 beats/min) and "captures" the myocardium	• TCP stimulus does not work through the normal cardiac conduction system but by a direct electrical stimulus of the myocardium • Therefore, a "capture," where TCP stimulus results in a myocardial contraction, will resemble a PVC • Electrical capture is characterized by a wide QRS complex, with the initial deflection and the terminal deflection *always* in opposite directions • A "mechanically captured beat" will produce effective myocardial contraction with production of some blood flow (usually assessed by a palpable carotid pulse)

| *FYI*

Pacing risk to healthcare providers? | There is no risk of electric injury (shock delivery) to healthcare providers during TCP. Power delivered during each impulse is less than 1/1000 of that delivered during defibrillation. Chest compressions can be administered directly over the insulated electrodes during pacing. Inadvertent contact with the active pacing surface during chest compressions results in only a mild tingling sensation if anything. Some pacers shut off when an electrode falls off the chest, but only some brands have this feature. |

Electrical Capture and Effective Myocardial Function: Excitation-Contraction Coupling

Myocardial depolarization and myocardial contraction involve a complex series of events that include the myocardial cells, electrolyte movement into and out of cells, calcium effects on actin and myosin filaments, and myocardial fiber shortening. These events are collectively referred to as excitation-contraction coupling. We know that electrical depolarization can occur without effective myocardial contraction—so-called *electromechanical dissociation*. This indicates ineffective excitation-contraction coupling. These patients will have electrical depolarization but ineffective cardiac output.

During pacing a pacer spike should be followed by myocardial depolarization (Figure 9). Implanted pacemakers can be atrial, ventricular, or a combination (Figure 10). Although a wide QRS complex following a pacer spike reflects electrical capture of the heart, the myocardial contraction (fiber shortening) and stroke volume associated with this depolarization may or may not be effective.

Echocardiographic and clinical evaluation may reveal ineffective ventricular contraction (so-called "mechanical capture" of the heart). For this reason the clinician must frequently evaluate both pulse and systemic perfusion during pacing to ensure that electrical capture is associated with effective myocardial function.

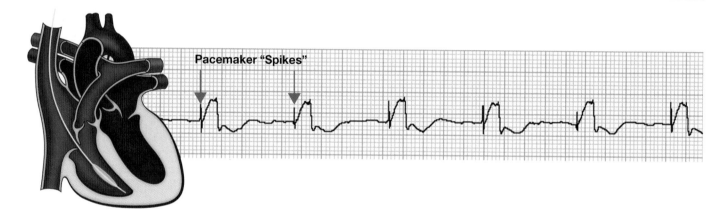

Pacemaker "Spikes"

Figure 9. Transcutaneous and single-chamber (ventricular) pacing. This rhythm strip is remarkable for a wide QRS complex. This can be mistaken for premature ventricular contractions and incorrectly interpreted as VT. But the rate is too slow. The wide QRS complex is preceded by pacemaker artifact ("spikes," blue arrows), indicating that this wide complex is due to pacing with abnormal ventricular activation.

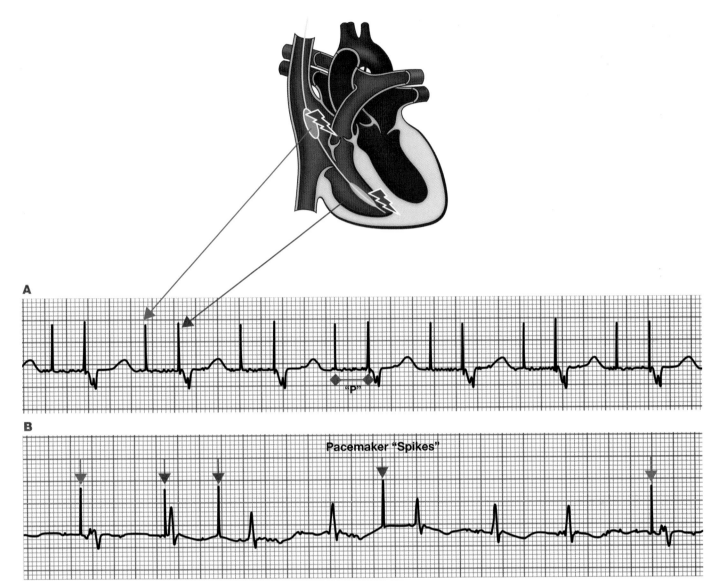

Figure 10. Dual-chamber (atrial and ventricular) pacing. **A,** The blue arrow demonstrates an atrial pacing stimulus with its atrial pacemaker artifact on the rhythm strip. The red arrow demonstrates an atrial pacing electrode and stimulus with ventricular capture. The artificial PR interval ("P") is set to allow physiologic loading of the ventricle by the atria. **B,** Pacemaker artifacts that fail to capture (small red arrows). Note that the first and last beats (small blue arrows) are followed by a captured beat. This is an example of intermittent capture or, alternatively, pacemaker malfunction with periods of failure to capture. Fortunately for this patient, the pacemaker is no longer needed because the patient's own rhythm has returned and only transiently is decreased below the preset pacer rate.

References

1. Smith I, Monk TG, White PF. Comparison of transesophageal atrial pacing with anticholinergic drugs for the treatment of intraoperative bradycardia. *Anesth Analg.* 1994;78:245-252.

2. Brady WJ, Swart G, DeBehnke DJ, Ma OJ, Aufderheide TP. The efficacy of atropine in the treatment of hemodynamically unstable bradycardia and atrioventricular block: prehospital and emergency department considerations. *Resuscitation.* 1999;41:47-55.

3. Chadda KD, Lichstein E, Gupta PK, Kourtesis P. Effects of atropine in patients with bradyarrhythmia complicating myocardial infarction: usefulness of an optimum dose for overdrive. *Am J Med.* 1977;63:503-510.

4. Errando CL, Peiro CM. An additional explanation for atrioventricular block after the administration of atropine. *Can J Anaesth.* 2004;51:88; author reply 88-89.

5. Maruyama K, Mochizuki N, Hara K. High-degree atrioventricular block after the administration of atropine for sinus arrest during anesthesia. *Can J Anaesth.* 2003;50:528-529.

6. Brunner-La Rocca HP, Kiowski W, Bracht C, Weilenmann D, Follath F. Atrioventricular block after administration of atropine in patients following cardiac transplantation. *Transplantation.* 1997;63:1838-1839.

7. Bernheim A, Fatio R, Kiowski W, Weilenmann D, Rickli H, Brunner-La Rocca HP. Atropine often results in complete atrioventricular block or sinus arrest after cardiac transplantation: an unpredictable and dose-independent phenomenon. *Transplantation.* 2004;77:1181-1185.

8. Dauchot P, Gravenstein JS. Effects of atropine on the electrocardiogram in different age groups. *Clin Pharmacol Ther.* 1971;12:274-280.

9. Dauchot P, Gravenstein JS. Bradycardia after myocardial ischemia and its treatment with atropine. *Anesthesiology.* 1976;44:501-518.

10. Ellenbogen KA, Thames MD, DiMarco JP, Sheehan H, Lerman BB. Electrophysiological effects of adenosine in the transplanted human heart: evidence of supersensitivity. *Circulation.* 1990;81:821-828.

11. Love JN, Sachdeva DK, Bessman ES, Curtis LA, Howell JM. A potential role for glucagon in the treatment of drug-induced symptomatic bradycardia. *Chest.* 1998;114:323-326.

12. Mangrum JM, DiMarco JP. The evaluation and management of bradycardia. *N Engl J Med.* 2000;342:703-709.

13. Barold SS, Hayes DL. Second-degree atrioventricular block: a reappraisal. *Mayo Clin Proc.* 2001;76:44-57.

14. Barold SS. Lingering misconceptions about type I second-degree atrioventricular block. *Am J Cardiol.* 2001;88:1018-1020.

15. Antman EM, Anbe DT, Armstrong PW, Bates ER, Green LA, Hand M, Hochman JS, Krumholz HM, Kushner FG, Lamas GA, Mullany CJ, Ornato JP, Pearle DL, Sloan MA, Smith SC Jr, Alpert JS, Anderson JL, Faxon DP, Fuster V, Gibbons RJ, Gregoratos G, Halperin JL, Hiratzka LF, Hunt SA, Jacobs AK. ACC/AHA guidelines for the management of patients with ST-elevation myocardial infarction: a report of the American College of Cardiology/American Heart Association Task Force on Practice Guidelines (Committee to Revise the 1999 Guidelines for the Management of Patients with Acute Myocardial Infarction). *Circulation.* 2004;110:e82-e293.

16. Hedges JR, Syverud SA, Dalsey WC. Developments in transcutaneous and transthoracic pacing during bradyasystolic arrest. *Ann Emerg Med.* 1984;13:822-827.

17. Gauss A, Hubner C, Radermacher P, Georgieff M, Schutz W. Perioperative risk of bradyarrhythmias in patients with asymptomatic chronic bifascicular block or left bundle branch block. *Anesthesiology.* 1998;88:679-687.

18. Gauss A, Hubner C, Meierhenrich R, Rohm HJ, Georgieff M, Schutz W. Perioperative transcutaneous pacemaker in patients with chronic bifascicular block or left bundle branch block and additional first-degree atrioventricular block. *Acta Anaesthesiol Scand.* 1999;43:731-736.

19. Dalsey WC, Syverud SA, Hedges JR. Emergency department use of transcutaneous pacing for cardiac arrests. *Crit Care Med.* 1985;13:399-401.

20. Eitel DR, Guzzardi LJ, Stein SE, Drawbaugh RE, Hess DR, Walton SL. Noninvasive transcutaneous cardiac pacing in prehospital cardiac arrest. *Ann Emerg Med.* 1987;16:531-534.

21. Cummins RO, Graves JR, Larsen MP, Hallstrom AP, Hearne TR, Ciliberti J, Nicola RM, Horan S. Out-of-hospital transcutaneous pacing by emergency medical technicians in patients with asystolic cardiac arrest. *N Engl J Med.* 1993;328:1377-1382.

22. Paris PM, Stewart RD, Kaplan RM, Whipkey R. Transcutaneous pacing for bradyasystolic cardiac arrests in prehospital care. *Ann Emerg Med.* 1985;14:320-323.

23. Proano L, Chiang WK, Wang RY. Calcium channel blocker overdose. *Am J Emerg Med.* 1995;13:444-450.

24. Watson NA, FitzGerald CP. Management of massive verapamil overdose. *Med J Aust.* 1991;155:124-125.

25. Gotz D, Pohle S, Barckow D. Primary and secondary detoxification in severe flecainide intoxication. *Intensive Care Med.* 1991;17:181-184.

26. Cummins R, Graves J, Haulman J, Quan L, Peterson D, Horan S. Near-fatal yew berry intoxication treated with external cardiac pacing and digoxin-specific FAB antibody fragments. *Ann Emerg Med.* 1991;19:38-43.

27. Quan L, Graves JR, Kinder DR, Horan S, Cummins RO. Transcutaneous cardiac pacing in the treatment of out-of-hospital pediatric cardiac arrests. *Ann Emerg Med.* 1992;21:905-909.

28. Beland MJ, Hesslein PS, Finlay CD, Faerron-Angel JE, Williams WG, Rowe RD. Noninvasive transcutaneous cardiac pacing in children. *Pacing Clin Electrophysiol.* 1987;10:1262-1270.

29. Zoll PM. Development of electric control of cardiac rhythm. *JAMA.* 1973;226:881-886.

30. Zoll PM, Belgard AH, Weintraub MJ, Frank HA. External mechanical cardiac stimulation. *N Engl J Med.* 1976;294:1274-1276.

31. Syverud SA, Hedges JR, Dalsey WC, Gabel M, Thomson DP, Engel PJ. Hemodynamics of transcutaneous cardiac pacing. *Am J Emerg Med.* 1986;4:17-20.

32. Pride HB, McKinley DF. Third-degree burns from the use of an external cardiac pacing device. *Crit Care Med.* 1990;18:572-573.

33. Kicklighter EJ, Syverud SA, Dalsey WC, Hedges JR, Van der Bel-Kahn JM. Pathological aspects of transcutaneous cardiac pacing. *Am J Emerg Med.* 1985;3:108-113.

34. Syverud SA, Dalsey WC, Hedges JR, Kicklighter E, Barsan WG, Joyce SM, van der Bel-Kahn JM, Levy RC. Transcutaneous cardiac pacing: determination of myocardial injury in a canine model. *Ann Emerg Med.* 1983;12:745-748.

35. Estes NA III, Deering TF, Manolis AS, Salem D, Zoll PM. External cardiac programmed stimulation for noninvasive termination of sustained supraventricular and ventricular tachycardia. *Am J Cardiol.* 1989;63:177-183.

36. Rosenthal ME, Stamato NJ, Marchlinski FE, Josephson ME. Noninvasive cardiac pacing for termination of sustained, uniform ventricular tachycardia. *Am J Cardiol.* 1986;58:561-562.

37. Sharkey SW, Chaffee V, Kapsner S. Prophylactic external pacing during cardioversion of atrial tachyarrhythmias. *Am J Cardiol.* 1985;55:1632-1634.

38. Schechter DC. *Exploring the Origins of Electrical Cardiac Stimulation.* Minneapolis, Minn: Medtronic Inc; 1983.

39. Sutton R, Bourgeois I. *The Foundations of Cardiac Pacing: An Illustrated Practical Guide to Basic Pacing.* Mount Kisco, NY: Futura Publishing Inc; 1991.

40. Dalsey WC, Syverud SA, Ross DS, Yeiser F, Carducci B. Transcutaneous cardiac pacing. *Ann Emerg Med.* 1984;13:410-411.

41. Jones M, Geddes LA. Strength-duration curves for cardiac pacemaking and ventricular fibrillation. *Cardiovasc Res Cent Bull.* 1977;15:101-112.

42. Voorhees WD III, Foster KS, Geddes LA, Babbs CF. Safety factor for precordial pacing: minimum current thresholds for pacing and for ventricular fibrillation by vulnerable-period stimulation. *Pacing Clin Electrophysiol.* 1984;7:356-360.

43. Falk RH, Zoll PM, Zoll RH. Safety and efficacy of noninvasive cardiac pacing. A preliminary report. *N Engl J Med.* 1983;309:1166-1168.

Chapter 8

Stable Tachycardias and Premature Contractions

This Chapter

- **When to treat fast heart rates in stable patients**

- **How to use vagotonic maneuvers and adenosine**

- **Do no harm and seek expert consultation when initial therapy fails or a wide-complex tachycardia is present**

- **What to do if patients become unstable**

Key Points

- *Stable* denotes a patient without signs or symptoms of impaired consciousness or hypoperfusion. With a *clinically stable* patient there is sufficient time to allow diagnosis of the rhythm (or transport to a facility where such a diagnosis can be made), a blood pressure sufficient to permit pharmacologic intervention, and no symptoms that mandate immediate electrical cardioversion.

- A stable tachycardia can initially be differentiated into one with a narrow or wide complex. The *width* of the complex (narrow vs wide) generally reflects the origin of the tachycardia (supraventricular vs ventricular). Exceptions to this rule, such as supraventricular tachycardias with aberrant conduction, are discussed where appropriate in this chapter. The width of the QRS complex is ≥0.12 second in wide-complex tachycardias and often ≤0.11 second in narrow-complex tachycardias.[1]

Introduction

This chapter reviews tachycardia with pulses for the ACLS provider. A tachyarrhythmia is a rhythm disorder with a heart rate faster than 100 per minute. These rhythms can be narrow-complex or wide-complex tachycardias. The ACLS provider requires the basic knowledge to initially differentiate narrow-complex from wide-complex tachycardias and symptomatic from asymptomatic arrhythmias. Initial therapy for narrow-complex tachycardias involves vagal maneuvers and use of adenosine, covered in the Advanced Cardiovascular Life Support (ACLS) Provider Course. If a patient with a wide-complex tachycardia is unstable, management follows the unstable tachycardia section of the Tachycardia With Pulses Algorithm (Figure 1). Management of wide-complex tachycardias is covered in the algorithm, but expert consultation is advised for these advanced arrhythmias. Part 2 of this text reviews the differential diagnosis of wide-complex tachycardias of uncertain etiology, concepts of aberrancy, and drug therapy.

Definition

For purposes of the ACLS Experienced Provider Course and instructor teaching, the term *tachycardia* is used for tachyarrhythmia. In this context a tachycardia can be sinus tachycardia or other supraventricular tachycardia, such as atrial fibrillation or flutter with a ventricular response rate faster than 100 per minute. The Tachycardia With Pulses Algorithm (Figure 1), like the Bradycardia Algorithm, can be implemented without the delay to initially identify the underlying rhythm disorder. The same initial considerations apply:

1. Identification of a tachycardia
2. Determination that signs or symptoms are due to the tachycardia

The next consideration involves identification and differential diagnosis of the rhythm disorder and "tailoring" and "titration" of therapy to the arrhythmia and patient.

ACLS instructors will note that the Tachycardia With Pulses Algorithm in this chapter emphasizes when expert consultation is advised. The tachycardia algorithms presented in the *ECC Guidelines 2000* were comprehensive and included both advanced and basic arrhythmias. Understanding the concepts for management of advanced arrhythmias requires expert knowledge about proarrhythmias and cardiac performance such as ejection fraction and left ventricular function. For this reason the current ACLS Provider Course deals with basic arrhythmias only.

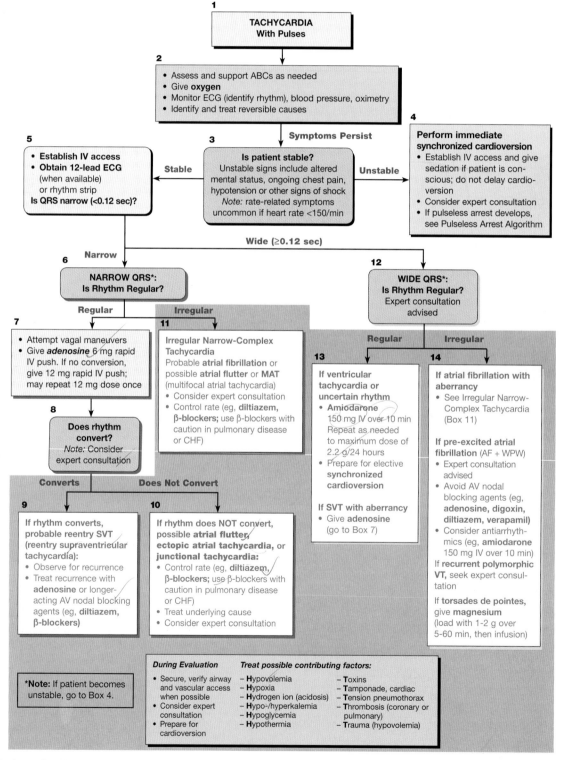

Figure 1. Tachycardia With Pulses Algorithm.

Tachycardia and *Symptoms*

Providers managing patients with a tachycardia must first evaluate whether the fast heart rate is symptomatic and hemodynamically significant. Does the tachycardia produce serious signs and symptoms that are the direct result of the heart's fast contractions or something else? Clinicians are required to emergently treat a tachycardia only when the rhythm disorder itself causes serious signs and symptoms.

Clinical *symptoms* that may be caused by tachycardia are similar to those caused by bradycardia and include angina or angina with exertion; shortness of breath or dyspnea on exertion; weakness; fatigue; exercise intolerance; lightheadedness, dizziness, syncope; and decreased level of consciousness. Clinical *signs* include the following:

- Hypotension, postural hypotension, or shock
- Pulmonary congestion (on physical exam or chest x-ray), congestive heart failure, or acute pulmonary edema
- Rate-related ischemic ventricular arrhythmias or ischemic ECG changes

Key Points for Interventions

Vagal Stimulation

Vagal maneuvers and adenosine are the preferred initial therapeutic choices for the termination of stable reentry supraventricular tachycardia (SVT). Vagal maneuvers alone (Valsalva maneuver or carotid sinus massage) will terminate about 20% to 25% of reentry SVT[2]; adenosine is required for the remainder.

Valsalva Maneuver

The Valsalva maneuver was named for Antonio Maria Valsalva (1666-1723), an Italian anatomist, surgeon, and pathologist who first described the procedure. The maneuver involves instructing a patient to exhale forcefully against a closed glottis so no air can escape.

Anatomy and Physiology

- The Valsalva maneuver produces an abrupt increase in intra-abdominal and intrathoracic pressure. The most common way to perform the Valsalva maneuver is to have the patient strain against a closed glottis during a held breath.
- The response to the Valsalva maneuver is complex:
  - First, the maneuver increases arterial pressure.

  - Second, the arterial pressure stimulates local arterial baroceptors.
  - Baroceptor signals travel to the brain, connecting with the parasympathetic and vagal nerve centers.
  - This response enhances vagal nerve output.
  - Vagal activation causes a reduction in heart rate in patients in sinus rhythm.
  - The heightened vagal tone may terminate reentrant rhythms or cause a brief atrioventricular (AV) block in automatic rhythms, allowing better diagnosis.
- Variable success rates (from 6% to 18%) have been reported in out-of-hospital settings and emergency departments.[2-4]
- Higher success rates have been achieved in electrophysiology laboratories for termination of induced paroxysmal supraventricular tachycardia (PSVT).[5]
- Additional factors may decrease the conversion success rate of vagal maneuvers in spontaneous PSVT.
  - The maneuver requires patient understanding and cooperation.
  - The response can be blunted in patients with common pathologic conditions (eg, congestive heart failure) and in patients taking chronotropic cardiovascular drugs.
- The Valsalva maneuver can be used in conjunction with carotid sinus massage (see next section). These 2 vagal stimulation techniques are equally effective in terminating spontaneous SVT; one method may succeed after the alternative intervention fails.

Technique of Valsalva Maneuver

- Position the patient in the erect or semierect position. As a precaution, consider placement of an intravenous (IV) catheter or have transcutaneous pacing readily available in case the maneuver provokes a symptomatic bradycardia requiring intervention.
  - Explain the procedure to the patient.
  - Instruct the patient to cough on command. The "vagolytic" effect of coughing can be helpful in terminating protracted bradyarrhythmias provoked by the Valsalva maneuver or carotid sinus massage.
  - Record baseline blood pressure and pulse, and obtain a rhythm strip.
  - Ask the patient to take a deep breath, hold it, and then bear down and strain. Alternatively the clinician can push firmly with 1 hand in the center of the patient's abdomen (short of causing discomfort) and

FYI

Guidelines 2005

Vagal maneuvers and adenosine are the preferred initial therapeutic choices for termination of stable reentry SVT.

then ask the patient to try to "push" the hand away with abdominal pressure.

— The patient should hold the breath and strain for 15 to 30 seconds. If equipment is available, the patient can breathe into a small tube or syringe connected to a mercury manometer or spirometer. Have the patient maintain a pressure of 30 mm Hg for 15 to 30 seconds.

— Record blood pressure and heart rate after 1 minute. Obtain a rhythm strip after performing the maneuver. Obtain a 12-lead ECG if the rhythm converts.

— Perform carotid sinus massage if the Valsalva maneuver fails.

Carotid Sinus Massage

Anatomy and Physiology

- The carotid sinus is a localized dilation in the common carotid artery at the branch point of the internal and external carotid arteries.
- The carotid sinus contains baroceptors that respond to pressure changes in the carotid artery.
- The carotid sinus contains nerve endings from the glossopharyngeal nerve; when stimulated, they convey impulses to the heart and vasomotor control centers in the brainstem.
  - These control centers in turn stimulate the efferent vagus nerve.
  - This increase in vagal tone inhibits impulse formation in the sinus node.
  - Inhibition of the sinus node produces a marked slowing of heart rate.

This classic feedback loop is called the *vasovagal reflex* because it starts in the carotid artery *(vaso)*, loops up to the brain and central nervous system, and then moves down the fibers of the vagus nerve *(vagal)* to the sinus node.

Preparation

Perform carotid sinus massage (CSM) after careful preparation. Be especially careful in older patients, paying close attention to exclusion criteria (eg, carotid bruit, history of stroke or transient ischemic attack; see below)

- Preparation for procedure:
  - Functional IV line is in place.
  - Atropine and lidocaine are available.
  - ECG monitor accurately displays the rhythm.
  - ECG is monitored continuously.
- Obtain patient history. Exclude patients with a history of stroke or transient cerebral ischemia, recent myocardial infarction, or life-threatening ventricular arrhythmias.
- Perform a physical examination. *Exclude patients with carotid bruits or carotid surgery*. As a precaution,

consider placement of an IV catheter or have transcutaneous pacing readily available in case CSM provokes a bradycardia requiring intervention.

- Explain the procedure to the patient.

Technique of Carotid Sinus Massage

- Turn the patient's head to the left.
- Locate the right carotid sinus immediately below the angle of the mandible and above the sternocleidomastoid muscle.
- Using 2 fingers of the right hand, press down with some force and begin a firm, up-and-down massage for 5 to 10 seconds.
- Massage the carotid sinus firmly in a longitudinal manner with posteromedial pressure, compressing the carotid sinus between your fingers and the cervical spine.
- Repeat this massage 2 to 3 times, pausing 5 to 10 seconds between each attempt.
- Monitor blood pressure and rhythm carefully; record a rhythm strip before and after CSM.
- Then move to the left carotid artery bifurcation near the angle of the jaw.
- Repeat CSM in the same manner as previously described.
- It takes time and repetition before you can conclude that CSM has no effect.
- Never attempt simultaneous, bilateral massage. This technique can compress the arteries and reduce blood flow to the brain.
- If CSM is successful, obtain a 12-lead ECG after conversion; if PSVT persists, repeat CSM on the opposite side when blood pressure and heart rate are at baseline levels.
- If CSM is ineffective, consider combining it with another vagal maneuver, such as the Valsalva maneuver or placement of an ice pack on the skin.

Possible Complications

Numerous complications of CSM have been reported, but the incidence of side effects and complications is low when close attention is given to exclusion criteria and the technique is performed carefully (0.28% to 0.45% of patients, 0.7% to 0.17% of CSM episodes) even in older patients.[6-8] Reported complications include the following:

- Cerebral emboli
- Stroke (embolic and occlusive)
- Syncope
- Sinus arrest
- Asystole
- Increased degree of AV block and paradoxical tachyarrhythmias in digoxin-toxic states

When CSM is properly performed in carefully selected patients (excluding those with known potential for complications), complications involving the central nervous system are rare (<1%). Complications are almost always transient, resolving in 24 hours. In rare cases CSM has induced ventricular tachycardia.[9]

Adenosine

If reentry SVT does not respond to vagal maneuvers, adenosine can be given as a rapid 6 mg IV push over 1 to 3 seconds through a large (eg, antecubital) vein, followed by a 20-mL saline flush and elevation of the arm. This treatment achieves initially high levels of adenosine in the heart.[10,11] If the arrhythmia does not convert within 1 to 2 minutes, a 12-mg bolus can be given. This second dose can be followed by another 12-mg bolus if the arrhythmia again fails to convert within 1 to 2 minutes. Several trials have demonstrated that adenosine is safe and effective in terminating reentry SVT.[12-16] **If the initial and subsequent doses are ineffective, further administration will likely not be effective, and the diagnosis and treatment now require expert consultation.**

Pharmacology

Adenosine has many cellular signaling effects. Adenosine acts on cardiac adenosine receptors to diminish automaticity and slow conduction in nodal tissue by opening inward potassium channels. These electrophysiologic effects can effectively terminate many episodes of PSVT. In the largest series reported in the literature, cumulative response rates after 6 mg of adenosine, followed by 12 mg if necessary, were 57% and 93%, respectively.[12] The effectiveness of adenosine is well established. It now stands as the drug of choice to terminate PSVT with AV nodal involvement. Adenosine has a very short half-life (10 to 30 seconds).

Diagnostic Value

In patients with atrial fibrillation or flutter without preexcitation, adenosine can provide valuable diagnostic information when it slows conduction through the AV node.[11,17] Atrial flutter waves, for example, are unaffected by adenosine. The slowed conduction through the AV node increases the RR interval, allowing a greater display of atrial activity on the ECG monitor.

Caution

Adenosine is safe and effective in pregnancy, effectively terminating reentry SVT with minimal effect on the fetus.[18-20] But adenosine does have several important drug-drug interactions. Larger doses may be required for patients with a significant blood level of theophylline, caffeine, or theobromine. The initial dose should be reduced to 3 mg in

patients taking dipyridamole or carbamazepine, in patients with transplanted hearts,[21,22] or if given by central venous access.[23] Patients taking verapamil, diltiazem, or β-blockers may also require dose reduction to avoid drug-drug interactions. Side effects with adenosine are common but transient; flushing, dyspnea, and chest pain are the most frequently observed.[24]

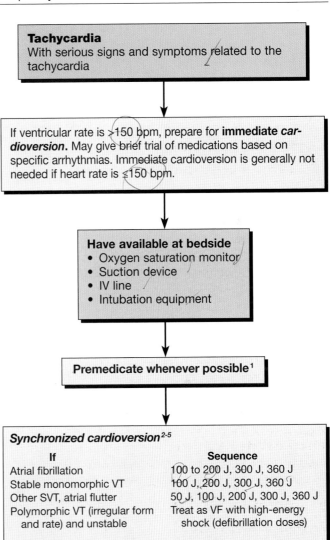

Figure 2. ACLS Electrical Cardioversion Algorithm.

Electrical Cardioversion for Stable and Unstable Tachycardias

Synchronized cardioversion is shock delivery that is timed (synchronized) with the QRS complex. This synchronization avoids shock delivery during the relative refractory period of the cardiac cycle (some call it the "vulnerable period"), when a shock could produce ventricular fibrillation (VF).[25] The energy (shock dose) used for synchronized cardioversion is lower than the doses used for unsynchronized shocks (ie, doses for attempted defibrillation). Low-energy shocks should always be delivered as synchronized shocks because delivery of low-energy unsynchronized shocks is likely to induce VF. If cardioversion is needed and it is impossible to synchronize a shock (eg, the patient's rhythm is irregular), use high-energy unsynchronized shocks (defibrillation doses).

Synchronized cardioversion is recommended to treat (1) unstable SVT due to reentry, (2) unstable atrial fibrillation, and (3) unstable atrial flutter. These arrhythmias are caused by *reentry,* an abnormal rhythm circuit that allows a wave of depolarization to travel in a circle. Delivery of a shock can stop these rhythms because the shock interrupts the circulating (reentry) pattern. Synchronized cardioversion is also recommended to treat unstable monomorphic (regular) VT. If possible, establish IV access before cardioversion and administer sedation if the patient is conscious. But do not delay cardioversion.

The recommended initial monophasic energy dose for cardioversion of atrial fibrillation is 100 to 200 J (Figure 2). Cardioversion of atrial flutter and other SVTs generally requires less energy. With a monophasic damped sine (MDS) waveform, an initial energy dose of 50 to 100 J is often sufficient. If the initial 50-J shock fails, increase the dose in a stepwise fashion.[26] Cardioversion with biphasic waveforms is now available, but more data is needed before specific comparative dosing recommendations can be made.

Cardioversion will not be effective for treatment of junctional tachycardia or ectopic or multifocal atrial tachycardia because these rhythms have an automatic focus, arising from cells that are spontaneously depolarizing at a rapid rate. Delivery of a shock cannot stop these rhythms. In fact,

shock delivery to a heart with a rapid automatic focus may increase the rate of the tachyarrhythmia.

The amount of energy required for cardioversion of VT is determined by the morphologic characteristics and the rate of the VT.[26] If the patient with monomorphic VT (regular form and rate) is unstable but has a pulse, treat with synchronized cardioversion. To treat monomorphic VT using a monophasic waveform, provide an initial shock of 100 J. If there is no response to the first shock, increase the dose in a stepwise fashion (eg, 100 J, 200 J, 300 J, 360 J) (Figure 2). There is insufficient data to recommend specific biphasic energy doses for treatment of VT.

Tachycardias—Refining the Diagnosis and Treatment
Premature Complexes

The ACLS Provider Course does not review premature complexes, but a few comments in this text are appropriate. Patients often report "palpitations." Palpitations are caused by frequent premature complexes, and they may herald or initiate both supraventricular and ventricular paroxysmal or sustained tachycardia. By themselves palpitations are usually benign, but their presence should prompt the clinician to search for structural heart disease and exacerbating factors that may require treatment.

Premature Atrial Contractions

Premature atrial contractions (PACs) are most common. They are identified on the ECG by the occurrence of a premature P wave with a PR interval greater than 120 ms except in preexcitation syndromes. PACs are also identified by an abnormal P wave contour, although this may not be readily apparent. The rhythm and pulse are irregular, but a complete compensatory pause is absent.

Pathophysiology

A PAC occurs as a result of atrial depolarization from a site that is not the sinus node. This premature contraction can initiate paroxysmal SVT. But alone PACs are usually benign.

Foundation Facts

Defibrillation for Polymorphic VT

If a patient has polymorphic VT and is unstable, treat the rhythm as VF and deliver high-energy (defibrillation dose) *unsynchronized* shocks. Although synchronized cardioversion is preferred for treatment of an organized ventricular rhythm, for some irregular rhythms, such as polymorphic VT, synchronization is not possible. If there is any doubt about whether monomorphic or polymorphic VT is present in the *unstable* patient, do not delay shock delivery to perform detailed rhythm analysis—provide defibrillation doses of energy.

Defining ECG Criteria

- The hallmark of a PAC is a P wave with the following characteristics:
  - Different morphology than a sinus-generated P wave
  - Occurs prematurely, before the next sinus depolarization
  - Is followed by a normal QRS complex (unless pre-existing bundle branch block)
  - The premature atrial event resets the sinus cycle
- The PR interval of the PAC may be normal or prolonged compared with a normal sinus complex.
  - When the PR interval is prolonged, the P wave may be superimposed on the previous T wave.
  - A PAC may occasionally result in an unexpected pause when a very early P wave is completely blocked and no ventricular complex results.

Clinical Manifestations

Patients are seldom aware of any symptom other than "palpitations" or their heart "skipping a beat."

Common Etiologies

PACs may be secondary to endogenous factors such as fever, hypovolemia, or hyperthyroidism. More often they are secondary to exogenous factors such as medications and various stimulants, such as caffeine, ephedrine-based or phenylpropanolamine-based products, and methamphetamines.

Treatment

PACs require no specific treatment. Clinicians should take the same therapeutic approach as for sinus tachycardia (see below), which is to identify the cause and treat the underlying condition.

Premature Ventricular Contractions

A premature ventricular complex (PVC) arises from depolarizations that occur in either ventricle before the next expected sinus impulse; hence the descriptor *premature* (Figure 3). Such impulses originate from either a focus of automaticity or from the reentry phenomenon. The following are general features and characteristics of PVCs:

- **QRS:** Abnormal in appearance, unusually broad, width ≥0.12 second.
- **Rhythm:** Irregular, usually with a complete compensatory pause.
- **P waves:** Seldom visible because they are obscured by the components of the PVC (QRS deflections, ST segment, and T wave).
  - P waves may become visible as a notching of the ST segment or T wave.
  - Retrograde P waves may be present.

PVCs Wide and Bizarre

PVCs will alter the normal pattern of ventricular depolarization. Conduction will take a different, slower course through the ventricles, bypassing normal conduction pathways through the specialized His-Purkinje cells.

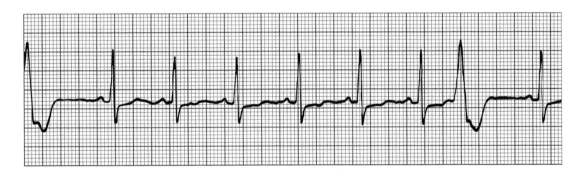

Figure 3. Premature ventricular complex (sometimes also called premature ventricular contraction).

Foundation Facts **Early PACs Confused With Pathologic AV Block**	When a P wave is not followed by a QRS, look closely at the preceding T wave for an abnormality that may be a P wave. When a P wave occurs early in diastole (eg, very prematurely), it may find the conduction system partially or completely refractory. This is sometimes called a blocked P wave but actually represents failure of impulse conduction to the ventricles. There may be no QRS, or the PR interval may be prolonged. The electrophysiologic principle notes that the shorter the RP interval (R wave to P' wave), the longer the PR interval (ie, they are inversely related). When the PR interval is prolonged or no QRS follows the P wave, confusion with pathologic AV block can occur.

The result is a wide (≥0.12 second) and bizarre-looking QRS complex. Ventricular repolarization is also altered, causing the ST segment and T wave to have the opposite polarity— and opposite direction—from the QRS complex.

Coupling Interval

The *coupling interval* is the interval between the preceding normal cycle and the PVC. In the past it was taught that fixed coupling resulted from a reentry mechanism and variable coupling resulted from a parasystolic focus. Although these are causes, the actual electrophysiologic mechanisms are complicated and multiple causes can be found, such as triggered activity and changing conduction in a reentrant or triggered circuit.

In general the coupling interval remains constant when the same reentry focus causes the PVCs (ie, they are unifocal in origin and uniform in appearance; Figure 4). When the coupling interval and QRS morphology vary, either different areas within the ventricles are generating the PVCs or the same focus of PVCs uses a variety of conduction pathways. Such PVCs are referred to as *multifocal* (Figure 5).

P Wave–PVC Relationships and "Compensatory Pauses"

PVCs occur independently of sinus node impulses. Sinus node activity is not disturbed by events occurring below the level of the AV node (such as PVCs), so the underlying sinus rhythm continues with regularity. Unless a retrograde impulse from the ventricles penetrates the AV node and conducts to the atria, sinus node impulses will continue completely undisturbed by ventricular events (Figure 6).

If the PVC is not conducted retrograde into the atria (which happens in some instances), resetting the sinus node, there is an apparent pause in rhythm before the next sinus impulse is generated and conducted to the ventricle. This pause is twice the interval of a normally conducted beat—or 2 RR intervals. This is called a *compensatory pause,* and such pauses *frequently* occur after PVCs. On occasion retrograde conduction from a PVC can spread to the atria and reset the sinoatrial node. In such instances the regularity of sinus node firing will be disrupted (reset) by the PVC.

Bigeminy and Trigeminy

Figure 7 displays a brief rhythm strip with several PVCs. Both the coupling interval and morphology remain constant. These PVCs therefore are unifocal. Because every second ventricular complex in this strip is a PVC, this rhythm can be called *ventricular bigeminy*. If every third ventricular complex is a PVC, the term *ventricular trigeminy* is used; if every fourth ventricular complex is a PVC, *ventricular quadrigeminy* is present; and so on.

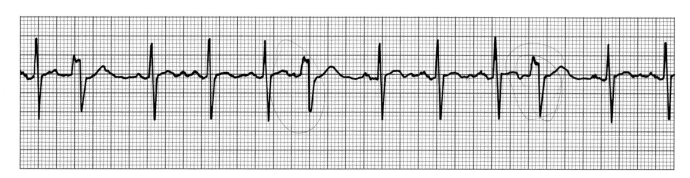

Figure 4. Uniform or unifocal PVCs. Note the occurrence of wide, premature QRS complexes. The interval between the preceding normal QRS and PVC (coupling interval) remains constant, and morphology remains the same.

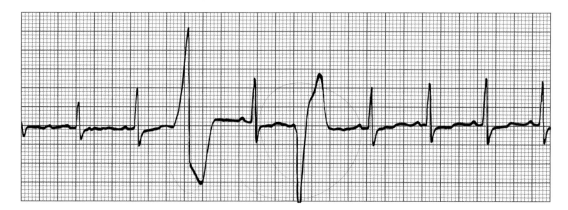

Figure 5. Multiform or multifocal PVCs. Note the variation in morphology and in the coupling interval of PVCs.

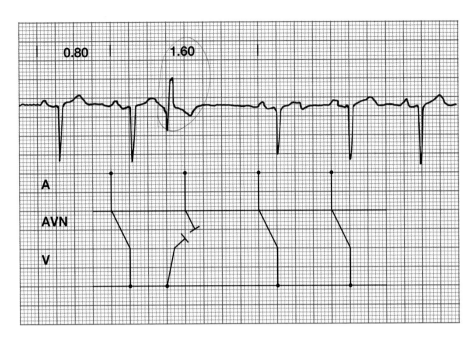

Figure 6. PVC with full compensatory pause. Two normal sinus-initiated cycles are followed by a premature, wide QRS complex without a preceding P wave. As illustrated in the accompanying "ladder diagram," firing of the sinus node (A, atrium) occurs undisturbed. Note that the sinus impulse that occurs shortly after the PVC depolarizes the atria. Neither the sinus impulse moving down nor the ventricular impulse moving up conducts through the AV node because each impulse is blocked by the refractory period of the other. The third sinus depolarization in the ladder diagram comes at the expected time. This timing makes the interval between the normal cycle preceding the PVC and the normal cycle following the PVC exactly equal to 2 normal sinus intervals. This interval is termed a full compensatory pause. Note that the RR interval preceding the PVC is 0.80 seconds and the RR interval including the premature complex is 1.60 – a complete compensatory pause twice the baseline RR interval because the sinus node is not reset.

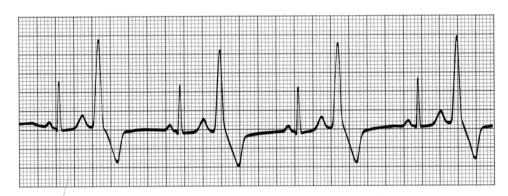

Figure 7. Ventricular bigeminy. Note that every other ventricular complex is a PVC. Both the coupling interval and morphology remain constant; hence the PVCs are unifocal. If every third ventricular complex is a PVC, the term *ventricular trigeminy* is used; if every fourth ventricular complex is a PVC, *ventricular quadrigeminy* is present; and so on.

Foundation Facts **PVCs Are Never Diagnosed With Certainty From the Rhythm Strip**	Although there are defining characteristics for PVCs, there are enough exceptions that PVCs can never be diagnosed with 100% certainty. • PVCs can be conducted retrograde into the atria, causing an "incomplete" compensatory pause. • PVCs can be "interpolated" between 2 normal beats without disrupting sinus rhythm. • Supraventricular beats can masquerade as PVCs. • A small percentage (4%) of PVCs can have a normal QRS width.[27]

The Vulnerable Period and the R-on-T Phenomenon

The T wave represents the period when the ventricles are *repolarizing* in preparation for the next cardiac impulse. The peak of the T wave serves as a rough dividing point between the *absolute refractory period* of the cardiac cycle and the *relative refractory period*. The relative refractory period is known to be a particularly unstable and *vulnerable period* of ventricular repolarization.

Historically it was thought that if a PVC fell on the T wave during the relative refractory period of ventricular repolarization, it might precipitate VT or VF (Figure 8).[28] More recently it has been found that late coupling of PVCs often initiates spontaneous VT and VF[29] (Figure 9). Conditions that cause a prolongation of the QT interval, such as drug overdoses and electrolyte abnormalities, can be associated with unstable rhythms, VT, VF, and even death. When these conditions are associated with bradycardia, a long RR interval followed by an early PVC with an R-on-T occurrence is particularly ominous.

Premature Junctional Contractions

Pathophysiology

A *premature junctional complex* (PJC) occurs when a premature impulse originates in the AV junction below the atria before the next expected sinus impulse (Figure 10). The exact site is unknown, and PJCs are the least common premature beats. From their location between the atria and ventricles, conduction is attempted both retrograde into the atria and anterograde into the ventricles. The retrograde P wave is abnormal and can occur before, after, or during the QRS, in which case it is obscured. The QRS is normal because of the antegrade conduction unless a preexisting bundle branch block or distal conduction system disease is present and strained by the premature complex.

Defining ECG Criteria

- **Abnormal P waves:** A PJC often results in an abnormal P wave because of retrograde atrial depolarization (negative P wave in leads II, III, and aVF).
  - The retrograde P wave may precede, coincide with, or follow the QRS.
  - The relation of a retrograde P wave to the QRS complex depends on the relative conduction times from the site of origin of the premature impulse within the junction to the atria and ventricles.
  - An impulse arising in the higher portion of the AV junction would result in a P wave appearing before or during the QRS complex, whereas one arising at a lower level would result in a P wave that appears within or after the QRS complex.
- **Normal QRS complexes:** The QRS complex is usually normal because conduction from the AV junction to the ventricles usually occurs along normal pathways.

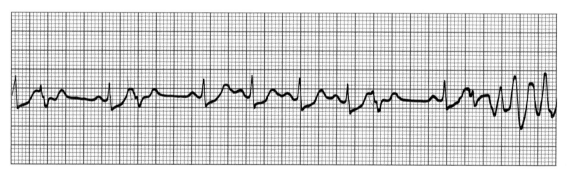

Figure 8. R-on-T phenomenon. Multiple PVCs are present. On the right a PVC falls on the downslope of the T wave during the relative refractory period (the vulnerable period), precipitating ventricular fibrillation.

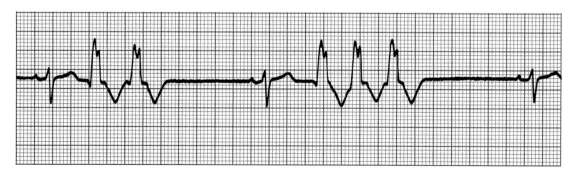

Figure 9. Initiation of ventricular tachycardia by a PVC. A late-cycle PVC, occurring well beyond the T wave, initiates a brief run of ventricular tachycardia.

— The QRS complex can be wide if either a bundle branch block or aberrant conduction is present.
- **Variable rhythm:** A PJC may or may not "reset" the sinus cycle depending on whether retrograde conduction to the atrium occurs.

Narrow-Complex Supraventricular Tachycardias
Attempt to Establish a Specific Diagnosis

If the patient is stable, try to establish a definitive arrhythmia diagnosis. The intent of this step is not to delay treatment but to give the patient a specific treatment for a specific diagnosis and to avoid therapy that may be ineffective or harmful.

Narrow-complex SVTs can be generally classified into 4 basic groups for purposes of initial assessment:

1. Sinus tachycardia
2. Reentry SVT
3. Atrial fibrillation
4. Atrial flutter

If the rhythm diagnosis is not immediately obvious, several features of the rhythm can be used to establish a specific diagnosis.

Assessment of Regularity, P Waves, and PR Intervals

In the case of narrow-complex QRS tachycardias (QRS <0.12, often ≤0.11 second), a rhythm diagnosis can be made by evaluation of the ECG for the features described below or by use of diagnostic maneuvers such as vagal stimulation or adenosine.

There are 3 important discriminating features of a narrow-complex tachycardia:

- Regularity of the rate
- Presence of P waves
- Appropriate PR interval preceding each QRS complex

A *regular* narrow-complex tachycardia is likely to be
- Sinus tachycardia or multifocal or ectopic atrial tachycardia if each QRS is preceded by a P wave and a relatively normal PR interval
- Atrial flutter (with a fixed degree of AV block) if flutter waves precede each QRS
- Reentry SVT or (less commonly) junctional tachycardia if P waves are indiscernible before each QRS or the PR interval is short (<0.12 second)

An *irregular* narrow-complex tachycardia is most often due to
- Atrial fibrillation
- Atrial flutter (with variable AV block)
- Multifocal atrial tachycardia (not discussed in the ACLS Provider Course)

Assessment of Response to Vagal Stimulation and Adenosine

In addition to ECG characteristics, the clinical and rhythmic responses to vagal maneuvers or adenosine can help establish a specific diagnosis for a regular narrow-complex tachycardia. Vagal stimulation and adenosine induce a characteristic response for each of the different supraventricular arrhythmias:

- For PSVT the response can be abrupt termination of the tachycardia.
- For atrial flutter or atrial tachycardia the response can be a transient AV block with slowing of the ventricular rate but no alteration of the atrial arrhythmia. These responses may unmask the "flutter" waves of atrial flutter or the altered P waves of ectopic atrial tachycardia.
- For sinus tachycardia the response can be a transient slowing of the sinus mechanism, occasionally with transient AV block.
- For junctional tachycardia the response can be a temporary slowing of the rate.
- These diagnostic maneuvers seldom establish the cause of irregular supraventricular tachycardia.

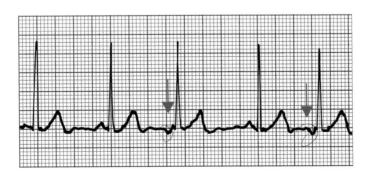

Figure 10. Premature junctional complexes. The third and fifth complexes occur early and are immediately preceded by inverted P waves (arrows). In lead II this pattern is consistent with retrograde atrial depolarization.

Assessment of Wide Complexes

- A wide-complex tachycardia known to be of *supraventricular* origin (with aberrancy) is approached in the same manner as narrow-complex SVT.
- Wide-complex tachycardias known to be of *ventricular origin* are treated according to the Stable Ventricular Tachycardia Algorithm. In most cases expert consultation is advised.
- Wide-complex tachycardias of *unknown etiology* require expert consultation to further assess the diagnosis and appropriate intervention. They should not be treated by trial and error with antiarrhythmic therapy as this could be dangerous because of an uncertain diagnosis and proarrhythmic effects of antiarrhythmics.

Sinus Tachycardia

Pathophysiology

Sinus tachycardia represents normal impulse formation and conduction at a rapid rate. It does not constitute a pathologic condition of and by itself. Sinus tachycardia is usually a physical sign of a problem or symptom. In rare cases inappropriate sinus tachycardia occurs in the absence of an obvious physiologic cause and in this context is regarded as a bona fide arrhythmia.

Defining ECG Criteria

- **Rate:** By definition >100 per minute.
- **Rhythm:** By definition always a sinus-originated rhythm.
- **PR interval:** ≤0.20 second.

- **QRS complex:** May be normal in width and configuration or abnormal if aberrant conduction to the ventricle is present (Figure 11).
- **Caution in diagnosis:** Clinicians will at times evaluate an unstable patient with an apparent rapid sinus tachycardia. The first question is whether the arrhythmia originates in the sinoatrial node or represents an ectopic atrial tachycardia. Careful examination of the P-wave configuration on a 12-lead ECG can often answer this question. P waves that originate from the sinus node will have a consistent, uniform appearance, whereas the P waves in ectopic atrial tachycardia will not.

Clinical Manifestations

Sinus tachycardia can cause a sensation of palpitations. In addition, the patient may develop symptoms secondary to the condition that is causing the tachycardia, such as fever, hypovolemia, or adrenergic stimulation.

Common Etiologies

Some of the more common causes of sinus tachycardia are

- Normal exercise
- Fever
- Hypovolemia
- Adrenergic stimulation, anxiety
- Hyperthyroidism
- Anemia

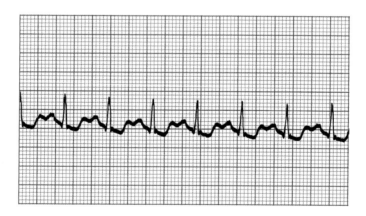

Figure 11. Sinus tachycardia. Note regular rhythm at the rate of 121 per minute. Each QRS is preceded by an upright P wave in lead II (also may be seen in leads I and aVF).

Critical Concept *Sinus Tachycardia*	• Sinus tachycardia represents normal impulse formation and conduction at a rapid rate and does not constitute a pathologic condition of and by itself. • Treatment is directed at the underlying cause. • β-Blockers may be contraindicated if the tachycardia is compensatory.

Recommended Therapy

Treatment of sinus tachycardia involves several important principles:

- There is no specific treatment for sinus tachycardia. (*Note:* A special type of sinus tachycardia called *inappropriate sinus tachycardia* does occur. It may require treatment with β-blockers, calcium channel blockers, or elective radiofrequency catheter ablation.)
- Treat the cause of the sinus tachycardia rather than the tachycardia itself.
- Never attempt cardioversion or defibrillation for sinus tachycardia. The goal of electrical cardioversion is to produce sinus rhythm. A person who is already in sinus tachycardia cannot be helped by electrical therapy.

Reentry Supraventricular Tachycardia

Narrow-Complex Tachycardias: General Nomenclature Categories

The narrow-complex tachycardias bear a variety of labels based on anatomic site of origin, width of the QRS complex, characteristics of onset and termination, and mechanism of formation.[17,30]

- These tachycardias are called *narrow-complex tachycardias* because the QRS complexes are typically

Sinus Tachycardia	
Pathophysiology	• None—more a physical sign than an arrhythmia or pathologic condition • Normal impulse formation and conduction
Defining Criteria and ECG Features	• **Rate:** >100 beats/min • **Rhythm:** sinus • **PR:** <0.20 sec • **QRS complex:** normal
Clinical Manifestations	• None specific for the tachycardia • Symptoms may be present due to the cause of the tachycardia (fever, hypovolemia, etc)
Common Etiologies	• Normal exercise • Fever • Hypovolemia • Adrenergic stimulation; anxiety • Hyperthyroidism
Recommended Therapy No specific treatment for sinus tachycardia	• Never treat the tachycardia itself • Treat only the causes of the tachycardia • Never countershock

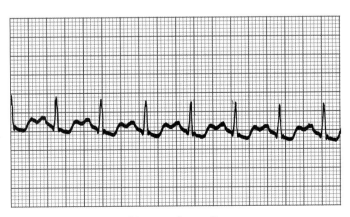

Sinus tachycardia

≤0.10 second unless bundle branch block or aberrancy is present.

- The rhythms are termed *supraventricular tachycardias* because they originate above the ventricles, in the AV node or above.
- The term *paroxysmal atrial tachycardia (PAT)* is now obsolete, because it implies events isolated to the atria.[17]
- Applied to these arrhythmias, the term *paroxysmal* refers to their *sudden,* often *single-beat onset*; *duration* of 30 seconds or more; and often equally sudden (within a single beat) *spontaneous termination* or abrupt interruption with treatment.
  - Some experts require documentation of the *paroxysmal* single-beat onset on an ECG monitor before applying the term *paroxysmal*.[31]
  - Paroxysmal arrhythmias may occur with increasing frequency over time, persist for progressively longer intervals, and eventually become permanent or chronic (at which time another descriptor, *incessant* or *persistent,* is used).
  - The most common narrow-complex tachycardia occurring in the paroxysmal manner described

above is labeled *paroxysmal supraventricular tachycardia*. PSVT most commonly involves reentry within the AV node and is more appropriately called AV nodal reentry tachycardia (AVNRT), or it may involve a reentry circuit that includes the AV node and an accessory pathway (AV reentry tachycardia or AVRT). We now understand that both forms of PSVT originate in or above the AV node and require the AV node for initiation and maintenance. The majority of episodes of reentry SVT in adults are due to AV nodal reentry, in which the AV node provides both the antegrade and retrograde portions of the circuit (Figure 12).

Nomenclature Based on Tachycardia Mechanism

Most supraventricular, narrow-complex, AV tachycardias originate from 1 of 2 mechanisms:

- **Automaticity** tachycardias (due to enhanced automaticity). Major examples of this mechanism are sinus, ectopic atrial, junctional, and multifocal (ectopic) atrial tachycardias. These arrhythmias are not responsive to DC cardioversion.

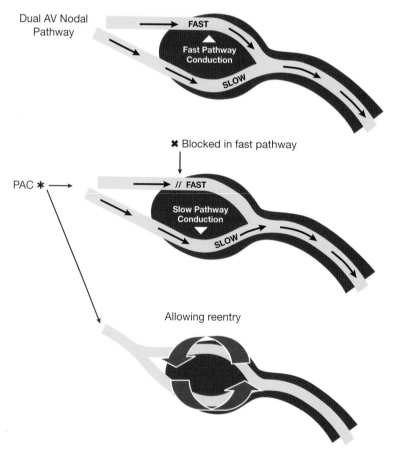

Should the QRS complex be narrow or wide?

Figure 12. The majority of episodes of reentry SVT are due to AV nodal reentry, in which the AV node provides both the antegrade and retrograde portions of the circuit. A premature atrial contraction (PAC) often provides the stimulus that incites the reentry cycle. Because conduction is through normal pathways into the ventricle, the QRS complex is normal unless a preexisting or rate-dependent bundle branch block is present.

- **Reentry** tachycardias (due to reentry mechanism). Major examples of this mechanism include atrial fibrillation, atrial flutter, and PSVT. These tachycardias are typically responsive to DC cardioversion. There are 3 common anatomic sites for reentry (Figure 13):

  — The active reentry site is *atrial,* occurring only in the atria and leading to atrial fibrillation and atrial flutter.

  — The active reentry site involves the AV node (termed AV nodal reentry tachycardia or AVNRT).
  — The active reentry site involves both the AV node and an *accessory* or *bypass conduction* pathway (AV reentry tachycardia or AVRT).

When PSVT is mediated by an accessory pathway, the AV node most commonly serves as the antegrade portion of

AV Reentry Tachycardia	AV Nodal Reentry Tachycardia	Atrial Tachycardia
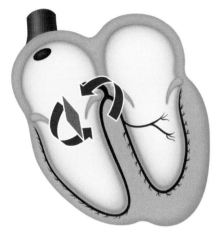	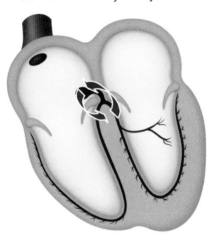	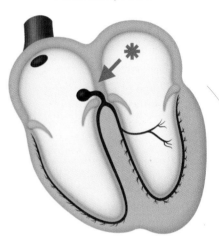
Connection between atria and ventricle	Uses dual pathway within AV node	Ectopic atrial focus

Figure 13. Example of 3 mechanisms for supraventricular arrhythmias. In AV reentry tachycardia there is an abnormal connection between the ventricles known as a bypass tract or accessory conduction pathway (eg, Wolff-Parkinson-White syndrome). In AV nodal reentry tachycardia there is a dual pathway within the AV node. In atrial tachycardia an automatic ectopic focus discharges.

AV Reentry Tachycardia

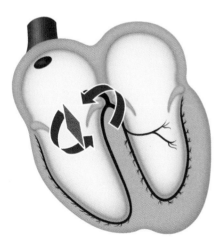

Connection between atria and ventricle

Antedromic Conduction
Wide QRS Complex

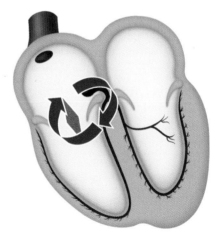

Connection between atria and ventricle

Orthodromic Conduction
Narrow QRS Complex

Figure 14. When PSVT is mediated by an accessory pathway, the AV node most commonly serves as the forward portion of the reentry circuit, and the accessory pathway serves as the retrograde portion (orthodromic reciprocating tachycardia), resulting in a narrow QRS complex because the conduction pathway to the ventricles is normal (right). When a reentry circuit circulates in the opposite direction (conducting antegrade down the accessory pathway and retrograde back to the atria via the AV node), a wide-complex (preexcited) PSVT (antidromic reciprocating tachycardia) results (left).

Reentry Supraventricular Tachycardia	
Pathophysiology	• **Reentry phenomenon:** impulses arise and recycle repeatedly in the AV node because of areas of unidirectional block in the Purkinje fibers
Defining Criteria and ECG Features **Key:** Regular, narrow-complex tachycardia without P-waves, and <u>sudden</u>, *paroxysmal* onset or cessation, or both **Note:** To merit the diagnosis some experts require capture of the paroxysmal onset or cessation on a monitor strip	• **Rate:** exceeds upper limit of sinus tachycardia (>120 beats/min); seldom <150 beats/min; up to 250 beats/min • **Rhythm:** regular • **P waves:** seldom seen because rapid rate causes P wave loss in preceding T waves or because the origin is low in the atrium • **QRS complex:** normal, narrow (≤0.10 sec usually)
Clinical Manifestations	• Palpitations felt by patient at the paroxysmal onset; becomes anxious, uncomfortable • Exercise tolerance low with very high rates • Symptoms of unstable tachycardia may occur
Common Etiologies	• Accessory conduction pathway in many PSVT patients • For such otherwise healthy people many factors can provoke the paroxysm, such as caffeine, hypoxia, cigarettes, stress, anxiety, sleep deprivation, numerous medications • Also increased frequency of PSVT in unhealthy patients with CAD, COPD, CHF

Recommended Therapy
 	
If specific diagnosis unknown, attempt therapeutic/diagnostic maneuver with
• Vagal stimulation
• *Adenosine . . .* THEN
	Preserved heart function:
	• AV nodal blockade
	  — *β-Blocker*
	  — *Calcium channel blocker*
	  — *Digoxin*
	• DC cardioversion
	• Parenteral antiarrhythmics:
	  — *Procainamide*
	  — *Amiodarone*
	  — *Sotalol* (not available in the United States)
	Impaired heart function:
	• *DC cardioversion*
	• *Digoxin*
	• *Amiodarone*
	• *Diltiazem*

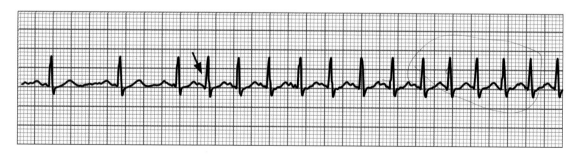

Sinus rhythm (3 complexes) with paroxysmal onset (arrow) of supraventricular tachycardia (PSVT)

the reentry circuit, and the accessory pathway serves as the retrograde portion (orthodromic reciprocating tachycardia). When a reentry circuit circulates in the opposite direction (conducting antegrade down the accessory pathway and retrograde back to the atria via the AV node), a wide-complex (preexcited) PSVT (antidromic reciprocating tachycardia) results (Figure 14).

Therapy

Vagal maneuvers are the initial indicated intervention for reentry SVT. Adenosine markedly decreases both antegrade and retrograde conduction through the AV node, interrupting any reentrant circuit that depends on conduction through the AV node for its perpetuation, including AVNRT and AVRT.

Atrial Fibrillation-Rate and Rhythm Control

The treatment approach for atrial fibrillation and atrial flutter includes the following steps, *listed in order of priority:*

1. Urgent treatment of unstable patients with synchronized cardioversion
2. Control of the ventricular rate (rate control)
3. Appropriate anticoagulation measures before and after cardioversion in stable patients with atrial fibrillation or flutter of longer than 48 hours' duration (rhythm control)
4. Consideration of electrical or pharmacologic conversion of the rhythm

Pathophysiology

Atrial fibrillation is the most common sustained cardiac rhythm disturbance. The basic mechanism continues to be defined, but atrial fibrillation is thought to result in part from multiple reentrant wavelets that circulate chaotically throughout the atria and drive the ventricular rate in a typically rapid and *irregularly irregular* fashion. The atrial electrical activity occurs at multiple sites of reentry within the atria, resulting in very rapid atrial depolarizations

(approximately 300 to 400 per minute or higher) that are too disorganized to result in effective atrial contraction. As a result, there is no contraction of the atria as a whole.

- Because there is no uniform atrial depolarization, no distinct P waves are visible on the ECG.
- The chaotic electrical activity produces a deflection on the ECG, referred to as fibrillation waves. Fibrillation waves vary in size and shape, and they are irregularly irregular in rhythm.
- Transmission of these multiple atrial impulses through the AV node is inconsistent, resulting in an irregularly irregular ventricular rate. Some impulses are conducted into but not through the AV node.
- These impulses, blocked in the AV node, constitute a form of "concealed conduction." Such nonconducted impulses contribute to an overall *refractoriness* of the AV node.
- The typical ventricular response rate in patients with atrial fibrillation averages 120 to 160 per minute or higher.

Defining ECG Criteria

- **Key:** The key feature of atrial fibrillation is the presence of irregularly irregular atrial and ventricular rhythms. The irregular variations in both atrial and ventricular rates are observed as virtually constant, rapid atrial activity without clearly organized P waves and no baseline between successive irregularly interspersed R waves (Figure 15).
- **Rate:** The atrial rate is irregular and as a rule is too rapid to be counted. The frequency of the atrial "fibrillation" impulses is 300 to 400 per minute or higher. The ventricular response to these impulses varies widely from beat to beat.
- **Rhythm:** Both the atrial and ventricular rhythms are irregular. The ubiquitous clinical expression is *irregularly irregular* (Figure 16).
- **P waves:** Organized P waves as such are not seen. The chaotic atrial fibrillation waves create an undulating baseline.
- **PR interval:** The absence of discernible P waves and no flat baseline precludes a PR interval.

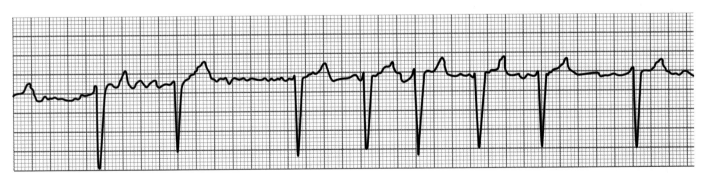

Figure 15. Atrial fibrillation with controlled ventricular response. Note irregular undulations of the baseline, which represent atrial electrical activity (fibrillation waves). The fibrillation waves vary in size and shape, and they are irregular in rhythm. Conduction through the AV node varies; hence the ventricular rhythm is irregular.

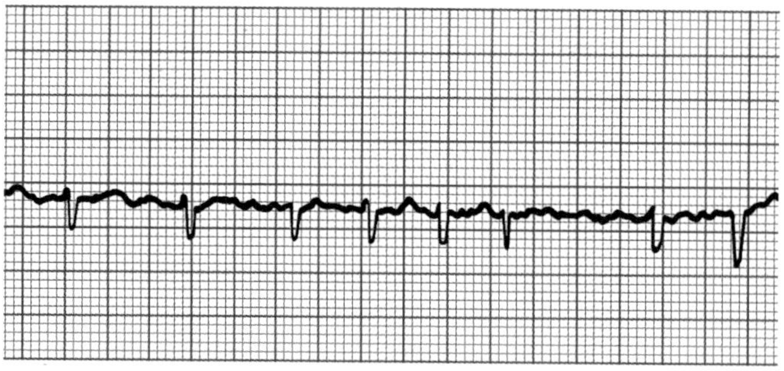

Figure 16. Atrial fibrillation with rapid ventricular response.

- **QRS complex:** The QRS complexes are normal (<0.12 second) in duration unless widened by conduction defects through the ventricles (*aberrant* conduction).

Clinical Manifestations

- Patients will often perceive or describe the irregular rhythm of atrial fibrillation as "palpitations." With coexisting disease and advancing age, patients may complain of lightheadedness, weakness, or presyncope. Exertional dyspnea may be a prominent feature.
- Atrial fibrillation may cause few if any symptoms in younger patients.
- **Ventricular rate and function:** The major signs and symptoms of atrial fibrillation are a function of the resulting ventricular rate, the effect on cardiac output, and the patient's underlying ventricular function. The ventricular rate is determined by the number of atrial fibrillation waves that pass through the AV node and stimulate a ventricular response:
  — If AV conduction allows numerous impulses through, a *rapid ventricular response* can occur.
  — This response can lead to a *symptomatic tachycardia* with serious signs and symptoms due to the tachycardia, such as hypotension, shortness of breath, angina, and even frank acute pulmonary edema. In general, rates exceeding 150 per minute are present when serious signs and symptoms are due to the ventricular rate unless another problem is present.
- **Loss of "atrial kick":** The absence of atrial contractions results in loss of the contribution of atrial contraction to ventricular filling. This "atrial kick" is responsible for approximately 25% of ventricular filling. Loss of the atrial kick can lead to a hemodynamically significant fall in stroke volume and cardiac output and a decrease in coronary perfusion.

- **Identification of coexistent Wolff-Parkinson-White (WPW) syndrome:** Atrial fibrillation or flutter occurring with preexcitation may be a medical emergency if rapid conduction occurs through an accessory pathway (Figure 14). Patients typically present with a very rapid, wide-complex tachycardia that may be difficult to distinguish from ventricular tachycardia unless there is a known history of WPW syndrome or there are discriminating features of the ECG (in the case of atrial fibrillation, varying degrees of QRS widening between successive irregularly irregular ventricular complexes).

Common Etiologies

- Although usually associated with some underlying form of heart disease, atrial fibrillation may be present in patients with no detectable heart disease (so-called lone atrial fibrillation).
- Atrial fibrillation can occur in these forms: paroxysmal (self-terminating), persistent (requiring treatment for termination), or permanent (unable to be terminated). When a patient has 2 or more episodes of atrial fibrillation, the arrhythmia is considered to be recurrent.
- Atrial fibrillation occurs most often in association with the following conditions:
  — Acute and chronic coronary syndromes, including coronary artery disease and congestive heart failure. Acute myocardial ischemia and infarction do not commonly cause atrial fibrillation, although atrial fibrillation frequently occurs in patients with chronic ischemic heart disease.
  — Structural heart disease, most commonly valvular, including disease at the mitral or tricuspid valve
  — Hyperthyroidism
  — Sick sinus syndrome
  — Acute pulmonary embolism

Critical Concept

Caution — Drug Use in AF With Preexcitation

Treatment of preexcited atrial fibrillation with drugs that block conduction through the AV node (adenosine, calcium channel blockers, digoxin, or β-blockers) is contraindicated because such agents may paradoxically accelerate the ventricular rate.

Critical Concept **Causes of Atrial Fibrillation**	Atrial fibrillation often occurs in the presence of atrial structural or electrophysiologic pathology. Excess sympathetic tone, however, frequently resets the threshold or triggers the onset of atrial fibrillation. Always search for a precipitating trigger or treatable comorbidity. • β-Blockers may be particularly useful in this group of patients.

— Hypoxia in general
— Increased atrial pressure from multiple causes
— Pericarditis

Reversible Causes

Reversible and underlying causes of atrial fibrillation should be identified and corrected if possible. The most commonly encountered reversible causes of atrial fibrillation are

- Hypoxemia
- Anemia
- Hypertension
- Congestive heart failure
- Mitral regurgitation
- Thyrotoxicosis
- Metabolic abnormalities (hypokalemia, hypomagnesemia)
- Drugs (alcohol, stimulants)

Recommended Therapy

Patients with atrial fibrillation who are stable require no additional therapy from an ACLS provider. Box 11 of the Tachycardia With Pulses Algorithm is shaded, indicating that expert consultation is recommended. The algorithm recommends expert consultation because optimal treatment of atrial fibrillation with pharmacologic or drug therapy requires additional pharmacologic knowledge, appreciation of the proarrhythmic effects of agents, understanding of rate and rhythm control strategies, and appreciation of ventricular function.

Selection of Therapy

Acute treatment of atrial fibrillation is directed by the answers to the following 4 questions:

1. Is this patient unstable and in need of urgent intervention?
2. Does this patient have significant impairment of ventricular function?
3. Is there evidence of preexcitation (WPW) syndrome?
4. Did this episode of atrial fibrillation or flutter start more than 48 hours ago?

For example, a patient who is clinically unstable requires immediate cardioversion. If the patient has impaired ventricular function, you should avoid the use of drugs with negative inotropic properties (eg, calcium channel blockers

and β-blockers) and most antiarrhythmic agents. Similarly, drugs that block conduction through the AV node, such as adenosine, digoxin, calcium channel blockers, and β-blockers, pose a significant hazard for patients with WPW syndrome. Finally, the 48-hour treatment window draws a sharp line between patients who need anticoagulation for several weeks before and after cardioversion and those who can safely undergo cardioversion without it.

Treatment Overview

Acute therapy for atrial fibrillation addresses the following issues, listed in order of clinical priority:

1. Treat unstable patients urgently.
2. Control the ventricular rate: control extremely rapid ventricular responses to atrial impulses.
3. Provide appropriate anticoagulation measures to patients at risk for thromboembolic complications before considering elective cardioversion.
4. Determine if conversion of the rhythm from atrial fibrillation to normal sinus rhythm is desirable or necessary.

Atrial Flutter

Pathophysiology

- Unlike atrial fibrillation, which results from multiple reentry circuits, atrial flutter is the result of a single reentry circuit within the right atrium. As a result of the single reentry circuit, the impulse takes a circular course around the atria.
- Atrial flutter is characterized by flutter waves that occur rapidly with a characteristic "sawtooth" pattern. These "flutter waves" are best observed in leads II, III, and aVF.

Defining ECG Criteria

- **Key:** The key defining feature of atrial flutter is a classic "sawtooth" pattern visible in the flutter waves.
- **Atrial rate:** The flutter waves usually occur at a rate of 300 per minute. But the rate can range from 220 to 350 per minute.
- **Ventricular rate:** This rate is a function of how often the AV node conducts or blocks the atrial impulses. At an atrial rate of 300 the AV node succeeds in blocking about half the impulses, resulting in a 2:1 AV block and a regular ventricular tachycardia of about 150 per minute (Figure 17). The ventricular rate may be faster or slower,

and regular or irregular, depending on conduction through the AV node.

- **Rhythm:** The atrial rhythm is regular (unlike atrial fibrillation). The ventricular rhythm is regular if a constant degree of AV block is present, such as 2:1 or 4:1 (Figure 18). The ventricular rhythm can be grossly irregular if variable block is present (Figure 19).
- **P waves:** Flutter waves resemble a "sawtooth" or "picket fence" pattern. They are best seen in leads II, III, or aVF, as well as in V_1 and V_2. In the presence of 2:1 or 1:1 conduction ratios, it may be difficult to identify the flutter waves. In this instance carotid sinus massage (or IV adenosine used diagnostically) may produce a transient delay in AV nodal conduction, increasing the degree

of AV block and slowing the ventricular response. This maneuver will "uncover" the flutter waves.
- **PR interval:** The PR interval is difficult to measure. It may be fixed or variable from beat to beat.
- **QRS complex:** The QRS complex appears normal with a duration of <0.12 second unless aberrant ventricular conduction occurs.

Clinical Manifestations

The clinical manifestations of atrial flutter are similar to those of atrial fibrillation.

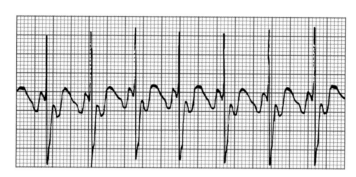

Figure 17. Atrial flutter. The atrial rate is 250 per minute, and the rhythm is regular. Every other flutter wave is conducted to ventricles (2:1 block), resulting in a regular ventricular rhythm at a rate of 125 per minute.

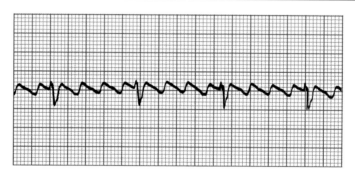

Figure 18. Atrial flutter with high-grade AV block. The atrial rhythm is regular (260 per minute), but only every fourth flutter wave is followed by a QRS (4:1 conduction).

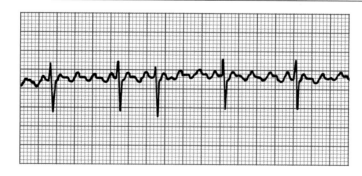

Figure 19. Atrial flutter with variable AV block. The atrial rhythm is regular, but variable AV block is present (2:1, 4:1 conduction ratios), resulting in an irregular ventricular rhythm.

Atrial Fibrillation/Atrial Flutter		
Pathophysiology	• Atrial impulses faster than SA node impulses • Atrial fibrillation → impulses take multiple, chaotic, random pathways through the atria • Atrial flutter → impulses take a circular course around the atria, setting up the flutter waves • Mechanism of impulse formation: reentry	

Defining Criteria and ECG Features (Distinctions here between atrial fibrillation vs atrial flutter; all other characteristics are the same) **Atrial Fibrillation Key:** A classic clinical axiom: *"Irregularly irregular rhythm—with variation in both interval and amplitude from R wave to R wave—is always atrial fibrillation."* This one is dependable. **Atrial Flutter Key:** Flutter waves seen in classic "sawtooth" pattern		**Atrial Fibrillation**	**Atrial Flutter**
	Rate	• Wide-ranging ventricular response to atrial rate of 300-400 beats/min	• Atrial rate 220-350 beats/min • Ventricular response = a function of AV node block or conduction of atrial impulses • Ventricular response rarely >150-180 beats because of AV node conduction limits
	Rhythm	• Irregular (classic "irregularly irregular")	• Regular (unlike atrial fibrillation) • Ventricular rhythm often regular • Set ratio to atrial rhythm, eg, 2-to-1 or 3-to-1
	P waves	• Chaotic atrial fibrillatory waves only • Creates disturbed baseline	• No true P waves seen • Flutter waves in "sawtooth" pattern is classic
	PR	• Cannot be measured	
	QRS	• No true P waves seen	

| **Clinical Manifestations** | • Signs and symptoms are function of the rate of ventricular response to atrial fibrillatory waves; *"atrial fibrillation with rapid ventricular response"* → DOE, SOB, acute pulmonary edema
• Loss of *"atrial kick"* may lead to drop in cardiac output and decreased coronary perfusion
• Irregular rhythm often perceived as *"palpitations"*
• Can be asymptomatic | | |

| **Common Etiologies** | • Acute coronary syndromes; CAD; CHF
• Disease at mitral or tricuspid valve
• Hypoxia; acute pulmonary embolism
• Drug-induced: *digoxin* or *quinidine* most common
• Hyperthyroidism | | |

Atrial Fibrillation/Atrial Flutter (continued)

Recommended Therapy		Control Rate	
Evaluation Focus:	**Treatment Focus:**	**Normal Heart**	**Impaired Heart**
1. Patient clinically unstable? 2. Cardiac function impaired? 3. WPW present? 4. Duration ≤48 or >48 hr?	1. Treat unstable patients urgently 2. Control the rate 3. Convert the rhythm 4. Provide anticoagulation	• Diltiazem or another calcium channel blocker **or** metoprolol or another β-blocker	• Digoxin **or** diltiazem **or** amiodarone
		Convert Rhythm	
		Normal Heart	**Impaired Heart**

		• If ≤48 hours:
		  − DC cardioversion or *amiodarone* or others
		
		• If >48 hours:
		  − Anticoagulate × 3 wk, **then**
		  − DC cardioversion, **then**
		  − Anticoagulate × 4 wk
		  or
		
		• IV *heparin* and TEE to rule out atrial clot, **then**
		
		• DC cardioversion within 24 hours, **then**
		
		• Anticoagulation × 4 more wk
			• If ≤48 hours:
			  − DC cardioversion **or** *amiodarone*
			
			• If >48 hours:
			  − Anticoagulate × 3 wk, **then**
			  − DC cardioversion, **then**
			  − Anticoagulate × 4 more wk

TEE indicates transesophageal echocardiogram.

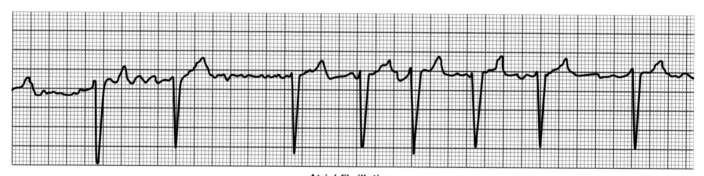

Atrial fibrillation

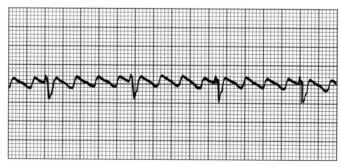

Atrial flutter

Common Etiologies

Atrial flutter typically occurs in association with organic heart disease. It is seen in association with mitral or tricuspid valvular heart disease, acute or chronic *cor pulmonale,* and coronary heart disease. Atrial flutter is rarely seen in the absence of organic heart disease.

Recommended Therapy

- Although acute atrial flutter differs somewhat in mechanism from atrial fibrillation, the initial management for rate control is the same.[32]
- Note that adenosine is not indicated for treatment of atrial fibrillation or flutter because of its ultrashort duration of action. But adenosine may be used diagnostically to induce brief AV block to search for atrial flutter waves. This step is seldom necessary, nor is it as helpful as ECG evaluation.

Stable Wide-Complex Tachycardia

A wide-complex tachycardia can be either ventricular or supraventricular in origin (Figure 20). The concept of aberrancy is not taught in the ACLS Provider Course. Basic providers should understand the following:

1. A wide-complex tachycardia is assumed to be ventricular until proven otherwise.

2. Unstable patients require immediate synchronized cardioversion if pulses are present.
3. Unstable pulseless patients are treated similarly to patients with VF.

Summary

Management of stable tachycardias can be challenging and the differential diagnosis uncertain. For the ACLS provider, initial assessment involves answering the following questions:

1. Are symptoms present and due to the tachycardia?
2. Is the patient stable or unstable?
3. Is the QRS complex wide or narrow?
4. If the QRS complex is narrow, is the rhythm regular or irregular?

If patients are stable and symptomatic with a narrow-complex QRS, you can use vagal maneuvers and adenosine to try to terminate the arrhythmia. If this strategy fails or the patient has a wide-complex stable tachycardia, expert consultation is advised. If the wide-complex tachycardia is thought to be VT, search for triggers or exacerbating factors. If there is concern about deterioration of the VT or development of hemodynamic instability, you can give amiodarone 150 mg IV over 10 minutes (may be repeated once) while expert consultation is obtained.

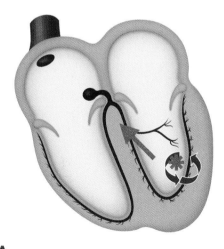

A

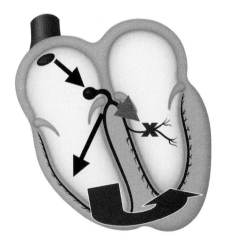

B

Figure 20. Wide-complex tachycardias can be ventricular or supraventricular in origin. **A,** An irritable ventricular focus excites the ventricular myocardium and spreads through the myocardium directly, causing a wide QRS complex typical of a PVC. **B,** The electrical impulse normally originates in the sinus node and is conducted through the AV node but is blocked when it enters the left bundle after passing through the bundle of His. Conduction through the right bundle occurs normally, but the left ventricle is then activated by this pathway, slowing conduction through the myocardium. This results in a wide QRS complex called, in this case, a left bundle branch block pattern. If a rapid supraventricular tachycardia is conducted in this manner, it results in a wide-QRS tachycardia resembling VT.

Example of Wide-Complex Tachycardia Due to Monomorphic Ventricular Tachycardia

Pathophysiology	• Impulse conduction is slowed around areas of ventricular injury, infarct, or ischemia • These areas also serve as source of ectopic impulses *(irritable foci)* • These areas of injury can cause the impulse to take a circular course, leading to the reentry phenomenon and rapid repetitive depolarizations
Defining Criteria per ECG **Key:** The same morphology, or shape, is seen in every QRS complex **Notes:** • 3 or more consecutive PVCs: VT • VT <30 sec duration → *nonsustained VT* • VT >30 sec duration → *sustained VT*	• **Rate:** ventricular rate >100 bpm; typically 120 to 250 bpm • **Rhythm:** no atrial activity seen, only regular ventricular • **PR:** nonexistent • **P waves:** seldom seen but present; VT is a form of AV dissociation (which is a defining characteristic for wide-complex tachycardias of ventricular origin vs supraventricular tachycardias with aberrant conduction) • **QRS complex:** wide and bizarre, "PVC-like" complexes >0.12 sec, with large T wave of opposite polarity from QRS
Clinical Manifestations	• Monomorphic VT can be asymptomatic, despite the widespread erroneous belief that sustained VT always produces symptoms • Majority of times, however, symptoms of decreased cardiac output (orthostasis, hypotension, syncope, exercise limitations, etc) are seen • Untreated and sustained will deteriorate to unstable VT, often VF
Common Etiologies	• An acute ischemic event (see pathophysiology) with areas of "ventricular irritability" leading to PVCs • PVCs that occur during the relative refractory period of the cardiac cycle ("R-on-T phenomenon") • Drug-induced, prolonged QT interval (tricyclic antidepressants, procainamide, digoxin, some long-acting antihistamines

Recommended Therapy	**Normal Heart**	**Impaired Heart**
	Any one of following parenteral antiarrhythmics: • *Procainamide* • *Sotalol* • *Amiodarone* • *Lidocaine*	• *Amiodarone* **or** • *Lidocaine* **then** • *DC cardioversion* if persists

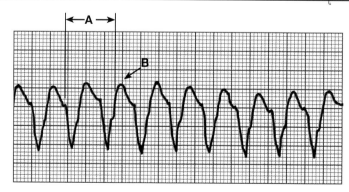

Monomorphic VT at rate of 150 bpm: wide QRS complexes (arrow A) with opposite polarity T waves (arrow B)

References

1. Atkins DL, Dorian P, Gonzalez ER, Gorgels AP, Kudenchuk PJ, Lurie KG, Morley PT, Robertson C, Samson RA, Silka MJ, Singh BN. Treatment of tachyarrhythmias. *Ann Emerg Med*. 2001;37: S91-S109.

2. Lim SH, Anantharaman V, Teo WS, Goh PP, Tan AT. Comparison of treatment of supraventricular tachycardia by Valsalva maneuver and carotid sinus massage. *Ann Emerg Med*. 1998;31:30-35.

3. Ornato JP, Hallagan LF, Reese WA, Clark RF, Tayal VS, Garnett AR, Gonzalez ER. Treatment of paroxysmal supraventricular tachycardia in the emergency department by clinical decision analysis. *Am J Emerg Med*. 1988;6:555-560.

4. O'Toole KS, Heller MB, Menegazzi JJ, Paris PM. Intravenous verapamil in the prehospital treatment of paroxysmal supraventricular tachycardia. *Ann Emerg Med*. 1990;19:291-294.

5. Mehta D, Wafa S, Ward DE, Camm AJ. Relative efficacy of various physical manoeuvres in the termination of junctional tachycardia. *Lancet*. 1988;1:1181-1185.

6. Davies AJ, Kenny RA. Frequency of neurologic complications following carotid sinus massage. *Am J Cardiol*. 1998;81:1256-1257.

7. Munro NC, McIntosh S, Lawson J, Morley CA, Sutton R, Kenny RA. Incidence of complications after carotid sinus massage in older patients with syncope. *J Am Geriatr Soc*. 1994;42:1248-1251.

8. Richardson DA, Bexton R, Shaw FE, Steen N, Bond J, Kenny RA. Complications of carotid sinus massage—a prospective series of older patients. *Age Ageing*. 2000;29:413-417.

9. Schweitzer P, Teichholz LE. Carotid sinus massage: its diagnostic and therapeutic value in arrhythmias. *Am J Med*. 1985;78:645-654.

10. DiMarco JP, Sellers TD, Berne RM, West GA, Belardinelli L. Adenosine: electrophysiologic effects and therapeutic use for terminating paroxysmal supraventricular tachycardia. *Circulation*. 1983;68:1254-1263.

11. DiMarco JP, Sellers TD, Lerman BB, Greenberg ML, Berne RM, Belardinelli L. Diagnostic and therapeutic use of adenosine in patients with supraventricular tachyarrhythmias. *J Am Coll Cardiol*. 1985;6:417-425.

12. DiMarco JP, Miles W, Akhtar M, Milstein S, Sharma AD, Platia E, McGovern B, Scheinman MM, Govier WC. Adenosine for paroxysmal supraventricular tachycardia: dose ranging and comparison with verapamil: assessment in placebo-controlled, multicenter trials. The Adenosine for PSVT Study Group [published correction appears in *Ann Intern Med*. 1990;113:996]. *Ann Intern Med*. 1990;113:104-110.

13. Brady WJ Jr, DeBehnke DJ, Wickman LL, Lindbeck G. Treatment of out-of-hospital supraventricular tachycardia: adenosine vs verapamil. *Acad Emerg Med*. 1996;3:574-585.

14. Furlong R, Gerhardt RT, Farber P, Schrank K, Willig R, Pittaluga J. Intravenous adenosine as first-line prehospital management of narrow-complex tachycardias by EMS personnel without direct physician control. *Am J Emerg Med*. 1995;13:383-388.

15. Madsen CD, Pointer JE, Lynch TG. A comparison of adenosine and verapamil for the treatment of supraventricular tachycardia in the prehospital setting. *Ann Emerg Med*. 1995;25:649-655.

16. Morrison LJ, Allan R, Vermeulen M, Dong SL, McCallum AL. Conversion rates for prehospital paroxysmal supraventricular tachycardia (PSVT) with the addition of adenosine: a before-and-after trial. *Prehosp Emerg Care*. 2001;5:353-359.

17. Ganz LI, Friedman PL. Supraventricular tachycardia. *N Engl J Med*. 1995;332:162-173.

18. Harrison JK, Greenfield RA, Wharton JM. Acute termination of supraventricular tachycardia by adenosine during pregnancy. *Am Heart J*. 1992;123:1386-1388.

19. Podolsky SM, Varon J. Adenosine use during pregnancy. *Ann Emerg Med*. 1991;20:1027-1028.

20. Leffler S, Johnson DR. Adenosine use in pregnancy: lack of effect on fetal heart rate. *Am J Emerg Med*. 1992;10:548-549.

21. Ellenbogen KA, Thames MD, DiMarco JP, Sheehan H, Lerman BB. Electrophysiological effects of adenosine in the transplanted human heart: evidence of supersensitivity. *Circulation*. 1990;81:821-828.

22. Anderson TJ, Ryan TJ Jr, Mudge GH, Selwyn AP, Ganz P, Yeung AC. Sinoatrial and atrioventricular block caused by intracoronary infusion of adenosine early after heart transplantation. *J Heart Lung Transplant*. 1993;12:522-524.

23. Chang M, Wrenn K. Adenosine dose should be less when administered through a central line. *J Emerg Med*. 2002;22:195-198.

24. Camm AJ, Garratt CJ. Adenosine and supraventricular tachycardia. *N Engl J Med*. 1991;325:1621-1629.

25. Lown B. Electrical reversion of cardiac arrhythmias. *Br Heart J*. 1967;29:469-489.

26. Kerber RE, Kienzle MG, Olshansky B, Waldo AL, Wilber D, Carlson MD, Aschoff AM, Birger S, Fugatt L, Walsh S, et al. Ventricular tachycardia rate and morphology determine energy and current requirements for transthoracic cardioversion. *Circulation*. 1992;85:158-163.

27. Hayes JJ, Stewart RB, Green HL, Bardy GH. Narrow QRS ventricular tachycardia. *Ann Intern Med*. 1991;114:460-463.

28. El-Sherif N, Myerburg RJ, Scherlag BJ, Befeler B, Aranda JM, Castellanos A, Lazzara R. Electrocardiographic antecedents of primary ventricular fibrillation: value of the R-on-T phenomenon in myocardial infarction. *Br Heart J*. 1976;38:415-422.

29. Kay GN, Plumb VJ, Arciniegas JG, Henthorn RW, Waldo AL. Torsade de pointes: the long-short initiating sequence and other clinical features: observations in 32 patients. *J Am Coll Cardiol*. 1983;2:806-817.

30. Delacretaz E. Clinical practice. Supraventricular tachycardia. *N Engl J Med*. 2006;354:1039-1051.

31. Akhtar M, Jazayeri MR, Sra J, Blanck Z, Deshpande S, Dhala A. Atrioventricular nodal reentry: clinical, electrophysiological, and therapeutic considerations. *Circulation*. 1993;88:282-295.

32. Waldo AL, Mackall JA, Biblo LA. Mechanisms and medical management of patients with atrial flutter. *Cardiol Clin*. 1997;15:661-676.

Stroke

Key Points

- Emergency Medical services (EMS) activation and transport results in faster hospital arrival and decreased emergency department (ED) evaluation time.
- EMS dispatchers can identify 50% of patients with stroke.
- Public education programs result in sustained identification and treatment of stroke patients.
- Designation of *primary stroke centers* for emergency stroke care is strongly recommended.

Introduction

Each year in the United States about 780 000 people suffer a new or repeat stroke. On average a new stroke occurs every 40 seconds. About 150 000 of these people will die, making stroke the third leading cause of death in the United States.[1] Many advances have been made in stroke prevention, treatment, and rehabilitation.[2,3] For example, fibrinolytic therapy can limit the extent of neurologic damage from stroke and improve outcome, but the time available for treatment is limited.[3,4]

Stroke Facts

- On average, every 40 seconds someone in the United States has a stroke; on average, every 3 to 4 minutes someone dies of a stroke.
- Each year about 780 000 people experience a new or recurrent stroke. About 600 000 of these are first attacks, and 180 000 are recurrent attacks.
- Men's stroke incidence rates are greater than women's at young er ages but not at older ages.
- Blacks have almost twice the risk of first-ever stroke compared with whites.

Healthcare providers, hospitals, and communities must develop systems to increase the efficiency and effectiveness of stroke care. The 7 "D's" of stroke care—detection, dispatch, delivery, door (arrival and urgent triage in the ED), data, decision, and drug administration—highlight the major steps in diagnosis and treatment and the key points at which delays can occur.[5,6]

This chapter describes the management of acute stroke in the adult patient. It summarizes out-of-hospital care through the first hours of therapy and focuses treatment on rapid identification of acute ischemic stroke while allowing evaluation for reperfusion therapy. Highlights and updates from the updated 2007 ischemic stroke guidelines are included. For additional information about the management of acute ischemic stroke and these guidelines, see the American Heart Association (AHA)/American Stroke Association (ASA) guidelines for the early management of adults with ischemic stroke.[7]

The Stroke Chain of Survival

The AHA and ASA have developed a community-oriented "Stroke Chain of Survival" that links specific actions to be taken by patients and family members with recommended actions by out-of-hospital healthcare responders, ED personnel, and in-hospital specialty services:

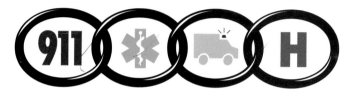

- Rapid recognition and reaction to stroke warning signs
- Rapid start of prehospital care
- Rapid EMS transport and hospital prenotification
- Rapid diagnosis and treatment in hospital

The 7 D's of Stroke Survival

In ST-segment elevation myocardial infarction time (STEMI) is muscle. When acute ischemic stroke occurs, time is brain, so the reperfusion concept was expanded to include not only patients with acute coronary syndromes (STEMI) but also highly selected stroke patients.[5] Hazinski was the first to describe an analogous series of linked actions to guide ACLS stroke care. Borrowing from the "door-to-drug" theme of the National Heart Attack Alert Program for fibrinolytic treatment of STEMI,[8] the "7 D's of Stroke Care" begin each step with the letter D: Detection, Dispatch, Delivery, Door, Data, Decision, and Drug administration. Table 1 lists the 7 steps of stroke care plus the major actions in each step. At each step care must be organized and efficient to avoid needless delays.

Definitions

Stroke refers to the acute neurologic impairment that follows an interruption in blood supply or a rupture of a blood vessel

Table 1. The 7 D's of ACLS Stroke Care in the Reperfusion Era

7 "D's"	Major Actions
✔ **Detection**	• Early recognition—onset of stroke signs and symptoms
✔ **Dispatch**	• Activation of the EMS system and prompt EMS response
✔ **Delivery**	• Transportation, with prearrival notification to receiving hospital • Provision of appropriate prehospital assessment and care
✔ **Door**	• Immediate general and neurologic assessment in the ED • Aim for predefined evaluation targets
✔ **Data**	• CT scan • Serial neurologic exams • Review for tPA exclusions • Review patient data

✔ **Decision**	• Patient remains candidate for tPA therapy? If "yes," then:
	  — Review risks and benefits with patient and family
	  — Obtain informed consent for tPA therapy

✔ **Drug**	• Begin tPA treatment within 3-hour time limit

CT indicates computed tomography; and tPA, tissue plasminogen activator.

to a specific region of the brain. Experts and clinicians most often classify strokes as either *ischemic* or *hemorrhagic* (Figure 1). The causes of stroke are numerous, but the initial therapy is based on the presence or absence of bleeding and a presumed ischemic stroke regardless of cause.

The distinction between ischemic and hemorrhagic stroke is important for 3 reasons:

- Reperfusion therapy using tissue plasminogen activator (tPA) is appropriate for ischemic stroke only.
- Hemorrhagic stroke is an absolute contraindication to tPA therapy.
- tPA can be fatal if given mistakenly to a patient having a hemorrhagic stroke.

Ischemic Stroke

Definition and Categories of Ischemic Stroke

In an ischemic stroke (87% of all strokes), interruption in blood supply is caused by occlusion of an artery to a region of the brain. Ischemic stroke rarely leads to death within the first hour.

Ischemic strokes can be defined on the basis of etiology and duration of symptoms. They are generally subdivided into the following categories:

- **Thrombotic stroke:** An acute clot that occludes an artery is superimposed on chronic arterial narrowing, acutely altered endothelial lining, or both. This pathophysiology parallels that for acute coronary syndromes (ACS) where a ruptured or eroded plaque is the proximate cause of most episodes of ACS.
- **Embolic stroke:** Intravascular material, most often a blood clot, separates from a proximal source and flows through an artery until it occludes an artery in the brain.

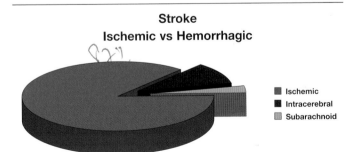

Stroke
Ischemic vs Hemorrhagic

■ Ischemic
■ Intracerebral
▨ Subarachnoid

Figure 1. Type of stroke. Eighty-seven percent of strokes are ischemic and potentially eligible for fibrinolytic therapy if patients otherwise qualify. Thirteen percent of strokes are hemorrhagic, and the majority of these are intracerebral. The male/female incidence ratio was 1.25 in those 55 to 64, 1.50 in those 65 to 74, 1.07 in those 75 to 84, and 0.76 in those 85 years of age and older, and blacks have almost twice the risk of first-ever stroke compared with whites.

Many of these are cardioembolic—originating from the heart—in patients with atrial fibrillation, valvular heart disease, acute myocardial infarction, or rarely endocarditis.

- **Transient ischemic attack (TIA) (sometimes called "mini-stroke"):** Any focal neurologic deficit that resolves completely and spontaneously within 1 hour. Formerly the time limit for resolution that defined the term *transient* was 24 hours. But TIAs frequently last for only 5 to 15 minutes, so the definition was refined.
- **Reversible ischemic neurologic deficit (RIND):** Any focal neurologic deficit that resolves completely and spontaneously within 24 hours. (RINDS were previously called TIAs.) Any patient with a persistent neurologic deficit beyond 24 hours is said to have suffered a stroke. New diagnostic techniques have shown that 60% of patients with a TIA or RIND have definite evidence of brain infarction.
- **Hypoperfusion stroke:** A more global pattern of brain infarction that results from low blood flow or intermittent periods of no flow. Hypoperfusion stroke often occurs in patients who recover cardiac function after sudden cardiac arrest.

Classification by Vascular Supply

Strokes are also classified by vascular supply and anatomic location:

- **Anterior circulation (carotid artery territory) stroke:** Stroke that follows occlusion of branches of the *carotid artery.* Such strokes usually involve the cerebral hemispheres.
- **Posterior circulation (vertebrobasilar artery territory) stroke:** Stroke that follows occlusion of branches of the *vertebrobasilar artery.* These strokes usually involve the brainstem or cerebellum.

Hemorrhagic Stroke

Hemorrhagic strokes (13% of all strokes) occur when a blood vessel in the brain suddenly ruptures with hemorrhage into the surrounding tissue. Damage results from direct trauma to brain cells; expanding mass effects, which lead to elevated intracranial pressure; release of damaging mediators; local vascular spasm; and loss of blood supply to brain tissue downstream from the ruptured vessel.

There are 2 types of hemorrhagic stroke, based on the location of the arterial rupture:

- **Intracerebral hemorrhagic stroke (10%):** Occurs when blood leaks directly into the brain parenchyma, usually from small intracerebral arterioles damaged by chronic hypertension.
  - Hypertension is the most common cause of intracerebral hemorrhage.

— Among the elderly, amyloid angiopathy appears to play a major role in intracerebral hemorrhage.

- **Subarachnoid hemorrhagic stroke (3%):** Occurs when blood leaks from a cerebral vessel into the subarachnoid space. If the rupture occurs in a cerebral artery, the blood is released at systemic arterial pressure, causing sudden, painful, and dramatic symptoms.
  — Aneurysms cause most subarachnoid hemorrhages.
  — Arteriovenous malformations cause approximately 5% of subarachnoid hemorrhages.

Pathophysiology

The Evolving "Ruptured Plaque" Concept

An ulcerated, ruptured plaque is the key mechanism of most thrombotic and embolic strokes in patients without valvular heart disease or atrial fibrillation. In thrombotic stroke complete occlusion develops at an atherosclerotic plaque. In embolic stroke the developing thrombus breaks off and heads downstream. Ruptured plaques occur not only in the intracranial branches of the carotid and vertebrobasilar arteries but also in the extracranial portions of the carotid arteries and in the ascending and transverse aorta.

The "ruptured plaque" concept, the pathophysiologic foundation of the ACS, explains many features of ischemic stroke[9-11] (see Chapter 10, Figure 1). Stroke effects result from interaction between blood vessels, the coagulation components of blood, inflammatory cells, and chemical mediators of inflammation.

- The most common cause of acute ischemic stroke is atherosclerosis of the carotid or vertebrobasilar artery. Varying degrees of inflammation in vulnerable atherosclerotic plaques predispose these arteries to endothelial erosion, plaque rupture, and platelet activation and aggregation.
- The ensuing development of a thrombus, composed of platelets, fibrin, and other elements, can completely occlude an artery already narrowed by atherosclerosis. This occlusion of blood flow leads to rapid infarction of downstream brain tissue cells, producing a thrombotic stroke.
- The thrombus, either before or immediately after it becomes completely occlusive, may dislodge and travel to more distal cerebral arteries, producing an embolic stroke (Figure 2).

Postocclusion Dynamics

Downstream from the thrombotic or embolic obstruction, brain cells begin to die and necrosis occurs. With persistent occlusion a central area of irreversible brain damage (infarction or necrosis) develops.

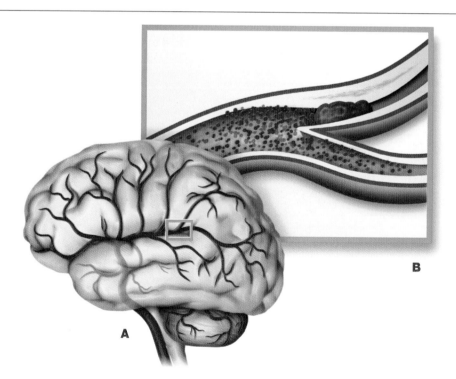

Figure 2. Occlusion in a cerebral artery by a thrombus: **A,** Area of infarction surrounding immediate site and distal portion of brain tissue after occlusion. **B,** Area of ischemic penumbra (ischemic, but not yet infarcted [dead] brain tissue) surrounding areas of infarction. This ischemic penumbra is alive but dysfunctional because of altered membrane potentials. The dysfunction is potentially reversible. Current stroke treatment tries to keep the area of permanent brain infarction as small as possible by preventing the areas of reversible brain ischemia in the penumbra from transforming into larger areas of irreversible brain infarction.

The recently coined term *brain attack* and the phrase *time is brain* convey the contemporary sense of urgency in stroke therapy.

- Once occlusion occurs, an inexorable countdown begins. There is only a limited time available to recognize, evaluate, and treat reversible brain damage.[12-14]

- Surrounding the central area of necrosis or infarction is an area of ischemia called the *ischemic penumbra* or *shadow*.
- This area of "threatened" brain tissue is an area of *potentially reversible* brain damage.
- Until the arrival of tPA therapy, practitioners had few effective methods to reduce the area of threatened brain tissue and to abort the progression from reversible brain damage to irreversible, permanent brain necrosis.

Other Pathophysiologic Processes

Atrial Fibrillation

Atrial fibrillation remains the most frequent cause of cardioembolic stroke.

- The noncontracting walls of the fibrillating left atrium and left atrial appendage serve as both a stimulus and a reservoir for small emboli.
- The risk of stroke in patients with nonvalvular atrial fibrillation averages 5% per year, 2 to 7 times that of people without atrial fibrillation.

Hypertension

Hypertension causes a thickening of the walls of small cerebral arteries, leading to reduced flow and a predisposition to thrombosis.

- Lacunar infarcts are one example of the type of thrombotic stroke caused by chronic hypertension. They are thought to result from occlusion of a small perforating artery to the subcortical areas of the brain.
- A major cerebrovascular burden imposed by chronic hypertension is hemorrhagic stroke.

Stroke Risk Factors

Risk factors can be identified in most stroke patients.[15] Stroke prevention requires identification of a patient's risk factors, followed by elimination, control, or treatment of as many factors as possible:

- Elimination (eg, smoking)
- Control (eg, hypertension, diabetes mellitus)
- Treatment (eg, antiplatelet therapy, carotid endarterectomy when indicated)

Table 2 lists the major stroke risk factors that are amenable to modification.

- A meta-analysis of reports of 31 observational studies conducted mainly in the United States and Europe found that moderate and high levels of leisure-time and occupational physical activity protected against total stroke, hemorrhagic stroke, and ischemic stroke.
- Physical activity reduces stroke risk. Results from the Physicians' Health Study showed a lower stroke risk associated with vigorous exercise among men. The Harvard Alumni Study also showed a decrease in total stroke risk in men who were highly physically active

Table 2. Stroke Risk: Factors That Can Be Modified

Risk Factor	Comments
Hypertension	• One of the most important modifiable risk factors for ischemic and spontaneous hemorrhagic stroke • Risk of hemorrhagic stroke increases markedly with elevations in systolic pressure • Control of hypertension significantly decreases the risk of stroke

Cigarette Smoking	• All of the following smoking effects have been linked to stroke:
	  — Accelerated atherosclerosis
	  — Transient elevations in blood pressure
	  — Release of toxic enzymes (linked to formation of aneurysms)
	  — Altered platelet function and reduced platelet survival
	• Cessation of cigarette smoking reduces the risk of stroke

Transient Ischemic Attack	• Highly significant indicator of a person at increased risk for stroke • 25% of stroke patients have had a previous TIA • 10% of patients presenting to an ED with TIA will have a completed stroke within 90 days; half of these within the first 2 days • Antiplatelet agents (eg, aspirin, ticlopidine) can reduce the risk of stroke in patients with TIA
Heart Disease	• Coronary artery disease and heart failure double the risk of stroke • Atrial fibrillation increases the risk of embolic stroke • Prophylactic warfarin, given to patients with atrial fibrillation, reduces the risk of embolic stroke
Diabetes Mellitus	• Highly associated with accelerated atherosclerosis • Careful monitoring and control of hyperglycemia reduce the risk of microvascular complications due to diabetes, and reduction of microvascular complications reduces stroke risk
Hypercoagulopathy	• Any hypercoagulative state (eg, protein S or C deficiency, cancer, pregnancy) increases the risk of stroke
High RBC Count and Sickle Cell Anemia	• A moderate increase in RBC count increases the risk of stroke • Increases in RBC count can be treated by removing blood and replacing it with intravenous fluid or by administering an anticoagulant • Sickle cell anemia increases the risk of stroke because "sickled" red blood cells can clump, causing arterial occlusion. Stroke risk from sickle cell anemia may be reduced by maintaining adequate oxygenation and hydration and by providing exchange transfusions
Carotid Bruit	• Carotid bruits often indicate partial obstruction (atherosclerosis) of an artery • Carotid bruits are associated with an increased risk of stroke • This risk is reduced by surgical endarterectomy but only in symptomatic patients with >70% stenosis • Some evidence suggests that carotid endarterectomy is beneficial in selected asymptomatic patients with high-grade stenosis

ED indicates emergency departments; RBC, red blood cell; and TIA, transient ischemic attack.

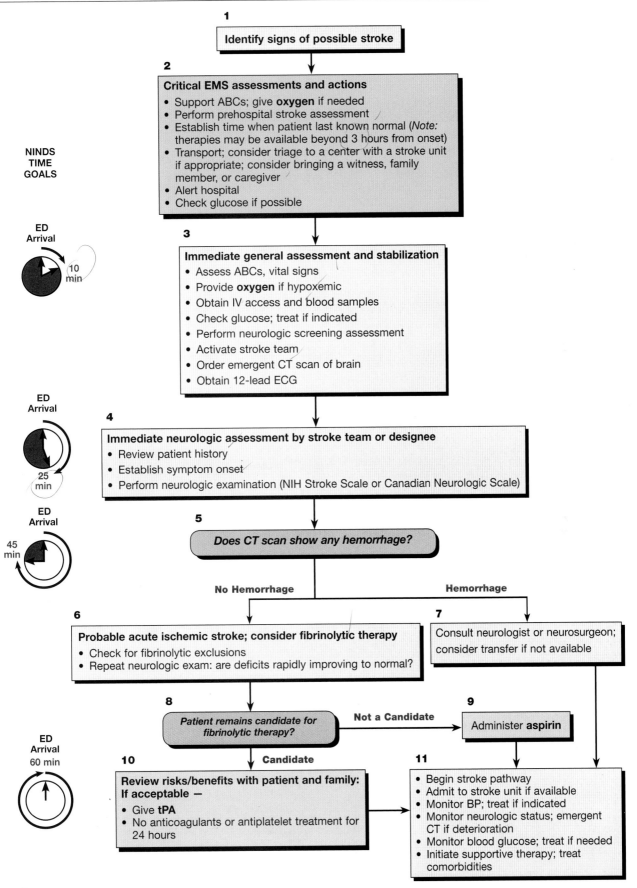

Figure 3. Suspected Stroke Algorithm.

Stroke Management

Stroke intervention begins with the recognition of the symptoms of stroke. An important component in this initial step is education—of the patient, family, community, and healthcare provider. Once recognition of potential stroke symptoms occurs, management involves expeditious transfer of the patient to an appropriate facility and rapid assessment of the patient for reperfusion therapy. Figure 3 is the Suspected Stroke Algorithm, which identifies treatment goals for these patients.

Ischemic Stroke Signs and Symptoms Box ❶

The warning signs of an ischemic stroke or TIA may be varied, subtle, and transient, but they foretell a potentially life-threatening neurologic illness. Similar to symptoms of ACS, symptoms of ischemic stroke can be misinterpreted and denied. Emergency healthcare providers should recognize the importance of these symptoms and respond quickly with medical or surgical measures with proven efficacy in stroke management. The signs and symptoms of a stroke may be subtle:

- Sudden weakness or numbness of the face, arm, or leg, especially on one side of the body
- Sudden confusion
- Trouble speaking or understanding
- Sudden trouble seeing in one or both eyes
- Sudden trouble walking
- Dizziness or loss of balance or coordination
- Sudden severe headache with no known cause

Out-of-Hospital Management Box ❷

The Important Role of the Community EMS System in Stroke Care

Three of the 4 links in the Stroke Chain of Survival and the first 3 of the 7 D's of ACLS Stroke Care (**D**etection, **D**ispatch, and **D**elivery) require effective operation of the EMS system. For this reason the *2005 AHA Guidelines for Cardiopulmonary Resuscitation and Emergency Cardiovascular Care* and the 2007 AHA/ASA Guidelines for the Early Management of Adults With Ischemic Stroke strongly emphasize the important role of these personnel and services. Recent data show that 29% to 65% of patients with signs and symptoms of stroke contact local

EMS, but only 14% to 32% of them arrive within 2 hours of symptom onset.[16,17] EMS use is strongly associated with decreased time to initial physician assessment, computed tomography (CT) imaging for stroke, and neurologic evaluation.[18,19]

✔ Detection: Early Recognition of Stroke Signs and Symptoms

Early treatment of stroke depends on the patient, family members, or other bystanders recognizing the event. Patients will often ignore the initial signs and symptoms of a stroke, and most delay access to care for several hours after the onset of symptoms. Because of these time delays, many patients with ischemic stroke cannot benefit from fibrinolytic treatment, which must be started within 3 hours of symptom onset.

In one study of 100 stroke patients, only 8% had received information about the signs of stroke, yet nearly half had previously had a TIA or stroke. Unlike a heart attack, in which chest pain can be a dramatic and unrelenting symptom, a stroke may have a subtle presentation with only mild facial paralysis or speech difficulty. Mild signs or symptoms may go unnoticed or be denied by the patient or bystander. Strokes that occur while the patient is asleep or when the patient is alone further hamper prompt recognition and action.

Public education, an essential part of any strategy to ensure timely access to care for stroke patients, has been successful in reducing the time to arrival in the ED. In the Temple Foundation Stroke Project (TLL), tPA use increased from 15% to 52% after patient and physician educational initiatives, and this increase was sustained at 6 months.[20,21]

EMS Assessments and Actions

EMS assessments and actions for patients with suspected stroke include the following steps:
- Rapid identification of patients with signs and symptoms of acute stroke
- Support of vital functions
- Prearrival notification of the receiving facility
- Rapid transport of the patient to the receiving facility

✔ Dispatch: Call 911 and Priority EMS Dispatch

Stroke patients and their families must understand the need to activate the EMS system as soon as they suspect stroke signs

Foundation Facts **Time to Stroke Treatment**	EMS use is strongly associated with *decreased* time to • Initial physician assessment • CT imaging for stroke • Neurologic evaluation

or symptoms. The EMS system provides the safest and most efficient method for transporting the patient to the hospital.[22]

Emergency medical dispatchers play a critical role in the timely treatment of potential stroke patients. Data show that dispatchers correctly identify stroke symptoms on the basis of just the initial phone description in more than half the cases of stroke.[16,23] Dispatchers can triage emergencies over the telephone and prioritize calls to ensure a rapid response by the EMS system. Specific educational efforts about stroke are encouraged, and stroke dispatch should be given a priority similar to that for acute myocardial infarction and trauma.

✔ Delivery: Prompt Transport and Prearrival Notification to Hospital

Leaders in EMS and emergency medicine must develop training programs and patient care protocols to guide the actions of prehospital care providers. After the BLS Primary and ACLS Secondary Surveys and appropriate actions have been performed for airway, breathing, and circulation, EMS providers should immediately obtain a focused history and patient assessment (Table 3). A key component of the patient's history is the *time of symptom onset*. The history *must* include this information. The provider may need to obtain this and other details of the patient's history from family or the appropriate bystander. Preferably this person should be transported with the patient. Prehospital providers can help establish the precise time of stroke onset or the last time the patient was noted to be neurologically normal. This time point is viewed as "time zero," a starting point that is critical for time-dependent treatment with fibrinolytic agents.

Out-of-Hospital Stroke Scales for Early Detection and Delivery

The assessment includes a brief and focused examination for stroke. Providers can conduct a rapid neurologic assessment using validated tools such as the Cincinnati Prehospital Stroke Scale[24,25] or the Los Angeles Prehospital Stroke Screen.[26,27] Studies have confirmed the sensitivity and specificity of these 2 scales for prehospital identification of patients with ischemic stroke.

Cincinnati Prehospital Stroke Scale (CPSS)

The CPSS (Table 4) is based on physical examination only, and it can be completed in 30 to 60 seconds.[24] The EMS responder checks for 3 physical findings:

- Facial droop (Figure 4)
- Arm weakness (Figure 5)
- Speech abnormalities

Los Angeles Prehospital Stroke Screen (LAPSS)

The LAPSS (Table 5) requires the examiner to rule out other causes of altered level of consciousness (eg, history of seizures, severe hyperglycemia or hypoglycemia) and then identify asymmetry (right vs left) in any of 3 exam categories:

- Facial smile or grimace
- Grip
- Arm strength

The LAPSS builds on the physical findings of the CPSS, adding criteria for age, history of seizures, symptom duration, blood glucose level, and ambulation. A person with positive findings for all 6 criteria has a 97% probability of stroke.

Table 3. Key Components of a Focused Stroke Patient History

- Time of symptom onset
- Recent past medical history
- Stroke
- Transient ischemic attack (TIA)
- Atrial fibrillation
- Acute coronary syndromes (myocardial infarction)
- Trauma or surgery
- Bleeding disorder
- Complicating disease
- Hypertension
- Diabetes mellitus
- Medication use
- Anticoagulants (warfarin)
- Antiplatelet agents (aspirin and clopidogrel)
- Antihypertensives

Foundation Facts

First Priorities in Stroke EMS Assessment

After the BLS Primary and ACLS Secondary Surveys and appropriate actions have been performed for airway, breathing, and circulation, EMS providers should immediately obtain a focused history and patient assessment.

- *Time of symptom onset* is the single most important component of the patient's history.

Out-of-hospital stroke scales provide objective, validated methods for early detection of stroke and enable prearrival notification of the receiving hospital. When EMS personnel obtain positive findings on either the CPSS or the LAPSS, they should notify the receiving hospital that they have a patient with possible acute stroke. This information allows the hospital to activate stroke protocols before the patient arrives to ensure rapid patient evaluation and possible therapy. Advanced planning and collaboration allow medical control physicians to direct EMS providers to transport the patient to a hospital designated and organized to provide the full range of acute stroke care.

Destination Hospital Protocols

Once a patient with probable stroke is identified, transport the patient to the nearest *most appropriate* facility. Prearrival notification of the facility is key to speeding patient evaluation, computated tomogaphy imaging, and reperfusion therapy. An ambulance may bypass a hospital that does not have the resources or the institutional commitment to treat patients with a stroke if a more appropriate hospital is available within a reasonable transport interval.

Air medical transport appears to be beneficial, but studies are limited. Helicopters may extend the range of reperfusion therapy to rural areas, delivering teams to administer tPA or rapidly transferring patients to appropriate facilities.[28-31] Helicopter transfer of patients has been shown to be cost-effective.[31]

Prehospital Initial Studies

Prehospital care and assessment beyond initial management should be completed during patient transport and should not delay departure for the hospital. Establish intravenous (IV) access with normal saline. Avoid glucose-containing fluids unless hypoglycemia is strongly suspected or present (excess glucose may be harmful to stroke patients). Checking blood glucose in suspected stroke patients is prudent. Also initiate cardiac monitoring. Obtain a 12-lead ECG if the patient has ongoing ischemic-type chest discomfort.

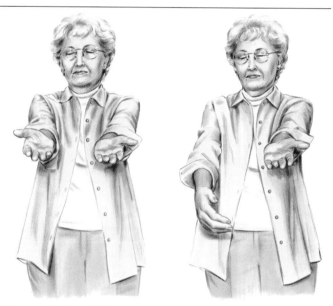

Figure 5. One-sided motor weakness (right arm).

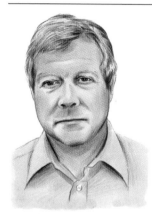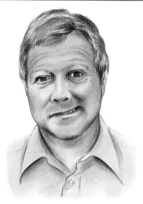

Figure 4. Facial droop.

Table 4. Cincinnati Prehospital Stroke Scale

Test	Findings
Facial Droop: Have the patient show teeth or smile (Figure 4)	❑ **Normal**—both sides of face move equally ❑ **Abnormal**—one side of face does not move as well as the other side
Arm Drift: Patient closes eyes and extends both arms straight out, with palms up, for 10 seconds (Figure 5)	❑ **Normal**—both arms move the same or both arms do not move at all (other findings, such as pronator drift, may be helpful) ❑ **Abnormal**—one arm does not move or one arm drifts down compared with the other
Abnormal Speech: Have the patient say "you can't teach an old dog new tricks"	❑ **Normal**—patient uses correct words with no slurring ❑ **Abnormal**—patient slurs words, uses the wrong words, or is unable to speak

Kothari R, Hall K, Brott T, Broderick J. Early stroke recognition: developing an out-of-hospital NIH Stroke Scale. *Acad Emerg Med.* 1997;4:986-990.

FYI **AHA/ASA 2007 Guidelines** **Hospital Bypass**	An ambulance may bypass a hospital if • The facility does not have the resources for acute stroke care • The facility lacks an institutional commitment to treat patients with a stroke • A more appropriate hospital is available within a reasonable transport interval

Table 5. Los Angeles Prehospital Stroke Screen

For *evaluation of acute, noncomatose, nontraumatic neurologic complaint.* If items 1 through 6 are *all* checked **"Yes"** (or "Unknown"), provide prearrival notification to hospital of potential stroke patient. If any item is checked "No," return to appropriate treatment protocol. *Interpretation:* 93% of patients with stroke will have a positive LAPSS score (sensitivity = 93%), and 97% of those with a positive LAPSS score will have a stroke (specificity = 97%). Note that the patient may still be experiencing a stroke if LAPSS criteria are not met.

Criteria	Yes	Unknown	No
1. Age >45 years	❑	❑	❑
2. History of seizures or epilepsy **absent**	❑	❑	❑
3. Symptom duration <24 hours	❑	❑	❑
4. At baseline, patient is **not** wheelchair bound or bedridden	❑	❑	❑
5. Blood glucose between 60 and 400	❑	❑	❑
6. *Obvious asymmetry* (right vs left) in *any* of the following 3 exam categories **(must be unilateral):**	❑	❑	❑

	Equal	R Weak	L Weak
Facial smile/grimace	❑	❑ Droop	❑ Droop
Grip	❑	❑ Weak grip ❑ No grip	❑ Weak grip ❑ No grip
Arm strength	❑	❑ Drifts down ❑ Falls rapidly	❑ Drifts down ❑ Falls rapidly

Kidwell CS, Saver JL, Schubert GB, Eckstein M, Starkman S. Design and retrospective analysis of the Los Angeles prehospital stroke screen (LAPSS). *Prehosp Emerg Care.* 1998;2:267-273. Kidwell CS, Starkman S, Eckstein M, Weems K, Saver JL. Identifying stroke in the field: prospective validation of the Los Angeles Prehospital Stroke Screen (LAPSS). *Stroke.* 2000;31:71-76.

In-Hospital Management

Critical Concept **ED Assessment Priorities**	Use protocols in the ED to minimize delay to definitive diagnosis and therapy.[32] Diagnostic studies ordered in the ED are aimed at 1. Establishing stroke as the cause of the patient's symptoms 2. Determining the exact time of onset 3. Differentiating ischemic from hemorrhagic stroke 4. Rapidly administering tPA to patients with ischemic stroke if no contraindications are present

✔ *Door: Immediate ED Triage*

Immediate General Assessment and Stabilization **Box ❸**

ED
Arrival

10
min

As a goal ED personnel should assess the patient with suspected stroke within 10 minutes of arrival in the ED. The ED physician should perform a neurologic screening assessment, order an emergent CT scan of the brain, and activate the stroke team or arrange consultation with a stroke expert. General care includes assessment and support of airway, breathing, and circulation and evaluation of baseline vital signs. Oxygen is administered to hypoxemic patients in the ED but is not recommended for patients without hypoxemia. Oxygen saturation should be monitored and maintained at ≥92%. A Cheyne-Stokes pattern of respirations can be reversed with oxygen supplementation. Establish (or confirm) IV access, and obtain blood samples for baseline studies (blood count, coagulation studies, blood glucose, etc). Treat hypoglycemia immediately if present.

A 12-lead ECG and other ancillary studies do not take priority over the CT scan and are performed as indicated and concomitant with expedited stroke care. The ECG may identify a recent acute myocardial infarction or arrhythmias (eg, atrial fibrillation) as the cause of a cardioembolic stroke. If the patient is hemodynamically stable, treatment of other arrhythmias, including bradycardia, premature atrial or ventricular contractions, or defects or blocks in atrioventricular conduction, may be unnecessary.[33] There is general agreement that cardiac monitoring should be done during the initial evaluation of patients with acute ischemic stroke to detect atrial fibrillation and potentially life-threatening arrhythmias.[34]

✔ *Data: ED Evaluation, Prompt Laboratory Studies, CT Imaging*

Immediately initiate diagnostic studies in all patients to assess conditions that may mimic stroke and comorbid problems that can complicate management. Consider the need for additional studies and perform them in selected patients as indicated. These tests may include the following:

All Patients	Selected Patients
• Noncontrast brain CT or MRI	• Chest x-ray
• Blood glucose	• Hepatic function
• Serum electrolytes	• Blood alcohol and toxicology screen
• Renal function	• Arterial blood gas
• CBC and platelet count	• Lumbar puncture
• Coagulation studies (PTT, PT, INR)	• EEG
• Oxygen saturation	• Pregnancy test
• ECG	

CT indicates computed tomography; MRI, magnetic resonance imaging; CBC, complete blood count; PPT, partial thromboplastin time; PT, prothrombin time; INR, international normalized ratio; ECG, electrocardiogram; and EEG, electroencephalogram.

Establish Time of Onset (<3 Hours Required for Fibrinolytics)

Protocols for EMS personnel should direct them to ask the patient and family about when they first noted any

---

Critical Concept **Diagnostic Studies— Do Not Delay CT Imaging or Fibrinolytic Therapy**	Routine and selected diagnostic studies are important, but they should not delay fibrinolytic therapy unless 1. There is clinical suspicion of a bleeding disorder 2. The patient has received heparin or warfarin 3. Anticoagulant status is uncertain

Critical Concept **Time of Symptom Onset Is Crucial**	*Inability to establish the time of symptom onset with accuracy is a contraindication to tPA therapy!* • If prehospital care personnel cannot reliably determine a specific time, ED personnel should continue the inquiries. Call or speak directly to a family member, coworker, or bystander.

stroke symptoms. Neither the patient nor family members may recall the exact hour and minute. But they may be able to relate the onset of symptoms to other events, such as a television or radio program that was playing, a telephone call, or someone's arrival or departure. Be aware that time of onset is difficult to establish for patients who are discovered unconscious or unable to communicate or for patients who awaken from sleep with neurologic abnormalities.

Immediate Neurologic Screening Assessment

The immediate neurologic stroke assessment should focus on 5 key assessments:

1. Onset of symptoms, or when the patient was last seen functioning normally
2. Level of consciousness
3. Level of stroke severity
4. Type of stroke: ischemic versus hemorrhagic
5. Location of stroke: anterior (carotid) versus posterior (vertebrobasilar)

The clinical status of stroke patients often fluctuates. Clinicians should perform several focused neurologic examinations to detect any deterioration or improvement.

Determine Level of Consciousness (Glasgow Coma Scale)

Altered consciousness or the appearance of confusion can complicate and delay evaluation. The Glasgow Coma Scale (GCS) (Table 6) provides a way to establish the severity of

Table 6. Glasgow Coma Scale

Eye opening	Score
Spontaneous	4
In response to speech	3
In response to pain	2
None	1
Best verbal response	
Oriented conversation	5
Confused conversation	4
Inappropriate words	3
Incomprehensible sounds	2
None	1
Best motor response	
Obeys	6
Localizes	5
Withdraws	4
Abnormal flexion	3
Abnormal extension	2
None	1

neurologic compromise in patients with altered consciousness and is a reliable tool to assess serial changes in function over time. The total score ranges from 3 to 15. It is the sum of the best response the patient displays for 3 functions: eye opening (1 through 4), verbal responses (1 through 5), and motor function (1 through 6).[35] The patient who has no verbal response, has no eye opening, and is flaccid has a GCS score of 3. In general a GCS score of 8 or less is associated with an ominous prognosis.

Immediate Neurologic Assessment by Stroke Team or Designee Box ❹

ED Arrival

25 min

The stroke team, another expert, or an emergency physician with access to remote stroke expert support will review the patient history and verify time of onset of symptoms (Box 4). This may require interviewing out-of-hospital providers, witnesses, and family members to establish the time that the patient was last known to be normal. Neurologic assessment is performed incorporating either the National Institutes of Health (NIH) Stroke Scale or Canadian Neurologic Scale.

Determine Severity of Stroke (NIH Stroke Scale)

The NIH Stroke Scale is a validated measure of stroke severity based on a detailed neurologic examination (cranial nerve and gait testing are omitted).[12] The NIH Stroke Scale allows either nurse stroke specialists or physicians to perform standardized neurologic evaluations of a patient.[12,36] The score correlates with long-term outcome in patients with ischemic stroke[36-38] and is designed to provide a reliable,[39] valid, and easy-to-perform alternative to the standard neurologic examination. The NIH Stroke Scale can be performed in fewer than 7 minutes. The NIH Stroke Scale received further validation during the landmark National Institute of Neurological Disorders and Stroke (NINDS) trial of tPA for acute ischemic stroke.[4]

The total score ranges from 0 (normal) to 42 points. The scale covers the following major areas[40]:

- Level of consciousness: alert, drowsy; knows month, age; performs tasks correctly
- Visual assessment: follows finger with or without gaze palsy, forced deviation; hemianopsia (none, partial, complete, bilateral)
- Motor function: face, arm, leg strength and movement
- Sensation: pin prick to face, arm, trunk, leg; compare side to side
- Cerebellar function: finger-nose; heel down shin
- Language: aphasia (name items, describe a picture, read sentences); dysarthria (evaluate speech clarity by having patient repeat listed words)

Table 7. NIH Stroke Scale: "Quick and Easy" Version

Category	Description	Score	Baseline Date/Time	Date/Time
1a. Level of consciousness (LOC) *(Alert, drowsy, etc)*	Alert Drowsy Stuporous Coma	0 1 2 3		
1b. LOC questions *(Month, age)*	Answers both correctly Answers 1 correctly Incorrect	0 1 2		
1c. LOC commands *(Open, close eyes; make fist, let go)*	Obeys both correctly Obeys 1 correctly Incorrect	0 1 2		
2. Best gaze *(Eyes open—patient follows examiner's finger or face)*	Normal Partial gaze palsy Forced deviation	0 1 2		
3. Visual *(Introduce visual stimulus/threat to patient's visual field quadrants)*	No visual loss Partial hemianopia Complete hemianopia Bilateral hemianopia	0 1 2 3		
4. Facial palsy *(Show teeth, raise eyebrows, and squeeze eyes shut)*	Normal Minor Partial Complete	0 1 2 3		
5a. Motor arm—left *(Elevate extremity to 90° and score drift/ movement)*	No drift Drift Can't resist gravity No effort against gravity No movement Amputation, joint fusion	0 1 2 3 4 UN		
5b. Motor arm—right *(Elevate extremity to 90° and score drift/ movement)*	No drift Drift Can't resist gravity No effort against gravity No movement Amputation, joint fusion	0 1 2 3 4 UN		
6a. Motor leg—left *(Elevate extremity to 30° and score drift/ movement)*	No drift Drift Can't resist gravity No effort against gravity No movement Amputation, joint fusion	0 1 2 3 4 UN		
6b. Motor leg—right *(Elevate extremity to 30° and score drift/ movement)*	No drift Drift Can't resist gravity No effort against gravity No movement Amputation, joint fusion	0 1 2 3 4 UN		

UN indicates undetermined.

Category	Description	Score	Baseline Date/Time	Date/Time
7. Limb ataxia *(Finger-nose, heel down shin)*	Absent Present in 1 limb Present in 2 limbs	0 1 2		
8. Sensory *(Pin prick to face, arm, trunk, and leg—compare side to side)*	Normal Partial loss Severe loss	0 1 2		
9. Best language *(Name items, describe a picture, and read sentences)*	No aphasia Mild to moderate aphasia Severe aphasia Mute	0 1 2 3		
10. Dysarthria *(Evaluate speech clarity by patient repeating listed words)*	Normal articulation Mild to moderate dysarthria Near to unintelligible or worse Intubated or other physical barrier	0 1 2 UN		
11. Extinction and inattention *(Use information from prior testing to identify neglect or double simultaneous stimuli testing)*	No neglect Partial neglect Complete neglect	0 1 2		
Individual administering scale:				

Adapted with permission from Spilker J, Kongable G. The NIH Stroke Scale: its importance and practical application in the clinical setting. *Stroke Intervent.* 2000;2:7-14. For further information, please refer to the website *www.stroke-site.org*.

An NIH Stroke Scale score of less than 4 usually indicates minor neurologic deficits, such as sensory losses, dysarthria, or some manual clumsiness. Fibrinolytic agents are not recommended for these patients because treatment offers minimal benefits relative to the risks. Some disabling neurologic deficits, such as isolated severe aphasia (score of 3) or the visual field losses of hemianopsia (score of 2 or 3), can be associated with a low score on the NIH Stroke Scale. Patients with these deficits may be exceptions to the recommendation against fibrinolytic agents for patients with an NIH Stroke Scale score of less than 4.

Severe deficits (score greater than 22) indicate large areas of ischemic damage. Patients with such deficits face an increased risk of brain hemorrhage. In general the use of fibrinolytic treatment in these patients should follow careful discussion with the patient, the patient's spouse and family, and the admitting physicians to ensure that everyone understands the risk and benefits. For some patients with severe deficits the probability of harm outweighs the potential for significant benefit. A favorable risk-benefit ratio varies from patient to patient. The responsible clinician should always evaluate therapeutic decisions on an individual basis in close collaboration with the patient and family.

Management of Hypertension

Management of hypertension in the stroke patient is controversial. For patients eligible for fibrinolytic therapy, however, control of blood pressure is required to reduce the risk of bleeding. If a patient who is otherwise eligible for treatment with tPA has elevated blood pressure, providers can try to lower it to a systolic pressure of <185 mm Hg and a diastolic blood pressure of <110 mm Hg. Because the maximum interval from onset of stroke until effective treatment of stroke with tPA is limited, most patients with sustained hypertension above these levels (ie, systolic blood pressure >185 mm Hg or diastolic blood pressure >110 mm Hg) cannot be treated with IV tPA (Table 8).[41-43]

Table 8. Approach to Arterial Hypertension in Acute Ischemic Stroke

Eligible for Treatment	During or After Treatment
Indication that patient is eligible for treatment with intravenous tPA or other acute reperfusion intervention	Management of blood pressure during and after treatment with tPA or other acute reperfusion intervention
Blood Pressure Level	Monitor blood pressure every 15 minutes during treatment and then for another 2 hours, then every 30 minutes for 6 hours, and then every hour for 16 hours
Systolic >185 mm Hg or diastolic >110 mm Hg	**Blood Pressure Level**
Labetalol 10 to 20 mg IV over 1 to 2 minutes, may repeat ×1;	**Systolic 180 to 230 mm Hg or diastolic 105 to 120 mm Hg**
or	Labetalol 10 mg IV over 1 to 2 minutes, may repeat every 10 to 20 minutes, maximum dose of 300 mg;
Nitropaste 1 to 2 inches;	or
or	Labetalol 10 mg IV followed by an infusion at 2 to 8 mg/min
Nicardipine infusion, 5 mg/h, titrate up by 2.5 mg/h at 5- to 15-minute intervals, maximum dose 15 mg/h; when desired blood pressure attained, reduce to 3 mg/h	**Systolic >230 mm Hg or diastolic 121 to 140 mm Hg**
	Labetalol 10 mg IV over 1 to 2 minutes, may repeat every 10 to 20 minutes, maximum dose of 300 mg;
If blood pressure does not decline and remains >185/110 mm Hg, do not administer tPA	or
	Labetalol 10 mg IV followed by an infusion at 2 to 8 mg/min;
	or
	Nicardipine infusion, 5 mg/h, titrate up to desired effect by increasing 2.5 mg/h every 5 minutes to maximum of 15 mg/h
	If blood pressure not controlled, consider sodium nitroprusside

Brain and Vascular Imaging Box ➎

The most commonly obtained brain imaging test is a non–contrast-enhanced CT scan, but some centers can now obtain a magnetic resonance imaging (MRI) scan with efficiency equal to CT scanning. The noncontrast CT scan accurately identifies most cases of intracranial hemorrhage and discriminates nonvascular causes of neurologic symptoms mimicking stroke (eg, brain tumor). Ongoing research is evaluating MRI, magnetic resonance angiography, and multimodal CT, which includes noncontrast CT, perfusion CT, and CT angiographic studies.

ED Arrival

45 min

Ideally the CT scan should be completed within 25 minutes of the patient's arrival in the ED and should be read within 45 minutes of ED arrival (Box 5). Emergent CT or MRI scans of patients with suspected stroke should be promptly evaluated by a physician with expertise in interpretation of these studies.[44,45] During the first few hours of an ischemic stroke, the noncontrast CT scan may not show signs of brain ischemia.

The CT scan is central to the triage and therapy of the stroke patient. If the CT scan shows no evidence of hemorrhage, the patient may be a candidate for fibrinolytic therapy (Boxes 6 and 8).

Foundation Facts **Treatment of Hypertension in Stroke**	Treatment of hypertension in acute ischemic stroke remains controversial. Administration of tPA with hypertension is associated with excess intracerebral hemorrhage. • Data suggests that prompt treatment should be initiated when systolic blood pressure exceeds 180 mm Hg or diastolic blood pressure exceeds 105 mm Hg. • A blood pressure >185 mm Hg systolic or >110 mm Hg diastolic is a contraindication for administration of tPA. • If blood pressure >185 mm Hg systolic or >110 mm Hg diastolic develops during or after tPA administration, begin immediate treatment.

The Initial Noncontrast CT Scan

On CT images blood from a hemorrhagic stroke has a density that is only about 3% greater than the density of brain tissue. On modern CT scanners this 3% difference in density can be manipulated so that the hemorrhage and free blood will appear distinctly white in comparison with surrounding tissues. Contrast agents also "light up" on CT scans. Because these agents would obscure the high-contrast areas of free blood, the initial CT scan is made without contrast enhancement. Acute intracranial complications of stroke, such as hydrocephalus, edema, mass effect, or shift of normal brain structures, can also be seen with CT.

Thrombotic Stroke

During the first few hours of a thrombotic or embolic stroke, the noncontrast CT scan will generally appear *normal*. Brain structures without normal blood flow appear initially the same as structures with good blood flow on the CT scan. For this reason the CT scan will continue to appear "normal" for a few hours after blood flow is blocked or reduced to an area of the brain. A well-defined area of hypodensity, purported to be caused by lack of blood flow past an occlusion, will rarely develop within the first 3 hours of a stroke. The brain tissue downstream from an occlusion is indeed ischemic and damaged. It soon begins to swell with edema and inflammation.

After 6 to 12 hours the edema and swelling are sufficient to produce a hypodense area that is usually visible on a CT scan. This well-defined hypodensity rarely develops within the 3-hour limit required for administration of tPA. In fact the time since stroke onset is likely to be more than 3 hours if a hypodensity is present on the CT scan. For this reason a hypodense area on the CT scan generally excludes a patient from fibrinolytic therapy. Larger infarctions can cause early CT changes. But these changes are often subtle, such as obscuration of the gray-white matter junction, sulcal effacement, or early hypodensity.

Hemorrhagic Stroke

If the initial noncontrast CT scan shows intracerebral or subarachnoid hemorrhage, the responsible physician should immediately consult a neurosurgeon and initiate appropriate actions for acute hemorrhage (see below and algorithm Boxes 7 and 11).

✔ Decision: Diagnosis and Decision: Appropriate Therapy

Risk Assessment and Administration of IV tPA Box ⑩

ED Arrival 60 min

When the CT scan shows no hemorrhage, the probability of acute ischemic stroke is high. The physician or stroke team should review the inclusion and exclusion criteria for IV fibrinolytic therapy (Table 9) and perform a repeat neurologic examination (incorporating the NIH Stroke Scale or Canadian Neurological Scale). If the patient's neurologic signs are spontaneously clearing (ie, function is rapidly improving toward normal) and are near baseline, fibrinolytic administration is not recommended (Box 6).

Critical Concept

Normal CT = Candidate for Fibrinolytic Therapy

An important, if somewhat counterintuitive, point to remember is that a completely normal CT scan—no sign of hemorrhage, no large areas of no flow, and no hypodense areas—is supportive of tPA administration in a stroke patient who otherwise meets the criteria for fibrinolytic therapy.

Table 9. Fibrinolytic Checklist

Use of tPA in Patients With Acute Ischemic Stroke

All boxes must be checked before tPA can be given.

Note: The following checklist includes FDA-approved indications and contraindications for tPA administration for acute ischemic stroke. A physician with expertise in acute stroke care may modify this list.

Inclusion Criteria (all Yes boxes in this section must be checked):

Yes

☐ Age 18 years or older?

☐ Clinical diagnosis of ischemic stroke with a measurable neurologic deficit?

☐ Time of symptom onset (when patient was last seen normal) well established as <180 minutes (3 hours) before treatment would begin?

Exclusion Criteria (all No boxes in "Contraindications" section must be checked):

Contraindications:

No

☐ Evidence of intracranial hemorrhage on pretreatment noncontrast head CT?

☐ Clinical presentation suggestive of subarachnoid hemorrhage even with normal CT?

☐ CT shows multilobar infarction (hypodensity greater than one third cerebral hemisphere)?

☐ History of intracranial hemorrhage?

☐ Uncontrolled hypertension: At the time treatment should begin, systolic pressure remains >185 mm Hg or diastolic pressure remains >110 mm Hg despite repeated measurements?

☐ Known arteriovenous malformation, neoplasm, or aneurysm?

☐ Seizure with post-ictal residual neurologic impairment? *Note:* Seizure alone at time of onset is not an absolute contraindication.

☐ Active internal bleeding or acute trauma (fracture)?

☐ Acute bleeding diathesis, including but not limited to

  — Platelet count <100 000/mm^3?

  — Heparin received within 48 hours, resulting in an activated partial thromboplastin time (aPTT) that is greater than upper limit of normal for laboratory?

  — Current use of anticoagulant (eg, warfarin sodium) that has produced an elevated international normalized ratio (INR) >1.7 or prothrombin time (PT) >15 seconds?*

☐ Within 3 months of intracranial or intraspinal surgery, serious head trauma, or previous stroke?

☐ Arterial puncture at a noncompressible site within past 7 days?

Relative Contraindications/Precautions:

Recent experience suggests that under some circumstances—with careful consideration and weighing of risk-to-benefit ratio—patients may receive fibrinolytic therapy despite one or more relative contraindications. Consider the pros and cons of tPA administration carefully if any of these relative contraindications is present:

- Only minor or rapidly improving stroke symptoms (clearing spontaneously)
- Within 14 days of major surgery or serious trauma
- Recent gastrointestinal or urinary tract hemorrhage (within previous 21 days)
- Recent acute myocardial infarction (within previous 3 months)
- Postmyocardial infarction pericarditis
- Abnormal blood glucose level (<50 or >400 mg/dL [<2.8 or >22.2 mmol/L])

---

*In patients without recent use of oral anticoagulants or heparin, treatment with tPA can be initiated before availability of coagulation study results but should be discontinued if the international normalized ratio (INR) is >1.7 or the partial thromboplastin time is elevated by local laboratory standards.

Major Benefit—Improved Neurologic Outcome Without Mortality

Several studies have documented a higher likelihood of good to excellent functional outcome when tPA is administered to adults with acute ischemic stroke within 3 hours of symptom onset. Such results are obtained when tPA is administered by physicians in hospitals with a stroke protocol that rigorously adheres to the eligibility criteria and therapeutic regimen of the NINDS protocol. These results have been supported by a subsequent 1-year follow-up study, reanalysis of the NINDS data, and a meta-analysis. Evidence from prospective, randomized studies in adults also documents a greater likelihood of benefit the earlier treatment is begun. Many physicians have emphasized the flaws in the NINDS trials. But additional analyses of the original NINDS data by an independent group of investigators confirmed the validity of the results, verifying that improved outcomes in the tPA treatment arm persist even when imbalances in baseline stroke severity among treatment groups are corrected.

Major Risk—Intracranial Hemorrhage and Death

Like all medications, fibrinolytics have potential adverse effects. The physician must verify that there are no exclusion criteria, consider the risks and benefits to the patient, and be prepared to monitor and treat any potential complications. The major complication of IV tPA for stroke is symptomatic intracranial hemorrhage. This complication occurred in 6.4% of the 312 patients treated in the NINDS trial[4] and 4.6% of the 1135 patients treated in 60 Canadian centers.[46] A meta-analysis of 15 published case series on the open-label use of tPA for acute ischemic stroke in general clinical practice shows a symptomatic hemorrhage rate of 5.2% of 2639 patients treated.[47] Other complications include orolingual angioedema (occurs in about 1.5% of patients), acute hypotension, and systemic bleeding. In one large prospective registry, major systemic bleeding was uncommon (0.4%) and usually occurred at the site of femoral groin puncture for acute angiography.[46,48]

How to Minimize Risks and Maximize Benefits of tPA for Acute Stroke

In the NINDS trial fatal intracranial hemorrhage occurred in approximately 3 of every 100 patients treated with tPA (3%) but only 3 of every 1000 (0.3%) receiving placebo. This means that the risk of fatal bleeding into the brain was 10 times greater in the tPA-treated patients. But it is important to note that overall mortality was not increased in the tPA-treated group. For a perspective on this risk, consider that the rate of fatal hemorrhagic stroke in patients given tPA within 12 hours of acute coronary artery occlusion averages less than 1%. To minimize the risks and maximize the benefits, responsible clinicians must adhere strictly to the inclusion and exclusion criteria (Table 9). tPA therapy is acceptable only with strict adherence to these criteria.

Strategies for Success

Administration of IV tPA to patients with acute ischemic stroke who meet the NINDS eligibility criteria is recommended if tPA is administered by physicians in the setting of a clearly defined protocol, a knowledgeable team, and institutional commitment. It is important to note that the superior outcomes reported in both community and tertiary care hospitals in the NINDS trials have been difficult to replicate in hospitals with less experience in, and institutional commitment to, acute stroke care.[49,50] Failure to adhere to protocol is associated with an increased rate of complications, particularly the risk of symptomatic intracranial hemorrhage.[51,52] There is also strong evidence to avoid all delays and treat patients as soon as possible.

Community hospitals have reported outcomes comparable to the results of the NINDS trials after implementing a stroke program with a focus on quality improvement.[46,53,54] The experience of the Cleveland Clinic system is instructive.[50,54] A quality improvement program increased compliance with the tPA treatment protocol in 9 community hospitals, and the rate of symptomatic intracerebral hemorrhage fell from 13.4% to 6.4%.[54]

There is a relationship between violations of the NINDS treatment protocol and increased risk of symptomatic intracerebral hemorrhage and death.[47] In Germany there was an increased risk of death after administration of tPA for acute ischemic stroke in hospitals that treated 5 or fewer patients per year, which suggests that clinical experience is an important factor in ensuring adherence to protocol.[48] Adding a dedicated stroke team to a community hospital can increase the number of patients with acute stroke treated with fibrinolytic therapy and produce excellent clinical outcomes.[55] These findings show that it is important to have an institutional commitment to ensure optimal patient outcomes.

FYI **AHA/ASA 2007 Guidelines**	New recommendations for stroke care include • Transport to closest facility with resources to care for stroke patients (ie, hospital bypass) • Development of primary stroke centers—strongly recommended • Certification of stroke centers by external agency—strongly encouraged

Critical Concept **Anticoagulants and Antiplatelet Therapy**	Neither anticoagulants nor antiplatelet treatment is administered for 24 hours after administration of tPA, typically until a follow-up CT scan at 24 hours shows no hemorrhage (Box 10). • If the patient has brain hemorrhage, DO NOT GIVE ASPIRIN (Box 7). • If the patient has ischemic stroke but is not a candidate for tPA, consider aspirin or another antiplatelet agent. • DO NOT administer heparin (unfractionated or low molecular weight). Heparin is associated with an increased risk of bleeding within the first 24 hours.

To provide standardized and comprehensive stroke care, the Brain Attack Coalition published criteria for primary stroke centers and comprehensive stroke centers—PSCs and CSCs. A PSC has resources to care for many patients with uncomplicated stroke. A CSC provides comprehensive and specialized care for patients with a complicated stroke and those requiring specialized care, such as surgery or stroke intensive care.[56]

✔ Drug: Administration of tPA and Other Therapies

Additional Actions Before Fibrinolytic Therapy

Review for CT Exclusions: Are Any Observed?

• Hemorrhage, either intracerebral or subarachnoid, must be excluded. Failure to identify a small area of hemorrhage could be a **fatal error.**

• Areas of well-defined hypodensity are generally CT exclusions because they indicate either that more than 3 hours have passed since the infarction or that a large area of the brain is threatened.

• CT indications of a large infarction (early hypodensity, obscured junction between gray and white matter, or sulcal effacement) are relative contraindications to tPA. Larger brain infarctions are prone to undergo hemorrhagic transformation, exposing a patient receiving a fibrinolytic agent to the risk of fatal intracerebral hemorrhage. These patients, however, have a poor outcome without intervention, so some authors have concluded that patients with severe deficit or CT findings of hypodensity or mass effect can be candidates for tPA therapy, with both greater possibility of benefit and greater risk of harm.

Repeat Neurologic Exam: Are Deficits Variable or Rapidly Improving?

• The risk of harm from tPA is not justified for patients with a TIA or rapidly improving deficits. These patients usually have lesions or partial occlusions that are not resolved by tPA. However, some stroke experts consider administration of tPA if there is a low NIHSS score or if the patient is aphasic.

Review Fibrinolytic Exclusions: Are Any Observed?

• Table 9 lists the major exclusions for the use of tPA. Such a checklist, in a form suitable for inclusion in a patient's medical record, should be available wherever stroke patients might be treated with fibrinolytics.

• One of the clinicians responsible for final decisions about tPA should personally complete this or a similar checklist, sign it, and make it a part of the formal medical record.

Review Patient Data: Is Time Since Symptom Onset Now More Than 3 Hours?

• This step reminds the clinician to make one last review of all the information gathered during the patient assessments. In particular, document the estimated length of time that has passed since the onset of the stroke.

• IV infusion of the tPA must begin within 180 minutes of the beginning of stroke symptoms.

✔ Drug: Administration and Monitoring of tPA Infusion

Fibrinolytic therapy is a Class I recommendation for a highly selected, well-defined subset of ischemic stroke patients. Treatment with IV tPA within 3 hours of the onset of ischemic stroke improved clinical outcome at 3 months. ED-based or hospital-based stroke specialists should aim to start the initial bolus within 60 minutes of arrival in the ED. Ten percent of a total dose of 0.9 mg/kg (maximum 90 mg) is given by bolus administration and the remainder over 60 minutes.

During tPA infusion:

• Monitor neurologic status; if any signs of deterioration develop, obtain an emergent CT scan.

• Monitor blood pressure, which may increase during fibrinolytic treatment. Initiate antihypertensive treatment with any increase over 185 mm Hg systolic or over 110 mm Hg diastolic (see above).

• Admit patient to the Critical Care Unit, Stroke Unit, or other skilled facility capable of careful observation, frequent neurologic assessments, and cardiovascular monitoring.

• Avoid anticoagulant or antiplatelet treatment for the next 24 hours.

Intra-arterial tPA

For patients with acute ischemic stroke who are not candidates for standard IV fibrinolysis, administration of intra-arterial fibrinolysis in centers that have the resources and expertise available may be considered within the first few hours after the onset of symptoms. Intra-arterial administration of tPA has not yet been approved by the US Food and Drug Administration (2007).

Transition to Critical Care and Rehabilitation

General Stroke Care

Additional stroke care includes support of the airway, oxygenation and ventilation, and nutritional support. Normal saline is administered at approximately 75 to 100 mL/h to maintain euvolemia if needed. The reported frequency of seizures during the first days of stroke ranges from 2% to 23%. Most seizures occur during the first day and can recur. Seizure prophylaxis is not recommended. Treatment of acute seizures followed by administration of anticonvulsants to prevent further seizures is recommended, consistent with the established management of seizures. Monitor the patient for signs of increased intracranial pressure. Continued control of blood pressure is required to reduce the risk of bleeding.

Hyperglycemia

Hyperglycemia is present in about one third of patients admitted with stroke. Hyperglycemia is associated with worse clinical outcome in patients with acute ischemic stroke than is normoglycemia, but there is no direct evidence that active glucose control improves clinical outcome.[57,58] There is evidence that insulin treatment of hyperglycemia in other critically ill patients improves survival rates. For this reason administration of IV or subcutaneous insulin may be considered to lower blood glucose in patients with acute ischemic stroke when the serum glucose level is >10 mmol/L (greater than about 200 mg/dL).[59,60]

Temperature Control

Increased temperature in stroke is associated with poor neurologic outcome. No data has demonstrated that lowering temperature improves outcome, but fever >37.5°C (99.5°F) should be treated and the source of fever identified and treated if possible.

Induced hypothermia can exert neuroprotective effects after a stroke. Hypothermia has been shown to improve survival and functional outcome in patients following resuscitation from ventricular fibrillation sudden cardiac arrest, but it has not been shown in controlled human trials to be effective for acute ischemic stroke. In some small human pilot studies and in animal models, hypothermia (33°C to 36°C [91.4°F to 96.8°F]) for acute ischemic stroke has been shown to be relatively safe and feasible (level of evidence 3 to 5). Although effects of hypothermia on both global and focal cerebral ischemia in animals have been promising, cooling to ≤33°C (91.4°F) appears to be associated with increased complications, including hypotension, cardiac arrhythmias, cardiac failure, pneumonia, thrombocytopenia, and a rebound increase in intracranial pressure during rewarming. At present there is insufficient scientific evidence to recommend for or against the use of hypothermia in the treatment of acute ischemic stroke (Class Indeterminate).

Stroke Units

Patients are admitted to a stroke unit (if available) for careful observation, including monitoring of blood pressure and neurologic status and treatment of hypertension if indicated. If the patient's neurologic status deteriorates, order an emergent CT scan to determine if cerebral edema or hemorrhage is responsible for the deterioration and treat if possible.

All patients with stroke should be screened for dysphagia before anything is given by mouth. A simple bedside screening evaluation involves asking the patient to sip water from a cup. If the patient can sip and swallow without difficulty, the patient is asked to take a large gulp of water and swallow. If there are no signs of coughing or aspiration after 30 seconds, then it is safe for the patient to have a thickened diet until formally assessed by a speech pathologist. Medications may be given in applesauce or jam. Any patient who fails a swallow test may be given medications such as aspirin rectally or if appropriate via the IV, intramuscular, or subcutaneous route.

References

1. American Heart Association. *Heart Disease and Stroke Statistics—2008 Update*. Dallas, Tex: American Heart Association; 2008.

2. Schwamm LH, Pancioli A, Acker JE III, Goldstein LB, Zorowitz RD, Shephard TJ, Moyer P, Gorman M, Johnston SC, Duncan PW, Gorelick P, Frank J, Stranne SK, Smith R, Federspiel W, Horton KB, Magnis E, Adams RJ. Recommendations for the establishment of stroke systems of care: recommendations from the American Stroke Association's Task Force on the Development of Stroke Systems. *Circulation*. 2005;111:1078-1091.

3. Dobkin BH. Clinical practice. Rehabilitation after stroke. *N Engl J Med*. 2005;352:1677-1684.

4. Tissue plasminogen activator for acute ischemic stroke. The National Institute of Neurological Disorders and Stroke rt-PA Stroke Study Group. *N Engl J Med*. 1995;333:1581-1587.

5. Hazinski M. D-mystifying recognition and management of stroke. *Currents in Emergency Cardiac Care*. 1996;7:8.

6. Acute stroke: current treatment and paradigms. In: Cummins R, Field J, Hazinski M, eds. *ACLS: Principles and Practice*. Dallas, Tex: American Heart Association; 2003:437-482.

7. Adams HP Jr, del Zoppo G, Alberts MJ, Bhatt DL, Brass L, Furlan A, Grubb RL, Higashida RT, Jauch EC, Kidwell C, Lyden PD, Morgenstern LB, Qureshi AI, Rosenwasser RH, Scott PA, Wijdicks EF. Guidelines for the early management of adults with ischemic stroke: a guideline from the American Heart Association/American Stroke Association Stroke Council, Clinical Cardiology Council, Cardiovascular Radiology and Intervention Council, and the Atherosclerotic Peripheral Vascular Disease and Quality of Care Outcomes in Research Interdisciplinary Working Groups: The American Academy of Neurology affirms the value of this guideline as an educational tool for neurologists. *Circulation*. 2007;115:e478-e534.

8. Emergency department: rapid identification and treatment of patients with acute myocardial infarction. National Heart Attack Alert Program Coordinating Committee, 60 Minutes to Treatment Working Group. *Ann Emerg Med*. 1994;23:311-329.

9. Carr S, Farb A, Pearce WH, Virmani R, Yao JS. Atherosclerotic plaque rupture in symptomatic carotid artery stenosis. *J Vasc Surg*. 1996;23:755-765; discussion 765-766.

10. Spagnoli LG, Mauriello A, Sangiorgi G, Fratoni S, Bonanno E, Schwartz RS, Piepgras DG, Pistolese R, Ippoliti A, Holmes DR Jr. Extracranial thrombotically active carotid plaque as a risk factor for ischemic stroke. *JAMA*. 2004;292:1845-1852.

11. Redgrave JN, Lovett JK, Gallagher PJ, Rothwell PM. Histological assessment of 526 symptomatic carotid plaques in relation to the nature and timing of ischemic symptoms: the Oxford plaque study. *Circulation*. 2006;113:2320-2328.

12. Brott T, Adams HP Jr, Olinger CP, Marler JR, Barsan WG, Biller J, Spilker J, Holleran R, Eberle R, Hertzberg V, et al. Measurements of acute cerebral infarction: a clinical examination scale. *Stroke*. 1989;20:864-870.

13. Brott T, Haley EC Jr, Levy DE, Barsan W, Broderick J, Sheppard GL, Spilker J, Kongable GL, Massey S, Reed R, et al. Urgent therapy for stroke, part I: pilot study of tissue plasminogen activator administered within 90 minutes. *Stroke*. 1992;23:632-640.

14. Zachariah BS, Pepe PE. The development of emergency medical dispatch in the USA: a historical perspective. *Eur J Emerg Med*. 1995;2:109-112.

15. Feldmann E, Gordon N, Brooks JM, Brass LM, Fayad PB, Sawaya KL, Nazareno F, Levine SR. Factors associated with early presentation of acute stroke. *Stroke*. 1993;24:1805-1810.

16. Handschu R, Poppe R, Rauss J, Neundorfer B, Erbguth F. Emergency calls in acute stroke. *Stroke*. 2003;34:1005-1009.

17. Williams JE, Rosamond WD, Morris DL. Stroke symptom attribution and time to emergency department arrival: the Delay in Accessing Stroke Healthcare Study. *Acad Emerg Med*. 2000;7:93-96.

18. Morris DL, Rosamond W, Madden K, Schultz C, Hamilton S. Prehospital and emergency department delays after acute stroke: the Genentech Stroke Presentation Survey. *Stroke*. 2000;31:2585-2590.

19. Schroeder EB, Rosamond WD, Morris DL, Evenson KR, Hinn AR. Determinants of use of emergency medical services in a population with stroke symptoms: the Second Delay in Accessing Stroke Healthcare (DASH II) Study. *Stroke*. 2000;31:2591-2596.

20. Morgenstern LB, Bartholomew LK, Grotta JC, Staub L, King M, Chan W. Sustained benefit of a community and profession-al intervention to increase acute stroke therapy. *Arch Intern Med*. 2003;163:2198-2202.

21. Morgenstern LB, Staub L, Chan W, Wein TH, Bartholomew LK, King M, Felberg RA, Burgin WS, Groff J, Hickenbottom SL, Saldin K, Demchuk AM, Kalra A, Dhingra A, Grotta JC. Improving delivery of acute stroke therapy: the TLL Temple Foundation Stroke Project. *Stroke*. 2002;33:160-166.

22. Barsan WG, Brott TG, Broderick JP, Haley EC, Levy DE, Marler JR. Time of hospital presentation in patients with acute stroke. *Arch Intern Med*. 1993;153:2558-2561.

23. Kothari R, Barsan W, Brott T, Broderick J, Ashbrock S. Frequency and accuracy of prehospital diagnosis of acute stroke. *Stroke*. 1995;26:937-941.

24. Kothari RU, Pancioli A, Liu T, Brott T, Broderick J. Cincinnati Prehospital Stroke Scale: reproducibility and validity. *Ann Emerg Med*. 1999;33:373-378.

25. Kothari R, Hall K, Brott T, Broderick J. Early stroke recognition: developing an out-of-hospital NIH Stroke Scale. *Acad Emerg Med*. 1997;4:986-990.

26. Kidwell CS, Saver JL, Schubert GB, Eckstein M, Starkman S. Design and retrospective analysis of the Los Angeles Prehospital Stroke Screen (LAPSS). *Prehosp Emerg Care*. 1998;2:267-273.

27. Kidwell CS, Starkman S, Eckstein M, Weems K, Saver JL. Identifying stroke in the field. Prospective validation of the Los Angeles prehospital stroke screen (LAPSS). *Stroke*. 2000;31:71-76.

28. Chalela JA, Kasner SE, Jauch EC, Pancioli AM. Safety of air medical transportation after tissue plasminogen activator administration in acute ischemic stroke. *Stroke*. 1999; 30:2366-2368.

29. Conroy MB, Rodriguez SU, Kimmel SE, Kasner SE. Helicopter transfer offers a potential benefit to patients with acute stroke. *Stroke*. 1999;30:2580-2584.

30. Silbergleit R, Scott PA. Thrombolysis for acute stroke: the incontrovertible, the controvertible, and the uncertain. *Acad Emerg Med*. 2005;12:348-351.

31. Silbergleit R, Scott PA, Lowell MJ, Silbergleit R. Cost-effectiveness of helicopter transport of stroke patients for thrombolysis. *Acad Emerg Med*. 2003;10:966-972.

32. A systems approach to immediate evaluation and management of hyperacute stroke. Experience at eight centers and implications for community practice and patient care. The National Institute of Neurological Disorders and Stroke (NINDS) rt-PA Stroke Study Group. *Stroke*. 1997;28:1530-1540.

33. Oppenheimer SM, Cechetto DF, Hachinski VC. Cerebrogenic cardiac arrhythmias: cerebral electrocardiographic influences and their role in sudden death. *Arch Neurol*. 1990;47:513-519.

34. Adams HJ, Brott T, Crowell R, Furlan A, Gomez C, Grotta J, Helgason C, Marler J, Woolson R, Zivin J, Feinberg W, Mayberg M. Guidelines for the management of patients with acute ischemic stroke: a statement for healthcare professionals from a special writing group of the Stroke Council, American Heart Association. *Stroke*. 1994;25:1901-1914.

35. Teasdale G, Jennett B. Assessment of coma and impaired consciousness: a practical scale. *Lancet*. 1974;2:81-84.

36. Lyden P, Rapp K, Babcock T, et al. Ultra-rapid identification, triage, and enrollment of stroke patients into clinical trials. *J Stroke Cerebrovasc Dis*. 1994;2:106-113.

37. Brott T. Utility of the NIH Stroke Scale. *Cerebrovasc Dis*. 1992;2:241-242.

38. Lyden P, Lu M, Jackson C, Marler J, Kothari R, Brott T, Zivin J. Underlying structure of the National Institutes of Health Stroke Scale: results of a factor analysis. NINDS rtPA tPA Stroke Trial Investigators. *Stroke*. 1999;30:2347-2354.

39. Goldstein LB, Bertels C, Davis JN. Interrater reliability of the NIH Stroke Scale. *Arch Neurol*. 1989;46:660-662.

40. Spilker J, Kongable GL. The NIH Stroke Scale: its importance and practical application in the clinical setting. *Stroke Intervent*. 2000;2:7-14. (For more information go to http://www.stroke-site.org).

41. Adams H, Adams R, Del Zoppo G, Goldstein LB. Guidelines for the early management of patients with ischemic stroke: 2005 guidelines update: a scientific statement from the Stroke Council of the American Heart Association/American Stroke Association. *Stroke*. 2005;36:916-923.

42. Part 6: Advanced cardiovascular life support—section 1: introduction to ACLS 2000: overview of recommended changes in ACLS from the Guidelines 2000 Conference. *Resuscitation*. 2000;46:103-107.

43. Adams HP Jr, Adams RJ, Brott T, del Zoppo GJ, Furlan A, Goldstein LB, Grubb RL, Higashida R, Kidwell C, Kwiatkowski TG, Marler JR, Hademenos GJ. Guidelines for the early management of patients with ischemic stroke: a scientific statement from the Stroke Council of the American Stroke Association. *Stroke*. 2003;34:1056-1083.

44. Connors JJ III, Sacks D, Furlan AJ, Selman WR, Russell EJ, Stieg PE, Hadley MN. Training, competency, and credentialing standards for diagnostic cervicocerebral angiography, carotid stenting, and cerebrovascular intervention: a joint statement from the American Academy of Neurology, American Association of Neurological Surgeons, American Society of Interventional and Therapeutic Radiology, American Society of Neuroradiology, Congress of Neurological Surgeons, AANS/CNS Cerebrovascular Section, and Society of Interventional Radiology. *Radiology*. 2005;234:26-34.

45. Schriger DL, Kalafut M, Starkman S, Krueger M, Saver JL. Cranial computed tomography interpretation in acute stroke: physician accuracy in determining eligibility for thrombolytic therapy. *JAMA*. 1998;279:1293-1297.

46. Hill MD, Buchan AM. Thrombolysis for acute ischemic stroke: results of the Canadian Alteplase for Stroke Effectiveness Study. Canadian Alteplase for Stroke Effectiveness Study (CASES) Investigators. *CMAJ*. 2005;172:1307-1312.

47. Graham GD. Tissue plasminogen activator for acute ischemic stroke in clinical practice: a meta-analysis of safety data. *Stroke*. 2003;34:2847-2850.

48. Heuschmann PU, Berger K, Misselwitz B, Hermanek P, Leffmann C, Adelmann M, Buecker-Nott HJ, Rother J, Neundoerfer B, Kolominsky-Rabas PL. Frequency of thrombolytic therapy in patients with acute ischemic stroke and the risk of in-hospital mortality: the German Stroke Registers Study Group. *Stroke*. 2003;34:1106-1113.

49. Bravata DM, Kim N, Concato J, Krumholz HM, Brass LM. Thrombolysis for acute stroke in routine clinical practice. *Arch Intern Med*. 2002;162:1994-2001.

50. Katzan IL, Furlan AJ, Lloyd LE, Frank JI, Harper DL, Hinchey JA, Hammel JP, Qu A, Sila CA. Use of tissue-type plasminogen activator for acute ischemic stroke: the Cleveland area experience. *JAMA*. 2000;283:1151-1158.

51. Katzan IL, Hammer MD, Hixson ED, Furlan AJ, Abou-Chebl A, Nadzam DM. Utilization of intravenous tissue plasminogen activator for acute ischemic stroke. *Arch Neurol*. 2004; 61:346-350.

52. Lopez-Yunez AM, Bruno A, Williams LS, Yilmaz E, Zurru C, Biller J. Protocol violations in community-based rTPA stroke treatment are associated with symptomatic intracerebral hemorrhage. *Stroke*. 2001;32:12-16.

53. Asimos AW, Norton HJ, Price MF, Cheek WM. Therapeutic yield and outcomes of a community teaching hospital code stroke protocol. *Acad Emerg Med*. 2004;11:361-370.

54. Katzan IL, Hammer MD, Furlan AJ, Hixson ED, Nadzam DM. Quality improvement and tissue-type plasminogen activator for acute ischemic stroke: a Cleveland update. *Stroke*. 2003;34:799-800.

55. Lattimore SU, Chalela J, Davis L, DeGraba T, Ezzeddine M, Haymore J, Nyquist P, Baird AE, Hallenbeck J, Warach S. Impact of establishing a primary stroke center at a community hospital on the use of thrombolytic therapy: the NINDS Suburban Hospital Stroke Center experience. *Stroke*. 2003; 34:e55-e57.

56. Alberts MJ, Hademenos G, Latchaw RE, Jagoda A, Marler JR, Mayberg MR, Starke RD, Todd HW, Viste KM, Girgus M, Shephard T, Emr M, Shwayder P, Walker MD. Recommendations for the establishment of primary stroke centers. Brain Attack Coalition. *JAMA*. 2000;283:3102-3109.

57. Scott JF, Robinson GM, French JM, O'Connell JE, Alberti KG, Gray CS. Glucose potassium insulin infusions in the treatment of acute stroke patients with mild to moderate hyperglycemia: the Glucose Insulin in Stroke Trial (GIST). *Stroke*. 1999; 30:793-799.

58. Gray CS, Hildreth AJ, Alberti GK, O'Connell JE. Poststroke hyperglycemia: natural history and immediate management. *Stroke*. 2004;35:122-126.

59. Van den Berghe G, Wouters PJ, Bouillon R, Weekers F, Verwaest C, Schetz M, Vlasselaers D, Ferdinande P, Lauwers P. Outcome benefit of intensive insulin therapy in the critically ill: insulin dose versus glycemic control. *Crit Care Med*. 2003;31:359-366.

60. Van den Berghe G, Wouters P, Weekers F, Verwaest C, Bruyninckx F, Schetz M, Vlasselaers D, Ferdinande P, Lauwers P, Bouillon R. Intensive insulin therapy in the critically ill patients. *N Engl J Med*. 2001;345:1359-1367.

Chapter 10

Acute Coronary Syndromes—STEMI

This Chapter

- **How to recognize ischemic chest pain**
- **Know why STEMI is a rapid fill reperfusion emergency**
- **How to identify patients with STEMI on the initial ECG**
- **Use initial treatments and recognize complications in ACS**

Key Points

The ACLS Provider Course discusses the initial management of patients with suspected ischemic pain and then focuses on patients with ST-segment elevation myocardial infarction (STEMI). STEMI patients need rapid identification and reperfusion by experienced centers and physicians. You should do the following:

- Rapidly identify chest discomfort that could be ischemic in origin.
- Perform and immediately interpret the 12-lead electrocardiogram (ECG) for acute ischemic syndromes.
- Use the ECG interpretation to place patients into 1 of 3 possible acute ischemic symptom categories: STEMI, non-STEMI (NSTEMI), and normal or nondiagnostic ECG.
- Evaluate *fast* for reperfusion therapy patients with STEMI and those with new or presumably new left bundle branch block. Treat eligible patients with fibrinolytic therapy within 30 minutes or with percutaneous coronary intervention (PCI) within 90 minutes of arrival at the Emergency Department (ED).
- Know how to use drugs for pain relief and as aids to reperfusion therapy.

Introduction to ACS and STEMI

This chapter reviews the evaluation of patients with possible ischemic chest discomfort. Rapid identification of patients with ST-segment elevation myocardial infarction (STEMI) is emphasized because patients with STEMI require fast reperfusion to save heart muscle and reduce the complications of MI. Out-of-hospital and early ED management are reviewed in detail. Discussions of non-

---

FYI

Major Recommendations

Guidelines 2005

- EMS dispatch—recommend aspirin 160 to 325 mg.
- EMS systems—implement 12-lead ECG programs.
- Prehospital care providers—transmit ECG or interpretation to receiving facility for rapid reperfusion identification and team activation.
- ED—rapidly triage STEMI patients to reperfusion strategy and risk stratification.
- Reperfusion goals—ED door-to-drug (fibrinolytic) within 30 minutes; ED door-to-balloon (angioplasty or stent) within 90 minutes.
- Transfer goal to another facility for PCI or cardiogenic shock—door-to-departure within 30 minutes.
- Clopidogrel as adjunctive therapy for fibrinolytic strategy or fibrinolytic ineligible patients.

STEMI (NSTEMI), chest pain triage, and the complications of acute myocardial infarction (AMI), such as cardiogenic shock and pulmonary edema, are presented in Part 2 of this text.

Acute Coronary Syndromes— A Spectrum

The formation and accumulation of lipid and oxidative byproducts in an arterial wall is called atherosclerosis. When this deposit involves the coronary arteries, it is called coronary atherosclerosis. This process is gradual (Figure 1) and can cause exertional symptoms when the lumen of the coronary artery is sufficiently occluded. An abrupt change in an atherosclerotic plaque of a diseased coronary arterial wall causes a spectrum of clinical conditions referred to as *acute coronary syndromes (ACS)*. Many of these plaque disruptions are asymptomatic and resolve spontaneously. Symptoms of this clinical spectrum can develop and are called angina pectoris. The resulting unstable syndromes are *unstable angina pectoris, NSTEMI,* and *STEMI. Sudden cardiac death* can complicate any of these clinical conditions and may be the first, only, and last presentation of the disease.

Angina Pectoris

Angina is a *symptom* often associated with chronic and gradual coronary artery narrowing. There are other causes of angina, and symptoms may occur in the absence of coronary artery narrowing as a result of other conditions. Typically discomfort is located in the *center of the lower chest (substernal)* and is described as *squeezing, heavy, or tight.* Two more features are characteristic. First, the discomfort is *precipitated by exertion or emotion;* second, it is *relieved by rest or nitroglycerin.* The definition of chest discomfort also includes typical, atypical, and noncardiac features. When an ACS occurs, these symptoms can occur at rest or with minimal exertion.

- Typical angina—all 3 features are present
- Atypical angina—only 2 features are present
- Noncardiac pain—1 or no features are present

Unstable Angina Pectoris

In some patients symptoms of angina become unstable, are prolonged, and may occur at rest or with minimal exertion, identifying patients at risk for serious complications of acute coronary syndromes. These serious complications are called **m**ajor **a**dverse **c**ardiac **e**vents, or **MACE.** Major adverse cardiac events usually include death, nonfatal MI, or the need for urgent coronary intervention, such as percutaneous coronary intervention (PCI: angioplasty and/or stent) or surgical revascularization. In general these symptoms are caused by a change in a segment of an artery significantly involved with coronary arteriosclerosis, usually plaque rupture or erosion. As a result symptoms or features indicating marginal blood flow due to obstructing disease develop abruptly. Features and symptoms of unstable angina include

- Prolonged or continuing chest discomfort (>15 to 20 minutes)
- An accelerating pattern over the past 48 hours
- Spontaneous discomfort at rest or discomfort that awakens a patient at night

Myocardial Infarction

Angina—either stable or unstable—does not cause heart damage. But if the reduction in blood flow is prolonged or complete, heart cells (called myocytes) die. When this happens their internal cellular contents are released and can be detected in blood samples. This process usually takes 20 to 30 minutes or longer to begin. Myocyte death is called necrosis, and cardiac markers of necrosis that are often measured clinically are the MB isoenzyme of

Critical Concept *Angina: A Symptom, Not a Diagnosis*	Angina pectoris is a symptom and not a diagnosis because it may be caused by several conditions. There are 4 emergency differential diagnoses of angina and possible acute coronary syndromes: • Aortic dissection • Pulmonary embolism • Pericardial effusion with tamponade • Tension pneumothorax
Foundation Facts *Chest Pain or Chest Discomfort*	• More recently descriptions of angina use the term chest (or neck, or arm) *discomfort* when describing symptoms. • When angina or discomfort is due to ACS, it is referred to as ischemic discomfort to distinguish the cause as cardiac and due to ischemia.

creatine kinase (CK-MB) and cardiac troponins. In contrast to more nonspecific changes of ischemia, infarction causes characteristic ECG changes. When myocyte necrosis is determined due to ACS, an MI is diagnosed. The diagnosis of myocardial infarction due to ACS requires a positive biomarker and either clinical symptoms or pathological confirmation.

Acute Coronary Syndromes— The Electrocardiogram

The electrocardiogram is central to the diagnosis and triage of patients with possible acute ischemic symptoms (Figure 2). Although it may be normal or have nonspecific changes, the ECG allows initial placement of patients into 3 categories that have diagnostic and treatment implications. When the patient presents with symptoms of a possible ACS, the senior clinician proficient in ECG interpretation rapidly reviews the ECG and places the patient into 1 of 3 categories:

1. **STEMI:** ST-segment elevation or new or presumably new left bundle branch block (LBBB) (Box 5 of Figure 2) is characterized by ST-segment elevation >1 mm (0.1 mV) in 2 or more contiguous precordial leads or 2 or more adjacent limb leads.

2. **High-risk unstable angina/NSTEMI:** This classification is characterized by ischemic ST-segment depression ≥0.5 mm (0.05 mV) or dynamic T-wave inversion with pain or discomfort (Box 9). Nonpersistent or transient ST-segment elevation ≥0.5 mm for <20 minutes is included in this category.

3. **Intermediate or low-risk unstable angina:** Normal or nondiagnostic changes in ST segment or T waves (Box 13) are inconclusive and require further risk stratification. This classification includes patients with normal ECGs and those with ST-segment deviation of <0.5 mm (0.05 mV) or T-wave inversion of ≤0.2 mV. Serial cardiac studies (and functional testing) are appropriate.

Chronology of Atherosclerotic Vascular Disease Process

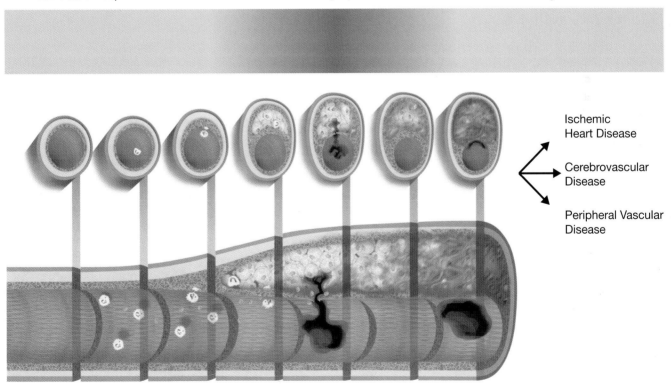

Development of Atherosclerosis and Vulnerable Plaque

Acute Coronary Syndrome

Secondary Prevention

Ischemic Heart Disease

Cerebrovascular Disease

Peripheral Vascular Disease

Figure 1. Timeline of atherosclerosis and acute coronary syndromes (ACSs). Slices through the coronary artery, each representing a decade of life, depict the development of coronary atherosclerosis. Gradual narrowing of the artery can cause the development of angina when a critical or "significant" narrowing develops, usually 90% cross-sectional narrowing of the artery. If plaque rupture or erosion occurs, an ACS can develop and result in STEMI, NSTEMI, or unstable angina. Sudden cardiac death can complicate any of these syndromes and can be the first, last, and only symptom. When this process occurs in other vascular beds, stroke or peripheral vacular disease may occur. Adapted with permission from Libby P. Current concepts of the pathogenesis of the acute coronary syndromes. *Circulation.* 2001;104;365-372.[1] © 2001 American Heart Association.

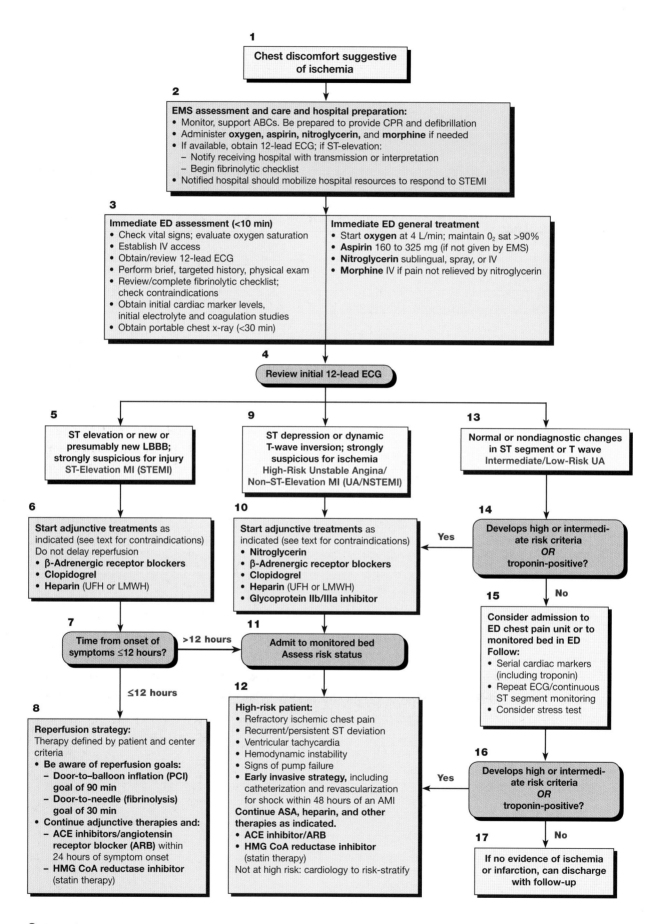

Figure 2. Acute Coronary Syndromes Algorithm.

Figure 3 shows characteristic ECG findings for the acute coronary syndromes.

If STEMI is present, immediately assess for reperfusion therapy and arrange for fibrinolytic therapy or primary PCI if the patient is a candidate and has no contraindications. Patients with ST-segment depression do not receive fibrinolytics (except true posterior MI); these agents may increase mortality and morbidity despite the magnitude and extent of ST-segment depression. Instead, antiplatelet and antithrombin therapy is indicated for these patients. Nonspecific or normal ECGs compose the largest group, and only a minority of patients have an ACS. Serial studies and risk stratification are appropriate if coronary artery disease is thought to be an intermediate or high probability. Aspirin is indicated for all ACS if no contraindications are present.

Older terminology labeled MIs as "Q wave" or "non–Q wave." These terms are pathological terms and are not helpful at the "front door" of the ED for risk stratification. Q waves generally are a late finding, and cardiac markers are necessary to distinguish unstable angina from MI.

ST-Segment Elevation Myocardial Infarction (STEMI)

When ischemia is prolonged and complete occlusion of a coronary artery occurs, myocytes die and the ST segment of the ECG becomes elevated. The majority of these patients will develop an MI. ST-segment elevation is an early ECG finding that identifies patients who may benefit from rapid reperfusion of the coronary artery. Confirmation of MI by detection of cardiac markers is variable, and elevation begins approximately 4 to 6 hours later. If the infarction process is not interrupted, Q waves, a later ECG finding consistent with a scar, will develop in many patients. Older terminology for this type of infarction included "transmural" or "Q-wave" MI.

Critical Concept **12-Lead ECG**	The ECG is central to the diagnosis of possible ischemic pain and initial triage and treatment of ACS. Obtain an ECG within 10 minutes of ED arrival if not already done by EMS.

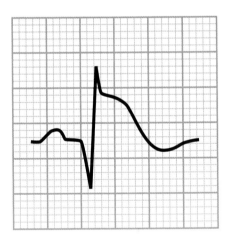

A. ST-segment elevation (STEMI)

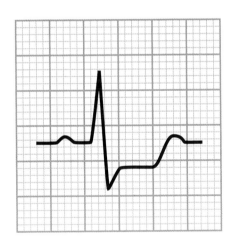

B. ST-segment depression

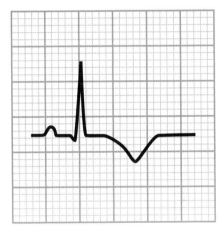

C. Nonspecific ECG abnormalities

Figure 3. ECG findings of the spectrum of acute coronary syndromes. **A,** This tracing shows >1 mm ST-segment elevation, measured 0.04 seconds after the J point (STEMI). **B,** This tracing shows ≥0.5 mm ST-segment depression, measured 0.04 seconds after the J point. **C,** The nonspecific ST-segment and T-wave changes on this tracing are consistent with either NSTEMI or unstable angina. Cardiac markers could be positive in any of these ECG tracings.

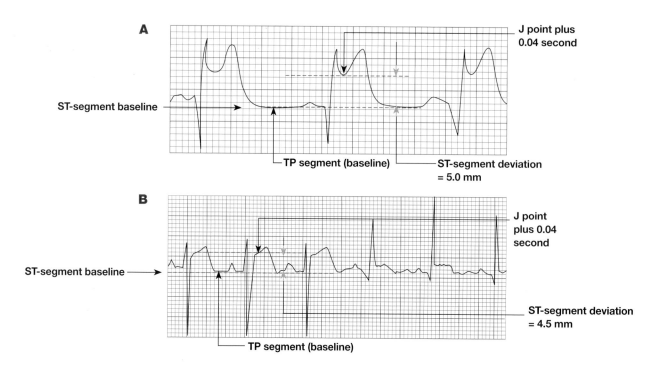

Figure 4. ECG findings of STEMI showing >1 mm ST-segment elevation, measured 0.04 second after the J point. **A,** Inferior myocardial infarction. ST segment has no low point (it is coved or concave). **B,** Anterior myocardial infarction.

How to Measure ST-Segment Deviation

ST-segment deviation (either elevation or depression) must be measured precisely and uniformly (Figure 4):

1. Draw the baseline ("zero ST deviation") from the *end* of the T wave to the *beginning* of the P wave (the TP segment).
   - The conventional baseline for measuring ST deviation has been the PR segment.
   - But a baseline drawn from the end of the T wave to the beginning of the P wave is considered to be *a more accurate baseline* for evaluation of ST deviation than the PR segment. The TP baseline is particularly helpful in ECGs with "coved" or "concave" ST segments or hyperacute T waves.
   - If the TP segment cannot be identified because of a rapid heart rate or artifact, use the PR *junction* as the baseline reference point. The PR junction is the intersection of the PR segment with the QRS complex.
2. Locate the J point, the position of juncture (angle change) between the QRS complex and the ST segment.
3. Locate 0.04 second (1 mm) after the J point. Measure the vertical deviation from this point (1 mm after the J point) either up or down to the baseline. This distance is the amount of ST deviation.

Other Causes of ST Elevation

Evaluation of the patient with acute chest pain includes a short list of emergency differential diagnoses and a long list of other non–life-threatening causes (see Part 2 of this text). Initial triage involves a determination of the likelihood of these causes. It may not be possible to rule out some of these causes, and the risk-benefit assessment involves estimating which additional causes are unlikely. This process requires integration of clinical and ECG data because time is crucial in early reperfusion. In general, reperfusion is not delayed to obtain diagnostic tests for these other conditions. Exceptions and reasonable delays in door-to-drug/balloon time include a chest x-ray or imaging study for suspected aortic dissection, a spiral computed tomography (CT) scan for suspected pulmonary embolism, and an echocardiogram for suspected pericardial effusion. These conditions may cause or be associated with ST elevation on the initial ECG and can be difficult to discriminate from acute injury. Healthcare providers must be aware that conditions other than acute ischemic injury can cause ST elevation[2,3] (Table 1), such as

- Pericarditis
- Old LBBB
- Paced beats with a pacemaker in the right ventricle
- Left ventricular (LV) hypertrophy
- Early repolarization

Table 1. Conditions Other Than STEMI That Can Cause Elevation of the ST Segment of the 12-Lead ECG

Condition	Features
Normal Variant (so-called male pattern)	• Seen in approximately 90% of healthy young men; therefore, normal • Elevation of 1 to 3 mm • Most marked in V_2 • Concave ST-segment
Early repolarization	• Most marked in V_4, with notching at J point • Tall, upright T waves • Reciprocal ST depression in aVR, not in aVL, when limb leads are involved
ST elevation of normal variant	• Seen in V_3 through V_5 with inverted T waves • Short QT, high QRS voltage
Left ventricular hypertrophy	• Concave • Other features of left ventricular hypertrophy
Left bundle branch block	• Concave • ST-segment deviation discordant from the QRS
Acute pericarditis	• Diffuse ST-segment elevation • Reciprocal ST-segment depression in aVR, not in aVL • Elevation seldom >5 mm • PR-segment depression
Hyperkalemia	Other features of hyperkalemia present: • Widened QRS and tall, peaked, tented T waves • Low-amplitude or absent P waves • ST segment usually downsloping
Brugada syndrome	• rSR′ in V_1 and V_2 • ST-segment elevation in V_1 and V_2, typically downsloping
Pulmonary embolism	• Changes simulating myocardial infarction seen often in both inferior and anteroseptal leads
Cardioversion	• Striking ST-segment elevation, often >10 mm, but lasting only a minute or two immediately after direct-current shock
Prinzmetal's angina	• Same as ST-segment elevation in infarction but transient

Adapted with permission from Wang K, Asinger RW, Marriott HJ. ST-segment elevation in conditions other than acute myocardial infarction. *N Engl J Med.* 2003;349:2128-2135.[3] © 2003 Massachusetts Medical Society.

Non–ST-Segment Elevation Myocardial Infarction

When ischemia is prolonged but the coronary artery is incompletely occluded, cardiac markers may increase but the ECG may demonstrate ST-segment depression, be normal, or show nonspecific changes. Detection of elevated cardiac markers in this setting defines non–ST-segment elevation myocardial infarction (NSTEMI).

Evolution of the 12-Lead ECG in ACS

The ECG changes and "evolves" during a process that initially involves ischemia, then injury, and finally necrosis of cardiac muscle cells. Not all phases may be present in every patient, and the findings vary on the basis of patient characteristics (eg, coronary anatomy), ECG sensitivity, and location of the infarct. Early in STEMI, T waves may be tented or "peaked"; these changes are referred to as hyperacute changes. Other ECGs may show changes that are nonspecific or nondiagnostic. Finally, Q waves generally represent necrosis and are a late finding, although they may be observed early in STEMI and may decrease or resolve contrary to the usual evolutionary pattern (Figure 5).

Sudden Cardiac Death

Acute ischemia or MI can cause electrical instability or catastrophic hemodynamic impairment. Sudden cardiac death results and is the major cause of out-of-hospital adult cardiac arrest in the hours after onset of symptoms. If an arrhythmia occurs as a primary event (not due to cardiogenic shock), *ventricular fibrillation* (VF) is the most common presentation. Defibrillation success depends on many factors, including high-quality CPR, early defibrillation, and the underlying acute coronary syndrome.

Resuscitation is more successful when VF occurs in the absence of an ACS, such as during cardiac rehabilitation or exercise stress testing.

Acute Coronary Syndromes— Pathophysiology

Stable and Unstable Plaques

Coronary atherosclerosis is a diffuse process with segmental lesions called *coronary plaques* that gradually enlarge and extend, causing variable degrees of coronary

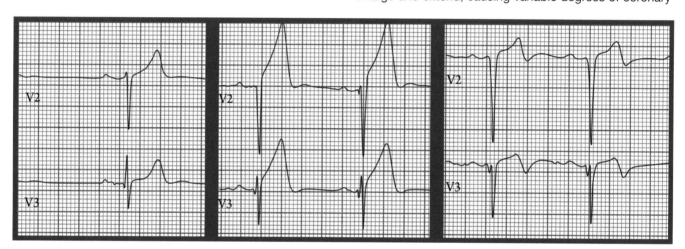

Figure 5A. This figure from left to right demonstrates the ST-segment changes of STEMI. The left panel shows minimal ST-segment elevation that is concave down, possibly due to early repolarization in the baseline tracing. This patient however was having symptoms of ischemic chest discomfort, and the ECG was repeated 10 minutes later. Clearly seen in the middle panel are tented and peaked ST segments. In the right panel, evolution of the ST segment and T-wave changes are seen in a tracing obtained one hour later, immediately after PCI. The ST segments are elevated but returning to normal and the T waves are biphasic. In addition, there is a QS complex in lead V_2 and further loss of R wave in V_3. Although Q waves are generally a later finding in STEMI evolution they may occur early in approximately 50% of patients.

Spectrum of Acute Coronary Syndromes: Laboratory Findings in Q-Wave AMI				
	Stable Angina	**Unstable Angina**	**Non–Q-Wave AMI**	**Q-Wave AMI**
Cardiac Marker Evidence of Necrosis		None	Positive	Positive
ECG Early		ST-segment depression and/or T-wave inversion	ST-segment depression and/or T-wave inversion	ST-segment elevation
ECG Late		No Q	No Q	Q develops

Figure 5B. Older terminology labeled myocardial infarctions as "Q-wave" and "non–Q wave." These terms are pathological terms and are not helpful at the "front door" of the ED for risk stratification. Q waves generally are a late finding, and cardiac markers are necessary to distinguish unstable angina from myocardial infarction. Reprinted with permission from Antman EM. In: Braunwald E, ed. *Heart Disease: A Textbook in Cardiovascular Medicine.* 5th ed. Philadelphia, Pa: WB Saunders; 1997.[4] © 1997 WB Saunders.

artery occlusion. Intravascular ultrasound of the coronary arteries has shown that the majority of the atheroma burden is subluminal and not visible by coronary angiography. Coronary arteries are usually closed about 70% (by angiography; 90% closed when viewed by a pathologist) before they cause symptoms and are considered for stenting or surgery.

Most plaques do not cause symptoms and are nonocclusive. But nonocclusive plaques are the ones most prone to cause acute coronary syndromes. They have little hemodynamic effect before rupture, and stress testing and angiography cannot predict which ones will rupture and cause an ACS. Plaques can be classified as *stable or vulnerable* on the basis of their lipid content, thickness of the cap that covers and separates them from the arterial lumen, and the degree of inflammation in the plaque itself.

1. A **"stable"** intracoronary plaque (Figure 6A) has a lipid core separated from the arterial lumen by a thick fibrous cap. Stable plaques have less lipid,

and the thick cap makes them resistant to fissuring and formation of thrombi. Over time the lumen of the vessel becomes progressively narrower, leading to flow limitations, supply-demand imbalance, and exertional angina.

2. A **"vulnerable"** intracoronary plaque (Figure 6B) has a lipid-rich core combined with an active inflammatory process that make the plaque soft and prone to rupture. These plaques infrequently restrict blood flow enough to cause clinical angina, and functional studies (eg, stress tests) often yield negative results. Imaging techniques such as cardiac CT and magnetic resonance imaging are being investigated as tools to identify unstable and inflamed plaques and may be helpful in the future.

3. Inflammation is often found in the plaque (Figure 6C). Inflammatory processes are concentrated in the leading edge impacted by coronary blood flow. It is here that most plaque ruptures occur. A plaque that is inflamed and prone to rupture is called **unstable**.

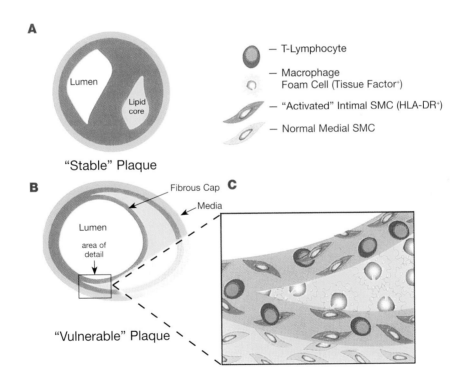

Figure 6. Stable and vulnerable plaques. **A**, Stable plaque. **B**, Vulnerable plaque. **C**, Area of detail of vulnerable plaque showing infiltration of inflammatory cells. SMC indicates smooth muscle cell. Reprinted from Libby P. Molecular bases of the acute coronary syndromes. *Circulation.* 1995;91:2844-2850.[5] © 1995 American Heart Association.

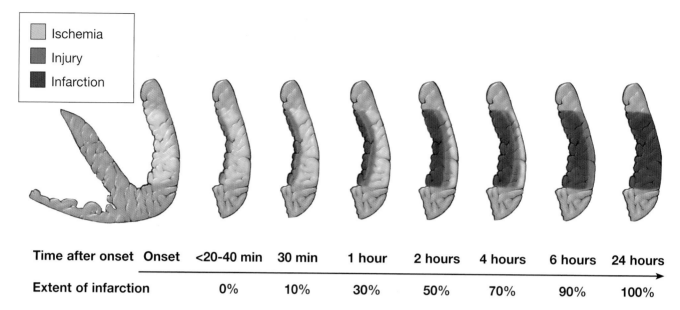

Time after onset	Onset	<20-40 min	30 min	1 hour	2 hours	4 hours	6 hours	24 hours
Extent of infarction		0%	10%	30%	50%	70%	90%	100%

Figure 7. After occlusion of a coronary artery, progressive cell death occurs. Note that the majority of myocardial infarction occurs by 4 hours after the onset of symptoms. After 6 hours the infarct is nearly complete. The extent and degree of myocardial infarction depends on several factors: the coronary artery involved, the amount of myocardium downstream, the degree and duration of occlusion, and the presence or absence of collateral supply.

STEMI—Goals of Therapy

The primary goals of reperfusion therapy in patients with STEMI are to

- Prevent or limit MI
- Prevent major adverse cardiac events—death, serious or fatal cardiac arrhythmias, congestive heart failure, and rupture of the heart or internal structures
- Anticipate and treat life-threatening complications

Complete occlusion of an epicardial coronary artery eventually produces elevation of the ST segment of the ECG in most patients. Myocardial cell death begins and proceeds rapidly from subendocardium to epicardium unless flow is reestablished (Figure 7). In a minority of patients the clot resolves spontaneously. In all others fibrinolytic therapy or mechanical reperfusion with PCI using balloons and stents is necessary to limit myocardial damage. Loss of heart muscle is time dependent—*time is muscle.* The majority of myocyte necrosis (MI) occurs within the first several hours. Reperfusion has been shown to reduce mortality, preserve LV function, and reduce or limit the development of congestive heart failure.

STEMI—Initial Management (Figure 8)

Community and Out-of-Hospital Management

Half of the patients who die of AMI do so before reaching the hospital. Ventricular fibrillation or pulseless ventricular tachycardia (VT) is the precipitating rhythm in most of

these deaths,[6-8] and sudden cardiac death is most likely to develop during the first 4 hours after onset of symptoms.[9-12] Communities should develop programs to respond to out-of-hospital cardiac arrest that include prompt recognition of symptoms of ACS, early activation of the emergency medical services (EMS) system, and if needed, early CPR and early defibrillation.

The major community and EMS issues in the management of ACS are

- Patient delay
- Potential need for early defibrillation
- Out-of-hospital 12-lead ECGs
- EMS notification of receiving facility
- EMS triage to appropriate facility

The Problem of Delay

Any delay in coronary reperfusion reduces the effectiveness of fibrinolytic-based or catheter-based therapy, increases mortality, and decreases myocardial salvage. Because the potential for myocardial salvage decreases with time and most benefit occurs in the first few hours, patients, family members, EMS personnel, and healthcare providers should operate with a sense of urgency—*time is muscle!* There are 3 major time intervals from the onset of ACS symptoms to the delivery of reperfusion therapy that provide opportunity for delay in treatment:

- Symptom onset to patient recognition and decision to act: accounts for 60% to 70% of delay
- Out-of-hospital transport: 5%
- Interval from ED arrival to treatment: 25% to 33%

Patient delay, the interval from the onset of symptoms to the patient's recognition of them, accounts for 60% to 70% of the delay to definitive therapy.[13] *EMS transport* accounts for the least amount of delay, and prehospital notification of ACS patients can speed the diagnosis and reduce the time to reperfusion. Unfortunately the majority of patients still arrive by private vehicle and not EMS. Physicians and healthcare providers should encourage patients, especially those with known coronary disease, to use their nitroglycerin and activate EMS if symptoms persist or worsen 5 minutes after using the *first* nitroglycerin dose. Over the past decade many EDs have reduced the average time from ED arrival to administration of fibrinolytics through education, improved patient triage, and development of multidisciplinary protocols.

Factors Associated With Delay

Chest discomfort is the major symptom in most patients (both men and women) with acute coronary syndromes. But patients frequently deny or misinterpret this and other symptoms. The elderly, women, diabetic patients, and hypertensive patients are most likely to delay, in part because they are more likely to have atypical symptoms or presentations. In the US Rapid Early Action for Coronary Treatment (REACT) trial, the median out-of-hospital delay was 2 hours or longer in non-Hispanic blacks, the elderly and disabled, homemakers, and Medicaid recipients. The decision to use an ambulance was an important variable that reduced out-of-hospital delay; this reduction persisted after correction for variables associated with severity of symptoms. Other factors that can affect the interval between symptom onset and presentation to hospital include time of day, location (eg, work or home), and presence of a family member.

Reducing Patient Delay

Patient Education

Education of patients with known coronary artery disease appears to be the only effective primary intervention to reduce denial or misinterpretation of symptoms. Public educational programs have had only transient effects. The physician and family members of patients with known coronary disease should reinforce the need to seek medical attention when symptoms recur because these patients paradoxically present later than patients with no known disease.

Initial EMS Care

Dispatchers and EMS providers must be trained to recognize symptoms of ACS. Dispatchers should advise patients with no history of aspirin allergy or signs of active or recent gastrointestinal bleeding to chew an aspirin (160 to 325 mg) while awaiting the arrival of EMS providers.[14,15]

Major EMS Assessments and Treatments (Box 2, Figure 8)

EMS and dispatch system personnel should be trained to

- Identify patients with acute ischemic chest pain
- Obtain an initial 12-lead ECG, provide prearrival notification to the receiving hospital, and transmit the ECG or their interpretation of the ECG
- Obtain a targeted history with a chest pain checklist to help determine eligibility for fibrinolytic therapy as appropriate
- Establish vascular access and measure vital signs and oxygen saturation
- Start initial medical treatment (oxygen, aspirin, nitroglycerin, and possibly morphine)
- Document initial rhythms and prepare for treatment of ischemic arrhythmias, in particular VF/VT
- Place transcutaneous patches for transcutaneous pacing if symptomatic sinus bradycardia or advanced atrioventricular block occurs

Critical Concept **Patient Use of Nitroglycerin for Acute Chest Discomfort**	Previously, patients with acute (not chronic) chest discomfort were instructed to take 3 doses of nitroglycerin and contact EMS if symptoms persisted. New guidelines recommend that healthcare providers instruct patients and family to activate EMS if symptoms persist or worsen **5 minutes after the first nitroglycerin dose.** These patients may have STEMI or prolonged ischemia and are at risk for sudden cardiac death.
Critical Concept **Community EMS Priority**	Half of the patients who die of an ACS die before reaching the hospital. VF or pulseless VT is the precipitating rhythm in most of these deaths.[6-8] VF is most likely to develop during the first 4 hours after symptom onset.[9-12] Communities should develop programs to respond to out-of-hospital cardiac arrest that include recognition of ACS symptoms, activation of the EMS system, and availability of high-quality CPR and an AED.[16] EMS and dispatch system personnel should be trained to respond to cardiac emergencies.

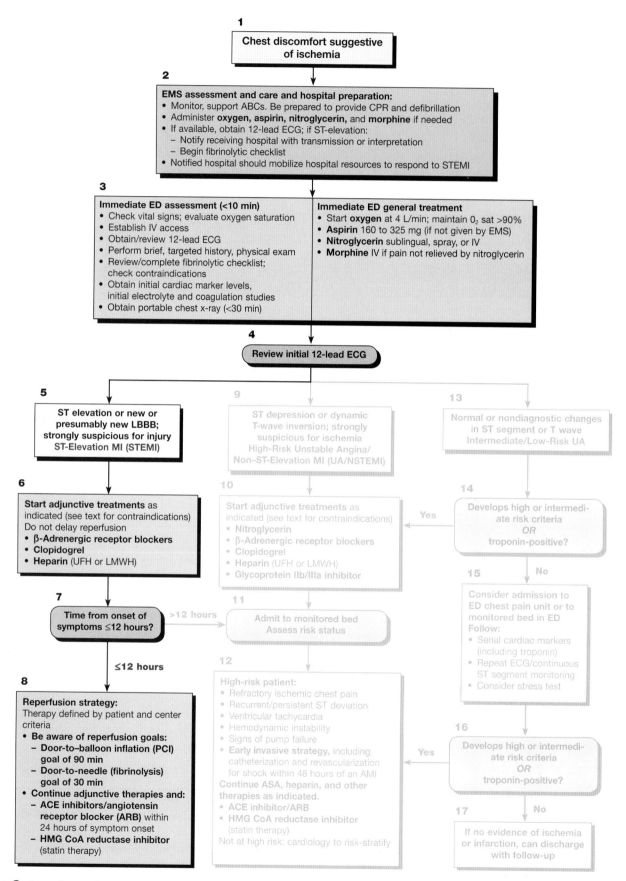

1
Chest discomfort suggestive
of ischemia

2
EMS assessment and care and hospital preparation:
- Monitor, support ABCs. Be prepared to provide CPR and defibrillation
- Administer **oxygen, aspirin, nitroglycerin,** and **morphine** if needed
- If available, obtain 12-lead ECG; if ST-elevation:
  – Notify receiving hospital with transmission or interpretation
  – Begin fibrinolytic checklist
- Notified hospital should mobilize hospital resources to respond to STEMI

3
Immediate ED assessment (<10 min)
- Check vital signs; evaluate oxygen saturation
- Establish IV access
- Obtain/review 12-lead ECG
- Perform brief, targeted history, physical exam
- Review/complete fibrinolytic checklist; check contraindications
- Obtain initial cardiac marker levels, initial electrolyte and coagulation studies
- Obtain portable chest x-ray (<30 min)

Immediate ED general treatment
- Start **oxygen** at 4 L/min; maintain O_2 sat >90%
- **Aspirin** 160 to 325 mg (if not given by EMS)
- **Nitroglycerin** sublingual, spray, or IV
- **Morphine** IV if pain not relieved by nitroglycerin

4
Review initial 12-lead ECG

5
ST elevation or new or presumably new LBBB; strongly suspicious for injury ST-Elevation MI (STEMI)

9
ST depression or dynamic T-wave inversion; strongly suspicious for ischemia High-Risk Unstable Angina/ Non–ST-Elevation MI (UA/NSTEMI)

13
Normal or nondiagnostic changes in ST segment or T wave Intermediate/Low-Risk UA

6
Start adjunctive treatments as indicated (see text for contraindications) Do not delay reperfusion
- **β-Adrenergic receptor blockers**
- **Clopidogrel**
- **Heparin** (UFH or LMWH)

10
Start adjunctive treatments as indicated (see text for contraindications)
- Nitroglycerin
- β-Adrenergic receptor blockers
- Clopidogrel
- Heparin (UFH or LMWH)
- Glycoprotein IIb/IIIa inhibitor

14
Develops high or intermediate risk criteria *OR* troponin-positive?

Yes

No

7
Time from onset of symptoms ≤12 hours?

>12 hours

11
Admit to monitored bed Assess risk status

15
Consider admission to ED chest pain unit or to monitored bed in ED Follow:
- Serial cardiac markers (including troponin)
- Repeat ECG/continuous ST segment monitoring
- Consider stress test

≤12 hours

12
High-risk patient:
- Refractory ischemic chest pain
- Recurrent/persistent ST deviation
- Ventricular tachycardia
- Hemodynamic instability
- Signs of pump failure
- Early invasive strategy, including catheterization and revascularization for shock within 48 hours of an AMI
Continue ASA, heparin, and other therapies as indicated.
- ACE inhibitor/ARB
- HMG CoA reductase inhibitor (statin therapy)
Not at high risk: cardiology to risk-stratify

16
Develops high or intermediate risk criteria *OR* troponin-positive?

Yes

No

8
Reperfusion strategy:
Therapy defined by patient and center criteria
- **Be aware of reperfusion goals:**
  – Door-to–balloon inflation (PCI) goal of 90 min
  – Door-to-needle (fibrinolysis) goal of 30 min
- **Continue adjunctive therapies and:**
  – **ACE inhibitors/angiotensin receptor blocker (ARB)** within 24 hours of symptom onset
  – **HMG CoA reductase inhibitor** (statin therapy)

17
If no evidence of ischemia or infarction, can discharge with follow-up

Figure 8. Acute Coronary Syndromes Algorithm—STEMI treatment pathway for reperfusion therapy.

Recognition of Possible Ischemic Discomfort (Box 1, Figure 8)

Chest discomfort of ischemic etiology is usually substernal and is often described as crushing, heavy, constricting, or oppressive. Symptoms suggestive of ACS include

- Uncomfortable pressure, fullness, squeezing, or pain in the center of the chest lasting several minutes (usually more than a few minutes)
- Chest discomfort spreading to the shoulders, neck, one or both arms, or jaw
- Chest discomfort spreading in the back or between the shoulder blades
- Chest discomfort with lightheadedness, fainting, sweating, or nausea
- Unexplained sudden shortness of breath with or without chest discomfort

Less commonly the discomfort occurs in the epigastrium and is described as indigestion. Just as a response to nitroglycerin is *not diagnostic* of cardiac ischemic pain, relief of pain with antacids in these patients is *not diagnostic* of a gastrointestinal cause.

- In one large study[17] only 54% of patients with typical ischemic symptoms developed an ACS. On the other hand, of all patients who developed an ACS, 43% had burning or indigestion, 32% had a chest ache, 20% had sharp or stabbing pain, and 42% could not describe their pain. The pain was *partially* pleuritic in 12%.
- In patients without a history of coronary disease, chest pain that was sharp or stabbing *and* pleuritic, positional, or reproducible with chest palpation was almost never due to ischemic syndromes, particularly when there was no history of coronary artery disease.

Prehospital ECGs

Out-of-hospital 12-lead ECGs and advance notification to the receiving facility speed diagnosis, shorten time to fibrinolysis, and may be associated with lower in-hospital mortality.[18-21] The reduction in door-to-reperfusion therapy interval in most studies ranges from 10 to 60 minutes. EMS providers can efficiently acquire and transmit diagnostic-quality ECGs to the ED[22,23] with a minimal increase in the on-scene time interval (0.2 to 5.6 minutes).[18,22-26]

Qualified and specially trained paramedics and prehospital nurses can accurately identify typical ST elevation (>1 mm in 2 or more contiguous leads) in the 12-lead ECG with a specificity of 91% to 100% and a sensitivity of 71% to 97% compared with emergency medicine physicians or cardiologists[27,28] and can provide advance notification by radio or cell phone to the receiving hospital.[29]

If EMS providers identify STEMI on the ECG, it is reasonable for them to begin assessment of the patient for fibrinolytic therapy (ie, the fibrinolytic checklist, Figure 9).

Immediate General Treatment

Four agents are routinely recommended for immediate general treatment of patients with possible ischemic-type chest pain unless allergies or other contraindications exist:

- **Oxygen**
- **Aspirin** 160 to 325 mg
- **Nitroglycerin** sublingual or spray
- **Morphine** IV 2 to 4 mg if chest discomfort is unrelieved by nitrates

Immediate Pain Relief

Healthcare professionals must place a high priority on alleviating acute ischemic pain during immediate general treatment. Ischemic pain produces complex neurohumoral activation, which in turn induces a heightened, anxiety-generating catecholamine state. As a result ischemic pain

FYI **Guidelines 2005** **Dispatch Recommendations**	Dispatchers must be trained to recognize ACS symptoms. If authorized by medical control and protocol, dispatchers should advise patients with no history of aspirin allergy or signs of active or recent gastrointestinal bleeding to chew an aspirin (160 to 325 mg) while awaiting arrival of EMS providers.[14,15]
FYI **Guidelines 2005** **Prehospital ECG: Receiving Facility Notification**	• Implementation of out-of-hospital 12-lead ECG diagnostic programs in EMS systems is recommended. • Transmission of the 12-lead ECG or interpretation and advance notification is recommended for patients exhibiting signs and symptoms of ACS. • A 12-lead out-of-hospital ECG with advanced ED notification may benefit patients with STEMI by reducing their time to reperfusion therapy.

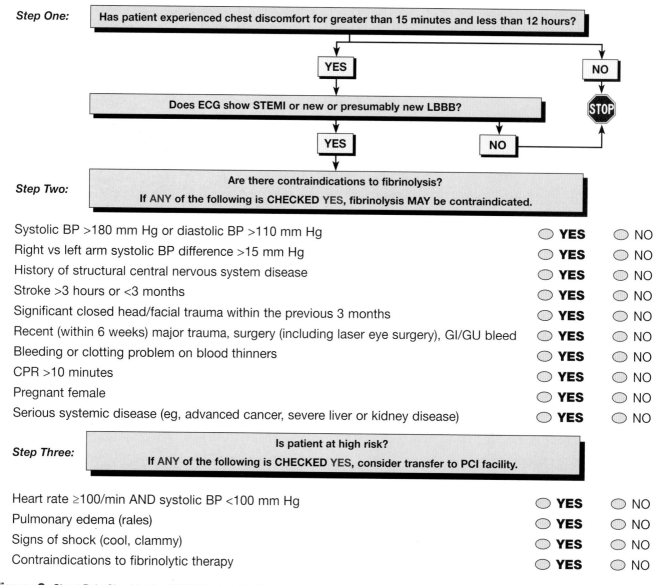

Step One: Has patient experienced chest discomfort for greater than 15 minutes and less than 12 hours?

YES → Does ECG show STEMI or new or presumably new LBBB?

NO → STOP

YES → NO → STOP

Step Two: Are there contraindications to fibrinolysis?
If ANY of the following is CHECKED YES, fibrinolysis MAY be contraindicated.

Systolic BP >180 mm Hg or diastolic BP >110 mm Hg	YES	NO
Right vs left arm systolic BP difference >15 mm Hg	YES	NO
History of structural central nervous system disease	YES	NO
Stroke >3 hours or <3 months	YES	NO
Significant closed head/facial trauma within the previous 3 months	YES	NO
Recent (within 6 weeks) major trauma, surgery (including laser eye surgery), GI/GU bleed	YES	NO
Bleeding or clotting problem on blood thinners	YES	NO
CPR >10 minutes	YES	NO
Pregnant female	YES	NO
Serious systemic disease (eg, advanced cancer, severe liver or kidney disease)	YES	NO

Step Three: Is patient at high risk?
If ANY of the following is CHECKED YES, consider transfer to PCI facility.

Heart rate ≥100/min AND systolic BP <100 mm Hg	YES	NO
Pulmonary edema (rales)	YES	NO
Signs of shock (cool, clammy)	YES	NO
Contraindications to fibrinolytic therapy	YES	NO

Figure 9. Chest Pain Checklist for STEMI Fibrinolytic Therapy

intensifies myocardial oxygen demand by accelerating heart rate, raising systolic blood pressure (SBP), and increasing contractility. This increased myocardial oxygen demand worsens existing ischemia and further impairs marginal hemodynamics.

Acute relief of pain will
- Reduce myocardial oxygen demand (morphine, nitrates, β-blockers)
- Attenuate the hyperactive catecholamine state (β-blockers)
- Reduce anxiety (morphine)

Oxygen

Rationale

Many patients with AMI (up to 70% in the first 24 hours[30]) demonstrate hypoxemia, due to either ventilation-perfusion mismatch or subclinical pulmonary edema from LV

dysfunction. Experimental studies have shown that oxygen administration can reduce ST elevation in anterior infarction.[31,32] The effects of hypoxemia and respiratory insufficiency on a heart already compromised by coronary occlusion can be profound. Increased demand on a heart with marginal blood flow and oxygen supply–demand can lead to increased infarct size and cardiovascular collapse. It is difficult, however, to document the effects of oxygen on morbidity or mortality. A small double-blind clinical trial in which investigators randomly assigned 200 patients to room air or oxygen by mask found no difference in mortality, incidence of arrhythmias, or use of pain medications. No clinical studies, including one prospective, randomized, controlled trial and a recent clinical trial evaluating hyperbaric oxygen, have shown a reduction in morbidity, mortality, or complications due to arrhythmias with routine use of supplementary oxygen.

Recommendations

It is reasonable to administer supplementary oxygen to all patients with ACS for the first 6 hours after presentation during initial evaluation and treatment. Supplementary oxygen limited ischemic myocardial injury in animals,[31] and oxygen therapy reduced the amount of ST-segment elevation in humans.[32] Short-term oxygen administration has no side effects and will be beneficial for the patient with unrecognized hypoxemia or unstable pulmonary function.

Aspirin

Administration of aspirin has been associated with reduced mortality in clinical trials, and multiple trials support the safety and efficacy of aspirin. Unless a true aspirin allergy or a recent history of gastrointestinal bleeding is present, aspirin should be given to all patients with possible ACS.

Rationale

A dose of 160 to 325 mg aspirin causes immediate and near-total inhibition of thromboxane-A_2 production by inhibiting platelet cyclooxygenase (COX-1). Platelets are one of the principle and earliest participants in thrombus formation. This rapid inhibition also reduces coronary reocclusion and other recurrent events independently and after fibrinolytic therapy. Platelet inhibitors are central to the prevention of acute stent thrombosis after placement in a coronary artery.

The importance of aspirin was demonstrated in early fibrinolytic trials. Aspirin alone reduced death from MI in the Second International Study of Infarct Survival (ISIS-2), and its effect was additive to the effect of streptokinase.[33] Clot lysis by fibrinolytics exposes free thrombin, a known platelet activator. Thus an antiplatelet effect is needed when fibrinolytic agents are administered. Patients can develop a paradoxical procoagulable state with fibrinolytic therapy unless platelet aggregation is reduced. In a review of 145 trials involving aspirin, investigators from the Antiplatelet Trialists' Collaboration reported a reduction in vascular events from 14% to 10% in patients with AMI. In high-risk patients aspirin reduced nonfatal AMI by 30% and vascular death by 17%.[34]

Precautions and Contraindications

Aspirin is contraindicated if patients have a history of true aspirin allergy, such as urticaria (hives) or systemic anaphylactic reaction. Patients with significant allergies or asthma may have an aspirin allergy—remember to ask!

Oral aspirin is relatively contraindicated for

- Patients with *active* peptic ulcer disease (use rectal suppositories)
- Patients with a history of intolerance to aspirin
- Patients with bleeding disorders or severe hepatic disease

Nitroglycerin

Rationale

Nitroglycerin is an effective analgesic for ischemic chest discomfort, and it has beneficial hemodynamic effects. The physiological effects of nitrates cause reduction in left and right ventricular preload through peripheral arterial and venous dilation. Nitroglycerin is an endothelium-independent vasodilator of the coronary arteries (particularly in the region of plaque disruption), the peripheral arterial bed, and venous capacitance vessels. Nitroglycerin sublingual or spray is the initial drug of choice for ischemic chest discomfort.

But the outcome benefits of nitroglycerin are limited, and no conclusive evidence supports routine use of intravenous, oral, or topical nitrate therapy in patients with AMI.[35] With this in mind, carefully consider use of these agents, especially when low blood pressure precludes the use of other agents shown to be effective in reducing morbidity and mortality (eg, angiotensin-converting enzyme [ACE] inhibitors).

Critical Concept **Pain Relief and STEMI**	Relief of pain is an important early goal for patients with STEMI or another ACS. Surges of catecholamines have been implicated in - Plaque fissuring - Thrombus propagation - Reduction in VF threshold
FYI **Guidelines 2005** **Oxygen**	Administer oxygen to - All patients initially suspected of having an acute ischemic syndrome - Patients with overt pulmonary congestion - Patients with oxygen saturation <90%

FYI **Guidelines 2005** **Aspirin**	• Administer aspirin to all patients initially suspected of having an acute ischemic syndrome. • Have the patient chew a dose of 160 to 325 mg. • Other formulations (soluble, IV) may be as effective. Consider rectal suppositories (300 mg) for patients unable to chew or swallow oral aspirin.

FAQ **What is a "true" aspirin allergy?**	Many patients will say they are allergic to aspirin when in fact they have had aspirin intolerance or a "side effect" in the past. That is, they may have had indigestion, nausea, or gastrointestinal upset. There is a dose-dependent increase in GI bleeding. Although this may preclude aspirin use on a chronic basis or require the addition of another medicine to aspirin for gastrointestinal prophylaxis, it does not preclude the use of aspirin in this life-threatening situation. Carefully review the history and weigh the risks and benefits. In patients with a true aspirin allergy, clopidogrel (300 mg) may be substituted for aspirin.

Treatment algorithm for potential STEMI patients who experience *non–trauma-related chest discomfort/pain.*

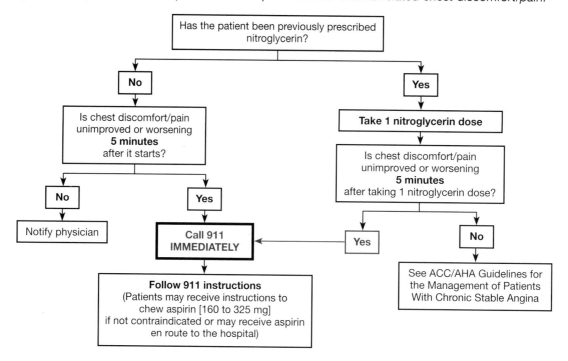

If patients have *not been previously prescribed nitroglycerin* (left side of algorithm), it is recommended that they call 911 if chest discomfort is unimproved or worsening 5 minutes after it starts. If the symptoms subside within 5 minutes of when they began, patients should notify their physician of the episode. For those patients with new onset chest discomfort who have not been prescribed nitroglycerin, it is appropriate to discourage them from seeking someone else's nitroglycerin (eg, from a neighbor, friend, or relative).

If patients experience chest discomfort and *have been previously prescribed nitroglycerin* and have it available (right side of algorithm), it is recommended that they be instructed (in advance) to take 1 nitroglycerin dose immediately in response to symptoms. If chest discomfort/pain is unimproved or worsening 5 minutes after taking 1 nitroglycerin dose, it is recommended that the patient call 911 immediately to access EMS. If the symptoms disappear after taking 1 nitroglycerin dose, the angina management recommendations in the *ACC/AHA Guidelines for the Management of Patients With Chronic Stable Angina* apply.

FYI **Guidelines 2005** **Nitroglycerin SL** **or Spray**	• Give nitroglycerin SL or spray to all patients with suspected ischemic chest discomfort unless contraindications are present. • Up to 3 doses at 5-minute intervals may be used. • Activate EMS if after 5 minutes symptoms do not resolve or are worsening.

Recommendations for Initial Administration

- Use nitroglycerin as the first drug (before morphine) to help relieve ischemic chest pain.
- Use 1 tablet (to 0.04 mg) SL or spray 1 metered dose (0.04 mg) under or onto the tongue; repeat 2 times at 5-minute intervals. Monitor clinical effects and blood pressure.

Precautions, Adverse Effects, and Contraindications

- **Recent phosphodiesterase inhibitor use.** If the patient has taken sildenafil or vardenafil within the previous 24 hours or tadalafil within 48 hours, nitrates may cause severe hypotension refractory to vasopressor agents.
- **Hypotension, bradycardia, or tachycardia.** Avoid use of nitroglycerin in patients with hypotension (SBP <90 mm Hg), marked bradycardia (heart rate <50 bpm), or tachycardia.
- **Right ventricular (RV) infarction.** Use nitroglycerin with caution in patients with inferior wall MI with possible RV involvement. Patients with RV dysfunction and acute infarction are very dependent on maintenance of RV filling pressures to maintain cardiac output and blood pressure. Until a 12-lead ECG confirms ST elevation or new LBBB ACS, it is prudent to avoid nitroglycerin for patients with borderline low blood pressure (SBP ≤100 mm Hg) or borderline sinus bradycardia (heart rate <60 per minute). Patients with excess vagal tone are unable to compensate when venodilation decreases blood pressure. Remember, cardiac output is the result of stroke volume and heart rate. If stroke volume falls because of decreased ventricular preload (caused by vasodilation), heart rate will be unable to compensate by increasing. Patients with a tachycardia may already be compensating (compensatory tachycardia) and unable to increase rate further. They also may become hypotensive.

Cardiac Output = Heart Rate × Stroke Volume

- Transdermal preparations are generally avoided; topical application results in variability in the amount of drug delivered and no predictable hemodynamic effect, and absorption is often erratic. Avoid long-acting oral preparations, especially in patients who may become hemodynamically unstable. The nitrate preparation is absorbed into the dermal skin layers and may not be completely removed by wiping to stop action.

Recommendations for IV Administration

IV nitroglycerin is not used *routinely* in patients with STEMI. A pooled analysis of more than 80 000 patients showed only a possible small effect of nitrates on mortality (odds reduction 7.7% to 7.4%). Do not administer IV nitroglycerin when it precludes the use of agents shown to have a greater treatment effect for STEMI (β-blockers, ACE inhibitors).

Dosing Recommendation for IV Nitroglycerin

The same cautions and contraindications exist for intravenous and oral nitrates. When intravenous nitrates are given, take care to frequently assess the patient and titrate the dose to avoid complications of therapy in the setting of STEMI/ACS. Drug-induced hypotension decreases coronary

FYI **Guidelines 2005** **IV Nitroglycerin**	STEMI Indications for IV Nitrates • Ongoing (after SL or spray) or recurrent ischemic discomfort • Preferred agent for hypertension and STEMI/ACS • Adjunct to treat pulmonary congestion (congestive heart failure)

FYI **ACC/AHA NSTEMI** **2007 Guidelines** **Dosing** **Regimen for IV** **Nitroglycerin**	• Begin infusion at 10 µg/min. • Increase dose by 10 µg/min every 3 to 5 minutes until symptom or blood pressure response is noted. • A ceiling dose of 200 µg/min is commonly used. • Systolic blood pressure (SBP) generally should not be reduced to less than 110 mm Hg in previously normotensive patients or 25% below the starting SBP in hypertensive patients. • Avoid nitroglycerin in SBP <90 mm Hg or 30 mm Hg or more below patient's baseline. • Avoid nitroglycerin if marked bradycardia or tachycardia exists.

perfusion and microvascular flow and has the potential to increase ischemia.

- Check vital signs and heart rate for contraindications before starting and before each increase in dose.

Morphine Sulfate

Rationale

Morphine is the analgesic of choice for patients with ischemic pain unresponsive to nitrates. Morphine is an important treatment, particularly for STEMI, because complete coronary occlusion is often associated with a hyperadrenergic state. Surges of catecholamines have been implicated with plaque fissuring, thrombus propagation, and a reduction in VF threshold. Morphine has the following effects:

- Produces central nervous system analgesia, which reduces the toxic effects of neurohumoral activation, catecholamine release, and heightened myocardial oxygen demand
- Produces venodilation, which reduces LV preload and oxygen requirements
- Decreases systemic vascular resistance, thereby reducing LV afterload
- Helps redistribute blood volume in patients with acute pulmonary edema

Similar to nitroglycerin, morphine is a vasodilator and is not to be used in patients with suspected hypovolemia or inadequate right or left ventricular preload.

Precautions, Adverse Effects, and Contraindications

- Avoid morphine in patients who are hypotensive and in patients with suspected hypovolemia.
- Morphine-induced hypotension is secondary to its vasodilative properties; it most often develops in volume-depleted patients.
- If hypotension develops in a supine patient in the absence of pulmonary congestion, elevate the patient's legs and administer a normal saline bolus of 200 to 500 mL IV. Assess the patient frequently.
- Avoid concomitant use of other vasodilators, such as IV nitroglycerin, in patients with continued, unresponsive pain. A β-blocker may be a better choice than nitroglycerin for refractory ischemic pain.
- The respiratory depression associated with morphine seldom presents a significant problem because the increased adrenergic state associated with infarction or pulmonary edema maintains respiratory drive.
  - If significant respiratory depression does occur, administer naloxone 0.4 mg IV at 3-minute intervals; repeat for 3 doses. Naloxone will reduce any morphine-induced respiratory depression that may occur. If hypoventilation persists, consider other causes.

Prehospital Fibrinolysis

Clinical trials have shown that the greatest potential for myocardial salvage comes from initiating fibrinolysis as soon as possible after the onset of ischemic-type chest pain. To reduce the time to treatment, a number of

---

FYI **ACC/AHA STEMI Guidelines 2007** **Morphine Dosing Change and New Caution for NSTEMI**	**Dose Titration for Morphine** - Initial dose 2 to 4 mg - Incremental dose 2 to 8 mg at 5-minute to 15-minute intervals The 2004 ACC/AHA guidelines for management of STEMI[15] issued a concern for underdosing patients with morphine and other analgesics. Pain, which is commonly severe early in STEMI, is associated with excess sympathetic activity and a hyperadrenergic state. Morphine is the agent of choice to treat this condition. Do not use pain relief or control to assess anti-ischemic or reperfusion therapy. For more information, see Chapter 12 in Part 2.

FAQ **What Happened To "MONA"?**	For years ACLS providers learned that "MONA (morphine, oxygen, nitrates, aspirin) greets all patients"—but not necessarily in that order. Concern about the administration of morphine *before* nitrates was addressed by the 2005 guidelines writing committee. By consensus recommendation the order for the first 4 agents administered for possible ACS was defined and "MONA" was retired. The order is - Aspirin - Oxygen - Nitrates (SL or spray) - Possibly morphine (if discomfort is unrelieved by nitrates)

researchers have proposed and evaluated out-of-hospital administration of fibrinolytics. Although several studies have demonstrated the feasibility and safety of out-of-hospital fibrinolytic administration, other trials have reached conflicting conclusions about the efficiency and efficacy of this strategy.

A meta-analysis of multiple out-of-hospital fibrinolytic trials found a 17% relative improvement in outcome associated with out-of-hospital fibrinolytic therapy.[36] The greatest improvement was observed when therapy was initiated 60 to 90 minutes earlier than in the hospital. More recently a meta-analysis evaluated time to therapy and impact of prehospital fibrinolysis on all-cause mortality.[37] Analysis of pooled results from 6 randomized trials with more than 6000 patients showed a significant 58-minute reduction in time to drug administration. This time reduction was associated with decreased all-cause hospital mortality. These studies concluded that out-of-hospital–initiated fibrinolytic therapy can definitely shorten the time to fibrinolytic treatment. But these time savings can be offset whenever effective ED triage results in a door-to-needle time of 30 minutes or less, obviating the need for implementation of special training and a rigorous out-of-hospital protocol.

However, persistent delay to fibrinolysis (2½ to 3 hours) after symptom onset has led to a reexamination of prehospital bolus fibrinolytic therapy. More recent trials have continued to show a reduction in treatment time when fibrinolytics are administered before arrival at the hospital. The Assessment of the Safety and Efficacy of a New Thrombolytic Regimen trial (ASSENT III Plus) showed reduced treatment delay (40 to 45 minutes) but increased cerebral hemorrhage (in patients aged >75 years).[38] The Early Retavase–Thrombolysis in Myocardial Infarction (ER-TIMI 19) trial and the Comparison of Angioplasty and Prehospital Thrombolysis in Acute Myocardial Infarction (CAPTIM) trial evaluated prehospital fibrinolysis and demonstrated a consistent decrease in time to treatment.[39,40] In the CAPTIM trial prehospital fibrinolysis was not inferior to primary angioplasty in patients presenting within 6 hours of onset of MI.

When prehospital personnel identify a patient with STEMI, it is appropriate for them to begin a fibrinolytic checklist when clinically indicated by protocol (Figure 9).

Destination Protocols

Prehospital Triage and Interfacility Transfer

Every community should have a written protocol that guides EMS system personnel where to take patients with possible STEMI. Patients in cardiogenic shock or with large MI with a high risk of dying should be taken primarily or transferred secondarily to a PCI facility. The goal for interfacility transfer is a door-to-departure time of 30 minutes or less.

Special Considerations

Patients in cardiogenic shock benefit from aggressive therapy, including intra-aortic balloon pump and percutaneous or surgical revascularization, when this can be accomplished within 36 hours of onset of MI and 18 hours from onset of shock. Patients in cardiogenic shock should be taken primarily or transferred secondarily to a PCI facility.

Emergency Department

The initial management and risk stratification of ACS patients is complex and requires additional training and experience beyond the ACLS Provider Course and demonstrated skills. In addition, the ACLS Provider Course was designed to focus on the initial management of ACS and early ED stratification and treatment, particularly early reperfusion. This chapter provides a brief overview. For

---

FYI

ACC/AHA STEMI Guidelines 2004 and 2007 Guidelines

Recommendation for Prehospital Fibrinolytic Therapy

Establishment of a prehospital fibrinolysis program is reasonable in the following settings:

1. EMS systems where physicians are present in the ambulance
2. A well-organized EMS system with full-time paramedics and
   - 12-lead ECGs with transmission capability
   - Initial and ongoing ECG training for paramedics
   - On-line medical command and a medical director with training and experience in STEMI management
   - Ongoing continuous quality-improvement program

The ACC/AHA Focused Update of the ACC/AHA 2004 Guidelines for the Management of STEMI recommends

- When EMS has fibrinolytic capability and the patient qualifies for treatment, a fibrinolytic should be administered within 30 minutes of EMS arrival

more detailed information, see the following sections in Part 2 of this text:

- Risk Stratification of ACS Patients—Selection of Reperfusion Strategy
- 12-Lead ECG in Ischemic Heart Disease—Infarct Localization
- Management of NSTEMI Patients and Cardiac Markers
- Evaluation of Life-Threatening Chest Pain and Nondiagnostic ECGs
- Cardiogenic Shock, Pulmonary Edema, and Hypotension

Early evaluation and management in the ED emphasizes efficient, focused evaluation of the patient with ischemic chest pain. The 4 "D's" of STEMI survival serve as benchmarks for time, evaluation, and treatment goals.

The 4 D's of STEMI Survival

Time is muscle. Limitation of infarct size historically relied on early reperfusion therapy with fibrinolytic drugs. Goals were developed on the basis of the open artery hypothesis—open the infarct-related artery, restore perfusion to the myocardium, limit infarct size, and reduce death and complications of MI (eg, congestive heart failure). The 4 D's represent benchmarks and time goals in the reperfusion strategy: **D**oor, **D**ata, **D**ecision, and **D**rug. The door-to-drug administration goal is 30 minutes.[41] As PCI became available the door-to-balloon goal became 90 minutes. According to the current ACC/AHA STEMI guidelines, when both fibrinolysis and PCI are available, PCI is generally preferred over fibrinolytic therapy when the expected delay for PCI is within 1 hour. However, if the patient has had symptoms for more that 3 hours, presumably making the clot more resistant to lysis and increasing the risks and decreasing the benefits from lytics, a delay of 90 minutes is considered acceptable.

Initial Risk Stratification

Part of the decision process is weighing the potential benefits of therapy against the risks. In patients receiving fibrinolytic therapy, the major risk is intracerebral hemorrhage (ICH). There is an early hazard of fibrinolysis, and the mortality rate in patients treated with fibrinolysis is paradoxically higher during the first 24 hours after treatment. Although the risk of ICH is minimal with PCI, patients who would receive no benefit from PCI assume the risk of the procedure and associated therapy. Because this risk is not offset by benefit, unnecessary PCI can have a net negative outcome.

Patients with ACS may receive a variety of treatments and evaluation strategies. In every case the physician must make a decision, weighing the risk versus the benefit for that patient. Evidence-based medicine can provide general data and recommendations for groups or types of patients. But the knowledgeable healthcare provider must in the end apply this data at the bedside to a single patient. Some decisions are easy, such as the use of aspirin in ACS. Others require a careful evaluation of the benefits, risks, and potential complications of therapy. Patients may meet eligibility criteria for a therapy, but the benefit may be small compared with the risk. For example, a small inferior STEMI presenting relatively late may be within the treatment time window for fibrinolytics, but an increased risk of ICH may favor conservative therapy or transfer for primary PCI.

The 12-Lead ECG in STEMI

The ACLS Provider Course does not require that students already know 12-lead ECG interpretation or learn it during the course. The skill of ECG interpretation takes years of training to acquire. But many students and healthcare providers can learn to recognize certain ECG patterns and features with basic training and some clinical experience. In the ACLS Provider Course the patterns of ST deviation

FYI **Guidelines 2005** **ACC/AHA STEMI** **Guidelines 2004**	Patients in cardiogenic shock or with a large MI with a high risk of dying should be taken primarily or transferred secondarily to an experienced PCI facility. • The goal for interfacility transfer is a door-to-departure time of 30 minutes or less.
Critical Concept **ECG Criteria** **for Fibrinolytic** **Therapy**	In addition to chest discomfort consistent with ongoing ischemia/infarction, the ECG must meet 1 of the following criteria to qualify the patient for acute reperfusion therapy: • More than 1 mm ST-segment elevation in 2 contiguous leads • New or presumably new LBBB • ST-segment depression if criteria for true posterior MI are present

are reviewed to allow the provider to recognize STEMI in most instances when present. The ACLS for Experienced Providers Course discusses the spectrum of ischemic ECGs and highlights complications associated with infarct location in core cases.

Basic ECG Measurements

Healthcare providers who may evaluate acute chest pain should be familiar with the basic concepts of ECG measurements and intervals from rhythm analysis. The ST segment is the cornerstone of decision making in the initial triage of patients into the 3 treatment categories. STEMI is emphasized in the ACLS Provider Course because of the

urgency of timely intervention. The majority of patients with ST-segment elevation will develop transmural or Q-wave MI unless an intervention or spontaneous reperfusion reopens the coronary artery.

Serial, Repeat, or Continuous 12-Lead ECGs?

If the initial ECG is nondiagnostic, serial ECGs are recommended. The clinician must determine the frequency of repeat ECGs, but perform at least 1 repeat ECG approximately 1 hour after the first. If the initial ECG is nondiagnostic but the patient is symptomatic and there is a high clinical suspicion for STEMI, obtain repeat ECGs at

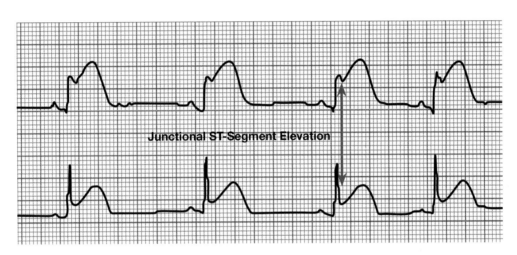

Figure 10. Leads III (top) and aVF (bottom) demonstrate significant ST-segment elevation typical of STEMI. In this instance leads III and aVF are contiguous inferior leads. A 12-lead ECG is required to confirm an inferior myocardial infarction.

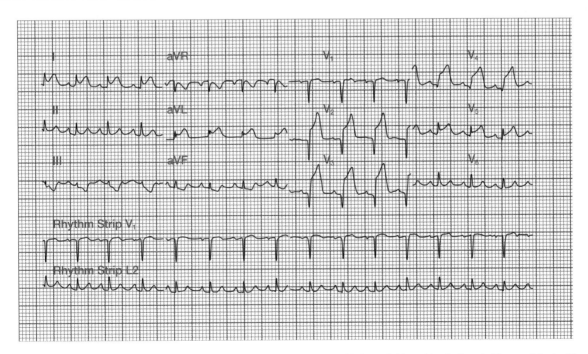

Figure 11. A 12-lead ECG demonstrating ST-segment elevation in anterior leads V₁ through V₅ and leads 1 and aVL, consistent with a large anterior wall myocardial infarction. Note the "reciprocal" ST-segment depression in the inferior leads III and aVF.

5-minute to 10-minute intervals or initiate continuous 12-lead ST-segment monitoring.

Dynamic ECG Changes

Repeat or serial ECGs often show *dynamic 12-lead changes,* meaning that the ST changes on the initial ECG normalize or a nondiagnostic initial ECG becomes abnormal. For example, ST elevation shown on an initial 12-lead ECG obtained in a satellite clinic or by EMS personnel in the field may be resolved minutes later on the ED ECG. It would be a serious error to base further management on the normalized ECG rather than on the initial abnormal recording.

New or Presumably New LBBB?

A *new* LBBB in the context of ischemic-like chest pain is an ominous event, indicating an occlusion in the left coronary artery system, usually above the septal branch of the left anterior descending artery. When an LBBB is present, the delayed LV depolarization of LBBB distorts the ST segment, preventing accurate identification of ST elevation. Thus the clinician operates without the ability to identify ST elevation. Because ST elevation has become the essential criterion for the use of fibrinolytics, its secondary repolarization change in patients with LBBB has posed difficulties in the many clinical trials of fibrinolytic therapy. In an excellent recent review of this problem, Kontos et al[42] observed that the fibrinolytic mega-trials were inconsistent and contradictory in regard to "new BBB." The trials used highly variable inclusion and exclusion criteria for chest pain patients presenting with "bundle branch block," "left bundle branch block," or "right bundle branch block."

Fibrinolytic trials have defined some changes in ECG morphology that increase the likelihood of MI in the presence of LBBB. But in most cases an experienced electrocardiographer is needed.

Determination of "New or Presumably New" BBB

This determination requires copies or reports of previous ECGs that may be difficult or impossible to obtain. This inability to determine whether the BBB is old or new forces the clinician to resort to unassisted clinical judgment and consideration of the benefits versus the risks of fibrinolytic therapy. In this clinical situation most clinicians let the patient's account of symptom onset and the degree of severity weigh heavily in the final decision about therapy. The more the pain and associated signs and symptoms match with an acute ischemic event, the more likely the patient has a new BBB. In a recent, thoughtful decision analysis, Gallagher[43] compared outcomes from a treatment strategy based on the Sgarbossa et al[44-46] ECG algorithm with outcomes from a treatment strategy of simply giving fibrinolytics to all symptomatic patients with LBBB. The analysis intentionally ignored the question of "new versus old" BBB and concluded that fibrinolytic administration was appropriate for all patients with BBB and ischemic-like chest pain.[43]

New or Presumably New RBBB?

A new right bundle branch block (RBBB) is also associated with increased mortality when associated with AMI. Acute ST-segment changes are more readily identified with RBBB and should not be overlooked. RBBB obscures the terminal portion of the QRS complex; significant or new Q waves can also be identified. But any BBB that obscures ST-segment evaluation in the setting of a high clinical suspicion of AMI may be an indication for reperfusion therapy. If fibrinolytic therapy is contraindicated, consider coronary angiography if suspicion remains high.

Cardiac Markers in STEMI

Previously called "cardiac enzymes," cardiac markers released from myocytes when they undergo necrosis are not used to identify patients with STEMI for reperfusion therapy. In many patients cardiac markers are not elevated within the first several hours after onset of chest pain. They may take 6 to 8 hours to reach detectable levels. The clinical markers used today are predominantly the creatine kinase subform found predominantly in the heart (CK-MB) and the cardiac specific troponins (cTn). See Figure 12.

STEMI—Adjunctive Therapy

After initial management and stabilization, additional drug therapy is administered. Although adjunctive therapy applies generally to many patients, the selection of drugs—and sometimes doses—is individualized on the basis of management strategies, local protocols, and the clinician's patient and data assessments. The following is an overview and is not to be viewed as routine recommendations for patients with ACS or STEMI. In addition, this area is fluid and clinical trials continue to evolve. There is no substitute for a knowledgeable physician applying this data to individual patients at the bedside. Some of this material is covered in more detail in Part 2 and is not core material for ACLS providers.

β-Adrenergic Receptor Blockers

In-hospital administration of β-blockers may reduce the size of the infarct, incidence of cardiac rupture, and mortality in patients who do not receive fibrinolytic therapy.[49-53] This data was largely observed during clinical trials before the "reperfusion era." β-Blockers also reduce the incidence of ventricular ectopy and fibrillation.[54] In patients who receive fibrinolytic agents, IV β-blockers decrease postinfarction ischemia and nonfatal AMI. A small but significant decrease in death and nonfatal infarction has been observed in patients treated with β-blockers very soon after the onset of symtpoms.[55] IV β-blockers may also be beneficial for NSTEMI.

Oral β-blockers should be administered in the ED for ACS of all types unless contraindications are present. They should be given irrespective of the need for revascularization therapies (Class I). IV β-blockers are often administered in the ED based on the results from the Metoprolol in Acute Myocardial Infarction (MIAMI) trial, but they are not "routine" and they require risk stratification. In the reperfusion era early administration of β-blockers decreased recurrent ischemia but did not appear to have a mortality benefit. To assess modern use, the Clopidogrel and Metoprolol in Myocardial Infarction Trial (COMMIT CCS2) trial used the MIAMI dosing schedule, administering 3 doses of metoprolol 5 mg IV over 15 minutes.[56] In this large trial there was no benefit of early administration of IV β-blockers. An analysis of prespecified subgroups showed that about 10 lives per 1000 were saved by a reduction in VF, but this benefit was offset by an increase in patient death from cardiogenic shock. Lives lost from cardiogenic shock increased with increasing Killip class, likely as a result of an increase in death from heart failure since LV

dysfunction increases with infarct size. For this reason careful attention should be given to treating patients with congestive heart failure. A tachycardia in these patients may be compensatory as heart rate compensates for impaired and decreased stroke volume due to infarction (Figure 12).

Contraindications to use of β-blockers are moderate to severe LV failure and pulmonary edema, bradycardia (heart rate <60 bpm), hypotension (SBP <100 mm Hg), signs of poor peripheral perfusion, second-degree or third-degree AV block, or reactive airway disease. In the presence of moderate or severe heart failure, oral β-blockers are preferred. They may need to be given in low and titrated doses after the patient is stabilized. This approach permits earlier administration of ACE inhibitors, which are documented to reduce 30-day mortality rates (see below). For more detailed recommendations for use early in STEMI see FYI on next page.

Heparins

Heparin is an indirect inhibitor of thrombin that has been widely used as adjunctive therapy for fibrinolysis and in combination with aspirin for the treatment of unstable angina.

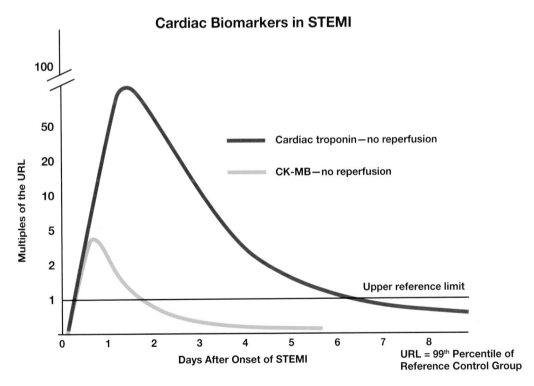

Figure 12. Cardiac biomarkers in STEMI. Typical cardiac biomarkers that are used to evaluate patients with STEMI include the MB isoenzyme of CK (CK-MB) and cardiac-specific troponins. The horizontal line depicts the upper reference limit (URL) for the cardiac biomarker in the clinical chemistry laboratory. The URL is that value representing the 99th percentile of a reference control group without STEMI. The kinetics of release of CK-MB and cardiac troponin in patients who do not undergo reperfusion are shown. Adapted with permission from Alpert JS, Thygesen K, Antman E, Bassand JP. Myocardial infarction redefined—a consensus document of The Joint European Society of Cardiology/American College of Cardiology Committee for the Redefinition of Myocardial Infarction. *J Am Coll Cardiol.* 2000;36:959-969[46] and Wu AH, Apple FS, Gibler WB, Jesse RL, Warshaw MM, Valdes R. National Academy of Clinical Biochemistry Standards of Laboratory Practice: recommendations for the use of cardiac markers in coronary artery diseases. *Clin Chem.* 1999;45:1104-1121.[47]

Unfractionated Heparin

Unfractionated heparin (UFH) is a heterogeneous mixture of sulfated glycosaminoglycans with varying chain lengths. UFH has several disadvantages, including an unpredictable anticoagulant response in individual patients, the need for IV administration, and the requirement for frequent monitoring of the activated partial thromboplastin time (aPTT). Heparin can also stimulate platelet activation, causing thrombocytopenia.

When UFH is used as adjunctive therapy with fibrin-specific lytics in STEMI, the current recommendations call for a bolus dose of 60 U/kg followed by infusion at a rate of 12 U/kg per hour (a maximum bolus of 4000 U and infusion of 1000 U/h for patients weighing >70 kg). An aPTT of 50 to 70 seconds is considered optimal.

The duration of therapy is 48 hours. The available data do not suggest a benefit from prolonging an infusion of heparin beyond this time in the absence of continuing indications for anticoagulation.

Low-Molecular-Weight Heparin

Low-molecular-weight heparins (LMWHs) have been found to be superior to UFH in patients with STEMI in terms of overall grade of flow (Thrombolysis in Myocardial Infarction [TIMI] grade)[57,58] and reducing the frequency of ischemic

---

FYI

ACC/AHA
Focused
Update

STEMI 2007
Guidelines

β-Adrenergic
Blockade Early in
STEMI

CAREFUL!

Recommendation for Oral β-Adrenergic Blockade Early in STEMI (Class I Recommendation; Level of Evidence Changed From A to B):

Oral β-blockade should be initiated within first 24 hours in STEMI to patients not at high risk* *without* any of the following:

- Signs of heart failure
- Evidence of low output state
- Increased risk for cardiogenic shock
- Other relative contraindications

Patients with early contraindication to β-blockade should be reevaluated for candidacy for secondary prevention before discharge

- Patients with moderate to severe heart failure should receive β-blockade as secondary prevention with a gradual titration scheme

Recommendation for IV β-Adrenergic Blockade Early in STEMI (Class II Recommendation; Level of Evidence Changed From A to B):

- Reasonable to administer IV β-blockade to patients who are hypertensive and who *do not* have
  - Signs of heart failure
  - Evidence of low output state
  - Increased risk for cardiogenic shock
  - Other relative contraindications

IV β-Adrenergic Blockade Class III (New 2007 Recommendation)

IV β-blockade should not be administered to patients who have any of the following:

- Signs of heart failure
- Evidence of low output state
- Risk factors for cardiogenic shock*
- Other relative contraindications: PR interval >0.24 second or higher AV block, active asthma or reactive airway disease

*Risk factors for cardiogenic shock include
- age >70 years
- SBP <120 mm Hg
- heart rate >110 or <60 per minute
- delayed presentation

complications,[59] with a trend to a 14% reduction in mortality rates in a meta-analysis.[60] No superiority was found in studies in which an invasive strategy (PCI) was used.

Two randomized, controlled trials have compared UFH with LMWH as ancillary treatment to fibrinolysis in the out-of-hospital setting.[38,61] Administration of LMWH for patients with STEMI showed superiority in composite end points compared with UFH. But this benefit must be balanced against the *increase in intracranial hemorrhage in patients >75 years of age* who received LMWH (enoxaparin).[38]

LMWH is an acceptable alternative to UFH in the ED as ancillary therapy for patients *<75 years of age* who are receiving fibrinolytic therapy, provided that significant renal dysfunction (serum creatinine >2.5 mg/dL in men or 2 mg/dL in women) is not present (Class IIb). UFH is recommended for patients >75 years of age as ancillary therapy to fibrinolysis (Class IIa) and for any STEMI patient who is undergoing revascularization. In patients with STEMI who are not receiving fibrinolysis or revascularization, LMWH (specifically enoxaparin) may be considered an acceptable alternative to UFH in the ED setting (Class IIb).

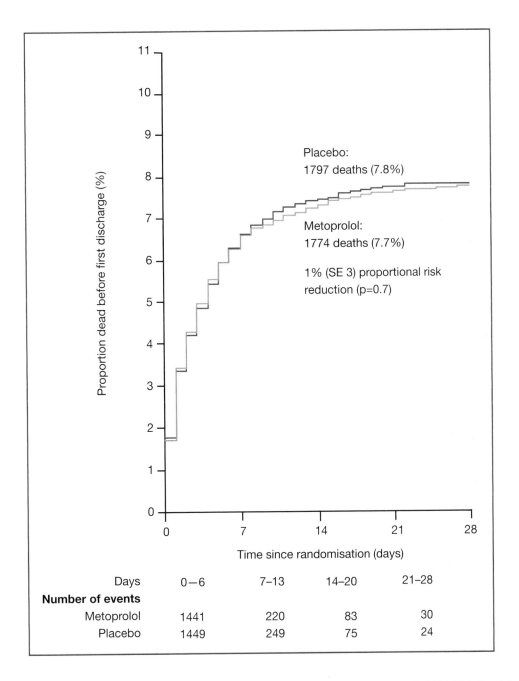

Days	0–6	7–13	14–20	21–28
Number of events				
Metoprolol	1441	220	83	30
Placebo	1449	249	75	24

Figure 12. Effects of metoprolol allocation on death before first discharge from hospital in the COMMITT CCS2 Trial. Reprinted with permission from Chen ZM, Pan HC, Chen YP, Peto R, Collins R, Jiang LX, Xie JX, Liu LS. Early intravenous then oral metoprolol in 45,852 patients with acute myocardial infarction: randomized placebo-controlled trial. *Lancet.* 2005;366:1622-1632.[55] © 2005 Lancet Publishing Group.

Table 2. Use of Heparin in ACS

Drug/Therapy	Indications/Precautions	Adult Dosage
Heparin Unfractionated (UFH) Concentrations range from 1000 to 40 000 IU/mL	**Indications** • Adjuvant therapy in AMI. • Begin heparin with fibrin-specific lytics (eg, alteplase, reteplase, tenecteplase). **Precautions/Contraindications** • Same contraindications as for fibrinolytic therapy: active bleeding; recent intracranial, intraspinal, or eye surgery; severe hypertension; bleeding disorders; gastrointestinal bleeding. • Doses and laboratory targets appropriate when used with fibrinolytic therapy. • Do not use if platelet count is or falls below <100 000 or with history of heparin-induced thrombocytopenia. For these patients consider direct antithrombins. See bivalirudin at the bottom of this column.	**UFH IV Infusion—STEMI** • Initial bolus 60 IU/kg (maximum bolus: 4000 IU). • Continue 12 IU/kg per hour, round to the nearest 50 IU (maximum: 1000 IU/hour for patients >70 kg). • Adjust to maintain aPTT 1.5 to 2 times the control values (50 to 70 seconds) for 48 hours or until angiography. • Check initial aPTT at 3 hours, then q 6 hours until stable, then daily. • Follow institutional heparin protocol. • Platelet count daily. **UFH IV Infusion—UA/NSTEMI** • Initial bolus 60 IU/kg. Maximum: 4000 IU. • 12 IU/kg per hour. Maximum: 1000 IU/h. • Follow institutional protocol.
Heparin Low Molecular Weight (LMWH)	**Indications** For use in acute coronary syndromes, specifically patients with UA/NSTEMI. These drugs inhibit thrombin generation by factor Xa inhibition and also inhibit thrombin indirectly by formation of a complex with antithrombin III. These drugs are **not** neutralized by heparin-binding proteins. **Precautions** • Hemorrhage may complicate any therapy with LMWH. Contraindicated in presence of hypersensitivity to heparin or pork products or history of sensitivity to drug. Use **enoxaparin** with extreme caution in patients with type II heparin-induced thrombocytopenia. • Adjust dose for renal insufficiency. • Contraindicated if platelet count <100 000. For these patients consider direct antithrombins: — **Bivalirudin** (Angiomax, FDA-approved for ACS patients undergoing PCI): Bolus with 0.1 mg/kg IV, then begin infusion of 0.25 mg/kg per hour.	**STEMI Protocol** • Enoxaparin — Age <75 years, normal creatinine clearance: initial bolus 30 mg IV with second bolus 15 minutes later of 1 mg/kg SQ, repeat q 12 hours. — Age ≥75 years: Eliminate initial IV bolus, give 0.75 mg/kg SQ q 12 hours. — If creatinine clearance <30 mL/min, give 1 mg/kg SQ q 24 hours. • Fondaparinux — Initial dose 2.5 mg/kg IV, then give 2.5 mg/kg SQ q 24 hours for up to 8 days. **UA/NSTEMI Protocol** • Enoxaparin: Loading dose 30 mg IV bolus. Maintenance dose 1 mg/kg SQ q 12 hours. If creatinine clearance <30 mL/min, reduce dosing interval to q 24 hours. • Fondaparinux: 2.5 mg SQ ONCE every 24 hours; avoid if creatinine clearance <30 mL/min. **Heparin Reversal** ICH or life-threatening bleed: Administer protamine, refer to package insert.

FYI

ACC/AHA Focused Update

STEMI 2007 Guidelines

Anticoagulation in STEMI

Heparin Therapy WITH Fibrinolytics

Patients undergoing reperfusion with *fibrinolytic agents* should receive anticoagulation therapy for a minimum of 48 hours with unfractionated heparin (UFH) and preferably for the duration of the hospitalization up to 8 days using another anticoagulation regimen (eg, enoxaparin), other LMWH, or antithrombin.

Recommendation for Unfractionated Heparin (UFH)

• Initial bolus unchanged 60 IU/kg (maximum 4000 IU)
• Target aPTT 1.5 to 2 times control (about 50 to 70 seconds)
• Treatment duration up to 48 hours unless other indications for anticoagulation

Recommendations for Enoxaparin

• Exclude men with serum creatinine 2.5 or greater (women 2.0 or greater)
• Give initial 30 mg IV bolus for patients <75 years of age
• Administer 1 mg/kg subcutaneously every 12 hours; reduce dose to 0.75 mg/kg if patient ≥75 years of age
• If creatinine clearance <30 mL/min (using the Cockcroft-Gault formula), decrease dose to 1 mg every 24 hours for all ages
• Maintain therapy for duration of hospitalization or up to 8 days

The use of heparin in ACS and as an adjunct to other treatments can increase major bleeding and cause mortality. Healthcare providers administering heparin should be familiar with its use in different ACS settings and strategies. Preferably the administration of heparin and other therapies should be protocol driven. Table 2, reproduced from the *ECC Handbook,* can serve as a general reference. The updated ACC/AHA Focused Guideline Recommendations for STEMI are presented in the FYI. Providers need to be aware of recent trials and new guidelines and recommendations as they emerge.

Clopidogrel in STEMI

Clopidogrel irreversibly inhibits the platelet adenosine diphosphate receptor (COX-1), resulting in a reduction in platelet aggregation through a different mechanism than aspirin. Since the publication of *ECC Guidelines 2005,* several important clopidogrel studies have been published and reviewed by the ACC/AHA STEMI writing group that document its efficacy for patients with STEMI. It was recently approved by the FDA for use in patients with STEMI, either with or without fibrinolytic therapy. Approval was based on results of the Clopidogrel as Adjunctive Reperfusion Therapy (CLARITY-TIMI 28) and COMMIT CCS-2 trials, which demonstrated increased efficacy of dual therapy with aspirin with no increase in intracerebral hemorrhage.

In patients up to 75 years of age with STEMI who are treated with fibrinolysis, aspirin, and heparin (LMWH or UFH), a 300-mg oral loading dose of clopidogrel given at the time of initial management (followed by a 75 mg daily dose for up to 8 days in hospital) improved coronary artery patency and reduced MACE.[62] The COMMITT trial,[63] which included more than 45 000 patients, found that those receiving clopidogrel 75 mg had a highly significant 9% reduction in death, reinfarction, or stroke, corresponding to 9 fewer events per 1000 patients treated for only about 2 weeks. There was also no increase in intracerebral hemorrhage. Based on these findings, providers should administer a 300-mg oral dose of clopidogrel to ED patients up to 75 years of age with STEMI who receive aspirin, heparin, and fibrinolysis. If a PCI strategy is planned, providers should rely on protocol recommendations or instructions from an interventional cardiologist. Clopidogrel should not be administered to patients in shock and those who may require urgent surgical procedures.

ACE Inhibitor Therapy

In general, ACE inhibitor therapy will not be initiated by ACLS providers. ACE inhibitor therapy is usually started in hospital after reperfusion therapy has been accomplished and the patient is hemodynamically stable. Administration of an oral ACE inhibitor is recommended within the first 24 hours after onset of symptoms in STEMI patients with pulmonary congestion or LV ejection fraction <40% in the absence of hypotension (SBP <100 mm Hg or >30 mm Hg below baseline) (Class IA). Additional Class IA indications from the 2007 Focused STEMI Update include patients with hypertension, chronic kidney disease, or diabetes. Oral ACE inhibitor therapy should be considered for all other patients with AMI with or without early reperfusion therapy (Class IB).

IV administration of ACE inhibitors is contraindicated in the first 24 hours because of the risk of hypotension (Class III).

HMG Coenzyme A Reductase Inhibitors (Statins)

A variety of studies document consistent reduction in incidence of major adverse cardiac events (reinfarction, recurrent angina, rehospitalization, stroke) when statin treatment is administered within a few days after onset of an ACS.[64-67] There is little data to suggest that this therapy should be initiated in the ED; but early initiation of statin therapy (within 24 hours of presentation) is safe and feasible in patients with an ACS or AMI (Class I). If patients are already on statin therapy, it should be continued.

Therapy for Cardiac Arrhythmias

Treatment of ventricular arrhythmias during and after AMI has been a controversial topic for 2 decades. Primary VF accounts for the majority of early deaths during AMI. The incidence of primary VF is highest during the first 4 hours after onset of symptoms but remains an important contributor to mortality during the first 24 hours. Secondary VF occurring in the setting of congestive heart failure or cardiogenic shock can also contribute to death from AMI. VF is a less common cause of death in the hospital with the early use of fibrinolytics in conjunction with β-blockers.

Although prophylaxis with lidocaine reduces the incidence of VF, an analysis of data from ISIS-3 and a meta-analysis suggest that lidocaine increased all-cause mortality rates.[68] For this reason the practice of prophylactic administration of lidocaine has been largely abandoned. Routine administration of magnesium to patients with MI has no significant clinical mortality benefit, particularly in patients receiving fibrinolytic therapy. The definitive studies on the subject are ISIS-4 and MAGIC.[35,69]

FYI

ACC/AHA Focused Update

STEMI 2007 Guidelines

Anticoagulation in STEMI

Clopidogrel Therapy

Patients undergoing reperfusion with *fibrinolytic agents and those not receiving reperfusion* should receive combination antiplatelet therapy with both aspirin and clopidogrel.

Recommendation for Adjunctive Use With Fibrinolytics

- Clopidogrel 75 mg oral daily maintenance dose
- A loading dose of 300 mg was administered in CLARITY TIMI 28, but
  - Efficacy and safety not demonstrated in patients >75 years of age
  - Patients receiving bolus 4000 IU heparin dose were excluded

Recommendation for Adjunctive Use Without Reperfusion

- Clopidogrel 75 mg oral daily maintenance dose
- A loading dose of 300 mg was administered in CLARITY TIMI 28, but
  - Efficacy and safety not demonstrated in patients ≥75 years of age
  - Patients receiving bolus 4000 IU heparin dose were excluded

No Recommendation for Adjunctive Use Upstream From PCI

No recommendation was made for upstream use prior to PCI, but it was noted:
- It appears that clopidogrel is beneficial when PCI is subsequently performed in patients receiving prior fibrinolytic therapy

Critical Concept

Out-of-Hospital Administration of Clopidogrel

Providers should refrain from administration of clopidogrel out-of-hospital unless and until a treatment strategy and reperfusion status have been determined by an experienced physician, planned protocol, or PCI team.

- Patients requiring urgent surgical intervention for complications of MI and left main or 3 vessel disease in shock should not receive clopidogrel.
- Patients *75 years of age and older* should not receive *a loading dose* (300 or 600 mg) of clopidogrel.

Foundation Facts

Use of ACE Inhibitors by ACLS Providers

ACE inhibitor therapy is usually started in-hospital after reperfusion therapy has been accomplished and the patient is stable hemodynamically.

- *IV ACE* inhibitor therapy is contraindicated within the first 24 hours of AMI and should not be used for control of hypertension early in the management of AMI patients.

Appendix: ACC-AHA Classification of Recommendation and Level of Evidence

	Class I **Benefit >>> Risk** Procedure/ Treatment SHOULD be performed/ administered	Class IIa **Benefit >> Risk** *Additional studies with focused objectives needed* IT IS REASONABLE to perform procedure/administer treatment	Class IIb **Benefit ≥ Risk** *Additional studies with broad objectives needed; additional registry data would be helpful* *Procedure/ Treatment MAY BE CONSIDERED*	Class III **Risk ≥ Benefit** *No additional studies needed* Procedure/ Treatment should NOT be performed/ administered SINCE IT IS NOT HELPFUL AND MAY BE HARMFUL
Level A *Multiple (3–5) population risk strata evaluated** *General consistency of direction and magnitude of effect*	• Recommendation procedure or treatment useful/ effective • Sufficient evidence multiple randomized meta-analyses	• Recommendation in favor of treatment or procedure being useful/effective • Some conflicting evidence from multiple randomized trials or meta-analyses	• Recommendation's usefulness/efficacy less well established • Greater conflicting evidence from multiple randomized trials or meta-analyses	• Recommendation that procedure or treatment is not useful/effective and may be harmful • Sufficient evidence from multiple randomized trials or meta-analyses
Level B *Limited (2–3) population risk strata evaluated**	• Recommendation that procedure or treatment is useful/ effective • Limited evidence from single randomized trial or nonrandomized studies	• Recommendation in favor of treatment or procedure being useful/effective • Some conflicting evidence from single randomized trial or nonrandomized studies	• Recommendation's usefulness/efficacy less well established • Greater conflicting evidence from single randomized trial or nonrandomized studies	• Recommendation that procedure or treatment is not useful/effective and may be harmful • Limited evidence from single randomized trial or nonrandomized studies
Level C *Very limited (1–2) population risk strata evaluated**	• Recommendation that procedure or treatment is useful/ effective • Only expert opinion, case studies, or standard-of-care	• Recommendation in of treatment or procedure being useful/effective • Only diverging expert opinion, case studies, or standard-of-care	• Recommendation's usefulness/efficacy less well established • Only diverging expert opinion, case studies, or standard-of-care	• Recommendation that procedure or treatment is not useful/effective and may be harmful • Only expert opinion, case studies, or standard-of-care

References

1. Libby P. Current concepts of the pathogenesis of the acute coronary syndromes. *Circulation*. 2001;104:365-372.

2. Spodick DH. Differential characteristics of the electrocardiogram in early repolarization and acute pericarditis. *N Engl J Med*. 1976;295:523-526.

3. Wang K, Asinger RW, Marriott HJ. ST-segment elevation in conditions other than acute myocardial infarction. *N Engl J Med*. 2003;349:2128-2135.

4. Antman EM. In: Braunwald E, ed. *Heart Disease: A Textbook in Cardiovascular Medicine*. 5th ed. Philadelphia, Pa: WB Saunders; 1997.

5. Libby P. Molecular bases of the acute coronary syndromes. *Circulation*. 1995;91:2844-2850.

6. Pantridge JF, Geddes JS. A mobile intensive-care unit in the management of myocardial infarction. *Lancet*. 1967;2:271-273.

7. Cohen MC, Rohtla KM, Lavery CE, Muller JE, Mittleman MA. Meta-analysis of the morning excess of acute myocardial infarction and sudden cardiac death [published correction appears in *Am J Cardiol*. 1998;81:260]. *Am J Cardiol*. 1997;79:1512-1516.

8. Colquhoun MC, Julien DG. Sudden death in the community—the arrhythmia causing cardiac arrest and results of immediate resuscitation. *Resuscitation*. 1992;24:177A.

9. Campbell RW, Murray A, Julian DG. Ventricular arrhythmias in first 12 hours of acute myocardial infarction: natural history study. *Br Heart J*. 1981;46:351-357.

10. O'Doherty M, Tayler DI, Quinn E, Vincent R, Chamberlain DA. Five hundred patients with myocardial infarction monitored within one hour of symptoms. *Br Med J (Clin Res Ed)*. 1983;286:1405-1408.

11. Lie KI, Wellens HJ, Downar E, Durrer D. Observations on patients with primary ventricular fibrillation complicating acute myocardial infarction. *Circulation*. 1975;52:755-759.

12. Chiriboga D, Yarzebski J, Goldberg RJ, Gore JM, Alpert JS. Temporal trends (1975 through 1990) in the incidence and case-fatality rates of primary ventricular fibrillation complicating acute myocardial infarction: a communitywide perspective. *Circulation*. 1994;89:998-1003.

13. Kereiakes DJ, Weaver WD, Anderson JL, Feldman T, Gibler B, Aufderheide T, Williams DO, Martin LH, Anderson LC, Martin JS, et al. Time delays in the diagnosis and treatment of acute myocardial infarction: a tale of eight cities. Report from the Pre-hospital Study Group and the Cincinnati Heart Project. *Am Heart J*. 1990;120:773-780.

14. Eisenberg MJ, Topol EJ. Prehospital administration of aspirin in patients with unstable angina and acute myocardial infarction. *Arch Intern Med*. 1996;156:1506-1510.

15. Antman EM, Anbe DT, Armstrong PW, Bates ER, Green LA, Hand M, Hochman JS, Krumholz HM, Kushner FG, Lamas GA, Mullany CJ, Ornato JP, Pearle DL, Sloan MA, Smith SC Jr, Alpert JS, Anderson JL, Faxon DP, Fuster V, Gibbons RJ, Gregoratos G, Halperin JL, Hiratzka LF, Hunt SA, Jacobs AK. ACC/AHA guidelines for the management of patients with ST-elevation myocardial infarction: a report of the American College of Cardiology/American Heart Association Task Force on Practice Guidelines (Committee to Revise the 1999 Guidelines for the Management of Patients With Acute Myocardial Infarction). *Circulation*. 2004;110:e82-e292.

16. The Public Access Defibrillation Trial Investigators. Public-access defibrillation and survival after out-of-hospital cardiac arrest. *N Engl J Med*. 2004;351:637-646.

17. Lee TH, Cook EF, Weisberg M, Sargent RK, Wilson C, Goldman L. Acute chest pain in the emergency room: identification and examination of low-risk patients. *Arch Intern Med*. 1985; 145:65-69.

18. Karagounis L, Ipsen SK, Jessop MR, Gilmore KM, Valenti DA, Clawson JJ, Teichman S, Anderson JL. Impact of field-transmitted electrocardiography on time to in-hospital thrombolytic therapy in acute myocardial infarction. *Am J Cardiol*. 1990;66:786-791.

19. Kudenchuk PJ, Ho MT, Weaver WD, Litwin PE, Martin JS, Eisenberg MS, Hallstrom AP, Cobb LA, Kennedy JW. Accuracy of computer-interpreted electrocardiography in selecting patients for thrombolytic therapy. MITI Project Investigators. *J Am Coll Cardiol*. 1991;17:1486-1491.

20. Kereiakes DJ, Gibler WB, Martin LH, Pieper KS, Anderson LC. Relative importance of emergency medical system transport and the prehospital electrocardiogram on reducing hospital time delay to therapy for acute myocardial infarction: a preliminary report from the Cincinnati Heart Project. *Am Heart J*. 1992;123(pt 1):835-840.

21. Aufderheide TP, Kereiakes DJ, Weaver WD, Gibler WB, Simoons ML. Planning, implementation, and process monitoring for prehospital 12-lead ECG diagnostic programs. *Prehospital Disaster Med*. 1996;11:162-171.

22. Aufderheide TP, Hendley GE, Thakur RK, Mateer JR, Stueven HA, Olson DW, Hargarten KM, Laitinen F, Robinson N, Preuss KC, et al. The diagnostic impact of prehospital 12-lead electrocardiography. *Ann Emerg Med*. 1990;19:1280-1287.

23. Grim PS, Feldman T, Childers RW. Evaluation of patients for the need of thrombolytic therapy in the prehospital setting. *Ann Emerg Med*. 1989;18:483-488.

24. Weaver WD, Cerqueira M, Hallstrom AP, Litwin PE, Martin JS, Kudenchuk PJ, Eisenberg M. Prehospital-initiated vs hospital-initiated thrombolytic therapy. The Myocardial Infarction Triage and Intervention Trial. *JAMA*. 1993;270:1211-1216.

25. Foster DB, Dufendach JH, Barkdoll CM, Mitchell BK. Prehospital recognition of AMI using independent nurse/paramedic 12-lead ECG evaluation: impact on in-hospital times to thrombolysis in a rural community hospital. *Am J Emerg Med*. 1994;12:25-31.

26. Aufderheide TP, Haselow WC, Hendley GE, Robinson NA, Armaganian L, Hargarten KM, Olson DW, Valley VT, Stueven HA. Feasibility of prehospital r-TPA therapy in chest pain patients. *Ann Emerg Med*. 1992;21:379-383.

27. Brinfield K. Identification of ST elevation AMI on prehospital 12 lead ECG: accuracy of unaided paramedic interpretation. *J Emerg Med*. 1998;16:22S.

28. Ioannidis JP, Salem D, Chew PW, Lau J. Accuracy and clinical effect of out-of-hospital electrocardiography in the diagnosis of acute cardiac ischemia: a meta-analysis. *Ann Emerg Med*. 2001;37:461-470.

29. Wall T, Albright J, Livingston B, Isley L, Young D, Nanny M, Jacobowitz S, Maynard C, Mayer N, Pierce K, Rathbone C, Stuckey T, Savona M, Leibrandt P, Brodie B, Wagner G. Prehospital ECG transmission speeds reperfusion for patients with acute myocardial infarction. *N C Med J*. 2000;61:104-108.

30. Rawles JM, Kenmure AC. Controlled trial of oxygen in uncomplicated myocardial infarction. *Br Med J*. 1976;1:1121-1123.

31. Maroko PR, Radvany P, Braunwald E, Hale SL. Reduction of infarct size by oxygen inhalation following acute coronary occlusion. *Circulation*. 1975;52:360-368.

32. Madias JE, Madias NE, Hood WB Jr. Precordial ST-segment mapping. 2. Effects of oxygen inhalation on ischemic injury in patients with acute myocardial infarction. Circulation. 1976;53:411-417.

33. Randomised trial of intravenous streptokinase, oral aspirin, both, or neither among 17,187 cases of suspected acute myocardial infarction: ISIS-2. ISIS-2 (Second International Study of Infarct Survival) Collaborative Group. *Lancet*. 1988;2:349-360.

34. Collaborative overview of randomised trials of antiplatelet therapy—I: prevention of death, myocardial infarction, and stroke by prolonged antiplatelet therapy in various categories of patients. Antiplatelet Trialists' Collaboration. *BMJ*. 1994;308:81-106.

35. ISIS-4: a randomised factorial trial assessing early oral captopril, oral mononitrate, and intravenous magnesium sulphate in 58,050 patients with suspected acute myocardial infarction. ISIS-4 (Fourth International Study of Infarct Survival) Collaborative Group. *Lancet*. 1995;345:669-685.

36. European Myocardial Infarction Project Group (EMIP). Prehospital thrombolytic therapy in patients with suspected acute myocardial infarction. The European Myocardial Infarction Project Group. *N Engl J Med*. 1993;329:383-389.

37. Morrison LJ, Verbeek PR, McDonald AC, Sawadsky BV, Cook DJ. Mortality and prehospital thrombolysis for acute myocardial infarction: a meta-analysis. *JAMA*. 2000;283:2686-2692.

38. Wallentin L, Goldstein P, Armstrong PW, Granger CB, Adgey AA, Arntz HR, Bogaerts K, Danays T, Lindahl B, Makijarvi M, Verheugt F, Van de Werf F. Efficacy and safety of tenecteplase in combination with the low-molecular-weight heparin enoxaparin or unfractionated heparin in the prehospital setting: the Assessment of the Safety and Efficacy of a New Thrombolytic Regimen (ASSENT)-3 PLUS randomized trial in acute myocardial infarction. *Circulation*. 2003;108:135-142.

39. Steg PG, Bonnefoy E, Chabaud S, Lapostolle F, Dubien PY, Cristofini P, Leizorovicz A, Touboul P. Impact of time to treatment on mortality after prehospital fibrinolysis or primary angioplasty: data from the CAPTIM randomized clinical trial. *Circulation.* 2003;108:2851-2856.

40. Morrow DA, Antman EM, Sayah A, Schuhwerk KC, Giugliano RP, deLemos JA, Waller M, Cohen SA, Rosenberg DG, Cutler SS, McCabe CH, Walls RM, Braunwald E. Evaluation of the time saved by prehospital initiation of reteplase for ST-elevation myocardial infarction: results of the Early Retavase—Thrombolysis in Myocardial Infarction (ER-TIMI) 19 trial. *J Am Coll Cardiol.* 2002;40:71-77.

41. Emergency department: rapid identification and treatment of patients with acute myocardial infarction. National Heart Attack Alert Program Coordinating Committee, 60 Minutes to Treatment Working Group. *Ann Emerg Med.* 1994;23:311-329.

42. Kontos MC, McQueen RH, Jesse RL, Tatum JL, Ornato JP. Can myocardial infarction be rapidly identified in emergency department patients who have left bundle-branch block? *Ann Emerg Med.* 2001;37:431-438.

43. Gallagher EJ. Which patients with suspected myocardial ischemia and left bundle-branch block should receive thrombolytic agents? *Ann Emerg Med.* 2001;37:439-444.

44. Sgarbossa EB, Pinski SL, Wagner GS. Left bundle-branch block and the ECG in diagnosis of acute myocardial infarction. *JAMA.* 1999;282:1224-1225.

45. Sgarbossa EB. Recent advances in the electrocardiographic diagnosis of myocardial infarction: left bundle branch block and pacing. *Pacing Clin Electrophysiol.* 1996;19:1370-1379.

46. Sgarbossa EB. Value of the ECG in suspected acute myocardial infarction with left bundle branch block. *J Electrocardiol.* 2000;33(suppl):87-92.

47. Alpert JS, Thygesen K, Antman E, Bassand JP. Myocardial infarction redefined—a consensus document of The Joint European Society of Cardiology/American College of Cardiology Committee for the Redefinition of Myocardial Infarction. *J Am Coll Cardiol.* 2000;36:959-969.

48. Wu AH, Apple FS, Gibler WB, Jesse RL, Warshaw MM, Valdes R. National Academy of Clinical Biochemistry Standards of Laboratory Practice: recommendations for the use of cardiac markers in coronary artery diseases. *Clin Chem.* 1999;45:1104-1121.

49. Hjalmarson A, Herlitz J, Holmberg S, Ryden L, Swedberg K, Vedin A, Waagstein F, Waldenstrom A, Waldenstrom J, Wedel H, Wilhelmsen L, Wilhelmsson C. The Göteborg metoprolol trial. Effects on mortality and morbidity in acute myocardial infarction. *Circulation.* 1983;67(6 pt 2):I26-I32.

50. Hjalmarson A, Herlitz J. Limitation of infarct size by beta blockers and its potential role for prognosis. *Circulation.* 1983;67(6 pt 2):I68-I71.

51. The MIAMI Trial Research Group. Metoprolol in acute myocardial infarction (MIAMI): a randomised placebo-controlled international trial. *Eur Heart J.* 1985;6:199-226.

52. Sleight P, Yusuf S, Peto R, Rossi P, Ramsdale D, Bennett D, Bray C, Furse L. Early intravenous atenolol treatment in suspected acute myocardial infarction. *Acta Med Scand Suppl.* 1981;210:185-192.

53. Randomised trial of intravenous atenolol among 16,027 cases of suspected acute myocardial infarction: ISIS-1. First International Study of Infarct Survival Collaborative Group. *Lancet.* 1986;2:57-66.

54. Rehnqvist N, Olsson G, Erhardt L, Ekman AM. Metoprolol in acute myocardial infarction reduces ventricular arrhythmias both in the early stage and after the acute event. *Int J Cardiol.* 1987;15:301-308.

55. Roberts R, Rogers WJ, Mueller HS, Lambrew CT, Diver DJ, Smith HC, Willerson JT, Knatterud GL, Forman S, Passamani E, et al. Immediate versus deferred beta-blockade following thrombolytic therapy in patients with acute myocardial infarction. Results of the Thrombolysis in Myocardial Infarction (TIMI) II-B study. *Circulation.* 1991;83:422-437.

56. Chen ZM, Pan HC, Chen YP, Peto R, Collins R, Jiang LX, Xie JX, Liu LS. Early intravenous then oral metoprolol in 45,852 patients with acute myocardial infarction: randomised placebo-controlled trial. *Lancet.* 2005;366:1622-1632.

57. Wallentin L, Bergstrand L, Dellborg M, Fellenius C, Granger CB, Lindahl B, Lins LE, Nilsson T, Pehrsson K, Siegbahn A, Swahn E. Low molecular weight heparin (dalteparin) compared to unfractionated heparin as an adjunct to rt-PA (alteplase) for improvement of coronary artery patency in acute myocardial infarction—the ASSENT Plus study. *Eur Heart J.* 2003;24:897-908.

58. Ross AM, Molhoek P, Lundergan C, Knudtson M, Draoui Y, Regalado L, Le Louer V, Bigonzi F, Schwartz W, De Jong E, Coyne K. Randomized comparison of enoxaparin, a low-molecular-weight heparin, with unfractionated heparin adjunctive to recombinant tissue plasminogen activator thrombolysis and aspirin: Second Trial of Heparin and Aspirin Reperfusion Therapy (HART II). *Circulation.* 2001;104:648-652.

59. Van de Werf FJ, Armstrong PW, Granger C, Wallentin L. Efficacy and safety of tenecteplase in combination with enoxaparin, abciximab, or unfractionated heparin: the ASSENT-3 randomised trial in acute myocardial infarction. *Lancet.* 2001;358:605-613.

60. Theroux P, Welsh RC. Meta-analysis of randomized trials comparing enoxaparin versus unfractionated heparin as adjunctive therapy to fibrinolysis in ST-elevation acute myocardial infarction. *Am J Cardiol.* 2003;91:860-864.

61. Baird SH, Menown IB, McBride SJ, Trouton TG, Wilson C. Randomized comparison of enoxaparin with unfractionated heparin following fibrinolytic therapy for acute myocardial infarction. *Eur Heart J.* 2002;23:627-632.

62. Sabatine MS, Cannon CP, Gibson CM, Lopez-Sendon JL, Montalescot G, Theroux P, Claeys MJ, Cools F, Hill KA, Skene AM, McCabe CH, Braunwald E. Addition of clopidogrel to aspirin and fibrinolytic therapy for myocardial infarction with ST-segment elevation. *N Engl J Med.* 2005;352:1179-1189.

63. Chen ZM, Jiang LX, Chen YP, Xie JX, Pan HC, Peto R, Collins R, Liu LS. Addition of clopidogrel to aspirin in 45,852 patients with acute myocardial infarction: randomised placebo-controlled trial. *Lancet.* 2005;366:1607-1621.

64. Correia LC, Sposito AC, Lima JC, Magalhaes LP, Passos LC, Rocha MS, D'Oliveira A, Esteves JP. Anti-inflammatory effect of atorvastatin (80 mg) in unstable angina pectoris and non-Q-wave acute myocardial infarction. *Am J Cardiol.* 2003;92:298-301.

65. Kayikcioglu M, Can L, Evrengul H, Payzin S, Kultursay H. The effect of statin therapy on ventricular late potentials in acute myocardial infarction. *Int J Cardiol.* 2003;90:63-72.

66. Kayikcioglu M, Can L, Kultursay H, Payzin S, Turkoglu C. Early use of pravastatin in patients with acute myocardial infarction undergoing coronary angioplasty. *Acta Cardiol.* 2002;57:295-302.

67. Kinlay S, Schwartz GG, Olsson AG, Rifai N, Leslie SJ, Sasiela WJ, Szarek M, Libby P, Ganz P. High-dose atorvastatin enhances the decline in inflammatory markers in patients with acute coronary syndromes in the MIRACL study. *Circulation.* 2003;108:1560-1566.

68. MacMahon S, Collins R, Peto R, Koster RW, Yusuf S. Effects of prophylactic lidocaine in suspected acute myocardial infarction. An overview of results from the randomized, controlled trials. *JAMA*. 1988;260:1910-1916.

69. Rationale and design of the magnesium in coronaries (MAGIC) study: A clinical trial to reevaluate the efficacy of early administration of magnesium in acute myocardial infarction. The MAGIC Steering Committee. *Am Heart J*. 2000;139:10-14.

Chapter (11)

Introduction to ACLS for Experienced Providers

ACLS for Experienced Providers: The Premise

The concept for ACLS for Experienced Providers (ACLS-EP) emerged while asking two simple questions:

- If you know the cause of a cardiac arrest, how will that knowledge change your approach to the attempted resuscitation? Will the ACLS core algorithms apply, or are special modifications required?
- If you encounter the potential patient with cardiac arrest *before* the cardiac arrest and you know or determine the cause, what rapid interventions or actions can you take to prevent the cardiac arrest?

The ACLS *Rhythm Approach*—used in the ACLS Provider Course—is effective for the treatment of many patients in cardiac arrest. But during some cardiovascular emergencies, the ACLS provider will need more resuscitation information and skills. In others, rapid assessment and intervention may prevent the arrest. Recently medical emergency teams, also known as rapid response teams, have been formed in many hospitals to respond to prearrest situations.

In the ACLS Provider Course providers learn a systematic method—the BLS Primary and ACLS Secondary ABCD Surveys—that is appropriate for nearly every cardiovascular emergency and resuscitation attempt. Experienced providers can expand the BLS Primary and ACLS Secondary Surveys into what is termed the *5 Quadrads Approach* (Figure). This approach can be applied to patients in cardiac arrest as well as to unstable patients at risk for development of cardiopulmonary arrest.

The Systematic Approach to ACLS for Experienced Providers

The 5 Quadrads Approach is a 5-step process that covers *assessments* and *actions* that apply to almost any emergency setting:

Critical Concept	
	Cardiac Arrest
	❶ BLS Primary ABCD Survey
	❷ ACLS Secondary ABCD Survey
The 5 Quadrads	**Periarrest**
	❸ Oxygen–IV–Monitor–Fluids (as needed)
	❹ Temperature–Heart Rate–Blood Pressure–Respirations
	❺ Tank Volume–Tank Resistance–Pump–Rate

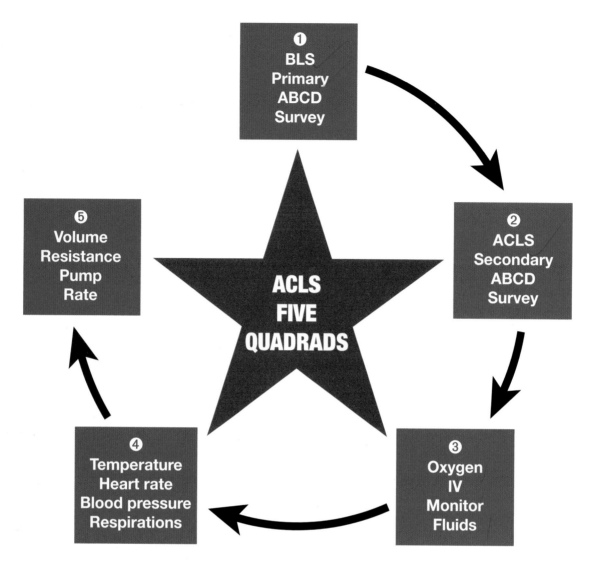

Figure. The 5 Quadrads of ACLS

- Patients in cardiac arrest
- Patients refractory to initial cardiac arrest interventions
- Prearrest: unstable patients who may progress to cardiac arrest if providers fail to identify specific problems and start appropriate treatments
- Patients with return of spontaneous circulation and those in the immediate postresuscitation period
- Any major clinical challenge or decision-making point in an unstable patient

Each step consists of 4 parameters. At each step the provider performs an assessment, manages problems detected, and evaluates the response to the therapy.

Important Points

- The first 2 steps, the BLS Primary and ACLS Secondary ABCD Surveys, usually apply to patients in cardiac arrest. But these 2 steps can also be used to highlight fundamental assessments and actions for all

patients. In unstable patients providers may identify serious abnormalities and may be able to correct them, preventing deterioration to cardiac arrest.

The 3rd, 4th, and 5th steps apply in general to patients experiencing a cardiopulmonary emergency but who have not yet developed cardiac arrest.

- Experienced clinicians need to tailor use of the 5 quadrads to the clinical situation. For example, cervical spine immobilization needs to be added to the Primary and Secondary ABCD Surveys when dealing with patients suffering from cardiac arrest associated with trauma, drowning, electric shock, or hypothermia. Modifications are also necessary when dealing with hypothermic cardiac arrest and cardiac arrest associated with pregnancy.

- Some redundancy exists among the 5 quadrads. For example, the pulse and breathing checks in the

Primary ABCD Survey may identify problems with heart rate, blood pressure, and respirations, which are components of the 4th quadrad (temperature–heart rate–blood pressure–respirations). Also, the support provided in the "C: Circulation" step in the Secondary ABCD Survey can include elements of the "oxygen–IV–monitor–fluids" components in the 3rd quadrad. As a memory aid the 5 Quadrads is not perfect, but it may be helpful.

Applying the 5 Quadrads

Cardiac Arrest Patients

Quadrad 1. BLS Primary ABCD Survey

This step covers basic CPR and defibrillation:

- **Airway:** Unresponsive (assessment); open airway (action).
- **Breathing:** Check breathing (assessment); if not breathing or if breathing is inadequate, provide 2 ventilations (action). If you cannot provide 2 ventilations (assessment), then correct a possible obstructed airway (action).
- **Circulation:** Check for pulse (assessment); if no pulse, provide chest compressions (action).
- **Defibrillation:** Check rhythm for presence of ventricular fibrillation/ventricular tachycardia (assessment); if VF or VT is present, provide 1 shock (action).

Quadrad 2. ACLS Secondary ABCD Survey

This step addresses advanced airways and pharmacologic treatment of arrhythmias. The experienced ACLS team leader also begins to think about the cause of the emergency, differential diagnoses, and alternative approaches to treatment.

- **Airway:** Determine if initial airway techniques and ventilations are adequate (assessment); if inadequate, establish advanced airway (action).
- **Breathing:** Check effectiveness of advanced airway and breathing support, including tube placement, oxygenation, and ventilation (assessment); provide positive-pressure ventilations through endotracheal tube or other advanced airway device (action).
- **Circulation:** Check heart rate and attach monitor leads to determine the rhythm (assessment); establish IV access to administer fluids and medications (treatment); administer rhythm-appropriate medications (treatment).
- **Differential diagnoses:** This critical part of the assessment of a cardiopulmonary emergency requires the experienced provider to *think*. Most other steps involve simple yes/no decision making. But at this time the provider should pause to think carefully and try to identify the cause of the cardiac arrest. As various causes are considered, think of the treatment for each cause.

The differential diagnoses become of paramount importance when dealing with *asystolic* and *pulseless electrical activity* cardiac arrest. As Table 1 shows, the "D" in the ACLS Secondary ABCD Survey can be expanded by using the *H's and T's*, a memory aid for the most common and potentially reversible causes of asystolic and pulseless electrical activity cardiac arrest. The table also shows how the steps of *assessment* and *action* are linked with each differential diagnosis.

Using the BLS Primary and ACLS Secondary ABCD Surveys: Key Principles

- The survey sequence addresses problems in their order of importance, using the alphabet as a memory aid.
- Whenever you identify a problem, *go no further* with the survey until the identified problem is resolved. For example, if you are unable to make the chest rise with ventilation ("B" of the ACLS Secondary Survey), you must solve that problem before you start an IV and administer medications.
- The survey assessments and actions can be followed only as far as personnel and equipment resources allow. A single provider, for example, would be limited to basic CPR and automated defibrillation until other help arrived.
- When additional personnel arrive, the survey sequence tells them exactly where to enter the resuscitative effort. To illustrate, personnel arriving to assist a lone provider doing CPR ("ABC" of the BLS Primary Survey) would assume responsibility for defibrillation, advanced airway management, IV access, and medications—and in that order.
- If a sufficient number of skilled personnel are available, they can proceed with the survey steps simultaneously. But the surveys supply a useful review to make sure someone has responsibility for every task.
- The ACLS Secondary Survey ends with *"D: Differential Diagnosis,"* a reminder to stop and *think*. This "D" directs providers, especially the team leader, to think about *why* the arrest occurred in the first place and *why* the person remains in arrest or remains unstable (see Table 1).

Periarrest Patients

Quadrad 3. Oxygen–IV–Monitor–Fluids

Experienced ACLS providers learn *oxygen–IV–monitor–fluids* as a single term. These assessments and actions are required in virtually every cardiopulmonary emergency and should be provided for every patient. Making these actions a core part of the 5 quadrads fosters a routine that will help prevent delays or omission of these actions.

Quadrad 4. Temperature–Heart Rate–Blood Pressure–Respirations

The vital signs are probably one of the most neglected areas in training for cardiopulmonary emergencies. But the vital signs provide critical information needed to manage these patients and evaluate their response to therapy.

Quadrad 5. Volume–Resistance–Pump–Rate

The 5th quadrad is the *cardiovascular quadrad.* The cardiovascular quadrad directs experienced ACLS providers

to consider whether patients with shock, hypotension, and acute pulmonary edema have a clinical problem dominated by

- Inadequate or excessive vascular volume (volume)
- Excessive or inadequate peripheral vascular resistance (resistance)
- Poor cardiac function as a pump (pump)
- Inadequate blood pressure and perfusion due to hemodynamically significant tachycardias or bradycardias (rate)

The next section provides more detail on this topic.

Table 1. "D" in the ACLS Secondary ABCD Survey: Developing Expanded Differential Diagnoses—"The H's and T's"*

The H's: Causes (Examples)	Assessments	Actions/Treatments
Hypovolemia • Occult bleeding • Anaphylaxis • Pregnancy with gravid uterus	• History, exam • Hematocrit • β-HCG test	• Administer volume • Administer blood if needed • If the patient has a large uterus, turn the patient to the left side (see Chapter 14, Part 6)
Hypoxia • Inadequate oxygenation	• Breath sounds • Tube placement? • Arterial blood gas	• Oxygen • Ventilation • Good CPR technique
Hydrogen ion • Acidosis • DKA • Drug overdoses • Renal failure	• Clinical setting • Arterial blood gas • Lab tests	• See Chapter 15 • Optimize perfusion • Establish effective oxygenation and ventilation • Tricyclic antidepressant overdose: bicarbonate • Other toxicologies: see Chapter 13
Hypo-/hyperelectrolytes • Potassium, sodium, magnesium, calcium	• History, exam • Risk factors	• Treat specific electrolyte balance: see Chapter 15 • Hyperkalemia: give calcium, bicarbonate, insulin, glucose
Hypo-/hyperglycemia • Low glucose = insulin reactions • DKA • Nonketotic, hyperosmolar coma	• History, exam • Lab tests	• See Chapter 15 • Fluids • Potassium • Hyperglycemia: insulin • Hypoglycemia: 50% glucose
Hypo-/hyperthermia • Profound hypothermia • Heat stroke	• Touch • Core body temperature	• Hypothermia: see Chapter 14, Part 1 • Hypothermia: active/passive, external/internal rewarming • Hyperthermia: surface cooling

β-HCG indicates human chorionic gonadotropin, beta subunit; CABG, coronary artery bypass graft; COPD, chronic obstructive pulmonary disease; DKA, diabetic ketoacidosis; PCI, percutaneous coronary intervention; STEMI, ST-elevation myocardial infarction; TCA, tricyclic antidepressant; tPA, tissue plasminogen activator.
*The "H's and T's" provide an expanded list of possible causes of asystolic or pulseless electrical activity cardiac arrest. The emphasis is on *reversible, treatable conditions.* The list contains examples and is not meant to be exhaustive or exclusive. The diagnostic test listed may not be useful during resuscitation, but results from recent studies or tests done after resuscitation may provide clinical clues or be diagnostic. Remember, diagnostic tests should never delay clinically indicated and necessary treatments and interventions. For example, fibrinolytics are administered on the basis of the patient's history, ECG, and clinical risk stratification. There is no delay waiting for cardiac biomarker results. Tension pneumothorax is treated on the basis of clinical examination, not the chest x-ray.

The T's: Causes (Examples)	Assessments	Actions/Treatments
Toxins (drug overdoses) • TCA, phenothiazines • β-Blockers, calcium channel blockers • Cocaine, digoxin, aspirin, acetaminophen	• Risk factors • History, toxidrome	• Specific antidotes and more comprehensive list of therapies: see Chapter 13 • Possible volume therapy (titrate carefully) and vasopressors for hypotension • TCA overdose: bicarbonate • Calcium channel blocker or β-blocker overdose: glucagon, calcium • Cocaine overdose: benzodiazepines; do not give β-blockers • Prolonged CPR may be justified • Cardiopulmonary bypass
Trauma • Massive trauma • Electrocution, lightning strike • Submersion	• History • Clinical setting • Physical exam	• See Chapter 14, Parts 2, 5, and 7 • Provider safety • Reverse triage (give priority to patients in cardiac arrest) • Early endotracheal intubation • In some situations (eg, small child submerged in icy water), prolonged resuscitation may be justified
Tamponade, cardiac • Trauma • Renal failure • Chest compressions • Carcinoma • Central line perforations	• Risk factors • History • Prearrest picture • Distended neck veins • Echo	• Administer volume • Pericardiocentesis • Thoracotomy
Tension pneumothorax • Asthma • Trauma • COPD, blebs • Ventilators + positive pressures	• Risk factors • Lung sounds diminished • Tracheal deviation • Neck vein distention	• Needle decompression • Chest tube
Thrombosis, heart • Acute STEMI • Other acute coronary syndromes	• Prearrest symptoms • ECG • Serum cardiac markers	• See Chapter 10 and Chapter 12 • Aspirin, oxygen, nitroglycerin, and morphine if no response to nitrates • Vasopressors • Emergent reperfusion (PCI or fibrinolytics) • Intra-aortic balloon pump (IABP), CABG
Thrombosis, lungs • Pulmonary embolus	• Risk factors • History • Diagnostic imaging	• Administer volume • Dopamine • Heparin • Consider tPA

The 5th (Cardiovascular) Quadrad

"Tank" Volume–"Tank" Resistance–Pump–Rate as an Aid to Diagnosis and Treatment

The *cardiovascular quadrad* is a conceptual aid to use when faced with a variety of prearrest cardiovascular emergencies and cardiac arrest unresponsive to actions in the BLS Primary and ACLS Secondary Surveys. The starting point for the Acute Pulmonary Edema, Hypotension, Shock Algorithm (see *ECC Handbook,* page 15, ACLS Figure 6, and Chapter 12, Part 2, in this volume) is *clinical signs of shock, hypoperfusion, congestive heart failure, and acute pulmonary edema.* Just below those signs is the question *"What is the most likely problem?"* This question asks the clinician to try to classify the patient's condition (if possible) into one or more categories of altered cardiovascular physiology: intravascular volume, peripheral vascular resistance, pump, and rate.

Quadrad 5 is based on the concept of the cardiovascular system as a hydraulic tank of a certain size with a certain (intravascular) *volume*. The heart acts as a variable-capacity *pump* that drives the flow of the intravascular volume. Each contraction of the pump injects a certain volume into the hydraulic system. The number of times per minute that the pump contracts affects the *rate* and volume of blood flow. The peripheral vascular *resistance* affects the size (capacity) of the tank and how much work the pump must do to perfuse the system.

The 5th quadrad asks whether a patient with low blood pressure, shock, vascular congestion, or pulmonary edema has a problem with 1 or more of these 4 determinants of cardiac output:

- "Tank" volume problem? (intravascular volume, fluid status): fluid loss, bleeding, gastrointestinal losses
- "Tank" resistance problem? (peripheral vascular resistance, vasomotor tone): vasodilation, vasoconstriction, redistribution of blood flow and cardiac output
- Pump problem? (contractility): either primary or secondary cardiac dysfunction
- Rate problem? (the electrical system): either too fast or too slow

Rules for Multiple or Overlapping Problems

Once the provider identifies the patient's problem, the provider can select the appropriate therapy. The following priority of actions is recommended:

- First, correct primary *rate* problems if present.
- Second, correct any *tank volume* problems with fluid or transfusions or diuresis. Always correct tank volume problems before treating tank resistance problems. Vasopressors will reduce tank size by increasing peripheral vascular resistance, and vasodilators will increase tank size by reducing peripheral vascular resistance.
- Third, treat *pump* problems with vasopressors, inotropic agents, or both.

Each patient requires individualized treatment. Three rules will help you avoid major errors:

1. Do not use fluids or vasopressors when the hypotension is caused by tachycardia or bradycardia (treat rate problems first).
2. Do not use vasopressors alone to treat hypotension caused by hypovolemia (eg, shock due to gastrointestinal bleeding). Treat tank volume problems before treating with vasopressors.
3. Do not use fluids when the tank is full and the problem is the pump. Pump problems can include acute myocardial infarction, congestive heart failure, or cardiomyopathy with acute pulmonary edema. Treat pump problems with vasopressors or inotropic agents rather than fluids. If the volume status is unclear during initial assessment, it may be prudent to administer a fluid bolus of 250 to 500 mL and serially evaluate the patient's clinical response.

Vasodilators may be needed to treat inadequate cardiac output with poor myocardial function. Ensure that intravascular volume is adequate before administering vasodilators, and be ready to administer additional volume if needed during vasodilator therapy.

Table 2 presents a comprehensive list of the assessments and actions involved in the 5 Quadrads Approach to ACLS.

Table 2. The ACLS 5 Quadrads Approach for Experienced Providers

Survey Step	Assessment	Action
Quadrad 1. BLS Primary ABCD Survey		
• **A**irway	• Open?	• Head tilt–chin lift or jaw thrust
(C-spine)	• Suspicious mechanism?	• Chin lift, jaw thrust with in-line stabilization, NO head tilt (unless ventilation cannot be achieved); immobilize head, neck, and torso; backboard
• **B**reathing	• Moving air?	• Give 2 breaths; follow obstructed airway protocols if needed
• **C**irculation	• Pulse?	• Chest compressions; continue CPR until AED is available
• **D**efibrillation	Attach AED, paddles, monitor	• Deliver shock for VF/pulseless VT
Quadrad 2. ACLS Secondary ABCD Survey		
• **A**irway (C-spine)	• Adequate? • Signs of airway protective mechanisms (cough/gag)? • Signs of obstruction (noisy breathing) or pooled secretions?	• Remove obstructions; suction — Insert oropharyngeal airway; nasal trumpet — Determine if advanced airway is needed: endotracheal tube/LMA/Combitube; nasotracheal intubation; surgical airway
• **B**reathing (oxygen)	• Cords visualized? tube in trachea and confirmed by clinical examination (5-point auscultation) and a device (eg, exhaled CO_2 detector)? • Chest x-ray: pneumothorax? flail chest? open chest? • Cyanosis? moving air? Order ABG; attach O_2 saturation monitor	• Support of airway and ventilation: see Chapter 4 • Provide oxygen by nasal cannula, face mask, Venturi mask, nonrebreathing mask at 15 L/min; with airway devices use high FiO_2 + hyperventilation + PEEP — Verify placement of advanced airway — Perform needle decompression; insert chest tube; cover/release sucking wounds as needed — Obtain mechanical ventilator
• **C**irculation (IV–monitor–fluids)	• Heart rate? Attach monitor; assess rhythm — Is blood pressure adequate or too high? • Send blood for type and crossmatch, lab tests (A-A-A-A-B-B-Tox)	• Establish IV access; administer volume as needed — Give rhythm-appropriate medications — For trauma, hemorrhage: order blood type and cross; stop visible hemorrhage; obtain serial hematocrits — If patient is pregnant with large uterus, place on left side (15° to 30° back from left lateral position)
• **D**ifferential **D**iagnosis **(THINK!)**	• Assess using the "D-(CP)-D-E-EE-F-F-F-G-G-H" system • Consider differential diagnoses using "H's and T's" (Table 1)	• Begin management of identified diagnoses

(continued)

Table 2. *Continued*

Survey Step	Assessment	Action
• **D**isability-**D**-(**CP**)-**D**	• Mental status? pupil response? • GCS score: best eye, vocal, motor response • For altered mental state, see Coma Protocol (right column) and reassess	• Coma Protocol (CP): give 50 mL of $D_{50}W$; give thiamine 100 mg IV; give Narcan 2 mg IV $D_{50}W$ • Assess response

• **E**xpose–**E**xamine–**E**xtremities	• Completely expose the patient; perform quick visual check for gross injuries, signs of pregnancy, skin lesions, skin temperature, medic alert
	• Check pulse in extremities
		• Stabilize obvious injuries
		  — Intervene if needed to restore pulse to compromised extremities
		  — Treat other wounds

• **F**ingers–**F**oley–**F**lip	• Rectal, vaginal exam; check for injuries of pelvis, perineum, and genitalia, then insert Foley catheter • "Flip" (logroll) patient to check back areas	• Insert Foley catheter for straight drainage; send urine specimen for analysis, including toxicology screen; observe rate of urine output
• **G**astric tube–"**G**unk"	• Check contraindications to nasal insertion of tubes • Observe aspirate for blood, pills, odors	• Instill "gunk" (activated charcoal 50 g + cathartic) down the gastric tube for suspected drug overdoses and *appropriate* indications
• **H**istory	• Document expanded history to increase differential diagnoses	• Delay history until patient is stable • Question family, friends, EMS personnel
Quadrad 3. O₂–IV–Monitor–Fluids	Assess response to 1st treatment; check lab tests, x-rays	• Continue management of identified diagnoses — Evaluate response
Quadrad 4. Temperature–HR–BP–Respirations	• Assess excessively low or high temperatures	• Continue management as indicated — Evaluate response
Quadrad 5. "Tank" Volume–"Tank" Resistance–Pump–Rate	• Consider problems in these categories	• Continue management as indicated — Evaluate response

A-A-A-A-B-B-Tox indicates alcohol, acetylsalicylic acid (aspirin), acetaminophen, amylase, β-human chorionic gonadotropin, bilirubin, and toxicology screen; ABG, arterial blood gas analysis; GCS, Glasgow Coma Scale; LMA, laryngeal mask airway; PEEP, positive end-expiratory pressure.

Summary: The 5 Quadrads

Quadrad 1. BLS Primary ABCD Survey

Airway:
- If unresponsive, open airway.

Breathing:
- If not breathing adequately, provide positive-pressure ventilations.

Circulation:
- If no pulse, perform chest compressions.

Defibrillation:
- Identify and shock VF/pulseless VT, attempt defibrillation.

Quadrad 2. ACLS Secondary ABCD Survey

Airway:
- Determine the effectiveness of the primary ventilation and airway techniques.
- Remove any airway obstruction.
- Achieve airway control and protection with advanced airway techniques if indicated.

Breathing:
- Confirm placement and function of advanced airway device, verify with exhaled CO_2 device.
- Provide positive-pressure ventilations through advanced airway device.
- Support oxygenation, verify with oxygen saturation measurement.
- Treat any condition that interferes with effective oxygenation and ventilation (eg, tension pneumothorax).
- Support ventilation that produces bilateral chest wall movement.

Circulation:
- Continue chest compressions.
- Establish IV access, administer volume if needed.
- Attach monitor leads.
- Identify rhythm and rate.
- Measure blood pressure.
- Administer medications appropriate for rhythm, rate, and blood pressure.

Differential Diagnosis:
- Identify and treat reversible causes of cardiovascular emergencies.
- Employ memory aids such as the *H's and the T's.*

Quadrad 3. Oxygen–IV–Monitor–Fluids

- Administer oxygen.
- Establish IV access, administer IV fluids as needed.
- Monitor heart rate and rhythm.

Quadrad 4. Temperature–Heart Rate–Blood Pressure–Respirations

- Evaluate vital signs.
- Treat any reversible problems identified (eg, hypothermia, bradycardia, hypotension, inadequate breathing).

Quadrad 5. The Cardiovascular Quadrad: "Tank" Volume–"Tank" Resistance–Pump–Rate

- Identify and support problems with
  - Heart rate
  - Intravascular volume ("tank" volume)
  - Vascular resistance ("tank" resistance)
  - Pump

Cardiovascular
Part 1: ACS, NSTEMI, and Unstable Angina

This Chapter

- **Differential diagnosis and risk stratification of chest pain**
- **Who is treated with heparin and glycoprotein IIb/IIIa inhibitors**
- **Markers of high-risk ACS**
- **Weighing the risks and benefits of ACS therapy**

Key Points

The ACLS Provider Course discusses the initial management of patients with suspected ischemic-type pain and then focuses on the patient with ST-segment elevation myocardial infarction (STEMI). Patients with STEMI need rapid identification and reperfusion by experienced physicians at experienced centers. This chapter discusses the patient with possible ischemic chest pain, unstable angina (UA), and non–ST-segment elevation MI (NSTEMI). Even though the underlying pathophysiologic process is usually similar to that of STEMI, these patients are managed differently. For example, fibrinolytics are contraindicated in patients with ST-segment *depression* MI because they are not beneficial and may be harmful.

The key initial steps in managing patients with ischemic-type pain are

- Rapidly identify chest discomfort that could be ischemic or life-threatening in origin
- Use the initial ECG interpretation to place patients into 1 of 3 acute ischemic symptom categories: STEMI, NSTEMI, or normal or nondiagnostic ECG
- Further risk stratify and treat patients with NSTEMI and high-risk unstable angina

Overview

Initially the patient who presents with chest pain is rapidly evaluated for life-threatening causes of chest discomfort. This evaluation plus the 12-lead ECG are used for initial assessment of the probability of an acute coronary syndrome (ACS) and other life-threatening causes of chest discomfort. If the clinical probability of other causes of chest discomfort is low, then the ECG is used to place the patient into an initial diagnostic and treatment category. This category may change or develop with time as additional tests and serial patient assessments are made (Figure 1).

Differential Diagnosis of Chest Pain

Patients presenting with chest pain are rapidly screened for life-threatening causes. The initial ECG and focused

Foundation Facts — ACS—First Question	The initial evaluation of the patient with chest discomfort begins with this question: *What is the likelihood that the presenting symptoms represent ischemia due to underlying coronary artery disease?*

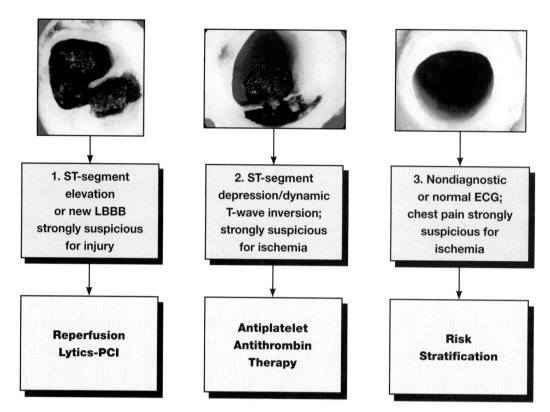

Figure 1. The 12-lead ECG is used to initially sort patients into 1 of 3 categories based on the presence or absence of ST-segment deviation and new or presumably new left bundle branch block (LBBB). Patients with ST-segment elevation or new LBBB (**1**) are evaluated for rapid reperfusion. Those with high-risk NSTEMI and an ACS (**2**) are treated with aggressive antiplatelet and antithrombin therapy. Patients with a low probability of ACS events (**3**) receive aspirin and undergo further risk stratification. PCI indicates percutaneous coronary intervention.

clinical assessment will identify patients with ST-segment deviation eligible for reperfusion or aggressive antiplatelet and antithrombin therapy. In other patients a noncardiac cause of chest pain is identified early, and appropriate additional diagnostic tests and treatment are initiated. But in many patients the question of whether the chest discomfort is ischemic persists, particularly when the initial ECG is nondiagnostic or normal. Many of these patients will be found to be at low risk for major adverse cardiac events (MACE) and to have noncardiac causes of chest discomfort.

Overview

Chapter 10 in Part 1 of this text discusses the initial management of patients with ischemic-type chest pain and STEMI. Ideally within 10 minutes of arrival at the emergency department (ED), providers should obtain a targeted history while a monitor is attached to the patient and a 12-lead ECG is obtained (if not done in the prehospital setting). If STEMI is present, the goals of reperfusion are to

- Administer fibrinolytics within 30 minutes of arrival (30-minute "door-to-drug" interval) or
- Provide percutaneous coronary intervention (PCI) within 90 minutes of arrival (90-minute "door-to–balloon inflation" interval in the catheterization suite)

Chest Pain Suggestive of Ischemia

A targeted history and physical examination are performed to aid diagnosis, evaluate and identify other causes of the patient's symptoms, and assess the patient for possible complications related to ACS or therapies. Although the use of clinical signs and symptoms may increase suspicion of ACS, no single sign or combination of clinical signs and symptoms alone can confirm the diagnosis prospectively.[1-4]

The "Rule Out" Process

During evaluation of a patient with chest pain, the responsible clinician attempts to assess and estimate the probability of life-threatening problems in the differential diagnosis. But none of these life threats can be "ruled out" with absolute confidence during initial triage and evaluation. This fact underscores an important point: *healthcare providers should focus on both risk stratification and continuing assessment and diagnosis during initial patient evaluation.* As the evaluation proceeds and an initial strategy is defined, the risks and benefits of testing and treatment are balanced against the probability and risk assessment of disease using clinical judgment and prudent assessment.

Healthcare providers initially use symptoms to estimate the likelihood of ACS and to assess the probability of other life-threatening causes of chest discomfort.

A differential diagnosis is developed and the probability of ACS and other life-threatening causes of chest discomfort is prioritized (Table 1).

Table 1. Immediate Life-Threatening Causes of Chest Pain

Acute coronary syndromes
Aortic dissection
Pulmonary embolism
Pericardial effusion with acute tamponade
Tension pneumothorax

Definition of Angina and Unstable Angina

Stable angina is a clinical syndrome usually characterized by deep, poorly localized chest discomfort. Stable angina is *reproducibly* associated with physical exertion or emotional stress and is *predictably* and promptly (<5 minutes) relieved with rest or sublingual nitroglycerin. Patients learn through experience how much physical exertion they can perform before the symptoms of angina begin. They also learn how soon and to what degree rest or nitroglycerin relieves the pain.

Unstable angina is an acute process of myocardial ischemia of insufficient severity and duration to cause myocardial necrosis. Patients with unstable angina typically do not present with ST-segment elevation on the ECG and do not release cardiac-specific biomarkers. Various terminology has been used in the past, originally when a change occurred in the predictable pattern of stable angina. These definitions have evolved over time, and unstable angina now indicates a period (usually over days or hours) of increasing symptoms precipitated by less exertion or prolonged episodes with minimal or no exertion. There are 3 principal presentations of unstable angina:

- **Rest angina:** Angina that occurs at rest, usually lasting less than 15 to 20 minutes.

- **Nocturnal angina:** Chest pain that awakens a patient at night.
- **Accelerating angina:** Angina that is distinctly more frequent, longer in duration, or lower in threshold. *Threshold* is the level of activity (or class of angina) that induces pain.

Classes of Angina

Angina can be graded according to the amount of physical activity that causes the pain:

- **Class I:** Ordinary physical activity does not cause the angina. Pain requires strenuous, rapid, or prolonged exercise.
- **Class II:** Slight limitation of ordinary activity. Pain occurs on (1) walking or climbing stairs rapidly, walking uphill, climbing stairs after meals, or walking in the wind or cold, or (2) walking more than 2 blocks or climbing more than 1 flight of stairs at a normal pace.
- **Class III:** Marked limitation of ordinary physical activity. Pain occurs after walking 1 or 2 blocks on the level or climbing 1 or 2 flights of stairs at a normal pace.
- **Class IV:** Inability to perform any physical exertion.

Symptom Clues and Limitations

Chapter 10 of Part 1 provides information about the most common symptomatic presentations of ACS. Approximately three quarters of patients with ACS—men and women—will present with chest discomfort. But some presentations are "atypical," and patients do not have chest discomfort as the presenting symptom.

To aid in the assessment of chest discomfort and link the presentation to adverse events, Braunwald classified patients *without* STEMI into 3 risk groups based on the likelihood that their symptoms were ischemic in origin (Table 2).[5,6] Note that patients with an intermediate or high likelihood that symptoms are ischemic in origin have chest discomfort or left arm pain as a *chief* symptom. In high-risk patients this pain reproduces prior anginal pain. Age older than 70, male sex, or diabetes mellitus also places a patient at intermediate risk. In men premature coronary disease by definition occurs by age 55 (65 in women). Physical findings largely involve evidence of left ventricular (LV) dysfunction (high risk) or evidence of other vascular disease, such

Foundation Facts **Unstable Angina— Pattern for MACE**	Unstable angina with a high likelihood of a major adverse cardiac event (MACE) is best defined by an accelerating tempo of symptoms over a period of 24 to 48 hours: • Symptoms increase in frequency or severity. • Symptoms occur with less and less exertion. • Symptoms occur at rest or awaken the patient at night.

Table 2. Likelihood of Ischemic Etiology in Chest Pain Patients Without ST-Segment Elevation

	A. High likelihood High likelihood that chest pain is of ischemic etiology if patient has *any* of the findings in the column below:	**B. Intermediate likelihood** Intermediate likelihood that chest pain is of ischemic etiology if patient has NO findings in column A and *any* of the findings in the column below:	**C. Low likelihood** Low likelihood that chest pain is of ischemic etiology if patient has NO findings in column A or B. Patients may have any of the findings in the column below:
History	• Chief symptom is chest or left arm pain or discomfort *plus* Current pain reproduces pain of prior documented angina *and* Known CAD, including MI	• Chief symptom is chest or left arm pain or discomfort • Age >70 years • Male sex • Diabetes mellitus	• Probable ischemic symptoms • Recent cocaine use
Physical exam	• Transient mitral regurgitation • Hypotension • Diaphoresis • Pulmonary edema or rales	• Extracardiac vascular disease	• Chest discomfort reproduced by palpation
ECG	• New (or presumed new) transient ST deviation (≥0.5 mm) *or* T-wave inversion (≥2 mm) with symptoms	• Fixed Q waves • Abnormal ST segments *or* T waves that are not new	• Normal ECG *or* T-wave flattening *or* T-wave inversion in leads with dominant R waves
Cardiac markers	• Elevated cardiac troponin I or T • Elevated CK-MB	*Any finding in column B above* PLUS • Normal	• Normal
	High (A) or Intermediate (B) Likelihood of Ischemia		

Modified from Braunwald et al. *Circulation.* 2002;106:1893-1900.[7]

as bruits (intermediate risk). ECG findings are grouped into degrees of ST-segment deviation (see "ST-Segment Deviation and Risk Stratification," later in this chapter).

Patients with atypical symptoms can be challenging, but adherence to an organized, evidence-based protocol makes the likelihood of a major adverse cardiac event very low. Clinical observation and research have identified several groups of patients who tend to experience an ACS in an "atypical" manner with "atypical" symptoms.

Chest discomfort is the predominant symptom of ACS in both men and women (Table 3). But women,[8-10] the elderly,[11] and insulin-dependent diabetics who develop ACS often do not present with the classic pattern of severe, crushing substernal chest pain or discomfort, nausea, diaphoresis, and pain radiating into the jaw, neck, or lateral aspect of the left arm. In fact, many middle-aged men with ACS do not

present with this pattern. For this reason the "typical" ACS symptom *complex* is not a particularly sensitive indicator for ACS. In a large study of all patients presenting to an ED with "typical" ischemic symptoms, only 54% developed an ACS. In addition, the patients who did develop an ACS described a variety of symptoms: 43% had burning or indigestion, 32% had a "chest ache," and 20% had "sharp" or "stabbing" pain; 42% could not provide specific descriptors of their pain. The pain was partially pleuritic in 12%.

The ACS symptom complex for women, the elderly, and diabetics may vary greatly. Chest discomfort or ache in itself may be minor. These patients may describe an ache or discomfort that may or may not be felt in the center of the chest but that seems to spread up to and across the shoulders, neck, arms, jaw, or back; between the shoulder blades; or into the epigastrium (upper left or right quadrant).

Table 3. Angina in Women and Men

	Women	Men
Presentation of CAD	Angina (65%)	ACS (63%)
Most common cause of angina	Noncardiac	CAD
Significant CAD	≤50%	80%
Follow-up	Increases with age	Plateau (55-65 y)

The discomfort in the chest is less troublesome to the patient than the pain in the areas of radiation. This pattern of symptom localization *outside* the chest was found to be the most common atypical symptom of women evaluated in the Women's Ischemia Syndrome Evaluation (WISE) study.[12] The patient may be bothered more by associated lightheadedness, fainting, sweating, nausea, or shortness of breath. This is another example of the dominance of symptoms outside the chest. A global feeling of distress, anxiety ("something is wrong" or "something is just not right"), or impending doom may be present.

Women

Women presenting with MI typically present about 1 hour later than men, in part because of their atypical symptoms, which include epigastric pain, shortness of breath, nausea, and fatigue. Several factors complicate evaluation of chest pain in women. Premenopausal women have a low likelihood of coronary artery disease (CAD) and commonly present with typical angina. The low incidence of positive angiograms in these women has led to a perception that their chest pain is benign and *nonischemic*. This misperception leads to underassessment of women with chest pain, so women with chest pain are less likely than men to be tested and treated for CAD. There is also a misperception that the course of CAD in women is more benign than it is in men. But the prognosis of women with CAD is similar to that of men, and women often have more angina and disability than men. Atypical symptoms in women often include the following:

- More angina at rest, occurring at night, or precipitated by mental rather than physical stress
- Shortness of breath, fatigue, palpitations, presyncope, sweating, nausea, or vomiting
- Atypical angina (in women with or without CAD)

Diabetics

Diabetic patients may present without chest pain but with complaints of weakness, fatigue, or severe prostration. Anginal equivalents such as shortness of breath, syncope, and lightheadedness may be their only symptoms. In diabetics with neuropathy these presentations have often been attributed to altered pain and neural perception.

Anginal Equivalents

Patients with ACS present with signs and symptoms that have been termed *ischemic equivalents* or *anginal equivalents*. It is important to note that these patients are *not* having atypical chest pain as described above. These patients seldom offer complaints of "pain" in the chest, below the sternum, or elsewhere, and the healthcare provider may not be able to elicit a report of such pain. Instead they may present with a symptom or sign that reflects the effects of the ischemia on LV function or electrical stability. Diabetic patients and the elderly are most likely to present with these symptoms. With advancing age the elderly are more likely to present with diaphoresis. Some of the more common chest pain equivalent symptoms experienced by these ACS patients are

- Ischemic LV dysfunction: shortness of breath, dyspnea on exertion
- Ischemic arrhythmias: palpitations, lightheadedness or near-syncope with exercise, syncope

The most common signs of anginal equivalents are acute pulmonary edema or pulmonary congestion, cardiomegaly, and a third heart sound. Ventricular arrhythmias can cause symptoms in these patients. Ventricular extrasystoles, nonsustained ventricular tachycardia, and symptomatic ventricular tachycardia or ventricular fibrillation have been documented. Ventricular ectopy that increases with activity (most benign ventricular premature contractions will suppress at increased sinus rates) is suspicious for ischemia. Atrial fibrillation is uncommonly an ischemic presentation. In most cases an anginal equivalent is diagnosed retrospectively when some objective evidence of ischemia has been linked to the patient's symptom complex. For example, left arm pain alone may raise suspicion of ACS in the appropriate clinical setting, but it is ischemic in origin only when definitely associated with ACS or reproduced with functional testing.

Differential Diagnosis of Nonischemic Life-Threatening Chest Pain

The ACLS provider may encounter patients who present with many of the typical chest pain signs and symptoms reported by ACS patients but who are in fact experiencing another problem altogether. Some of these "ACS mimics" are relatively benign (eg, costochondritis or gastroesophageal reflux disease). But several are severe and life-threatening, and the ACLS provider must be able to identify them. There are numerous non-ACS causes of chest pain. The 4 most frequent potentially fatal non-ACS causes of chest pain are

- Aortic dissection
- Acute pulmonary embolism
- Pericardial effusion and acute tamponade
- Tension pneumothorax

Aortic Dissection

Signs and Symptoms

Aortic dissection is rare in comparison with ACS. The incidence of aortic dissection has been estimated at 5 to 30 per 1 million people per year; about 4400 MIs occur per 1 million people per year. Severe pain is the most common presenting symptom of aortic dissection. Untreated aortic dissection is a lethal disease; 25% of patients die in the first 24 hours and 75% in 2 weeks.

Risk factors for aortic dissection include hypertension (70% to 90% of patients), chest trauma, male sex, advancing age (usually 6th or 7th decade), bicuspid aortic valve, Marfan syndrome, aortitis, and cocaine use. Cardiac catheterization is the most common cause of iatrogenic aortic dissection.

The typical patient is a man in his 70s with a history of hypertension, a predisposing factor in 70% to 90% of patients. Although hypertension is a predisposing factor, it does not help in the differential diagnosis because many more patients with ACS have hypertension. Chest pain is the most frequent initial complaint caused by aortic dissection. The onset of the pain of aortic dissection is abrupt, and the pain is most severe at onset. Think *aortic dissection* when patients report sudden or abrupt pain that

is most severe at the start. But remember that such pain neither confirms dissection nor rules out ACS.

The pain of aortic dissection may be migratory or may change in severity and location with time. The initial location of pain provides a valuable clue about the origin and extension of the dissection. This pain may be similar to that of ACS. In ascending and transverse aortic dissection, anterior chest pain is typical. Anterior chest pain also occurs in descending aortic dissection, but these patients also have more back and abdominal pain.

More often, though, the pain is described as sharp. Classically the pain of aortic dissection is described as "ripping" or "tearing" and migratory (as the dissection plane advances). The International Registry of Aortic Dissection has found a classic symptom complex only in a minority of patients. Tearing or ripping pain occurred in 50% of patients. Thirty-two percent of patients had a murmur of aortic regurgitation, and 15% had a pulse deficit.[13] Table 4 lists contemporary signs and symptoms of patients with acute aortic dissection.

12-Lead ECG in Aortic Dissection

The majority of patients will have nondiagnostic ECGs with nonspecific changes. About 25% of patients will have left ventricular hypertrophy (LVH) on their ECG due to a history of hypertension. ST-segment and T-wave changes suggesting ischemia are often secondary repolarization changes due to LVH as well, although ischemia with associated CAD cannot be excluded. In rare cases a patient has ST-segment elevation. This elevation may be due to compression of the origin of a coronary artery in the proximal aortic root, most often the right coronary artery. For this reason the ECG has little value in differentiating these 2 causes of chest pain. If the acute aortic dissection occludes a coronary artery, it will produce ECG changes that closely mimic the ECG changes of ACS.

Pulmonary Embolism

Pulmonary embolism (PE) is a life-threatening complication of venous thrombosis, usually of the lower extremities. PE occurs when microthrombi manage to evade the body's intrinsic fibrinolytic system, and they enlarge, spread, and embolize. As these thrombi propagate they become so

Foundation Facts	The most common signs and symptoms of PE are[15]
Most Common Symptoms of PE	• Tachypnea (96%) • Shortness of breath (82%) • Chest pain (49%) • Cough (20%) • Hemoptysis (7%)

Table 4. Presenting Symptoms and Physical Examination of Patients With Acute Aortic Dissection (N = 464)

Category	Present, No. Reported (%)	Type A,* No. (%)	Type B,* No. (%)	P Value, Type A vs B
Presenting symptoms				
Any pain reported	443/464 (95.5)	271 (93.8)	172 (98.3)	.02
Abrupt onset	379/447 (84.8)	234 (85.4)	145 (83.8)	.65
Chest pain	331/455 (72.7)	221 (78.9)	110 (62.9)	<.001
Anterior chest pain	262/430 (60.9)	191 (71.0)	71 (44.1)	<.001
Posterior chest pain	149/415 (35.9)	85 (32.8)	64 (41)	.09
Back pain	240/451 (53.2)	129 (46.6)	111 (63.8)	<.001
Abdominal pain	133/449 (29.6)	60 (21.6)	73 (42.7)	<.001
Severity of pain: severe or worst ever	346/382 (90.6)	211 (90.1)	135 (90)	NA
Quality of pain: sharp	174/270 (64.4)	103 (62)	71 (68.3)	NA
Quality of pain: tearing or ripping	135/267 (50.6)	78 (49.4)	57 (52.3)	NA
Radiating	127/449 (28.3)	75 (27.2)	52 (30.1)	.51
Migrating	74/446 (16.6)	41 (14.9)	33 (19.3)	.22
Syncope	42/447 (9.4)	35 (12.7)	7 (4.1)	.002
Physical examination findings				
Hemodynamics (n = 451)†				
Hypertensive (SBP ≥150 mm Hg)	221 (49.0)	99 (35.7)	122 (70.1)	
Normotensive (SBP 100-149 mm Hg)	156 (34.6)	110 (39.7)	46 (26.4)	<.001
Hypotensive (SBP <100 mm Hg)	36 (8.0)	32 (11.6)	4 (2.3)	
Shock or tamponade (SBP ≤80 mm Hg)	38 (8.4)	36 (13.0)	2 (1.5)	
Auscultated murmur of aortic insufficiency	137/434 (31.6)	117 (44)	20 (12)	<.001
Pulse deficit	69/457 (15.1)	53 (18.7)	16 (9.2)	.006
Cerebrovascular accident	21/447 (4.7)	17 (6.1)	4 (2.3)	.07
Congestive heart failure	29/440 (6.6)	24 (8.8)	5 (3.0)	.02

SBP indicates systolic blood pressure; NA, not applicable.
*Type A dissections involve the aorta; type B dissections occur distal to the left subclavian artery.
†Systolic blood pressure is reported for 277 patients with type A and 174 patients with type B acute aortic dissection.
Reprinted with permission from Hagan et al.[13] *JAMA.* 2000;283:897-903.

large that they eventually break loose, traveling to the right heart and then into the pulmonary artery. Depending on the size and fragmentation of the thrombus, the patient can be asymptomatic or in cardiac arrest due to acute right heart failure. An interruption in pulmonary blood flow produces effects both downstream (ventilation-perfusion mismatch, atelectasis, pain) and upstream (cor pulmonale, right ventricular [RV] failure due to pulmonary hypertension).[14] An international cooperative registry of pulmonary embolism, ICOPER, documented the serious nature of pulmonary thromboembolism, showing a 3-month mortality rate of 15%.[15] Among symptomatic patients with PE, the initial clinical presentation is sudden death in 25%.[16] Massive PE is rare, occurring in less than 5% of patients with PE, but 30-day mortality exceeds 50%.[17,18]

Signs and Symptoms

The symptoms and manifestations of PE are often nonspecific, and the differential diagnosis is extensive. The diagnosis is difficult, and both underdiagnosis and overdiagnosis occur. As with aortic dissection, the classic triad of PE (hemoptysis, shortness of breath, and pleuritic chest pain) has limited diagnostic value, occurring in less than 20% of confirmed cases. This symptom complex is usually observed with smaller emboli that migrate to the lung periphery and cause pulmonary infarction and pleuritis. A small effusion may be present on chest x-ray. Dyspnea is the most common presenting symptom, and tachypnea is the most frequent presenting sign. In the ICOPER study 89% of patients were symptomatic and hemodynamically stable, and only 4% were unstable.[15] The only consistent finding in the majority of patients with PE is tachypnea, present in 96%.

12-Lead ECG in Pulmonary Embolism

The ECG is nonspecific or nondiagnostic in patients with PE. It is useful in the sense that it may suggest alternative diagnoses. Tachycardia and nonspecific ST-T-wave changes are the most common finding. Because of RV pressure overload and acute failure, right bundle branch block and atrial fibrillation were present in about 15% of patients in ICOPER.

Why Are Troponins Positive in Some Patients With PE?

During the course of evaluation for ACS, patients have been identified with elevated cardiac markers but negative coronary angiograms. Investigation has found that troponins and occasionally CK-MB (the MB isoenzyme of creatine kinase) will elevate with PE. This finding correlates with a large PE and RV dysfunction. The acute increase in RV afterload imposed by submassive and massive PE causes right heart ischemia that can lead to subendocardial infarction.

Remember to revisit the differential diagnosis of chest pain as discussed above. If troponin-positive patients have normal coronary angiograms, consider the possibility of PE.

What Can Early Recognition and Triage by ACLS Providers Do to Improve Outcome Beyond Traditional Therapy (Heparin)?

Risk stratification with echocardiography has now been introduced for patients with PE. Clinically about 5% of patients with PE present in shock and are candidates for fibrinolytic therapy or mechanical fragmentation techniques where available. About 40% of patients with PE have RV dysfunction demonstrated by transthoracic echocardiography. This RV dysfunction is manifest as RV hypokinesis of variable degrees and normal arterial pressure. Some studies have shown that fibrinolytic therapy can rapidly improve RV function and lower the incidence of recurrent PE. Treatment of these patients is currently controversial, but most experts would seriously weigh the risks and benefits of the treatment options if hemodynamics are borderline or tenuous cardiopulmonary comorbidity exists. At the very least the finding of RV dysfunction alerts

Rapid Response Interventions **Fibrinolysis for Massive PE**	Primary fibrinolytic therapy with tissue plasminogen activator for massive pulmonary embolism presenting with arterial hypotension is approved by the FDA. But this therapy remains controversial because there are few randomized trials and because <ul><li>The risk of intracranial hemorrhage may be as high as 3%[19]</li><li>Although the therapy may be lifesaving, the extent of clinical benefit (risk-benefit) remains unclear[17]</li></ul>

FYI **More Information**	For a complete discussion on the diagnosis and management of deep venous thrombosis and pulmonary embolism, see **CLINICIAN UPDATE** Acute Pulmonary Embolism, Parts I and II, in *Circulation*.[20,21]

the provider to pay close attention to anticoagulation parameters and adjunctive therapy.

Pericarditis With Acute Tamponade

This disease complex is often confused with ACS because it produces pain and ECG abnormalities that can be similar to those caused by ACS. It is important to differentiate pericarditis from ACS because fibrinolytic administration to patients with pericarditis can produce fatal hemorrhage because the inflamed pericardium can bleed easily. Heparin is also contraindicated except in a special form of post-infarction focal pericarditis. Cardiac tamponade refers to the hemodynamic effects of fluid accumulation in the pericardial sac. The most common causes of pericardial effusions with tamponade are pericarditis, malignancy, uremia associated with renal failure, and tuberculosis (in areas where it is endemic).[22] Hemopericardium is increasing in frequency, and tuberculous effusions are rare in developed countries.

The pericardial complex around the heart comprises the outer fibrous pericardium and a thin serous layer that adheres to the surface of the heart. Because of the close proximity of the serous pericardium to the heart, most instances of pericarditis are actually myopericarditis. This can further confuse the diagnosis because the myopericarditis may produce elevation of cardiac markers. A potential space exists between the fibrous and serous pericardial layers. Normally the space contains around 20 mL of plasmalike fluid. It can accommodate roughly 120 mL before pericardial pressure increases. If fluid accumulation continues, the pericardial pressure can rise sharply. This increased pressure results in a significant decrease in cardiac output and blood pressure. But it is the *rate* of accumulation rather than the absolute *volume* that is most important. Acute effusions, including hemopericardium from penetrating trauma, occur rapidly and can produce rapid decompensation. Cardiac rupture of the left ventricle following acute myocardial infarction (AMI) also causes immediate fatal hemopericardium. The patient usually presents with a sudden onset of pulseless electrical activity. Survival is rare even with immediate pericardiocentesis and cardiac surgery.

Right ventricular perforation can occur after temporary pacer placement, pulmonary artery catheter insertion, and right ventricular biopsy. Right ventricular pressures are lower than left ventricular pressures, so survival from RV perforation is possible with prompt recognition and drainage. Previously, idiopathic pericarditis was considered the primary cause of pericardial effusion and tamponade. But with the recent increase in the number of cardiology interventions performed, the provider following these in-hospital patients must be able to detect and treat pericardial effusion as a potential complication of cardiac catheterization. Small guidewires are used to track angioplasty balloons for dilation and stent placement. Microperforation of a coronary artery or dissection of the vessel may present with delayed tamponade after patients leave the catheterization suite, particularly if platelet inhibitors are administered after the procedure.

Signs and Symptoms

Chest pain is the most frequent symptom of acute pericarditis.[23] Patients may describe pericarditis with the same terms used to describe ACS, or the description may differ. Patients will describe the pain as sharp or stabbing. The pain is localized in the middle of the chest or below the sternum. Onset may be sudden or gradual. The pain may radiate to the back, neck, left arm, or left shoulder. Inspiration or movement can aggravate the pain. This is called a respirophasic component. A unique feature of pericardial pain is that it typically increases when the patient lies supine and decreases when the patient sits and leans forward. This is believed to occur because the diaphragmatic surface of the pericardium is richly innervated. When the patient lies supine, the diaphragmatic surface of the heart comes into contact with this pericardial segment, creating more pain. Patients often have fever (low grade or intermittent), shortness of breath, cough, or painful swallowing. Patients with tuberculous pericarditis commonly have the fever, night sweats, and weight loss of tuberculosis infection.

A *pericardial friction rub* is present in about half of patients with pericarditis. The character of the rub often changes from

Foundation Facts **ECG in Tamponade Complicating Pericarditis**	Cardiac tamponade may produce a diagnostic ECG pattern of *electrical alternans*. The amplitude (voltage) of each ECG complex (the P wave, QRS, and T wave) alternates from complex to complex. This pattern is caused by motion of the heart toward and away from the precordial leads. The motion is exacerbated by the large effusion. The heart "bobs" in the fluid, similar to a boat bobbing on the water.

one hour to the next, from heartbeat to heartbeat, and with changes in position. Many clinicians describe it as sounding like footsteps in crunchy snow or sandpaper rubbed together. It is loudest along the lower left border of the sternum and at the apex of the heart. The rub is best heard when the patient sits and leans forward or assumes the "hands-and-knees" position, bringing the anterior epicardium into contact with the inflamed pericardial segment. Patients may have occasional premature atrial or ventricular beats, tachypnea and dyspnea, ascites, or hepatomegaly.

Cardiac Tamponade

As fluid accumulates in the pericardial sac, the patient may develop dyspnea, easy fatigue, anxiety, and other signs of hemodynamic compromise. The volume of fluid, the rate of fluid accumulation, and the compliance of the pericardial sac all affect the onset and severity of clinical consequences. Rapid or substantial fluid accumulation or a constrictive pericardium will produce more acute cardiovascular deterioration than gradual fluid accumulation in the presence of a distensible pericardial sac.

Very few patients with pericardial tamponade demonstrate the 3 symptoms associated with tamponade that are known as *Beck's triad:* jugular venous distention, hypotension, and muffled or distant heart sounds.[24] The finding of clear lungs, hypotension, and jugular venous distention alerts trauma teams to the possible presence of traumatic hemopericardium with effusion.

Pulsus paradoxus is commonly present with tamponade. Pulsus paradoxus is a fall in systolic blood pressure (SBP) $\geq$8 to 10 mm Hg during spontaneous inspiration. A fall in SBP of more than 10 mm Hg is significant.[23] But providers need to know that acute airway disorders—rather than tamponade—are the most common causes of pulsus paradoxus. The name itself, *paradoxus, is* a misnomer. The pulse is actually not a paradox but an accentuation of the normal fall in SBP with inspiration. The difference is that the normal fall is not more than 10 mm Hg.

12-Lead ECG in Pericardial Tamponade

The 12-lead ECG can yield pathognomonic findings in both pericarditis and ACS. Four stages of ECG findings have been reported to occur in pericarditis, but all 4 stages occur in only about half of involved patients. The clinical clue involves the finding of ST-segment elevation in multiple leads, in contrast to the regional elevation observed in acute coronary artery occlusion in STEMI. When combined with depression of the P-R interval, the ECG is highly suggestive of acute pericarditis. But it is important to remember that pericarditis and pericardial effusion may present with nonspecific ECG changes. Echocardiography can be a useful bedside tool to aid in the diagnosis, especially in the ED. In addition, ACS can mimic pericarditis and vice versa.

The 4 stages of pericarditis are

- Stage 1: ST-segment elevation with ST segments that concave upward. This stage occurs within hours of the onset of pericarditis-associated chest pain. The elevation is frequently noted in all leads except V_1. ST-segment elevation may last several days.
- Stage 2: T waves flatten as the ST elevation returns to baseline.
- Stage 3: T waves become inverted, but Q waves do not form.
- Stage 4: The ECG gradually returns to normal.

Tension Pneumothorax

An injury to the lung parenchyma or a bronchus that produces an air leak can cause a tension pneumothorax. When a tension pneumothorax develops, air accumulates in the chest and pressure in the pleural space increases, compressing the lung on the involved side and pushing the heart and mediastinum to the opposite side. The mediastinum can compress the opposite lung, causing collapse and worsening hypoxia. The pneumothorax compresses the heart and great vessels, impeding venous return and cardiac output. Hypotension and hypoxia can combine to produce hemodynamic collapse, shock, and death.

A pneumothorax can be primary or secondary. A primary pneumothorax is also called a spontaneous pneumothorax; it rarely causes tension pneumothorax, although it can cause acute chest pain.

Clinical circumstances raise suspicion of a tension pneumothorax in certain patient groups. These include patients with a recently inserted central venous catheter; those who have had any recent diagnostic procedure in the chest, lower neck, or upper abdomen; ventilated patients with underlying pulmonary disease or high peak inspiratory airway pressures; and patients with chest or multisystem trauma. Tension pneumothorax may also follow removal of chest tubes.

Signs and Symptoms

Shortness of breath, progressing in some patients to acute respiratory distress, is the most common presenting symptom. The classic signs of tension pneumothorax are

- Decreased breath sounds, decreased chest expansion, and hyperresonance on the involved side.
- Shift of the mediastinum away from the side of the pneumothorax. This shift can cause decreased breath sounds in the chest opposite the side of the pneumothorax.
- Hypoxemia.

Table 5. Risk of Death or Nonfatal MI Over the Short Term in Patients With Chest Pain With High or Intermediate Likelihood of Ischemia*

	High risk: Risk is high if patient has *any* of the following findings:	Intermediate risk: Risk is intermediate if patient has *any* of the following findings:	Low risk: Risk is low if patient has NO high- or intermediate-risk features; may have any of the following:
History	• Accelerating tempo of ischemic symptoms over prior 48 hours	• Prior MI *or* • Peripheral artery disease *or* • Cerebrovascular disease *or* • CABG, prior aspirin use	
Character of pain	• Prolonged, continuing (>20 min) rest pain	• Prolonged (>20 min) rest angina is now resolved (moderate to high likelihood of CAD) • Rest angina (<20 min) or relieved by rest or sublingual nitrates	• New-onset functional angina (Class III or IV) in past 2 weeks without prolonged rest pain (but with moderate or high likelihood of CAD)
Physical exam	• Pulmonary edema secondary to ischemia • New or worse mitral regurgitation murmur • Hypotension, bradycardia, tachycardia • S$_3$ gallop or new or worsening rales • Age >75 years	• Age >70 years	
ECG	• Transient ST-segment deviation (≥0.5 mm) with rest angina • New or presumably new bundle branch block • Sustained VT	• T-wave inversion ≥2 mm • Pathologic Q waves or T waves that are not new	• Normal or unchanged ECG during an episode of chest discomfort
Cardiac markers	• Elevated cardiac troponin I or T • Elevated CK-MB	*Any of the above findings PLUS* • Normal	• Normal

*See columns A and B in Table 2 for definitions of high and intermediate likelihood of ischemia.
Modified from Braunwald et al. *Circulation.* 2002;106:1893-1900.

The diagnosis of a tension pneumothorax is a clinical, not a radiographic, diagnosis. The ACLS provider should not wait to obtain a chest radiograph to make the diagnosis. The following clinical signs and symptoms of extreme compromise in cardiopulmonary function indicate the need for empiric needle decompression:

• Lung sounds that are decreased or even absent on one side
• Tracheal deviation (a very late finding)
• Jugular vein distention
• Hypotension
• Pulsus paradoxus
• Respiratory distress or arrest
• Cyanosis

12-Lead ECG in Tension Pneumothorax

The 12-lead ECG is nonspecific, and tachycardia is the most common finding. Depending on whether a right or left pneumothorax has developed, clockwise or counterclockwise rotation of the electrical axis occurs as the heart is repositioned in the thorax.

> ### Foundation Facts
>
> ### Ischemic T-Wave Changes
>
> T-wave inversion is a nonspecific finding on the ECG. The mean QRS vector and the mean T-wave vector are related and called the QRS-T angle (normally about 45 to 60 degrees). In pattern recognition terms this results in T waves that are upright in leads with predominantly upright or "dominant" R waves (≥2 mm and inverted in leads with domintant R waves).
>
> - Ischemia causes a widening of the QRS-T angle. In pattern recognition terms this causes T-wave inversion in leads with dominant R waves.
> - This T-wave inversion is nonspecific with other causes.
> - But if dynamic T-wave inversion occurs and is associated with symptoms, it is strongly suggestive of ischemia.

Risk Stratification—Matching the Right Patient, the Right Therapy, at the Right Time: ECG and Troponin

Once a patient is thought to have an intermediate or high probability that chest discomfort is likely due to CAD (Table 2), a second question is asked. This involves estimating the probability that a major adverse cardiac event will occur. These events include death, nonfatal MI, and urgent need for coronary revascularization (Table 5).

Clinical indicators of high risk include an accelerating tempo of symptoms, such as occurrence with less exertion or at rest and prolonged episodes of pain or discomfort. Again, any evidence of LV dysfunction, or worsening LV failure, is serious. Troponin indicates myocyte necrosis and predicts high risk as well.

ST-Segment Deviation and Risk Stratification

The ECG is not a perfect test for myocardial ischemia or infarction and has limitations. Cardiac ischemia is identified when horizontal ST-segment depression is present. In the past consensus limits of ST-segment deviation were based on clinical data or trials with thresholds established to obtain adequate sensitivity (to detect patients with disease) and specificity (to identify patients who likely do not have the disease and will not benefit from therapy).

Measurement of ST-Segment Deviation

ST-segment depression often represents ischemia, and 1 mm of horizontal (flat) depression persisting for 0.08 second after the J point is used to define this abnormality in exercise stress testing. Some clinical ACS trials have used earlier measurements (0.02 second after the J point) to increase sensitivity. Compared to these ACS trials, others have used less (0.06 second after the J point) to increase specificity. Clinical algorithms for acute chest pain in ACS have used ST-segment depression measured 0.04 second after the J point as representative and easy to measure (it is one horizontal small box on the ECG).

Clinical trials have found that only 0.5 mm of ST depression is as predictive as 1 mm. Although this 0.5-mm ST-deviation threshold has not been subjected to the ECC evidence evaluation process, it is the threshold recommended in the American College of Cardiology (ACC)/American Heart Association (AHA) guidelines[25] and the ACC/AHA guidelines update,[7] and the material in this text has been changed to reflect this threshold. Measurements of this small magnitude and ischemic characterization (horizontal flat depression) require careful review and interpretation by experienced ECG readers.

Dynamic T-Wave Changes

T waves may normally be inverted in lead III (and occasionally in lead II), and these T waves are often incorrectly interpreted as indicating ischemia. T-wave inversions that do reflect ischemia involve a widening of the normal QRS axis and T-wave vector for an individual ECG. This change occurs with ischemia and may also be associated with a prolonged QTc interval. This diagnosis may be difficult for pattern ECG readers to make. But remember that T waves are normally upright in the leads that have dominant R waves (more of the QRS above baseline than below it). T-wave abnormalities may be difficult to identify unless a previous tracing is available for comparison. In outcome studies of ACS, T-wave abnormalities alone are not helpful in diagnosis or prognosis.

Dynamic T-wave changes are important indicators of ischemia in patients with acute chest pain. In such patients the finding of widening of the angle between the QRS axis and the T-wave axis and resolution of this abnormality with rest or nitroglycerin is indicative of ischemia. To detect these dynamic changes, you must obtain an ECG *before* administration of nitroglycerin in patients with suspected ACS. Typical response to nitrates (in several minutes) is suggestive but not diagnostic of cardiac ischemia. If you fail to obtain an ECG tracing when the patient is in pain and a repeat ECG after resolution of the pain, you may miss a diagnostic abnormality and opportunity. T waves suspicious for ischemia are defined in the ACC/AHA guidelines.[25] These T waves that are ≥2 mm and inverted in leads with

Prognostic Value of ECG Changes in ACS Patients: Gusto IIb

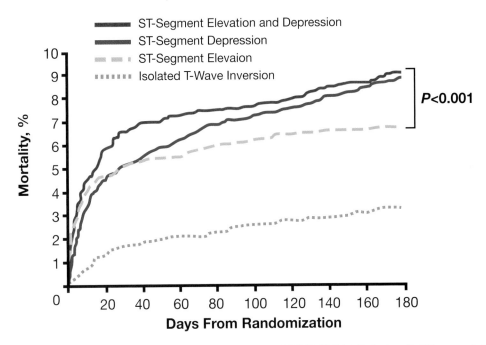

Figure 2. Percent mortality at 6 months based on initial ECG findings in the GUSTO IIB Trial. Patients with ST-segment depression have a higher mortality than "routine" patients with ST-segment elevation and rival STEMI patients with "reciprocal" ST-segment depression. These patients have reciprocal depression as a marker of large infarction or multivessel coronary disease. Isolated T-wave inversion has a lower prognostic value because it is nonspecific and includes patients without ACS. Reprinted with permission from Savonitto et al.[26] *JAMA.* 1999;281:707-713.

dominant R waves are suggestive of ischemia (indicate a widened QRS-T angle).

Nondiagnostic and Normal ECGs

Cardiologists vary in their criteria for diagnosis of nonspecific ST-segment and T-wave changes. Also, criteria may differ for some clinical situations. For example, ST-segment deviation in ACS is measured 0.04 second after the J point. A cardiologist performing a treadmill test measures ST-segment deviation at a point that is 0.08 second after the J point and does not count T waves at all.

A nonspecific or nondiagnostic ECG has the following characteristics:

- ST depression <0.5 mm, measured 0.04 second after the J point
- Upright T waves in leads with dominant R waves (normal) *or*
- T-wave inversion <2 mm in leads with dominant R waves

Prognostic Significance of ST-Segment Deviation and Prognosis

Although it can be nonspecific and has limitations, the ST segment can be a powerful prognostic and triage marker for patients with possible ACS. Important and appropriate, STEMI patients have a time-dependent critical factor

inherent in the priority for rapid reperfusion. This does not and should not imply that patients with ST-segment depression have a better prognosis or can be the focus of casual evaluation and treatment. In fact, patients with NSTEMI may have a worse outcome and higher mortality than STEMI patients without reciprocal ST-segment depression (Figure 2).

Cardiac Biomarkers

New cardiac biomarkers—troponins—are more sensitive than CK-MB and are useful in diagnosis, risk stratification, and determination of prognosis. An elevated level of *troponin* correlates with an increased risk of death, and greater elevations predict greater risk of adverse outcome.[27] Patients with increased troponin levels have increased thrombus burden and microvascular embolization to the distal coronary circulation.

Cardiac biomarkers should be obtained during the initial evaluation of the patient, but therapeutic decisions and reperfusion therapy for patients with STEMI should not be delayed pending the results of these tests. These tests are insensitive during the first 4 to 6 hours of presentation unless continuous, persistent pain has been present for 6 to 8 hours. For this reason cardiac biomarkers are not useful in the prehospital setting.[28,29] But over time serial marker testing (CK-MB and cardiac troponin) has better sensitivity for detection of myocardial ischemia.

Early Invasive vs Early Conservative Strategies

By 2002 treatment strategies had been developed using evidence-based trials and clinical bedside risk stratification of patients. An *early invasive strategy* recommends *routinely* taking patients with unstable angina or NSTEMI to cardiac catheterization and performing angiographically indicated revascularization. This could be PCI, coronary artery bypass grafting (CABG), or continued medical therapy, depending on the results of coronary angiography. The *early conservative strategy* recommends initial management of stable patients with antiplatelet, antithrombin, and antianginal therapy as indicated. The recurrence of symptoms despite adequate therapy or the finding of high-risk features (based on clinical criteria or stress testing) is then an indication for coronary angiography. The ACC/AHA Task Force on the Management of Patients With Unstable Angina recently concluded that the latest clinical trials comparing early conservative and early invasive strategies showed an improved outcome for patients at intermediate or high risk when assigned to the invasive strategy. For this reason the task force made the early invasive strategy a Class I recommendation in the 2002 update of the guidelines for patients with unstable angina and NSTEMI at intermediate or high risk of MACE.[25]

Indicators for Early Invasive Strategies

Risk stratification (Figure 3, Box 12) helps the clinician identify patients with NSTEMI and unstable angina who should be managed with an invasive strategy. Coronary angiography then allows the clinician to determine whether patients are appropriate candidates for revascularization with PCI or CABG.

The following clinical indicators identify patients at increased risk:

- New ST-segment depression or positive troponins
- Persistent or recurrent ischemic symptoms
- Hemodynamic instability or ventricular tachycardia
- Depressed LV function (ejection fraction <40%)
- ECG or functional study that suggests multivessel CAD

TIMI Risk Score

The risk of MACE has been further studied and refined. Researchers who derived the important Thrombolysis in Myocardial Ischemia (TIMI) risk score used data from the TIMI-IIB and ESSENCE (Efficacy and Safety of Subcutaneous Enoxaparin in Non–Q-Wave Coronary Events) trials for NSTEMI and UA[30] and from the In-TIME trial for STEMI. The TIMI risk score comprises 7 independent prognostic variables (Table 6). These 7 variables were significantly associated with the occurrence within 14 days of at least 1 of the primary end points: death, new or recurrent MI, or need for urgent revascularization. The score is derived from complex multivariate logistic regression analysis and includes variables that seem historically counterintuitive. For example, it is useful to note that traditional cardiac risk factors are only weakly associated with MACE. Use of aspirin within the previous 7 days, for example, would not seem to be an indicator of a bad outcome. But aspirin use was found to be one of the most powerful predictors. It is possible that aspirin use identified a subgroup of patients at higher risk or on active but failed therapy for CAD.

The creators of the TIMI risk score validated it with 3 groups of patients, and 4 clinical trials showed a significant interaction between the TIMI risk score and outcome. These findings confirm the value of the TIMI risk score as a guide to therapeutic decisions. A PDA download of the TIMI Risk Calculator is available at www.TIMI.org.

The Braunwald (Table 2) and TIMI (Table 6) risk scores serve as the dominant clinical guides for predicting the risk of MACE in patients with ACS. It is important to note that risk stratification is applicable to patients with an intermediate or high risk of symptoms due to CAD, not the larger general population of patients presenting with chest pain or symptoms possibly due to anginal equivalents. Risk stratification enables clinicians to direct therapy to those patients at intermediate or high risk of MACE and to avoid unnecessary therapy and the potential for adverse consequences in patients at lower risk.

The TIMI risk score has become the primary tool for evaluating therapeutic recommendations. Some of the newer therapies may provide incrementally greater benefit for patients with higher risk scores.

One additional product of the TIMI trials is the TIMI grading system of coronary artery blood flow. TIMI investigators developed and validated a coronary artery perfusion scoring system, characterizing the degree of reperfusion of a coronary artery on a scale of 0 (no flow) to 3 (complete, brisk flow). This grading system is now used as an outcome measure in many studies of ACS interventions.

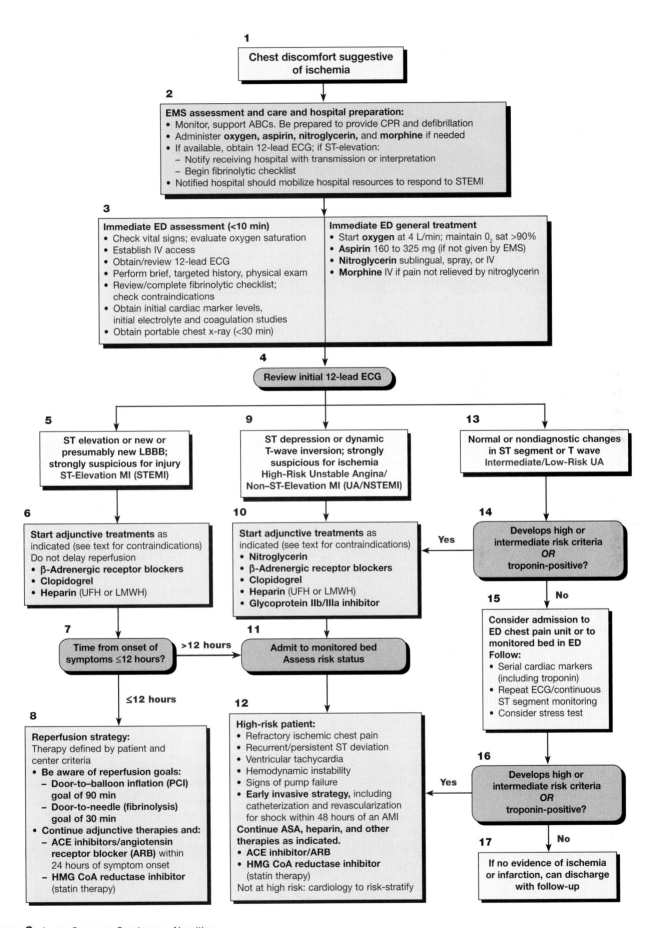

Figure 3. Acute Coronary Syndromes Algorithm.

Table 6. TIMI Risk Score for Patients With Unstable Angina and NSTEMI: Predictor Variables

Predictor Variable	Point Value of Variable	Definition
Age ≥65 years	1	
≥3 Risk factors for CAD	1	Risk factors • Family history of CAD • Hypertension • Hypercholesterolemia • Diabetes • Current smoker
Aspirin use in last 7 days	1	
Recent, severe symptoms of angina	1	≥2 anginal events in last 24 hours
Elevated cardiac markers	1	CK-MB or cardiac-specific troponin level
ST deviation ≥0.5 mm	1	ST depession ≥0.5 mm is significant; transient ST elevation >0.5 mm for <20 minutes is treated as ST-segment depression and is high risk; ST elevation ≥1 mm for >20 minutes places these patients in the STEMI treatment category
Prior coronary artery stenosis ≥50%	1	Risk predictor remains valid even if this information is unknown

Calculated TIMI Risk Score	Risk of ≥1 Primary End Point* in ≤14 Days	Risk Status
0 or 1	5%	Low
2	8%	Low
3	13%	Intermediate
4	20%	Intermediate
5	26%	High
6 or 7	41%	High

*Primary end points: death, new or recurrent MI, or need for urgent revascularization.

Foundation Facts

Integration of Cardiac Troponins With ECG Parameters

Serial cardiac biomarkers are diagnostic and prognostic, and they guide therapy.

- If troponin is positive on presentation, NSTEMI is present and the patient is already at high risk.
- If serial markers become positive, the patient has NSTEMI and an early invasive strategy is preferred.
- If serial markers remain negative in the patient with ST-segment depression, the patient has unstable angina unless ST-segment depression has another cause, such as secondary repolarization changes due to left ventricular hypertrophy.
- Some patients with positive serial markers will develop Q-wave MI.
- If patients with a normal or nondiagnostic ECG develop positive troponin, they have NSTEMI. These patients are now candidates for an invasive strategy rather than functional testing.

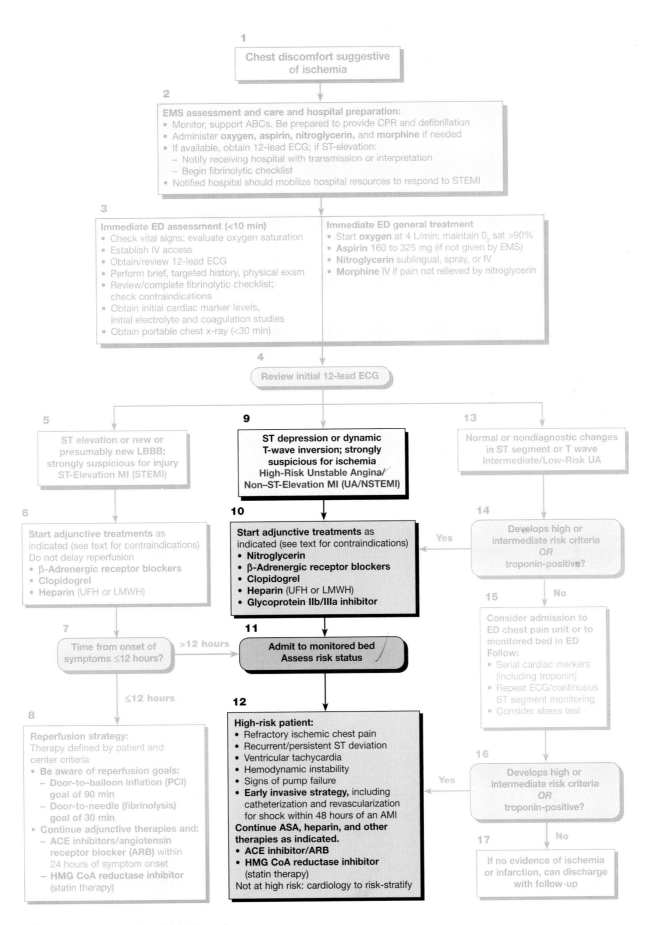

Figure 4. Non–ST-elevation MI and high-risk angina.

ECG: ST-Segment Depression or Dynamic T-Wave Inversion

When the patient presents with signs of ACS, the clinician uses the acute chest pain algorithm (Figure 3) to initially assess the patient and then the ECG findings (Figure 3, Box 4) to classify the patient into 1 of 3 groups:

- ST-segment elevation or presumed new LBBB (Box 5) is characterized by ST-segment elevation >1 mm (0.1 mV) in 2 or more contiguous precordial leads or 2 or more adjacent limb leads and is classified as **STEMI.**
- Ischemic ST-segment depression ≥0.5 mm (0.05 mV) or dynamic T-wave inversion with pain or discomfort (Box 9) is classified as *high-risk UA/NSTEMI.* Nonpersistent or transient ST-segment elevation ≥0.5 mm for <20 minutes is also included in this category.
- Normal or nondiagnostic changes in the ST segment or T waves (Box 13) are inconclusive and require further risk stratification. This classification includes patients with normal ECGs and those with ST-segment deviation of <0.5 mm (0.05 mV) or T-wave inversion less than 2 mm (<0.2 mV). Serial cardiac studies (and functional testing) are appropriate.

When patients have ischemic ST depression or dynamic T-wave inversion, they are considered high risk (Figure 4, Boxes 9-12) and are candidates for intensive management with an early invasive strategy of cardiac catheterization and PCI (Figure 4, Box 12).

General Management—Start Adjunctive Treatments (Box 10)

Patients who are at high risk for complications of ACS receive intensive antiplatelet and antithrombotic therapy. *Healthcare providers need to be aware that data is continually evolving, and individualization of therapy is necessary in the context of the risk-benefit assessment and a time-dependent strategy. If available, use an institutional protocol and consult with cardiology teams.*

Treatment options include aspirin, clopidogrel, heparin (unfractionated [UFH] or low molecular weight [LMWH]), glycoprotein IIb/IIIa receptor inhibitors, parenteral nitroglycerin for recurrent or persistent discomfort, and β-adrenergic receptor blockers.

Antiplatelet and Antithrombin Therapy— Aspirin and Beyond

Aspirin

Although a time-dependent effect of aspirin in unstable angina and NSTEMI is not supported by evidence, aspirin (160 to 325 mg PO) should be given as soon as possible to all patients with suspected ACS unless the patient has aspirin allergy or sensitivity, an active bleeding disorder, active peptic ulcer disease, or recent or acute gastrointestinal bleeding. A dose of 160 to 325 mg causes rapid and near-total inhibition of thromboxane A_2 production, so it reduces platelet aggregation. It can reduce death and vascular events. In high-risk patients aspirin can reduce nonfatal MI and vascular death, and it is effective in patients with unstable angina. Aspirin is often administered as four 81-mg tablets. Enteric-coated formulations are not used. An aspirin suppository is given if oral administration is not effective (eg, with nausea or vomiting).

If patients are to be considered for an interventional strategy, it is customary to give 325 mg PO to achieve complete platelet inhibition. This dose will be continued in conjunction with clopidogrel if a stent is placed.

Clopidogrel

Clopidogrel is a thienopyridine, or an adenosine diphosphate antagonist, that is used for antiplatelet therapy. Clopidogrel irreversibly inhibits the platelet adenosine diphosphate receptor, reducing platelet aggregation through a different mechanism than aspirin. Since 2000 several important studies of clopidogrel have been published documenting its efficacy for both patients with UA/NSTEMI and those with STEMI. In these studies patients with an ACS and a rise in serum levels of cardiac biomarkers or ECG changes consistent with ischemia had reduced stroke and MACE if clopidogrel was added to aspirin and heparin within 4 hours of hospital presentation.[31] One study confirmed that clopidogrel did not increase the risk of bleeding in comparison with aspirin.[32] Clopidogrel given 6 hours or more before elective PCI for patients with ACS without ST elevation has been shown to reduce adverse ischemic events at 28 days (level of evidence 1).[33]

The appropriate timing and dose of clopidogrel remain uncertain and are the subject of continuing investigation. The Clopidogrel for the Reduction of Events During Observation

FAQ

Is the Clopidogrel Dose Changing?

Studies have shown that some patients may have a resistance to clopidogrel similar to the phenomenon of aspirin resistance. In addition, the current loading dose of clopidogrel (300 mg) is not effective in most patients until >6 hours after administration. Studies are evaluating a 600-mg loading dose.[35,36]

(CREDO) trial (post hoc analysis) found only a small clinical benefit unless the current loading dose of 300 mg was administered >15 hours before PCI. Clopidogrel resistance was present in about 25% of the patients.[34] Another trial used a 600-mg loading dose of clopidogrel given >12 hours before PCI and found an increased antiplatelet effect and fewer major adverse cardiac events at 1 month.[35]

On the basis of these findings, providers should administer a 300-mg loading dose of clopidogrel in addition to standard care (aspirin, UFH or LMWH, and glycoprotein IIb/IIIa inhibitors if indicated) to ED patients with ACS and elevated cardiac markers or new ECG changes consistent with ischemia in whom a medical approach or PCI is planned. It is also reasonable to administer a 300-mg oral dose of clopidogrel to ED patients with suspected ACS (without ECG or cardiac marker changes) who are unable to take aspirin because of hypersensitivity or major gastrointestinal intolerance.

Glycoprotein IIb/IIIa Inhibitors

After plaque rupture in the coronary artery, tissue factor in the lipid-rich core is exposed and forms complexes with or triggers other coagulation factors. Platelet adhesion, activation, and aggregation may result in formation of an arterial thrombus, and these processes are pivotal in the pathogenesis of ACS. The integrin glycoprotein IIb/IIIa (GP IIb/IIIa) receptor is the final common pathway to platelet aggregation, leading to binding of circulating adhesive macromolecules. Administration of a GP IIb/IIIa receptor antagonist (inhibitor) is one way of reducing acute ischemic complications after plaque fissure or rupture.

Several large studies of GP IIb/IIIa inhibitors in UA/NSTEMI have shown a clear benefit of these agents when combined with standard aspirin and heparin and a strategy of mechanical reperfusion (PCI).[37] Severe bleeding complications in a minority of patients (but no increase in intracranial hemorrhage) in the GP IIb/IIIa group were offset by the large benefit of these agents. This benefit extends to high-risk patients with UA/NSTEMI treated with PCI.[38]

In UA/NSTEMI patients not treated with PCI, the effect of GP IIb/IIIa inhibitors has been mixed. One large meta-analysis[38] showed that GP IIb/IIIa inhibitors produced no mortality advantage and only a slight reduction in recurrent ischemic events, but a later, equally large meta-analysis showed a reduction in 30-day mortality.[39] Of note, the benefit of GP IIb/IIIa inhibitors was dependent on coadministration of UFH or LMWH. Interestingly abciximab appears to behave differently from the other 2 GP IIb/IIIa inhibitors. In the Global Utilization of Streptokinase and Tissue Plasminogen Activator for Occluded Coronary Arteries (GUSTO) IV ACS trial and 1-year follow-up involving 7800 patients,[40,41] abciximab showed a lack of treatment effect compared with placebo in patients treated medically only.

On the basis of these findings, GP IIb/IIIa inhibitors should be used in patients with high-risk UA/NSTEMI as soon as possible in conjunction with aspirin, heparin, and clopidogrel and a strategy of early PCI (Class I). Patients with positive biomarkers benefit the most. Extrapolation from efficacy studies suggests that this therapy may be administered in the ED once a decision has been made to proceed to PCI.

If PCI is not planned, the GP IIb/IIIa inhibitors tirofiban and eptifibatide may be used in conjunction with standard therapy in selected patients with high-risk UA/NSTEMI. But data is inconclusive at this time, and a careful risk-benefit assessment should be performed, especially for older patients and those with renal dysfunction since increased bleeding is seen. Because of the lack of benefit demonstrated in the GUSTO IV ACS trial, abciximab should not be given unless PCI is planned.

Precautions and contraindications to use of GP IIb/IIIa inhibitors include the following:

- Active internal bleeding or bleeding disorder in the past 30 days (thrombocytopenia, platelets <150 000)
- History of intracranial hemorrhage, neoplasm, arteriovenous malformation, or aneurysm, or stroke or major surgical procedure or trauma within the past 30 days
- Aortic dissection, pericarditis, and severe hypertension
- Hypersensitivity

Heparins

Heparin, an indirect inhibitor of thrombin, has been widely used as adjunctive therapy for fibrinolysis and in combination with aspirin for the treatment of UA. UFH is a heterogeneous mixture of sulfated glycosaminoglycans of various chain lengths. UFH has several disadvantages, including an unpredictable anticoagulant response in individual patients, the need for IV administration, and the requirement for frequent monitoring of the activated partial thromboplastin time (aPTT). Heparin can also stimulate platelet activation, causing thrombocytopenia.

Six in-hospital randomized, controlled trials and additional studies (including 7 meta-analyses) have documented similar or improved composite outcomes (death, MI and/or recurrent angina, or recurrent ischemia or revascularization) when LMWH is given instead of UFH to patients with UA/NSTEMI within the first 24 to 36 hours after onset of symptoms. Although major bleeding events are not significantly different with LMWH, there is a consistent increase in minor and postoperative bleeding with LMWH.

Four trials have compared UFH and LMWH in patients with NSTEMI who were treated with a GP IIb/IIIa inhibitor. In terms of efficacy LMWH compared favorably with UFH. In terms of safety there were similar or less frequent major bleeding events with LMWH, but again there was an increased frequency of minor bleeding complications.

Overall, ED administration of LMWH (specifically enoxaparin) is beneficial compared with UFH when given in addition to antiplatelet therapy such as aspirin for patients with UA/NSTEMI. UFH should be considered if reperfusion is planned in the first 24 to 36 hours after onset of symptoms. Changing from one form of heparin to another (crossover of antithrombin therapy) during an acute event is not recommended because it may lead to increased bleeding complications.[42,43]

Antianginal Therapy

Nitroglycerin IV Infusion

Nitroglycerin reduces myocardial oxygen demand while enhancing myocardial oxygen delivery. Nitroglycerin, an endothelium-independent vasodilator, has both peripheral and coronary vascular effects that contribute to increased oxygen delivery and reduced oxygen demand. By dilating the capacitance vessels (ie, the venous beds), it increases venous pooling to decrease myocardial preload and myocardial oxygen consumption. More modest effects on the arterial circulation decrease afterload, contributing to further reduction in myocardial oxygen consumption and increased oxygen delivery. IV rather than long-acting preparations should be used acutely to enable titration.

Nitroglycerin is an effective analgesic for ischemic chest discomfort. It also has beneficial hemodynamic effects, including dilation of the coronary arteries (particularly in the region of plaque disruption), the peripheral arterial bed, and venous capacitance vessels. But the treatment benefits of nitroglycerin are limited, and no conclusive evidence supports *routine* use of IV, oral, or topical nitrate therapy in patients with AMI.[44] With this in mind, providers should carefully consider use of these agents, especially when low blood pressure precludes the use of other agents shown to be effective in reducing morbidity and mortality (eg, β-blockers and angiotensin-converting enzyme inhibitors).

Nitrates are contraindicated in patients with hypotension (SBP <90 mm Hg or >30 mm Hg below baseline), extreme bradycardia (<50 per minute), or tachycardia (>100 per minute). Nitrates should be given with extreme caution, if at all, to patients with inferior wall MI and suspected RV involvement because these patients require adequate RV preload. Nitrates are also contraindicated if patients have taken a phosphodiesterase inhibitor for erectile dysfunction within the last 24 hours (longer for some preparations).

β-Adrenoceptor Blocking Agents (β-Blockers)

β-Blockers block sympathetic nervous system stimulation of heart rate and contractility, resulting in vasodilation and reduced ventricular afterload. They can reduce infarct size, decrease postinfarction ischemia, and reduce the incidence of ventricular ectopy and fibrillation.

Oral β-blockers should be administered in the ED for ACS of all types unless contraindications are present (see Chapter 10, page 202). They should be given irrespective of the need for revascularization therapies. IV β-blockers can be used to treat tachyarrhythmias or hypertension in the absence of moderate to severe congestive heart failure. Contraindications to β-blockers are moderate to severe LV failure and pulmonary edema, bradycardia (<50 per minute), hypotension (SBP <100 mm Hg), signs of poor peripheral perfusion, second-degree or third-degree heart block, or reactive airway disease. In the presence of heart failure, oral β-blockers are used with caution, and they are given in low and titrated doses after the patient is stabilized.

The following are absolute contraindications to β-blocker therapy:

- Acute moderate or severe LV failure and pulmonary edema
- Bradycardia (heart rate <50 per minute)
- Low blood pressure in acute setting (SBP <100 mm Hg)
- Signs of poor peripheral perfusion
- Second-degree or third-degree heart block

Foundation Facts

IV Nitroglycerin (or Topical Nitrates) Not "Routine"

Nitroglycerin is indicated for the initial management of pain and ischemia with ACS but without hypotension (SBP <90 mm Hg) except in patients with RV infarction. Evidence does not support routine administration of nitroglycerin in patients with uncomplicated AMI.

Give IV nitroglycerin in the following circumstances:

- If pain is not controlled with up to 3 sublingual nitroglycerin tablets, 3 metered spray doses, or nitroglycerin paste
- If pain recurs after initial relief
- As an adjunct for blood pressure control after giving β-blockers
- As an adjunct for treatment of congestive heart failure with ACS

Cardiac Catheterization (Box 12)

Coronary angiography identifies lesions at risk for occlusion or with a high level of ischemic potential. These are called "target lesions." When technically feasible angioplasty is performed to dilate these target lesions. The majority of patients today also receive a stent to maintain vessel patency. This is possible in most patients with single-vessel disease and in some patients with more than one lesion. Coronary artery bypass surgery, if not contraindicated, is performed for patients with multiple target lesions, particularly diabetic patients.

Revascularization (Box 12)

When indicated PCI or surgical revascularization may reduce the incidence of MACE and decrease the incidence of recurrent ischemia. CABG is indicated primarily for patients with stenosis of the left main coronary artery, severe multivessel disease, or when PCI is not an option.

Normal or Nondiagnostic ECG: Absence of Diagnostic Changes in ST Segment or T Waves (Intermediate/Low-Risk Unstable Angina) (Box 13)

Patients who present with possible or probable angina, or noncardiac chest pain, who may have ischemia but have a normal or nondiagnostic ECG are rendered pain free and then administered an aspirin if not already given. These patients are then further evaluated, and serial studies and functional testing are performed as indicated (Figure 5).

Patients who develop clinical indicators of instability or high risk, such as ECG changes with pain or positive troponin or CK-MB tests, are then managed similarly to patients initially presenting with ST-segment depression or dynamic T-wave inversion. Intensive medical therapy is indicated, as is an invasive strategy. Functional testing is contraindicated in these patients, who are unstable. If a conservative strategy is selected for indicated reasons or patient preference, functional testing is deferred until the patient has been pain free and stable for at least 24 hours on medical therapy.

Adjunctive treatments should continue or be started on the basis of specific indications (Box 14). Serial cardiac studies are obtained. If serial ECGs reveal development of persistent ST *elevation,* immediate reperfusion therapy is indicated. An exercise or perfusion imaging study (radionuclide or 2D echocardiography) is obtained in the majority of patients to identify ischemia, determine prognosis, and further risk stratify the patient.

Patients presenting with chest pain syndromes require continuous risk stratification during evaluation. In isolation neither the history nor the ECG will identify patients at risk or free of disease. But once a noncardiac etiology is identified during the evaluation, patients are treated for this diagnosis and the chest pain evaluation protocol is no longer followed. A few clinical pearls assist in evaluation:

- Although the presence of ACS is low, a normal ECG does not rule out an ACS. For this reason a second ECG is indicated if the chest pain persists or recurs to *any degree* during observation. A repeat ECG is obtained about 1 hour after admission or upon anticipated discharge from the ED or transfer to another unit if ACS is suspected. If the pain recurs, obtain an ECG, preferably before administration of nitroglycerin. But do not significantly delay nitroglycerin administration solely for an "ECG during pain."

- Cardiac-specific markers of MI do not begin to become positive until several hours after damage to myocardial cells occurs. The ACC/AHA guidelines recommend obtaining a *second* set of cardiac markers (troponin I or T and CK-MB) when initial levels are not elevated. This testing is usually done 6 to 8 hours after admission. Timing is important. The first ED sample may be equivalent to a 6-hour to 8-hour sample if the patient has had prolonged and continuous pain before ED presentation. It is important to note the time relationships, duration of discomfort, and episodic nature of the discomfort if present.

- An institutional protocol is encouraged to define the type and time of testing in patients at low risk for ACS. Patients at low risk for symptoms due to CAD and for MACE can be discharged and undergo functional testing within 48 to 72 hours if they are pain free, have normal ECGs, and have no elevation of cardiac markers (including "gray zone" troponin). Patients at high risk for MACE and those with positive markers do not usually undergo stress testing. Whether and when an individual patient at intermediate risk for ACS undergoes functional testing requires careful assessment and clinical judgment.

| **Critical Concept**

 "Rule Out" Is Now Ruled Out and ACS Is Now "Ruled In" | Recently published consensus guidelines clearly establish that clinicians cannot rule out an ACS in patients with typical ischemic chest pain symptoms on the basis of history, physical examination, traditional risk factor evaluation, or clinical judgment alone.

 An institutional interdisciplinary protocol applied *routinely* to patients with chest discomfort suspicious for ischemia is recommended to guide the care of patients with possible ACS. |

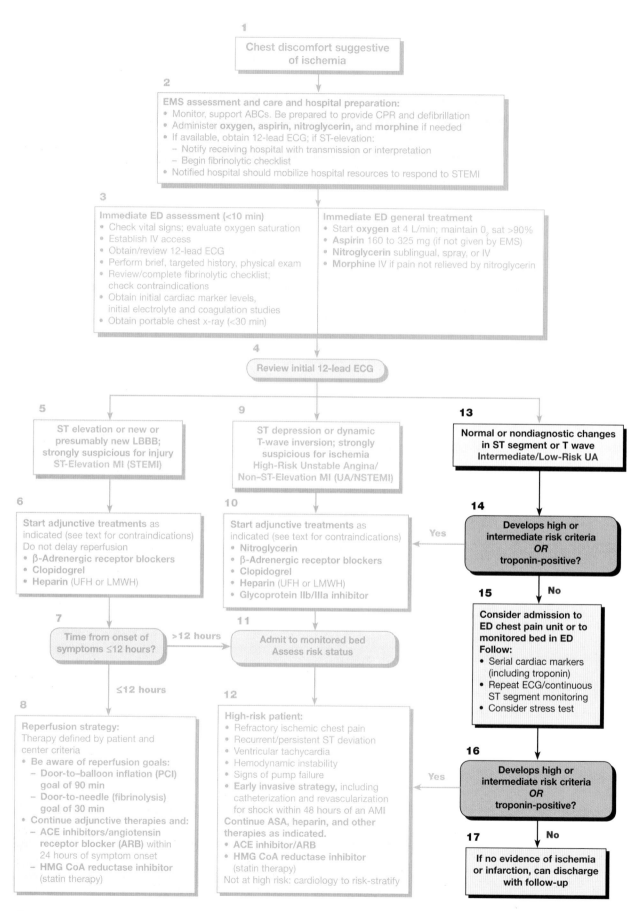

1
Chest discomfort suggestive of ischemia

2
EMS assessment and care and hospital preparation:
- Monitor, support ABCs. Be prepared to provide CPR and defibrillation
- Administer **oxygen, aspirin, nitroglycerin,** and **morphine** if needed
- If available, obtain 12-lead ECG; if ST-elevation:
  – Notify receiving hospital with transmission or interpretation
  – Begin fibrinolytic checklist
- Notified hospital should mobilize hospital resources to respond to STEMI

3
Immediate ED assessment (<10 min)
- Check vital signs; evaluate oxygen saturation
- Establish IV access
- Obtain/review 12-lead ECG
- Perform brief, targeted history, physical exam
- Review/complete fibrinolytic checklist; check contraindications
- Obtain initial cardiac marker levels, initial electrolyte and coagulation studies
- Obtain portable chest x-ray (<30 min)

Immediate ED general treatment
- Start **oxygen** at 4 L/min; maintain O$_2$ sat >90%
- **Aspirin** 160 to 325 mg (if not given by EMS)
- **Nitroglycerin** sublingual, spray, or IV
- **Morphine** IV if pain not relieved by nitroglycerin

4
Review initial 12-lead ECG

5
ST elevation or new or presumably new LBBB; strongly suspicious for injury ST-Elevation MI (STEMI)

9
ST depression or dynamic T-wave inversion; strongly suspicious for ischemia High-Risk Unstable Angina/ Non–ST-Elevation MI (UA/NSTEMI)

13
Normal or nondiagnostic changes in ST segment or T wave Intermediate/Low-Risk UA

6
Start adjunctive treatments as indicated (see text for contraindications) Do not delay reperfusion
- β-Adrenergic receptor blockers
- Clopidogrel
- Heparin (UFH or LMWH)

10
Start adjunctive treatments as indicated (see text for contraindications)
- Nitroglycerin
- β-Adrenergic receptor blockers
- Clopidogrel
- Heparin (UFH or LMWH)
- Glycoprotein IIb/IIIa inhibitor

14
Develops high or intermediate risk criteria *OR* troponin-positive?

Yes

No

15
Consider admission to ED chest pain unit or to monitored bed in ED Follow:
- Serial cardiac markers (including troponin)
- Repeat ECG/continuous ST segment monitoring
- Consider stress test

7
Time from onset of symptoms ≤12 hours?

>12 hours

≤12 hours

11
Admit to monitored bed Assess risk status

8
Reperfusion strategy:
Therapy defined by patient and center criteria
- Be aware of reperfusion goals:
  – Door-to–balloon inflation (PCI) goal of 90 min
  – Door-to-needle (fibrinolysis) goal of 30 min
- Continue adjunctive therapies and:
  – ACE inhibitors/angiotensin receptor blocker (ARB) within 24 hours of symptom onset
  – HMG CoA reductase inhibitor (statin therapy)

12
High-risk patient:
- Refractory ischemic chest pain
- Recurrent/persistent ST deviation
- Ventricular tachycardia
- Hemodynamic instability
- Signs of pump failure
- Early invasive strategy, including catheterization and revascularization for shock within 48 hours of an AMI
Continue ASA, heparin, and other therapies as indicated.
- ACE inhibitor/ARB
- HMG CoA reductase inhibitor (statin therapy)
Not at high risk: cardiology to risk-stratify

16
Develops high or intermediate risk criteria *OR* troponin-positive?

Yes

No

17
If no evidence of ischemia or infarction, can discharge with follow-up

Figure 5. Normal or nondiagnostic ECG.

Discharge Acceptable (Box 17)

Patients to be discharged should have experienced complete relief of pain early after presenting to the ED unless a noncardiac cause of pain has been identified. If the pain was not quickly eliminated soon after ED presentation or if possible ischemic pain recurs during evaluation, then the patient is considered at least intermediate risk.

If objective evidence (minimum of 2 normal ECGs with no ST-segment deviation or significant changes plus 2 sets of normal cardiac markers obtained 6 or more hours apart) excludes myocardial necrosis and stratifies the patient as low risk for MACE, the patient can be discharged with specific instructions and follow-up. These actions not only constitute appropriate clinical care but also are prudent risk management for ED physicians.

- The responsible physician should arrange for timely follow-up of the patient. Document these arrangements in writing in the medical record. If practical, communicate directly (voice to voice) with the physician who will take responsibility for the patient's continued evaluation.
- Ask the patient to sign a statement confirming the patient's understanding and acceptance of the follow-up plans, and place the statement in the medical record. In contemporary emergency medicine practice this statement most conveniently takes the form of a copy of the signed discharge instructions to the patient.
- Instruct patients to phone 911 and request EMS transport to return to the ED if any of their symptoms recur.

References

1. Goodacre S, Locker T, Morris F, Campbell S. How useful are clinical features in the diagnosis of acute, undifferentiated chest pain? *Acad Emerg Med*. 2002;9:203-208.

2. Goodacre SW, Angelini K, Arnold J, Revill S, Morris F. Clinical predictors of acute coronary syndromes in patients with undifferentiated chest pain. *QJM*. 2003;96:893-898.

3. Everts B, Karlson BW, Wahrborg P, Hedner T, Herlitz J. Localization of pain in suspected acute myocardial infarction in relation to final diagnosis, age and sex, and site and type of infarction. *Heart Lung*. 1996;25:430-437.

4. McSweeney JC, Cody M, O'Sullivan P, Elberson K, Moser DK, Garvin BJ. Women's early warning symptoms of acute myocardial infarction. *Circulation*. 2003;108:2619-2623.

5. Braunwald E. Unstable angina: an etiologic approach to management [editorial]. *Circulation*. 1998;98:2219-2222.

6. Braunwald E, Antman EM, Beasley JW, Califf RM, Cheitlin MD, Hochman JS, Jones RH, Kereiakes D, Kupersmith J, Levin TN, Pepine CJ, Schaeffer JW, Smith EE III, Steward DE, Theroux P, Gibbons RJ, Alpert JS, Eagle KA, Faxon DP, Fuster V, Gardner TJ, Gregoratos G, Russell RO, Smith SC Jr. ACC/AHA guidelines for the management of patients with unstable angina and non-ST-segment elevation myocardial infarction: executive summary and recommendations. A report of the American College of Cardiology/American Heart Association Task Force on Practice Guidelines (Committee on the Management of

Patients With Unstable Angina). *Circulation*. 2000; 102:1193-1209.

7. Braunwald E, Antman EM, Beasley JW, Califf RM, Cheitlin MD, Hochman JS, Jones RH, Kereiakes D, Kupersmith J, Levin TN, Pepine CJ, Schaeffer JW, Smith EE III, Steward DE, Theroux P, Gibbons RJ, Alpert JS, Faxon DP, Fuster V, Gregoratos G, Hiratzka LF, Jacobs AK, Smith SC Jr. ACC/AHA guideline update for the management of patients with unstable angina and non-ST-segment elevation myocardial infarction—2002: summary article: a report of the American College of Cardiology/American Heart Association Task Force on Practice Guidelines (Committee on the Management of Patients With Unstable Angina). *Circulation*. 2002;106:1893-1900.

8. Peberdy MA, Ornato JP. Coronary artery disease in women. *Heart Dis Stroke*. 1992;1:315-319.

9. Douglas PS, Ginsburg GS. The evaluation of chest pain in women. *N Engl J Med*. 1996;334:1311-1315.

10. Sullivan AK, Holdright DR, Wright CA, Sparrow JL, Cunningham D, Fox KM. Chest pain in women: clinical, investigative, and prognostic features. *BMJ*. 1994;308:883-886.

11. Solomon CG, Lee TH, Cook EF, Weisberg MC, Brand DA, Rouan GW, Goldman L. Comparison of clinical presentation of acute myocardial infarction in patients older than 65 years of age to younger patients: the Multicenter Chest Pain Study experience. *Am J Cardiol*. 1989;63:772-776.

12. Sizemore C, Lewis JF. Clinical relevance of chest pain during dobutamine stress echocardiography in women. *Clin Cardiol*. 1999;22:715-718.

13. Hagan PG, Nienaber CA, Isselbacher EM, Bruckman D, Karavite DJ, Russman PL, Evangelista A, Fattori R, Suzuki T, Oh JK, Moore AG, Malouf JF, Pape LA, Gaca C, Sechtem U, Lenferink S, Deutsch HJ, Diedrichs H, Marcos y Robles J, Llovet A, Gilon D, Das SK, Armstrong WF, Deeb GM, Eagle KA. The International Registry of Acute Aortic Dissection (IRAD): new insights into an old disease. *JAMA*. 2000;283:897-903.

14. Podbregar M, Krivec B, Voga G. Impact of morphologic characteristics of central pulmonary thromboemboli in massive pulmonary embolism. *Chest*. 2002;122:973-979.

15. Goldhaber SZ, Visani L, De Rosa M. Acute pulmonary embolism: clinical outcomes in the International Cooperative Pulmonary Embolism Registry (ICOPER). *Lancet*. 1999;353:1386-1389.

16. Heit JA. The epidemiology of venous thromboembolism in the community: implications for prevention and management. *J Thromb Thrombolysis*. 2006;21:23-29.

17. Kucher N, Rossi E, De Rosa M, Goldhaber SZ. Massive pulmonary embolism. *Circulation*. 2006;113:577-582.

18. Miller AC. Suspected pulmonary embolism. *Clin Med*. 2004;4:215-219.

19. Thabut G, Thabut D, Myers RP, Bernard-Chabert B, Marrash-Chahla R, Mal H, Fournier M. Thrombolytic therapy of pulmonary embolism: a meta-analysis. *J Am Coll Cardiol*. 2002;40:1660-1667.

20. Piazza G, Goldhaber SZ. Acute pulmonary embolism: part I: epidemiology and diagnosis. *Circulation*. 2006;114:e28-e32.

21. Piazza G, Goldhaber SZ. Acute pulmonary embolism: part II: treatment and prophylaxis. *Circulation*. 2006;114:e42-e47.

22. Aikat S, Ghaffari S. A review of pericardial diseases: clinical, ECG and hemodynamic features and management. *Cleve Clin J Med*. 2000;67:903-914.

23. Bilchick KC, Wise RA. Paradoxical physical findings described by Kussmaul: pulsus paradoxus and Kussmaul's sign. *Lancet.* 2002;359:1940-1942.

24. Spittell J Jr. Chest pain in patients with normal findings on angiography. *Mayo Clin Proc.* 2002;77:296.

25. Braunwald E, Antman EM, Beasley JW, Califf RM, Cheitlin MD, Hochman JS, Jones RH, Kereiakes D, Kupersmith J, Levin TN, Pepine CJ, Schaeffer JW, Smith EE III, Steward DE, Theroux P, Alpert JS, Eagle KA, Faxon DP, Fuster V, Gardner TJ, Gregoratos G, Russell RO, Smith SC Jr. ACC/AHA guidelines for the management of patients with unstable angina and non-ST-segment elevation myocardial infarction. A report of the American College of Cardiology/American Heart Association Task Force on Practice Guidelines (Committee on the Management of Patients With Unstable Angina). *J Am Coll Cardiol.* 2000;36:970-1062.

26. Savonitto S, Ardissino D, Granger CB, Morando G, Prando MD, Mafrici A, Cavallini C, Melandri G, Thompson TD, Vahanian A, Ohman EM, Califf RM, Van de Werf F, Topol EJ. Prognostic value of the admission electrocardiogram in acute coronary syndromes. *JAMA.* 1999;281:707-713.

27. Antman EM, Tanasijevic MJ, Thompson B, Schactman M, McCabe CH, Cannon CP, Fischer GA, Fung AY, Thompson C, Wybenga D, Braunwald E. Cardiac-specific troponin I levels to predict the risk of mortality in patients with acute coronary syndromes. *N Engl J Med.* 1996;335:1342-1349.

28. Gust R, Gust A, Bottiger BW, Bohrer H, Martin E. Bedside troponin T testing is not useful for early out-of-hospital diagnosis of myocardial infarction. *Acta Anaesthesiol Scand.* 1998;42:414-417.

29. Newman J, Aulick N, Cheng T, Faynor S, Curtis R, Mercer D, Williams J, Hobbs G. Prehospital identification of acute coronary ischemia using a troponin T rapid assay. *Prehosp Emerg Care.* 1999;3:97-101.

30. Antman EM, Cohen M, Bernink PJ, McCabe CH, Horacek T, Papuchis G, Mautner B, Corbalan R, Radley D, Braunwald E. The TIMI risk score for unstable angina/non-ST elevation MI: a method for prognostication and therapeutic decision making. *JAMA.* 2000;284:835-842.

31. Yusuf S, Zhao F, Mehta SR, Chrolavicius S, Tognoni G, Fox KK. Effects of clopidogrel in addition to aspirin in patients with acute coronary syndromes without ST-segment elevation. *N Engl J Med.* 2001;345:494-502.

32. A randomised, blinded, trial of clopidogrel versus aspirin in patients at risk of ischaemic events (CAPRIE). CAPRIE Steering Committee. *Lancet.* 1996;348:1329-1339.

33. Steinhubl SR, Berger PB, Mann JT III, Fry ET, DeLago A, Wilmer C, Topol EJ. Early and sustained dual oral antiplatelet therapy following percutaneous coronary intervention: a randomized controlled trial. *JAMA.* 2002;288:2411-2420.

34. Steinhubl SR, Berger PB, Brennan DM, Topol EJ. Optimal timing for the initiation of pre-treatment with 300 mg clopidogrel before percutaneous coronary intervention. *J Am Coll Cardiol.* 2006;47:939-943.

35. Cuisset T, Frere C, Quilici J, Morange PE, Nait-Saidi L, Carvajal J, Lehmann A, Lambert M, Bonnet JL, Alessi MC. Benefit of a 600-mg loading dose of clopidogrel on platelet reactivity and clinical outcomes in patients with non-ST-segment elevation acute coronary syndrome undergoing coronary stenting. *J Am Coll Cardiol.* 2006;48:1339-1345.

36. Hochholzer W, Trenk D, Frundi D, Blanke P, Fischer B, Andris K, Bestehorn HP, Buttner HJ, Neumann FJ. Time dependence of platelet inhibition after a 600-mg loading dose of clopidogrel

in a large, unselected cohort of candidates for percutaneous coronary intervention. *Circulation.* 2005;111:2560-2564.

37. Bosch X, Marrugat J. Platelet glycoprotein IIb/IIIa blockers for percutaneous coronary revascularization, and unstable angina and non-ST-segment elevation myocardial infarction. *Cochrane Database Syst Rev.* 2001:CD002130.

38. Roffi M, Chew DP, Mukherjee D, Bhatt DL, White JA, Heeschen C, Hamm CW, Moliterno DJ, Califf RM, White HD, Kleiman NS, Theroux P, Topol EJ. Platelet glycoprotein IIb/IIIa inhibitors reduce mortality in diabetic patients with non-ST-segment-elevation acute coronary syndromes. *Circulation.* 2001;104:2767-2771.

39. Boersma E, Harrington RA, Moliterno DJ, White H, Theroux P, Van de Werf F, de Torbal A, Armstrong PW, Wallentin LC, Wilcox RG, Simes J, Califf RM, Topol EJ, Simoons ML. Platelet glycoprotein IIb/IIIa inhibitors in acute coronary syndromes: a meta-analysis of all major randomised clinical trials [published correction appears in *Lancet.* 2002.;359:2120]. *Lancet.* 2002;359:189-198.

40. Simoons ML. Effect of glycoprotein IIb/IIIa receptor blocker abciximab on outcome in patients with acute coronary syndromes without early coronary revascularisation: the GUSTO IV-ACS randomised trial. *Lancet.* 2001;357:1915-1924.

41. Ottervanger JP, Armstrong P, Barnathan ES, Boersma E, Cooper JS, Ohman EM, James S, Topol E, Wallentin L, Simoons ML. Long-term results after the glycoprotein IIb/IIIa inhibitor abciximab in unstable angina: one-year survival in the GUSTO IV-ACS (Global Use of Strategies To Open Occluded Coronary Arteries IV--Acute Coronary Syndrome) Trial. *Circulation.* 2003;107:437-442.

42. Ferguson J. Low-molecular-weight heparins and glycoprotein IIb/IIIa antagonists in acute coronary syndromes. *J Invasive Cardiol.* 2004;16:136-144.

43. Ferguson JJ, Califf RM, Antman EM, Cohen M, Grines CL, Goodman S, Kereiakes DJ, Langer A, Mahaffey KW, Nessel CC, Armstrong PW, Avezum A, Aylward P, Becker RC, Biasucci L, Borzak S, Col J, Frey MJ, Fry E, Gulba DC, Guneri S, Gurfinkel E, Harrington R, Hochman JS, Kleiman NS, Leon MB, Lopez-Sendon JL, Pepine CJ, Ruzyllo W, Steinhubl SR, Teirstein PS, Toro-Figueroa L, White H. Enoxaparin vs unfractionated heparin in high-risk patients with non-ST-segment elevation acute coronary syndromes managed with an intended early invasive strategy: primary results of the SYNERGY randomized trial. *JAMA.* 2004;292:45-54.

44. ISIS-4: a randomised factorial trial assessing early oral captopril, oral mononitrate, and intravenous magnesium sulphate in 58,050 patients with suspected acute myocardial infarction. ISIS-4 (Fourth International Study of Infarct Survival) Collaborative Group. *Lancet.* 1995;345:669-685.

Chapter 12

Cardiovascular
Part 2: Heart Failure and Shock Complicating ACS

This chapter of the cardiovascular section describes complications of acute coronary syndromes (ACS): shock, pulmonary edema, and hypotension. The first section discusses a general approach to the patient presenting in shock. The second section summarizes the pathophysiology and treatment of cardiogenic shock associated with ST-elevation myocardial infarction (STEMI) and other ACSs, emphasizing therapy unique to these patients. The last section reviews the Acute Pulmonary Edema, Hypotension, and Shock Algorithm and details initial evaluation and stabilization of any patient with pulmonary edema and shock or hypertensive urgency. This section contains more information about treatment decisions based on the initial response to therapy.

Key Points

- Cardiogenic shock is the leading cause of death in patients with acute myocardial infarction (AMI) who survive to reach the hospital.
- The incidence of cardiogenic shock has largely remained unchanged, and mortality is high, about 50% in published trials.

- RV shock (usually found in association with inferior wall MI) has a high mortality rate similar to that of LV shock.
- Patients with cardiogenic shock and STEMI should be primarily transported or secondarily transferred (with a door-to-departure time of ≤30 minutes) to facilities capable of invasive strategies such as insertion of an intra-aortic balloon pump (IABP), percutaneous coronary intervention (PCI), and coronary artery bypass grafting (CABG).
- An invasive strategy is recommended for patients <75 years of age; carefully selected patients age 75 and older also can receive aggressive early revascularization.
- If heart failure and shock develop after hospital admission, the patient should undergo diagnostic angiography and PCI or CABG if possible if shock develops within the first 36 hours of onset of MI.

Shock

Shock is a clinical condition characterized by a sustained and significant reduction in blood flow and oxygen delivery to organs and tissues. It is important to realize that shock and low blood pressure, although related, are not the same. In basic terms shock is a condition in which tissue oxygenation (and cellular ventilation and nutrition) is inadequate for demand.

Patients frequently present with shock and no immediately obvious etiology. Blood pressure alone can be misleading or "normal" for a variety of reasons. Hence the diagnosis of shock is a clinical one characterized by several of the following findings:

- Clinically ill appearance or altered mental status
- Low blood pressure (defined as a systolic blood pressure [SBP] <80 or 90 mm Hg)
- Tachycardia (heart rate >100)
- Tachypnea (respiratory rate >22 breaths/min or $PaCO_2$ <32 mm Hg)
- Systemic acidosis (serum lactate >4 mmol/L)
- Decreased urine output (<0.5 mL/kg per hour)

Differential Diagnosis of Shock

Not all of these criteria may be present. For example, patients on β-blockers may not have tachycardia. In early shock blood pressure may be normal or only slightly low because of excess adrenergic drive, and it may not drop significantly until late in the process.

Blalock initially divided shock into 4 general categories,[1] and variations of these are still useful today during initial assessment of the patient in shock. Blalock's categories were hematologic, neurologic, vasogenic, and cardiogenic. Today we initially classify patients as those with volume problems, cardiac problems, or "distributive" problems. Recall the 5th quadrad in the Introduction: Tank Volume, Tank Resistance, Pump, and Rhythm.

- Tank Volume—Inadequate intravascular volume relative to the vascular space (eg, hemorrhage, dehydration)
- Tank Resistance—Inappropriate vascular resistance or maldistribution of blood flow (eg, septic shock)
- Pump—Inadequate cardiac output due to pump failure or obstruction (eg, cardiogenic shock, pulmonary embolism, tamponade)
- Rate—Bradycardia or tachycardia reducing cardiac output (eg, complete atrioventricular block, ventricular tachycardia)

The clinician can use these provisional etiologic mechanisms to characterize shock and to identify the appropriate initial focus of therapy:

- Arrhythmic shock → Antiarrhythmic therapy
- Hypovolemic shock → Volume therapy
- Cardiogenic shock → Support of pump function
- Distributive shock → Vasoactive drug therapy

An etiologic approach to shock often oversimplifies the problem. Any patient with severe or sustained shock will likely require some support of heart rate and rhythm, titration of fluid therapy to optimize intravascular volume, support of pump function, and manipulation of vascular resistance and distribution of blood flow. All patients with severe or sustained shock will have some myocardial failure or even necrosis. In fact, patients in intensive care units (ICUs) with elevation of troponin in the absence of coronary artery disease have a worse prognosis.

Determinants of Cardiac Output

A more detailed diagnostic approach that defines the variable of cardiac output and allows for a more targeted approach to therapy is often required. Recall from Chapter 10 that BP is only a surrogate for cardiac output. And cardiac output is determined by stroke volume and heart rate. So 3 variables determine cardiac output and distribution of blood to the periphery: stroke volume (pump function), heart rate (rhythm), and vascular resistance (systemic).

$$\text{Arterial Pressure} = \textbf{Cardiac Output} \times \text{Total (Systemic) Vascular Resistance}$$

$$\textbf{Cardiac Output} = \text{Stroke Volume} \times \text{Heart Rate}$$

Cardiac function and other variables influencing cardiac output are complex. But one major determinant relevant to the initial assessment is the volume loading conditions of the heart. At normal volume loading conditions, cardiac output is optimal at rest and in the absence of pathologic conditions. As venous return decreases (low filling pressure), cardiac output falls. At the patient's bedside a pulmonary arterial catheter can measure these filling pressures (central venous and pulmonary capillary wedge pressures) and cardiac output, using these measures to calculate systemic vascular resistance when necessary and indicated.

With 3 variables there are 27 possible combinations, so interpretation can be complex. But 3 general divisions improve diagnostic accuracy (Table 1) and allow general classification into hypovolemic, cardiogenic, and vasogenic shock. It should be remembered that insertion of a pulmonary artery catheter is a diagnostic, not a therapeutic, procedure with associated complications. In most patients clinical assessment of filling pressure (central venous pressure, rales) and clinical circumstances are diagnostic.

Cardiogenic Shock Complicating AMI

Infarction of 40% or more of the LV myocardium in acute STEMI usually results in cardiogenic shock and death. Although the mortality rate of cardiogenic shock has decreased in selected recent trials, death rates still average 50% to 70%,[2] and the overall incidence has not declined appreciably.[3,4]

Cardiogenic Shock in NSTEMI ACS

It should also be appreciated that shock can occur in patients with non–ST-elevation myocardial infarction (NSTEMI), and even a small or modest infarct can cause hemodynamic instability if prior MI or LV dysfunction is present at the time of recurrent ACS. Patients with NSTEMI are significantly older and have more prior MI, heart failure, and 3-vessel disease. They also have more comorbidities, including renal dysfunction, bypass surgery, and peripheral vascular disease, than patients with STEMI.[5,6]

Pathophysiology and Hemodynamics of Cardiogenic Shock

MI may result in hemodynamic instability and congestive heart failure (CHF). As described above, cardiogenic shock classically has been defined as a pump problem due to "massive" heart attack. Cardiac output and ventricular ejection fraction fall and heart rate increases to compensate for the fall in stroke volume in a reflex effort to maintain cardiac output. The damaged ventricle dilates, and the amount of blood ejected with each contraction decreases (ejection fraction or EF).

β-Blockade and Heart Failure

As noted, tachycardia may help maintain cardiac output despite the fall in ejection fraction and stroke volume. But all compensatory changes are likely to increase myocardial oxygen consumption. They also can worsen ischemia in viable or distant myocardium and extend infarction. In some cases (eg, large anterior MI without CHF), a reduction in heart rate with β-blockade improves outcome. Blockade of excess sympathetic and neurohumoral stimulation reduces myocardial oxygen consumption. But in compensatory tachycardia, β-blockade can be life-threatening, such as in cardiogenic shock or severe heart failure, when the stroke volume is critically dependent on the tachycardia.

The Clopidogrel and Metoprolol in Myocardial Infarction Trial (COMMIT) trial evaluated the Metoprolol in Acute Myocardial Infarction (MIAMI) trial protocol for early intravenous (IV) blockade in 45,852 patients with STEMI.[8] The primary outcomes of (1) death, reinfarction, or cardiac arrest and (2) death from any cause during the scheduled treatment period were not reduced by treatment with IV metoprolol. In this prospective study decreases in reinfarction and ventricular fibrillation were offset by an increase in cardiogenic shock, largely occurring within the first day of treatment. The authors concluded that early use of β-blocker therapy in AMI reduces the risks of reinfarction and ventricular fibrillation but increases the risk of cardiogenic shock, especially during the first day or two after admission. Cardiogenic shock and moderate to severe heart failure are contraindications to β-blockade. In patients with a large MI and who are at risk for heart failure, early IV β-blockade should be withheld and started orally after the patient is stable and angiotensin-converting enzyme (ACE) inhibitors have been started to attenuate LV remodeling.

Foundation Facts Cardiogenic Shock and "Small MI"	Patients with a small or modest MI can develop cardiogenic shock or severe LV failure. • Prior MI and poor LV function decrease cardiac reserve. • Patients are older with more comorbidities. • The mortality rate rivals that of large MI because of delayed diagnosis and comorbidities. • ECG findings for the circumflex distribution can be limited, and the circumflex artery is the cause in about one third of patients.

Table 1. Hemodynamic Parameters in the 3 Major Categories of Shock*

Hypovolemic	Cardiogenic	Vasogenic
Low CVP/PCWP	High CVP/PCWP	Low CVP/PCWP
Low CO	Low CO	High CO
High SVR	High SVR	Low SVR

*In hypovolemic shock, filling pressure (central venous pressure [CVP], pulmonary capillary wedge pressure [PCWP]) is low, reducing cardiac output. In an attempt to compensate and maintain arterial pressure, systemic vascular resistance (SVR) increases. In cardiogenic shock the pump is damaged and cardiac output is low, raising filling pressures (CVP, PCWP) and decreasing cardiac output. Because cardiac output is low, SVR also increases to maintain arterial pressure. In vasogenic shock, seen in sepsis for example, vasodilation occurs, lowering SVR. This vasodilation causes a fall in vascular volume, and cardiac output increases in an attempt to compensate and "fill the tank." (CVP estimates right atrial pressure, and PCWP estimates left atrial pressure. CO indicates cardiac output.

FYI

More Information on Cardiogenic Shock

For a complete discussion of the diagnosis and management of deep venous thrombosis and pulmonary embolism, see

CLINICIAN UPDATE

Cardiogenic Shock Complicating Myocardial Infarction: Expanding the Paradigm, by Judith S Hochman[9]

Hemodynamic Parameters of Cardiogenic Shock

When LV end-diastolic pressure increases substantially (>25 to 30 mm Hg), interstitial and then pulmonary edema develops. If RV end-diastolic pressure increases, peripheral edema will be observed. A fall in cardiac output also triggers an adrenergic response, producing tachycardia and peripheral vasoregulatory changes that try to redistribute blood flow. Constriction of arteries to the skin, kidneys, and gut redistributes blood flow away from these tissues to maintain blood flow to the brain and heart. But this systemic vasoconstriction may create increased LV *afterload,* impeding LV ejection. As cardiac output continues to fall, hypotension and lactic acidosis develop. This combination of pulmonary edema with signs of inadequate systemic perfusion is the hallmark of cardiogenic shock.

The patient with LV dysfunction classically has been described as one with a cardiac index (cardiac output corrected for body surface area) ≤ 2.2 L/min per m^2, PCWP >18 mm Hg, and SBP <90 mm Hg. When the cardiac index falls to 2.2 L/min per m^2 and SBP falls to 90 mm Hg, frank signs of poor peripheral perfusion are usually present.

Changing the Paradigm of Cardiogenic Shock

The changes described above for cardiogenic shock result from severe depression of myocardial contractility due to MI. Cardiogenic shock remains the leading cause of in-hospital mortality from MI. In the shock trial, the classic assumption that acute reduction in cardiac output leads to compensatory vasoconstriction in all patients was not confirmed, and a subgroup of patients was identified with low SVR.[11] New insights suggest that an inflammatory response and inappropriate vasodilation may play a role in these patients (Figure 1).[9]

Treatment of Cardiogenic Shock Associated With AMI

The mortality rate of AMI associated with cardiogenic shock is 50% or more in virtually every outcome report, and half of the deaths occur within the first 48 hours. Initial therapy for LV dysfunction without shock includes oxygen administration, IV administration of nitrates to reduce cardiac preload and afterload, and diuresis. Morphine is an excellent adjunct agent if the patient has continuing ischemia. If SBP is <100 mm Hg, nitrates and morphine should be used with caution if at all. When SBP is <90 mm Hg, they are contraindicated.

If the patient presents or becomes markedly hypotensive, avoid or discontinue vasodilators and administer vasoactive drugs based on SBP to increase arterial tone (vasopressors), improve blood pressure, and redistribute cardiac output. If the patient does not respond to these initial therapies, be prepared to perform additional diagnostic studies, initiate advanced hemodynamic monitoring, and provide advanced therapies. In selected patients mechanical circulatory assistance with intra-aortic balloon counterpulsation is an effective adjunct with reperfusion therapy. Results from the Global Utilization of Streptokinase and Tissue Plasminogen Activator for Occluded Coronary Arteries (GUSTO-I) and SHOCK (**SH**ould We Emergently Revascularize **O**ccluded Coronaries for **C**ardiogenic Shoc**K**) trials[3] found that an aggressive, early invasive approach increases survival for patients with cardiogenic shock and AMI (see below).

With increasing use of both fibrinolytic therapy and PCI, controversy arose over which technique was the better method of reperfusion. Retrospective and registry trial evidence has shown that for patients with AMI and cardiogenic shock, an aggressive early strategy of PCI is superior to medical therapy with fibrinolytics:

Foundation Facts

Classic Hemodynamic Definition of Cardiogenic Shock

Cardiogenic shock is defined[10] as SBP ≤ 90 mm Hg for ≥ 1 hour that is

- Not responsive to fluid administration alone
- Secondary to cardiac dysfunction
- Associated with signs of hypoperfusion or a cardiac index ≤ 2.2 L/min per m^2 and a pulmonary capillary wedge pressure >18 mm Hg

- The GUSTO-I investigators reported that mortality was lower in patients with cardiogenic shock treated with an aggressive PCI strategy than in similar patients given fibrinolytic therapy.[13]
- Investigators have reported higher survival rates for cardiogenic shock patients who undergo revascularization instead of fibrinolysis.[14]
- In the US Second National Registry of Myocardial Infarction, the mortality rate in patients with AMI and shock was lower in those treated with PCI as a primary strategy than in those treated with fibrinolytics.[14]
- In a large registry of patients with shock, mortality was lower in AMI patients who received early revascularization with either PCI or CABG.[15]
- Multiple investigators have reported reduced mortality in patients with cardiogenic shock and AMI who received intra-aortic balloon pumping followed by cardiac catheterization and revascularization with PCI or CABG (when anatomy was suitable).[16,17]

Rapid Response Interventions **Destination Hospital Protocol for Cardiogenic Shock**	When possible, transfer patients at high risk for mortality or severe LV dysfunction with signs of shock, pulmonary congestion, heart rate >100 *and* SBP <100 mm Hg to a facility capable of performing cardiac catheterization and rapid revascularization (PCI or CABG). • Also consider triage or transfer for patients with a large anterior wall infarct, CHF, or pulmonary edema. • Defer fibrinolytic therapy if PCI is *rapidly* available and anticipated door-to-balloon-inflation time is ≤60 minutes. If you cannot ensure transfer within a time that would allow rapid PCI, administer fibrinolytics if there are no contraindications to their use. Then transfer the patient with a door-to-departure time of 30 minutes or less.

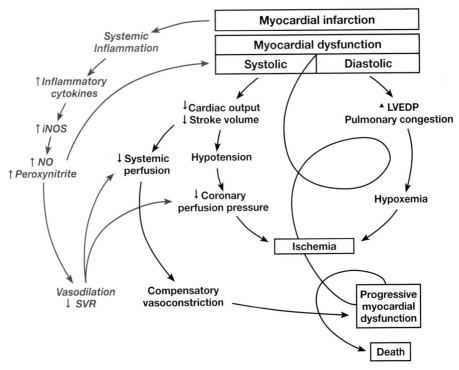

Figure 1. Classic shock paradigm, as illustrated by S Hollenberg, is shown in black. The influence of the inflammatory response syndrome initiated by a large MI is illustrated in red. LVEDP indicates left ventricular end-diastolic pressure. Reprinted with permission from *Harrison's Principles of Internal Medicine.*[12]

Figure 2 gives recommendations for initial reperfusion therapy when cardiogenic shock complicates AMI.

The best method and timing of revascularization as well as optimal therapy for shock was a topic of controversy until evaluated and resolved by the randomized, controlled SHOCK trial. This study compared early revascularization using IABP plus percutaneous transluminal coronary angioplasty or CABG with early medical stabilization using fibrinolytic therapy. Mortality at 6 months and at 1 year of follow-up was significantly lower in the early revascularization group than in the early medical therapy group (number needed to treat was approximately 8 at both time points). Follow-up data through 6 years is now available from this randomized trial. Almost two thirds of hospital survivors with cardiogenic shock who were treated with early revascularization were alive 6 years later. A strategy of early revascularization resulted in a 13.2% absolute and a 67% relative improvement in 6-year survival compared with initial medical stabilization.[18]

In hospitals without interventional capabilities or an on-site intervention team, proceed with administration of fibrinolytics. If the patient fails to reperfuse or remains clinically unstable, or has persistent shock and CHF,

transfer the patient for coronary angiography and PCI (or CABG) for failed lysis, a procedure often referred to as "rescue PCI."

In 2004 the American College of Cardiology (ACC)/American Heart Association (AHA) Committee on Management of Acute Myocardial Infarction updated prior guidelines, and PCI remained a Class I recommendation for patients with ACS and shock who are <75 years old. Resuscitation experts reviewed and endorsed these recommendations at the 2000 and 2005 International Consensus Conferences. The current recommendations from the updated ACC/AHA STEMI guidelines[19] are as follows:

- Provide early triage or transfer to cardiovascular facilities with cardiac catheterization suites and interventional capability.
- When possible, transfer patients at high risk for mortality or severe LV dysfunction with signs of shock, pulmonary congestion, heart rate >100, *and* SBP <100 mm Hg to a facility capable of performing cardiac catheterization and rapid revascularization (PCI or CABG). For patients younger than 75 years, this is a Class I recommendation.

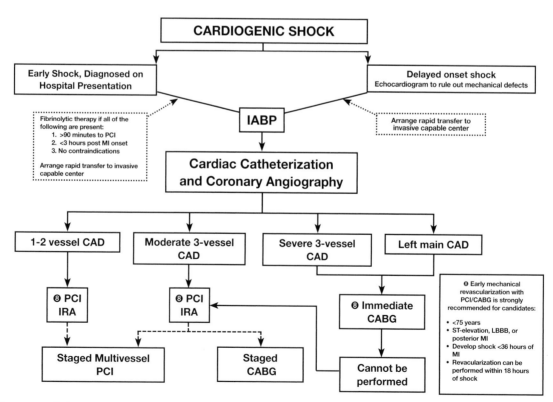

Figure 2. Recommendations for initial reperfusion therapy when cardiogenic shock complicates acute MI. Early mechanical revascularization with PCI or CABG is strongly recommended for suitable candidates <75 years of age and for selected elderly patients. Eighty-five percent of shock cases are diagnosed after initial therapy for acute MI, but most patients develop shock within 24 hours. IABP is recommended when shock is not quickly reversed with pharmacological therapy, as a stabilizing measure for patients who are candidates for further invasive care. Dashed lines indicate that the procedure should be performed in patients with specific indications only. LBBB indicates left bundle-branch block; and IRA, infarct-related artery. Reprinted with permission from Hochman.[9]

<table>
<tr>
<td>

FYI

Management Guidelines for Cardiogenic Shock Complicating STEMI

</td>
<td>

For a complete discussion of the diagnosis and management of Cardiogenic Shock complicating STEMI, see

ACC/AHA Guidelines for the Management of Patients With ST-Elevation Myocardial Infarction. A Report of the American College of Cardiology/American Heart Association Task Force on Practice Guidelines (Committee to Revise the 1999 Guidelines for the Management of Patients With Acute Myocardial Infarction).
Developed in Collaboration With the Canadian Cardiovascular Society.[19]

</td>
</tr>
</table>

- PCI, including angioplasty with stent placement, is a Class I recommendation for patients <75 years of age with ACS and signs of shock.
- Use of IABP and diagnostic cardiac catheterization and coronary revascularization with PCI or CABG (if anatomy is suitable) may reduce mortality.
- The healthcare provider can use a checklist to identify patients who have contraindications to fibrinolytic therapy (see Chapter 10, Figure 9). If contraindications to fibrinolytic therapy exist, consider transfer to a cardiac intervention facility for reperfusion.

Right Ventricular Shock

In the majority of persons the right coronary artery supplies blood to the inferior wall and right ventricle (Figure 3). When a thrombus occludes the proximal right coronary artery, ischemia and infarction of the right ventricle occur. The RV marginal branch is involved in about one third of patients

with inferior infarction, and in one half of these patients occlusion is hemodynamically significant. Infarction of the right ventricle has a favorable *long-term* prognosis, but hemodynamic infarction of the right ventricle at the time of infarction more than doubles mortality. The right ventricle is fairly resistant to infarction; most acute dysfunction is due to ischemic but viable myocardium that can recover.

The SHOCK trial evaluated 933 patients in cardiogenic shock due to predominant RV (n = 49) or LV failure (n = 884). Patients with predominant RV shock were younger and had a lower prevalence of previous MI and multivessel disease. Despite the younger age, lower rate of anterior MI, and higher prevalence of single-vessel coronary disease of patients with RV shock, and the similar benefit they eceive from revascularization, mortality in these patients is unexpectedly high, similar to that in patients with LV shock.[20]

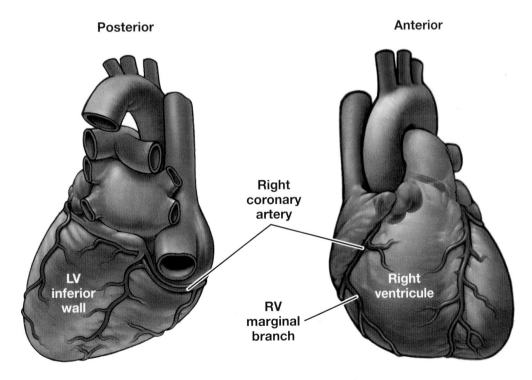

Posterior　　　　**Anterior**

Right coronary artery

LV inferior wall

Right ventricule

RV marginal branch

Figure 3. Anatomy of the heart showing the right coronary artery and RV marginal branch that supplies blood to the right ventricle. A thrombus occluding the right coronary artery proximal to the RV marginal branch causes infarction of the inferior and posterior walls of the heart (if not supplied by the circumflex coronary artery) and the right ventricle. In about 50% of patients, RV involvement leads to hemodynamic instability.

These patients have difficulty filling the lungs and returning blood to the left heart. Only a small area of left ventricular myocardium may be involved (inferior and posterior walls), and shock is due to inadequate filling of the left ventricle, which is due to RV dysfunction. In patients with an inferior wall MI (Figure 4), RV involvement should be suspected and a right sided 12-lead ECG performed (Figure 5). A 1 mm

ST-segment elevation in lead V_4 is 88% sensitive and 78% specific for RV involvement.

Clinical findings are different in RV and LV shock. Lungs may be relatively clear because of the inability of the right ventricle to pump blood to the pulmonary vasculature and the absence of LV dysfunction, causing increased pulmonary capillary pressures. Paradoxically neck veins

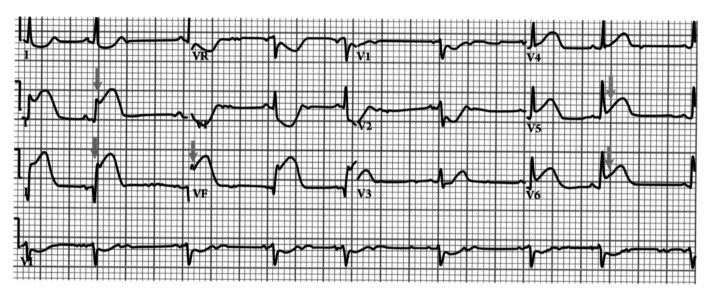

Figure 4. Twelve-lead ECG showing junctional ST-segment elevation in inferior leads II, III, and aVF. Note the ST-segment elevation in lateral leads V_5 and V_6, indicating lateral wall involvement (inferolateral wall), and the ST-segment depression in precordial leads V_1 and V_2. These findings are not due to anterior wall ischemia but to infarction of the posterior wall of the ventricle.

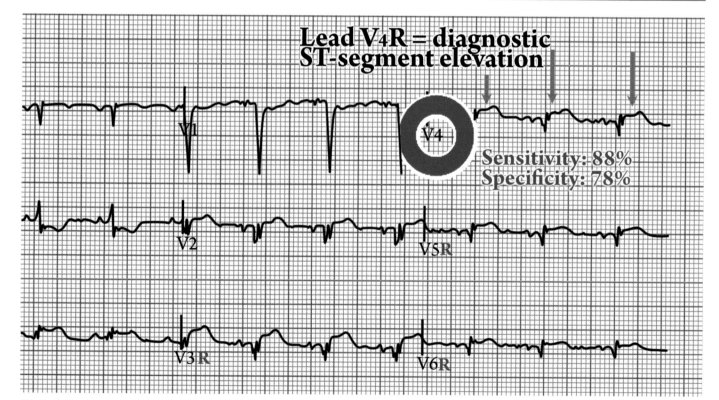

Figure 5. *Right-sided* 12-lead ECG showing junctional ST-segment elevation in leads over the right ventricle. Lead V_4R (blue circle) has 1 mm ST-segment elevation. This elevation is 88% sensitive and 78% specific for right ventricular involvement.

may be distended because of high right atrial pressures. The triad of clear lungs, elevated jugular venous distention, and hypotension is present in only about 25% of patients.

Both RV and LV cardiogenic shock require emergent reperfusion. However, adjunctive medical management is different for each type. Vasodilation and low filling pressures are to be avoided in RV shock. The impaired right ventricle requires optimal preload. Treatments that decrease preload, including nitrates, morphine, diuretics, and ACE inhibitors, may increase mortality and are avoided. Optimal preload should be achieved with cautious and monitored volume replacement. Initially 1 to 2 L of fluid may be required. This should be given in a 250 to 500 mL bolus, and vital signs and clinical assessment should be repeated. The rapid and injudicious administration of large amounts of fluid without clinical benefit should also be avoided because high pressures and large amounts of volume will further impair RV function and recovery. In patients with multivessel involvement or prior MI, significant LV dysfunction may require additional measures such as IABP support. When initial measures do not improve hemodynamics, inotropic

support of the right ventricle with dobutamine may be beneficial. Dopamine can be added to augment arterial perfusion pressure if indicated.

The Acute Pulmonary Edema, Hypotension, and Shock Algorithm

The Acute Pulmonary Edema, Hypotension, and Shock Algorithm (Figure 6) illustrates the management of patients who present with these complications of AMI. Based on clinical assessment and judgment, some of these recommendations will also be applicable to patients without MI or applicable during the early evaluation for ACS. The following sections explain management of these patients in greater detail.

Clinical Signs

Shock and pulmonary edema are medical emergencies. Signs of shock include inadequate tissue perfusion (diminished peripheral pulses, cool extremities, delayed capillary refill, decreased urine output, and lactic acidosis). With CHF, signs of systemic and pulmonary venous

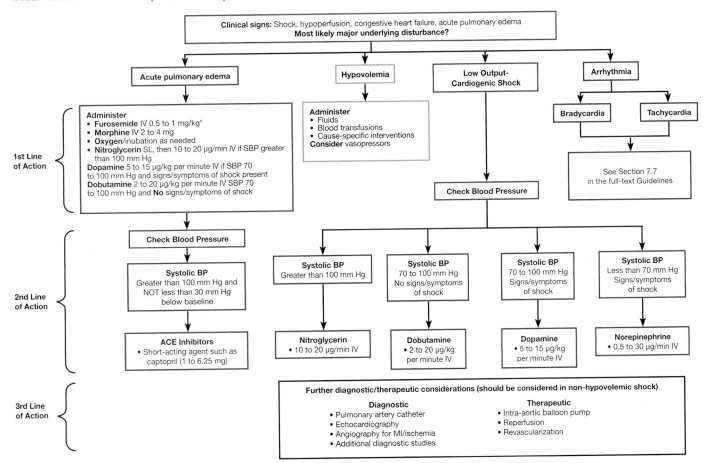

Figure 6. Emergency management of complicated STEMI. The emergency management of patients with cardiogenic shock or acute pulmonary edema, or both, is outlined. Give *furosemide <0.5 mg/kg for new onset acute pulmonary edema without hypovolemia; 1 mg/kg for acute or chronic volume overload, renal insufficiency. Nesiritide has not been studied adequately in patients with STEMI. Combinations of medications (eg, dobutamine and dopamine) may be used. Modified with permission from *Guidelines 2000 for Cardiopulmonary Resuscitation and Emergency Cardiovascular Care. Part 7: The Era of Reperfusion. Section 1: Acute Coronary Syndromes (Acute Myocardial Infarction).*[21]

congestion are present. Pulmonary edema produces tachypnea, labored respirations, rales, dyspnea, cyanosis, and hypoxemia. Frothy sputum may also be present. Providers should identify these conditions and begin treatment as soon as possible.

First-Line Actions

If signs of acute pulmonary edema are present, proceed with first-line actions if *low blood pressure and shock are absent*:

- Oxygen and intubation as needed
- Nitroglycerin SL or IV
- Furosemide IV 0.5 to 1 mg/kg
- Morphine IV 2 to 4 mg

If the patient's blood pressure is adequate, help the patient sit upright with the legs dependent. This position increases lung volume and vital capacity, diminishes the work of breathing, and decreases venous return to the heart. Administer morphine to dilate veins and arteries and to reduce cardiac preload and afterload.

Provide oxygen, establish IV access, and begin cardiac monitoring (ACLS providers treat "oxygen-IV-monitor" as a single word). Monitor oxyhemoglobin saturation with pulse oximetry, although results may be inaccurate and misleading if peripheral perfusion is poor. Oxyhemoglobin saturation does not provide information about hemoglobin concentration, oxygen content, ventilation, or acid-base status. Additional laboratory studies are ordered to evaluate any significant comorbidity or complicating factors, such as anemia, renal dysfunction, or electrolyte imbalance.

Oxygen and Possible Intubation

Deliver oxygen at high flow rates, starting at 5 or 6 L/min by mask. Nonrebreathing masks with reservoir bags can provide oxygen concentrations of 90% to near 100%. A bag-mask may be used to provide assisted ventilation if the patient's ventilation is inadequate. If the patient is breathing spontaneously, consider continuous positive airway pressure by mask (BiPAP).

Be prepared to intubate the patient who has significant respiratory distress or respiratory failure. A need for intubation is particularly likely in situations that indicate progressive or imminent respiratory failure despite initial measures:

- PaO_2 cannot be maintained above 60 mm Hg despite 100% oxygen.
- Signs of cerebral hypoxia (eg, lethargy or confusion) develop.
- PCO_2 increases progressively.
- Respiratory acidosis develops.

Always verify successful intubation using both clinical confirmation and a device.

Nitroglycerin

If SBP is adequate (usually >100 mm Hg) and the patient has no serious signs or symptoms of shock, then IV nitroglycerin is the drug of choice for acute pulmonary edema. Nitroglycerin reduces pulmonary congestion by dilating the venous capacitance vessels, reducing preload. It also dilates systemic arteries, decreasing systemic vascular resistance. This effect can reduce afterload and increase cardiac output.

Nitroglycerin may initially be administered by sublingual tablets, oral spray (isosorbide oral spray is an acceptable alternative), or the IV route. A standard 0.4 mg tablet can be given every 5 to 10 minutes provided SBP remains >90 to 100 mm Hg and the patient has no clinical signs of tissue hypoperfusion (shock).

FYI **Endotracheal Tube Confirmation in the Presence of Pulmonary Edema**	Pulmonary edema should not interfere with detection of exhaled CO_2 in the trachea, but • If copious respiratory secretions are present, an esophageal detector device may fail to reinflate despite correct placement of the tube in the trachea. This failure may lead to the inaccurate conclusion that the tube is in the esophagus when it is accurately placed in the trachea.

Foundation Facts **Use of Nitrates in Patients With Impaired Ventricular Function**	Nitroglycerin is contraindicated in hypotensive patients with signs of shock. • Typically these patients cannot tolerate vasodilatation because of impaired cardiac output. • They cannot compensate for the nitrate-induced tachycardia with increased stroke volume—one of the reasons why tachycardia is a contraindication to nitroglycerin. • Patients with RV infarction are preload dependent.

Nitrates are also contraindicated in patients who have used phosphodiesterase inhibitors (eg, sildenafil citrate) within the previous 24 hours. In these patients nitroglycerin may cause severe hypotension refractory to vasopressors. Use nitroglycerin with caution (if at all) if the patient has an inferior wall AMI with possible RV involvement.[27] Patients with RV dysfunction are very dependent on maintenance of RV filling pressures to maintain cardiac output and blood pressure.

Furosemide

Furosemide has long been a mainstay in the treatment of acute pulmonary edema. It has a biphasic action. First, within approximately 5 minutes it causes an immediate decrease in venous tone and an increase in venous capacitance. These changes lead to a fall in LV filling pressure (preload) that may improve clinical symptoms. Second, furosemide produces diuresis within 5 to 10 minutes of IV administration. The diuresis need not be marked to be effective. If the patient is not already taking furosemide, a typical dose is 0.5 to 1 mg/kg given as a slow IV bolus over 1 to 2 minutes. If the response to this dose is inadequate after about 20 minutes, another bolus of 2 mg/kg is administered. If the patient is already taking oral furosemide, the clinical rule of thumb is to administer an initial dose that is twice the daily oral dose. If no effect occurs within about 20 minutes, double the initial dose. You may need to use higher doses if the patient has significant fluid retention, refractory heart failure, or renal insufficiency.

Clinical trials have been conducted with nesiritide, a recombinant human brain natriuretic peptide, in patients hospitalized with decompensated CHF. Compared with placebo and "standard therapy," nesiritide was associated with improved hemodynamic function, decreased dyspnea and fatigue, and better global clinical status.[22]

Morphine Sulfate

Morphine sulfate remains a part of the therapy for acute pulmonary edema, although recent research questions its effectiveness, especially outside the hospital. Morphine dilates the capacitance vessels of the peripheral venous bed. This dilatation reduces venous return to the central circulation and diminishes ventricular preload. Morphine also reduces afterload by causing mild arterial vasodilatation. It also has a sedative effect. More effective vaso-

dilators are now available, so morphine is considered an acceptable adjunct rather than a drug of choice for acute pulmonary edema. In selected patients ACE inhibitors may also be a useful adjunct and are presently under clinical study and review.

Agents to Optimize Initial Blood Pressure

First-line actions also include the administration of agents to optimize blood pressure. Patients with acute pulmonary edema have excess adrenergic drive, and many have preexisting hypertension. These patients can present with high blood pressures or accelerated hypertension. Often treatment of the pulmonary edema itself will resolve high blood pressure. But initial therapy may include the use of IV nitroglycerin as an antihypertensive agent as well as a venodilator. Nitrates will reduce both preload and afterload to achieve this goal. In these patients the goal is to reduce blood pressure by no more than 30 mm Hg below the presentation blood pressure by titration of nitrates. IV nitroglycerin is initiated at 10 µg/kg and titrated to this target goal. As mentioned, patients may respond to initial therapy with resolution of their elevated blood pressure, decreasing or eliminating the need for IV nitrates. Use caution to avoid precipitating hypotension, because this may aggravate cardiac ischemia or precipitate organ ischemia in other vascular beds (eg, brain, kidneys, or gut).

Second-Line Actions

- Dopamine if SBP is 70 to 100 mm Hg with signs or symptoms of shock
- Dobutamine if SBP is 70 to 100 mm Hg with no signs or symptoms of shock
- ACE inhibitors if SBP is >100 mm Hg and not <30 mm Hg below baseline

Patients who respond to first-line actions for pulmonary edema may not require additional therapy unless otherwise indicated. If additional therapy is indicated, second-line actions are based on the patient's SBP and clinical response.

Patients Not in Shock With SBP >100 mm Hg

If SBP is >100 mm Hg and not less than 30 mm Hg below baseline, an ACE inhibitor is given to reduce afterload and attenuate LV remodeling in STEMI patients. Other agents

Foundation Facts **Furosemide Dosing for Acute Pulmonary Edema**	• Administer furosemide <0.5 mg/kg for new onset acute pulmonary edema without hypovolemia. • Give 1 mg/kg for acute or chronic volume overload. • Give 1 mg/kg to patients with underlying renal insufficiency.

can be used as indicated and tailored to the patient's clinical profile.

Nitrates can be continued with the precautions noted under first-line actions. Tachyphylaxis (tolerance) to nitrates occurs in about 24 hours, so other agents are considered once the patient is stable. Avoid long-acting and topical preparations in hemodynamically unstable or potentially unstable patients. Avoid use of nitroglycerin in patients who have taken phosphodiesterase inhibitors within the previous 24 to 48 hours, with hypotension (SBP <90 mm Hg), with extreme bradycardia (heart rate <50), or with tachycardia. Use with caution in patients with an inferior wall AMI with possible RV involvement. Nitroprusside is an alternative drug to treat hypertension.

IV nitroglycerin may be initiated at a rate of 10 µg/min through continuous infusion with nonabsorbing tubing. Increase by 5 to 10 µg every 3 to 5 minutes until a symptom or blood pressure response is noted. If no response is seen at 20 µg/min, incremental increases of 10 µg/min and later 20 µg/min can be used. As the symptoms and signs of acute pulmonary edema or cardiac ischemia begin to resolve, there is no need to continue upward titration of nitroglycerin simply to obtain a fall in blood pressure. When blood pressure reduction is a therapeutic goal, reduce the dosage when the blood pressure begins to fall. Frequently recommended limits for blood pressure reduction are 10% of baseline level in normotensive patients and 30% (or 30 mm Hg below baseline) in hypertensive patients.

Patients With SBP 70 to 100 mm Hg

If SBP is between 70 and 100 mm Hg and signs of shock *are* present, a dopamine infusion is recommended. If SBP is 70 to 100 mm Hg and the patient has *no signs of shock,* a dobutamine infusion is recommended as an inotropic agent to improve cardiac output or distribution of blood flow.

Third-Line Actions

Although called third-line actions, these diagnostic and therapeutic considerations or interventions may occur concurrently with first-line and second-line actions. For example, reperfusion in patients with pulmonary edema and STEMI is pursued without delay while treatment is initiated. An ECG is obtained within 10 minutes of presentation in patients with pulmonary edema to assess STEMI as a cause or complication. Any reversible or complicating conditions are identified and treated if possible. For example, mechanical complications of MI occur as the second leading cause of in-hospital mortality. Patients with acute mitral regurgitation due to rupture of a papillary muscle or chordae are surgical emergencies. The use of echocardiography in the ICU or ED on an emergent basis can identify these patients early. Patients at bed rest and

those with heart failure are at increased risk for pulmonary embolism. An ED and hospital plan for rapid activation of cardiology and ancillary personnel and for IABP should be in place. Hospitals without IABP, PCI, or cardiac surgery should also have an action plan to mobilize personnel and equipment for rapid transfer of STEMI patients to facilities with these capabilities.

References

1. Blalock A. *Principles of Surgical Care: Shock and Other Problems*. St Louis, Mo: Mosby; 1940.

2. GUSTO Investigators, Hasdai D, Holmes DR Jr, Califf RM, Thompson TD, Hochman JS, Pfisterer M, Topol EJ. Cardiogenic shock complicating acute myocardial infarction: predictors of death. GUSTO Investigators. Global Utilization of Streptokinase and Tissue-Plasminogen Activator for Occluded Coronary Arteries. *Am Heart J*. 1999;138:21-31.

3. Goldberg RJ, Samad NA, Yarzebski J, Gurwitz J, Bigelow C, Gore JM. Temporal trends in cardiogenic shock complicating acute myocardial infarction. *N Engl J Med*. 1999;340:1162-1168.

4. Goldberg RJ, Gore JM, Alpert JS, Osganian V, de Groot J, Bade J, Chen Z, Frid D, Dalen JE. Cardiogenic shock after acute myocardial infarction. Incidence and mortality from a community-wide perspective, 1975 to 1988. *N Engl J Med*. 1991;325:1117-1122.

5. Jacobs AK, French JK, Col J, Sleeper LA, Slater JN, Carnendran L, Boland J, Jiang X, LeJemtel T, Hochman JS. Cardiogenic shock with non-ST-segment elevation myocardial infarction: a report from the SHOCK trial registry. Should we emergently revascularize occluded coronaries for cardiogenic shock? *J Am Coll Cardiol*. 2000;36:1091-1096.

6. Holmes DR Jr, Berger PB, Hochman JS, Granger CB, Thompson TD, Califf RM, Vahanian A, Bates ER, Topol EJ. Cardiogenic shock in patients with acute ischemic syndromes with and without ST-segment elevation. *Circulation*. 1999;100:2067-2073.

7. Parrillo JE, Burch C, Shelhamer JH, Parker MM, Natanson C, Schuette W. A circulating myocardial depressant substance in humans with septic shock. Septic shock patients with a reduced ejection fraction have a circulating factor that depresses in vitro myocardial cell performance. *J Clin Invest*. 1985;76:1539-1553.

8. Chen ZM, Pan HC, Chen YP, Peto R, Collins R, Jiang LX, Xie JX, Liu LS. Early intravenous then oral metoprolol in 45,852 patients with acute myocardial infarction: randomised placebo-controlled trial. *Lancet*. 2005;366:1622-1632.

9. Hochman JS. Cardiogenic shock complicating acute myocardial infarction: expanding the paradigm. *Circulation*. 2003;107:2998-3002.

10. Hasdai D, Topol EJ, Califf RM, Berger PB, Holmes DR Jr. Cardiogenic shock complicating acute coronary syndromes. *Lancet*. 2000;356:749-756.

11. Menon V, Slater JN, White HD, Sleeper LA, Cocke T, Hochman JS. Acute myocardial infarction complicated by systemic hypoperfusion without hypotension: report of the SHOCK trial registry. *Am J Med*. 2000;108:374-380.

12. Antman EM, Braunwald E. Acute myocardial infarction. In: Braunwald E, Fauci A, Kasper D, et al, eds. *Harrison's Principles of Internal Medicine*. 15th ed. New York, NY: McGraw-Hill; 2001.

13. Berger PB, Holmes DR Jr, Stebbins AL, Bates ER, Califf RM, Topol EJ. Impact of an aggressive invasive catheterization and revascularization strategy on mortality in patients with cardiogenic shock in the Global Utilization of Streptokinase and Tissue Plasminogen Activator for Occluded Coronary Arteries (GUSTO-I) trial. An observational study. *Circulation.* 1997;96:122-127.

14. Tiefenbrunn AJ, Chandra NC, French WJ, Gore JM, Rogers WJ. Clinical experience with primary percutaneous transluminal coronary angioplasty compared with alteplase (recombinant tissue-type plasminogen activator) in patients with acute myocardial infarction: a report from the Second National Registry of Myocardial Infarction (NRMI-2). *J Am Coll Cardiol.* 1998;31:1240-1245.

15. Lee L, Erbel R, Brown TM, Laufer N, Meyer J, O'Neill WW. Multicenter registry of angioplasty therapy of cardiogenic shock: initial and long-term survival. *J Am Coll Cardiol.* 1991;17:599-603.

16. Ohman EM, Califf RM, Topol EJ, Stack RS, George BS. Intra-aortic balloon pumping: benefits after thrombolytic therapy. *Cardiol Board Rev.* 1991;8:41-56.

17. Grines CL. Aggressive intervention for myocardial infarction: angioplasty, stents, and intra-aortic balloon pumping. *Am J Cardiol.* 1996;78:29-34.

18. Hochman JS, Sleeper LA, Webb JG, Dzavik V, Buller CE, Aylward P, Col J, White HD. Early revascularization and long-term survival in cardiogenic shock complicating acute myocardial infarction. *JAMA.* 2006;295:2511-2515.

19. Antman EM, Anbe DT, Armstrong PW, Bates ER, Green LA, Hand M, Hochman JS, Krumholz HM, Kushner FG, Lamas GA, Mullany CJ, Ornato JP, Pearle DL, Sloan MA, Smith SC Jr, Alpert JS, Anderson JL, Faxon DP, Fuster V, Gibbons RJ, Gregoratos G, Halperin JL, Hiratzka LF, Hunt SA, Jacobs AK. ACC/AHA guidelines for the management of patients with ST-elevation myocardial infarction: a report of the American College of Cardiology/American Heart Association Task Force on Practice Guidelines (Committee to Revise the 1999 Guidelines for the Management of Patients With Acute Myocardial Infarction). *Circulation.* 2004;110:e82-e292.

20. Jacobs AK, Leopold JA, Bates E, Mendes LA, Sleeper LA, White H, Davidoff R, Boland J, Modur S, Forman R, Hochman JS. Cardiogenic shock caused by right ventricular infarction: a report from the SHOCK registry. *J Am Coll Cardiol.* 2003;41:1273-1279.

21. Guidelines 2000 for cardiopulmonary resuscitation and emergency cardiovascular care. Part 7: the era of reperfusion. Section 1: acute coronary syndromes (acute myocardial infarction). The American Heart Association in collaboration with the International Liaison Committee on Resuscitation. *Circulation.* 2000;102:I172-I203.

22. Colucci WS, Elkayam U, Horton DP, Abraham WT, Bourge RC, Johnson AD, Wagoner LE, Givertz MM, Liang CS, Neibaur M, Haught WH, LeJemtel TH. Intravenous nesiritide, a natriuretic peptide, in the treatment of decompensated congestive heart failure. Nesiritide Study Group. *N Engl J Med.* 2000;343:246-253.

Chapter (13)

Toxicology in Emergency Cardiovascular Care

This Chapter

- **Poisoning—A leading cause of cardiac arrest in persons younger than 40**
- **Emergency cardiovascular care for the poisoned patient—Are standard guidelines optimal?**
- **Common toxidromes and complications in patients with known and unknown poisonings**
- **When to consult with a medical toxicologist or regional poison center**

General Considerations

ACLS providers frequently encounter cardiopulmonary problems and imminent cardiac or pulmonary arrest situations due to poisoning, either intentional or accidental. Today exposure to chemical or biological agents is another threat that must be considered. Immediate identification of a specific poison is not always possible, yet patients require immediate

treatment. In these situations it is helpful to look for a *toxidrome*. A toxidrome is a set of signs and symptoms commonly caused by a particular toxin (eg, cocaine) or group of toxins (eg, calcium channel blockers). Identification of a toxidrome allows provision of symptom-based general therapy until the specific toxin is known.

To identify a toxidrome:

- First, have an index of suspicion for poisonings in appropriate clinical situations. A toxidrome is often suggested by the history and presenting findings.
- Look for a constellation of signs and symptoms usually observed after exposure to a toxic substance.
- Physiologically group abnormalities according to the following physical findings:
  — Vital signs.
  — Skin and mucous membranes.
  — Pupils.
  — Cardiovascular system.
  — Gastrointestinal and genitourinary systems.
  — Neurologic findings/mental status.

Use of standard ACLS protocols for all patients who are critically poisoned may not result in an optimal outcome. Care of patients with severe poisoning can be enhanced by consultation with a medical toxicologist or regional poison center. Alternative approaches that may be effective in severely poisoned patients include

Critical Concept Be Suspicious for Poisoning	Suspect poisoning in appropriate or suspicious clinical settings. Look for groups of symptoms and signs that may be markers of a toxin and toxidrome. If a toxidrome is identified, begin treatment immediately while attempting to identify the specific toxin. Keep in mind that multiple or mass exposure may occur with some toxins.

- Higher doses of medication than used in standard protocols
- Nonstandard drug therapies, including inamrinone, calcium chloride, glucagon, insulin, labetalol, phenylephrine, physostigmine, and sodium bicarbonate
- Use of specific antagonists or antidotes
- Extraordinary measures, such as prolonged CPR and possibly use of circulatory assist devices (eg, extracorporeal membrane oxygenation)

Major Toxidromes

This section reviews the major toxidromes (Table 1). If you suspect a toxidrome, initiate the following general treatment measures:

- Identify need for decontamination and personal protective measures.
- Begin BLS Primary and ACLS Secondary ABCD Surveys and support.
- During the differential diagnosis, attempt to identify a possible toxidrome and a specific antidote or therapy.
- Gastrointestinal decontamination generally is not effective more than 1 hour after ingestion. Follow local protocols for use of this therapy.

Prehospital providers must ensure scene safety before approaching patients, particularly if multiple patients or an unknown toxin is involved or if airborne or topical contamination is thought to be present. The BLS Primary and ACLS Secondary ABCD Surveys provide an excellent initial approach to any life-threatening problem. Be

Table 1. Common Toxidromes

Sympathomimetic
Cholinergic
Anticholinergic
Opiates
Cocaine
Cardiac toxins
Salicylates

prepared to support airway, oxygenation, ventilation, and circulation as needed. Establishment of vascular access and vasoactive and rhythm support may be critical. Attempt to determine the presence of a common toxidrome or history of ingestion or exposure that would explain the clinical findings or failure to respond to initial therapy. If a toxidrome is identified or suspected during consideration of the differential diagnosis, therapy can be modified to include a specific treatment or antidote.

Gastrointestinal decontamination is controversial and is generally reserved for the emergency department. Activated charcoal and gastric lavage are not likely to be effective beyond 1 hour after ingestion. Whole bowel irrigation may be effective, but more research is needed. At this time there is no evidence that gastrointestinal decontamination changes outcome. Follow local protocols, consulting the poison control center for recommendations.

Symptom-Based Therapy for Toxidromes

Example: Airway and Respiratory Management in Opiate Poisoning

Poisoned patients may deteriorate rapidly. Frequent assessment of the airway, breathing, and circulation are required. In patients who are obtunded or comatose, perform rapid sequence intubation *before* gastric lavage if lavage is indicated. Lethal opiate poisoning eliminates airway protective reflexes and directly suppresses respiratory drive. Opiate poisoning provides the "default" model for a general approach to drug-induced airway and respiratory compromise. Although this chapter focuses on the effects of poisonings and drug overdoses on the cardiovascular system, respiratory failure is the most common cause of death in cases of overdose and poisoning.

Opiate Reversal

Opiate poisoning commonly causes respiratory depression followed by respiratory insufficiency and arrest. Heroin overdose may also cause respiratory depression, and it frequently causes noncardiogenic pulmonary edema. The respiratory effects of opiates are rapidly reversed by the opiate antagonist naloxone.

Critical Concept

ACLS Toxidrome Management Principles

- Identify need for decontamination.
- Begin BLS Primary and ACLS Secondary ABCD Surveys and support.
- During the differential diagnosis, attempt to identify a possible toxidrome and a specific antidote or therapy.
- Gastrointestinal decontamination is generally not effective more than 1 hour after ingestion. Follow local protocols for use of this therapy.

Foundation Facts **Opiate Toxidrome**	Major Findings: • Central nervous system depression • Respiratory depression • Miosis (small pupils) Examples: • Heroin • Morphine • Fentanyl derivatives ("China white") Possible Specific Therapy: • Naloxone • Supportive care

Before or After Endotracheal Intubation?

In a patient with a clinically significant opiate overdose, healthcare providers have long taken the practical approach of performing endotracheal intubation before giving naloxone. This sequence allowed the narcotizing effects of the opiate to serve as an intubation adjunct. In addition, intubation and ventilation allowed correction of hypercarbia before administration of naloxone. There is some data from animals and limited clinical experience[1,2] that if ventilation normalizes the arterial carbon dioxide tension *before* naloxone administration, the potential rise in epinephrine concentration associated with naloxone administration and its attendant potentially toxic effects are blunted.

But in the hospital setting the administration of naloxone for acute opiate exposure without prior ventilation has been successful in otherwise healthy adults with no chronic exposure and a normal cardiovascular system if the airway was maintained and the patient received high-flow oxygen.[3] The practice of *routine intubation* before naloxone administration for treatment of severe opiate overdose is no longer recommended.

Specific ACLS recommendations for naloxone administration, endotracheal intubation, and support of ventilation for opiate toxicity include the following:

- When patients with suspected opiate overdose have *respiratory insufficiency plus a detectable pulse,* attempt opiate reversal *before* endotracheal intubation.
- Support ventilation with a bag and mask while preparing to administer naloxone. Existing evidence does not justify withholding naloxone until endotracheal intubation is performed. In the United States opiates are associated with more drug-induced cardiopulmonary arrests than any other drug. But the incidence of severe complications after opiate reversal is less than 2%.
- Naloxone is the preferred reversal agent for opiate toxicity even though it has a shorter duration of effect (45 to 70 minutes) than heroin (4 to 5 hours).

Critical Concept **Benzodiazepine Reversal and Flumazenil**	• Reversal of benzodiazepine intoxication with flumazenil is associated with significant toxicity in patients with benzodiazepine dependence or coingestion of proconvulsant medications such as tricyclic antidepressants. • Flumazenil is not recommended for routine use or inclusion in a "coma cocktail." It may be useful for reversal of respiratory depression when benzodiazepines have been used for procedural sedation.

Foundation Facts **Opiate Reversal: General Recommendations**	• As a general practice providers should try to support ventilation with a bag mask before administering naloxone. • Naloxone may be administered before intubation because significant complications are uncommon. In addition, reversal of opiate effects may eliminate the need for intubation. • Use naloxone with caution in patients suspected of opiate dependency to avoid precipitating acute withdrawal symptoms.

Critical Concept

Evaluation and Management After Naloxone Administration

- It is recommended that opiate-intoxicated patients aroused with naloxone be transported to the hospital. Some EMS systems, especially in Europe, allow selected patients aroused with naloxone to refuse transport to the hospital.

  — Although the incidence of severe complications after opiate reversal is less than 2%, the duration of action of naloxone is shorter than the duration of action of most opiates. In very severe poisonings failure to continue care has occasionally led to serious consequences, such as severe renarcotization or delayed pulmonary edema.[4,5]

  — For this reason it is recommended that after arousal, all patients be observed beyond the duration of the naloxone effect to ensure their safety.

- Some experts note the theoretical advantages of the intramuscular (IM) and subcutaneous (SC) routes of naloxone administration over the intravenous (IV) route (ease of administration, reduced risk of needle puncture for healthcare personnel, and less severe withdrawal for opiate addicts). But others contend that all such patients should have IV access when possible because of the severity of their illness.

End Points for Opiate Reversal

- The end point objectives for opiate reversal are adequate airway reflexes and ventilation, not complete arousal.
- Acute, abrupt opiate withdrawal increases the likelihood of severe complications, such as pulmonary edema, ventricular arrhythmias, and severe agitation and hostility.

Naloxone: Dose and Route

- In emergencies a slow incremental rate of administration is less satisfactory. For these cases the recommended initial dose of naloxone is 0.4 to 0.8 mg IV or 0.8 mg IM or SC.
- The IM and SC routes have theoretical advantages over the IV route: ease of administration, reduced risk of needle puncture for healthcare providers, and less severe withdrawal for opiate addicts.
- In communities where abuse of naloxone-resistant opiates is prevalent, larger initial doses of naloxone may be appropriate.
- When opiate overdose is strongly suspected or in locations where "China white" (ie, fentanyl and its derivatives) abuse is prevalent, titration to total naloxone doses of 6 to 10 mg over a short period of time may be necessary.

Management of Cardiovascular Compromise Caused by Drugs or Toxins

Table 2 summarizes the altered vital signs that may be observed with drug-induced cardiovascular emergencies and lists both indicated and contraindicated therapies.

Hemodynamically Significant Bradycardia

Hemodynamically significant bradycardia from poisoning or drug overdose may be refractory to standard ACLS protocols because some toxins bind receptors or produce direct cellular toxicity. In these cases specific antidote therapy may be needed.

Treatment

Atropine

Atropine is neither helpful nor harmful in the treatment of most drug-induced hemodynamically significant bradycardias. But administration of atropine may be lifesaving in poisoning from cholinesterase inhibitors such as organophosphate, carbamate, or nerve agents. The recommended starting adult dose for insecticide poisoning from cholinesterase inhibitors is 2 to 4 mg. In these cases doses well in excess of accepted maximums may be required. Providers should notify the pharmacy to obtain a large amount (eg, 20 to 40 mg or higher) of atropine for use if needed.

Pacing

Transcutaneous cardiac pacing is often effective in cases of mild to moderate drug-induced bradycardia. Prophylactic transvenous pacing is not recommended because the tip of the transvenous catheter may trigger ventricular arrhythmias when the myocardium is irritable (eg, as in digoxin toxicity). However, transvenous pacing is needed if transcutaneous pacing fails or is poorly tolerated or if electrical capture is difficult to maintain. In very severe poisonings failure to capture may occur despite proper pacer electrode location and the highest pacemaker voltage output settings.

Table 2. Drug-Induced Cardiovascular Emergencies or Altered Vital Signs*: Therapies to Consider[†] and Contraindicated Interventions

Drug-Induced Cardiovascular Emergency or Altered Vital Signs*	Therapies to Consider[†]	Contraindicated Interventions (or Use With Caution)
Bradycardia	• Pacemaker (transcutaneous or transvenous) • Toxic drug—*calcium channel blocker*: epinephrine, calcium salt? glucose/insulin? glucagon? NS (if hypotensive) • Toxic drug—*β-blocker*: NS, epinephrine, calcium salt? glucose/insulin? glucagon?	• Atropine (seldom helpful except for cholinesterase inhibitor poisonings) • Isoproterenol if hypotensive • Prophylactic transvenous pacing
Tachycardia	• Toxic drug—*sympathomimetics*: benzodiazepines, lidocaine, sodium bicarbonate, nitroglycerin, nitroprusside, labetalol • Toxic drug—*tricyclic antidepressants*: sodium bicarbonate, hyperventilation, NS, magnesium sulfate, lidocaine • Toxic drug—*anticholinergics*: physostigmine	• β-Blockers (not generally useful in drug-induced tachycardia) • Do not use propranolol for cocaine intoxication • Cardioversion (rarely indicated) • Adenosine (rarely indicated) • Calcium channel blockers (rarely indicated) • Physostigmine for TCA overdose
Impaired conduction/ ventricular arrhythmias	• Sodium bicarbonate • Lidocaine	• If TCA overdose: amiodarone or type I$_{VW}$ antiarrhythmics (eg, procainamide)
Hypertensive emergencies	• Toxic drug—*sympathomimetics*: benzodiazepines, lidocaine, sodium bicarbonate, nitroglycerin, nitroprusside, phentolamine	• β-Blockers
Acute coronary syndrome	• Benzodiazepines • Lidocaine • Sodium bicarbonate • Nitroglycerin • Aspirin, heparin • Base reperfusion strategy on cardiac catheterization data	• β-Blockers
Shock	• Toxic drug—*calcium channel blocker*: NS, epinephrine, norepinephrine, dopamine, calcium salt? glucose/insulin? glucagon? • Toxic drug—*β-blocker*: NS, epinephrine, norepinephrine, dopamine, calcium salt? glucose/insulin? glucagon? • If refractory to *maximal* medical therapy: consider circulatory assist devices	• Isoproterenol • Avoid calcium salts if digoxin toxicity is suspected
Acute cholinergic syndrome	• Atropine • Pralidoxime/obidoxime	• Succinylcholine
Acute anticholinergic syndrome	• Benzodiazepine • Physostigmine (not for TCA overdose)	• Antipsychotics • Other anticholinergic agents

(continued)

Table 2. *Continued*

Drug-Induced Cardiovascular Emergency or Altered Vital Signs*	Therapies to Consider†	Contraindicated Interventions (or Use With Caution)
Opioid poisoning	• Assisted ventilation • Naloxone • Endotracheal intubation	• Do not use naloxone for meperidine-induced seizures

*Unless stated otherwise, listed alterations of vital signs (bradycardia, tachycardia, tachypnea) are "hemodynamically significant."
†Therapies to consider should be based on specific indications. Therapies followed by "?" are *Class Indeterminate*.
NS indicates normal saline; TCA, tricyclic antidepressant; and VW, Vaughan Williams.

Vasopressors

In drug-induced bradycardia resistant to atropine and pacing, vasopressors with β-adrenergic agonist activity are indicated. See "Shock" (later in this chapter) for more information about the use of vasopressors in the management of drug-induced cardiovascular dysfunction.

Isoproterenol

Isoproterenol is contraindicated in most drug-induced bradycardias, including acetylcholinesterase-induced bradycardias, because it may induce or aggravate hypotension and ventricular arrhythmias. In massive β-blocker poisoning, however, very-high-dose isoproterenol therapy has been reported to be effective. It may be useful at high doses in refractory bradycardia induced by β-antagonist receptor blockade.

Digoxin-Specific Fab Antibody Fragments

This therapy is extremely effective for life-threatening ventricular arrhythmias and atrioventricular (AV) block due to digoxin and cardiac glycoside poisoning. AV block and ventricular arrhythmias associated with digoxin or digitalis glycoside poisoning may be effectively treated with digoxin-specific antibody fragment therapy (level of evidence 5).[6] Antibody-specific therapy may also be effective in poisonings caused by plants and Chinese herbal medications containing digitalis glycosides.[7,8]

Hemodynamically Significant Tachycardia

Drug-induced hemodynamically significant tachycardia may cause myocardial ischemia, myocardial infarction, or ventricular arrhythmias and may lead to high-output heart failure and shock. Adenosine and synchronized cardioversion are unlikely to be of benefit in this context given the ongoing presence of a toxin, although some drug-induced tachyarrhythmias may be successfully treated with adenosine.[9] In patients with borderline hypotension, diltiazem and verapamil are contraindicated because they may further lower blood pressure.

Treatment

Benzodiazepines

Benzodiazepines such as diazepam or lorazepam are generally safe and effective for the treatment of symptomatic drug-induced tachycardia resulting from sympathomimetic agents. Benzodiazepines are particularly helpful in the treatment of cocaine toxicity because they appear to attenuate the toxic myocardial and central nervous system (CNS) effects of cocaine.[10,11] When large quantities of benzodiazepines are used to treat poisoning or overdose, providers must closely monitor the patient's level of consciousness, ventilatory effort, and respiratory function because the sedative effects of benzodiazepines may produce respiratory depression and loss of protective airway reflexes.

Physostigmine

Physostigmine is a specific antidote that may be preferable for drug-induced hemodynamically significant tachycardia and central anticholinergic syndrome caused by pure anticholinergic poisoning.[12] Physostigmine must be used with caution because it can produce symptoms of cholinergic crisis, such as copious tracheobronchial

Foundation Facts Treatment of Drug-Induced Tachycardia	Drug-induced tachycardia may induce myocardial ischemia, myocardial infarction, or ventricular arrhythmias and may lead to high-output heart failure and shock. • Avoid the more common therapies for supraventricular tachycardia, such as adenosine and synchronized cardioversion; drug-induced supraventricular tachycardia is commonly recurrent or refractory because of the ongoing presence of the toxin. • Avoid diltiazem and verapamil in poisoned patients with borderline hypotension; these drugs may precipitate more severe shock.

Critical Concept **Emergency Treatment for Acute Decompensation**	Boluses of sodium bicarbonate are used without prior determination of serum pH for acute decompensation if the QRS duration is >100 milliseconds or if hypotension develops.

secretions (frequent suctioning will be required), seizures, bradycardia, and even asystole if given in excessive doses or if given too rapidly. Often patients with anticholinergic intoxication can be managed with benzodiazepines alone, but at least 1 clinical study suggests that physostigmine used appropriately may offer superior results.[12] Physostigmine should not be administered for anticholinergic symptoms associated with tricyclic antidepressant (TCA) overdose. Consultation with a medical toxicologist or regional poison center is recommended.

Propranolol

A nonselective β-blocker such as propranolol may be effective in drug-induced tachycardia due to some poisonings, but β-blockers should not be used in cocaine intoxication or amphetamine or ephedrine poisoning.

Drug-Induced Impaired Conduction

Poisonings with sodium channel antagonists (membrane-stabilizing agents such as flecainide and procainamide) and tricyclic antidepressants can result in prolonged ventricular conduction (increased QRS interval). Prolonged QRS and QT intervals predispose the heart to ventricular and other wide-complex tachycardias.

Treatment

Hypertonic Saline and Systemic Alkalinization

Hypertonic saline and systemic alkalinization may prevent or terminate ventricular tachycardia (VT) secondary to poisoning from sodium channel blocking agents (eg,

procainamide, flecainide) and tricyclic antidepressants.[13-15] *Hypertonic sodium bicarbonate* provides both hypertonic saline and systemic alkalinization. This therapy appears to provide benefit in several types of sodium channel blocker poisoning, such as TCA overdose and cocaine intoxication.

There is insufficient evidence to recommend for or against the use of sodium bicarbonate in adults with calcium channel blocker overdose. Calcium channel antagonist and β-adrenergic antagonist overdose may lead to seriously impaired conduction. These patients may require chronotropic adrenergic agents such as epinephrine, high-dose glucagon (although data to support this is inadequate and primarily limited to animal studies),[16] or possibly pacing.[17]

Ventricular Tachycardia/Fibrillation

Drug-induced VT and ventricular fibrillation (VF) may be difficult to distinguish from drug-induced wide-complex conduction impairments. When a patient develops sudden conversion to a wide-complex rhythm with hypotension, drug-induced VT is likely and cardioversion is indicated.

Treatment

Cardioversion or Defibrillation

Treatment of patients with drug-induced VT is determined by the presence or absence of hemodynamic stability. Perform immediate shock for VF or VT without pulses. Perform electrical cardioversion for hemodynamically unstable VT with pulses according to ACLS algorithms.

FYI **Treatment Goals for Systemic Alkalinization for Arrhythmias and Hypotension**	In severe poisonings the goal of alkalinization therapy is an arterial pH of 7.45 to 7.55. • Respiratory alkalosis can be induced as a temporizing measure. • Use repeated boluses of 1 to 2 mEq/kg of sodium bicarbonate to reach target pH. • Then maintain alkalinization by infusion of an alkaline solution consisting of 3 ampules of sodium bicarbonate (150 mEq) plus 30 mEq KCl mixed in 850 mL of D_5W.

Critical Concept **Drug-Induced Ventricular Tachycardia**	Suspect the development of a drug-induced VT whenever a poisoned patient demonstrates a sudden conversion to a wide-complex rhythm with hypotension. If the patient is unstable and polymorphic VT is present, use high-energy unsynchronized shocks (defibrillation doses).

In sympathomimetic poisonings with refractory VF, the risk-beneift ratio of epinephrine in management is unknown. If epinephrine is used, increase the interval between doses and use only standard dose amounts (1 mg IV). Avoid high-dose epinephrine.

Antiarrhythmics

Antiarrhythmics are indicated for most cases of hemodynamically stable drug-induced VT, although only a few published reports can guide therapy. Lidocaine is the initial antiarrhythmic of choice for drug-induced monomorphic VT. Types I_A and I_C and other antiarrhythmics that block the fast sodium channel (eg, sotalol) are contraindicated in cases of poisoning with tricyclic antidepressants or other fast sodium channel blockers because of the risk of synergistic toxicity. The efficacy and safety of phenytoin for TCA poisoning has been questioned and is no longer recommended.[18,19] Magnesium has beneficial effects in certain cases of drug-induced VT, but it may also aggravate drug-induced hypotension.[20,21]

Lidocaine

For most types of drug-induced monomorphic VT or VF, and for VT/VF associated with cocaine-induced myocardial ischemia, lidocaine is the antiarrhythmic of choice. This consensus is based on limited published studies but extensive clinical experience.[22] When VF/VT develops immediately after cocaine use, most experts favor early use of sodium bicarbonate.

Propranolol

In sympathomimetic poisonings (especially with cocaine), propranolol is contraindicated. This guideline is based on limited human studies in the cardiac catheterization suite and on animal survival studies.

Procainamide

Procainamide is contraindicated in poisonings from tricyclic antidepressants and other drugs with similar antiarrhythmic (Vaughan Williams type Ia_{vw}) properties.

Phenytoin

Phenytoin was previously recommended for VT induced by TCA overdose. But subsequent studies have questioned the efficacy and safety of this agent.[18,19]

Magnesium

Magnesium has demonstrated beneficial effects for drug-induced VT. But magnesium may aggravate drug-induced hypotension.[20,21]

Amiodarone

A handful of cases of refractory drug-induced VT or VF have been reported to respond to amiodarone. Because data is limited and amiodarone may worsen drug-induced hypotension and may have proarrhythmic effects, it should be used with caution if at all.

Torsades de Pointes

Torsades de pointes can occur with either therapeutic or toxic exposure to many drugs. Contributing factors for torsades de pointes include hypoxemia, hypokalemia, and hypomagnesemia. The safety and efficacy of many of these recommended therapies for drug-induced polymorphic VT have not been established by high levels of research, and most therapies are Class Indeterminate. However, administration of magnesium is recommended for patients with torsades de pointes even when the serum magnesium concentration is normal. A reasonable strategy for the management of torsades de pointes due to drug exposure is:

- Correct hypoxia, hypokalemia, and hypomagnesemia if present.
- Administer magnesium 1 to 2 g diluted in 10 mL D_5W IV push, even when the serum magnesium concentration is normal.
- Consider lidocaine. But keep in mind that the effectiveness of lidocaine in the treatment of torsades de pointes has not been demonstrated.
- Consider electrical overdrive pacing at rates of 100 to 120 beats.
- Consider pharmacologic overdrive pacing with isoproterenol at 2 to 10 µg/kg per minute; titrate to increase heart rate until VT is suppressed.[23]

- Drug-induced hypertensive emergencies are frequently short lived. Therapy is often not indicated because the hypertension rapidly resolves and may be followed by hypotension.
- Hypertensive emergencies frequently develop in patients with cocaine toxicity.

Propranolol (a nonselective β-blocker) is contraindicated for drug-induced hypertension. It may block only β receptors, leaving unopposed α-adrenergic stimulation and worsening hypertension.

- Some toxicologists recommend potassium supplementation even when the serum potassium concentration is normal.

Hypertensive Emergencies

Drug-induced hypertensive emergencies are frequently short lived. Therapy is often not indicated because the hypertension rapidly resolves and may be followed by hypotension. When treatment is indicated, benzodiazepines are the drug class of choice because they decrease the effects of endogenous catecholamine release. Hypertensive emergencies frequently develop in patients with cocaine toxicity.

Treatment

Antihypertensive therapy should be initiated when hypertension is severe or coexisting conditions require lowering of blood pressure. If the high blood pressure is refractory to adequate treatment with benzodiazepines, begin treatment with antihypertensive agents. Short-acting antihypertensive agents should be used because of the short-lived nature of many hypertensive episodes and the possible occurrence of hypotension after resolution. Aggressive control of blood pressure may not be warranted.

Benzodiazepines

Most toxicology experts consider benzodiazepines the first-line therapy for hypertension in cases of sympathomimetic overdose (eg, cocaine intoxication).

Nitroprusside

In drug-induced hypertensive emergencies refractory to benzodiazepines, use a short-acting antihypertensive such as nitroprusside as the second line of therapy.

Combined α-/β-Blockade

A combination of α- and β-blockade can be achieved using phentolamine and a nonselective α-antagonist, such as labetalol. But most experts now recommend against the use of *any* β-blocker if the hypertensive emergency is suspected to be caused by a sympathomimetic such as cocaine.

Shock

Drug-induced shock may produce a decrease in intravascular volume, a decrease in systemic vascular resistance (SVR), diminished myocardial contractility, or a combination of these factors. In addition, drugs can disable normal compensatory mechanisms. These combined aspects of cardiovascular dysfunction render drug-induced shock refractory to many standard therapies.

Drug-Induced Hypovolemic Shock With Normal Systemic Vascular Resistance

Overdose of some drugs or chemicals (eg, zinc salts) can cause excessive fluid loss through the gastrointestinal tract, resulting in pure hypovolemia. But drug-induced shock typically includes cardiovascular dysfunction with decreased myocardial contractility and low SVR, necessitating a combination of volume therapy and myocardial support.

Although an initial clinical impression may identify a likely cause of hypotension, many drugs cause multiple problems superimposed upon various patient comorbidities. The following sections describe a general approach to the patient with drug-induced shock.

Fluid Challenge

Initial treatment must include a fluid challenge (250 to 500 mL normal saline) to correct hypovolemia and optimize cardiac preload. If the offending agent is cardiotoxic, it will reduce the patient's ability to tolerate excess intravascular volume, and volume therapy may lead to iatrogenic congestive heart failure with pulmonary edema. Be prepared to support oxygenation and ventilation.

Drug-induced shock results from 1 of 3 mechanisms or from a combination of these factors:

- The drug induces a *decrease in intravascular volume.*
- The drug induces a *fall in systemic vascular resistance.*
- The drug induces *diminished myocardial contractility.*

Critical Concept **Drug-Induced Distributive Shock**	Distributive shock is associated with normal or even high cardiac output and low SVR. Treatment with α-adrenergic drugs such as norepinephrine or phenylephrine may be needed.

- Avoid dobutamine and isoproterenol, which may worsen hypotension by further decreasing SVR.

Vasopressors (Dopamine)

If shock persists after an adequate fluid challenge, start a vasopressor. Evidence supports dopamine as an effective vasopressor in mild to moderate poisonings.[24,25] But most patients with drug-induced shock have decreased myocardial contractility and decreased SVR, so more potent vasoconstrictors may be needed.

Higher-Dose Vasopressors

Other vasopressors in higher doses may be required if dopamine is not effective. Higher-dose vasopressors are indicated when drug-induced shock is unresponsive to volume loading and conventional doses of dopamine. If possible establish central hemodynamic monitoring with a pulmonary artery or central venous catheter, but do not delay treatment of hypotension. Optimize cardiac preload quickly; then use calculated cardiac output and SVR to guide selection and titration of a vasopressor and inotropic agent.

Drug-Induced Distributive Shock (Normal Volume With Decreased Systemic Vascular Resistance)

Distributive shock is associated with normal or even high cardiac output and low SVR. Treatment with α-adrenergic drugs such as norepinephrine or phenylephrine may be needed. Case reports suggest that vasopressin may also be useful.[26] More powerful vasoconstrictors such as endothelin are not yet available in the United States and have not been well studied. Watch for the development of ventricular arrhythmias with the use of these agents.

Norepinephrine or Phenylephrine

With normal volume plus decreased SVR (distributive shock), use more potent vasoconstrictive agents with greater α-adrenergic effect (norepinephrine or phenylephrine). Increase the dose of the α-adrenergic vasopressor until the shock is adequately treated or adverse effects (eg, ventricular arrhythmias) begin to appear. Some poisoned patients require doses of vasopressors far above conventional doses, so-called "high-dose vasopressor therapy." Consider use of powerful vasoconstrictors such as *vasopressin* or *endothelin* in severely poisoned patients if other adrenergic agents produce ventricular arrhythmias before the shock is adequately treated. Note that little formal evidence supports this recommendation.

Drug-Induced Cardiogenic Shock (Low Cardiac Output, Low Systemic Vascular Resistance)

Drug-induced cardiogenic shock can be associated with low cardiac output and low SVR. Cardiac ischemia may also be present in these patients. In addition to volume titration and use of sympathomimetic drugs such as dobutamine, inotropic support may be provided by agents such as inamrinone, calcium, glucagon, insulin, or even isoproterenol depending on the toxic agent(s) identified.[27,28] Concurrent vasopressor therapy is often required.[29]

Inotropic and Vasopressor Agents

Agents used successfully in some studies include *inamrinone* and *dobutamine,* as well as *calcium, glucose,* and *insulin.*[30-32] In some patients more than one agent is necessary. Although these agents can increase contractility and cardiac output, they may also further decrease SVR. Often a concomitant vasopressor such as *norepinephrine* is required.[29]

Drug-Induced Cardiac Arrest

Cardiac arrest associated with drugs or poisonings may be associated with any of the arrest rhythms: asystole, pulseless electrical activity, or VF/pulseless VT.

Cardioversion/Defibrillation

Electric defibrillation is appropriate for pulseless patients with drug-induced VT or VF and for unstable patients with polymorphic VT. In cases of sympathomimetic poisoning with refractory VF, increase the interval between doses of epinephrine and use only standard dosing. Propranolol is contraindicated in cocaine overdose. It was thought to be contraindicated in sympathomimetic poisoning, but some case reports suggest that it may be useful in the treatment of ephedrine and pseudoephedrine overdose.[33]

Prolonged CPR and Resuscitation

More prolonged CPR and resuscitation may be warranted in patients with poisoning or overdose, especially those with calcium channel blocker poisoning.[34] In cases of severe poisoning, recovery with good neurologic outcomes has been reported in patients who received prolonged CPR (eg, 3 to 5 hours).[27,28] Cardiopulmonary bypass (extracorporeal membrane oxygenation) has been used successfully in resuscitation of patients with severe poisoning.[35]

Intra-aortic Balloon Pumps and Cardiopulmonary Bypass

These circulatory assist devices have been used successfully in critical poisonings refractory to maximal medical care. These techniques, however, are expensive and manpower intensive and have significant associated morbidity. To be effective these devices must be employed early in the resuscitative effort, before the irreversible effects of severe shock or cardiac arrest develop. If intra-aortic balloon pump support is planned, the patient must have an intrinsic cardiac rhythm because balloon inflation is synchronized with the electrocardiogram (ECG) to provide diastolic augmentation. Emergency cardiopulmonary bypass does not require an intrinsic rhythm, and recent technologic advancements have made rapid application possible through peripheral vessels.

Brain Death and Organ Donation Criteria

Brain death criteria based on an electroencephalogram and neurologic examination only are invalid during acute toxic encephalopathy. These brain death criteria apply only when drug levels are no longer toxic. In the presence of toxic drug levels, the only valid confirmatory test for brain death is absent cerebral blood flow.

Organ transplantation after a fatal poisoning from agents capable of causing severe end-organ damage, such as carbon monoxide, cocaine, and iron, is controversial. When organ function is carefully evaluated, successful transplantation of some organs from patients of fatal poisoning with *acetaminophen, cyanide, methanol,* and *carbon monoxide* is possible.[36] However, transplantation of known *target* organs following a fatal poisoning is unlikely to succeed. These target organs include the heart in carbon monoxide poisoning, the heart and liver in cocaine and iron poisonings, and the liver and kidneys in acetaminophen poisonings.

Acute Coronary Syndromes

In adults the most frequent cause of cocaine-induced hospitalization is an acute coronary syndrome (ACS) producing chest pain and a variety of cardiac rhythm disturbances. ACS results from ischemia caused by the combined effects of cocaine: stimulation of β-adrenergic myocardial receptors increases myocardial oxygen demand, and the α-adrenergic and 5-HT agonist actions of cocaine cause coronary artery constriction.

Treatment

Treatment is directed at the direct effects of cocaine and their secondary complications, such as ischemia, coronary vasospasm, and arrhythmias. In cases of prolonged coronary vasospasm with or without underlying coronary artery disease, acute coronary thrombosis may develop in situ in affected arteries (see below).

Benzodiazepines and Nitroglycerin

These agents are the first-line agents for treatment of cocaine-induced ACS.[37] Nitroglycerin has been shown to reverse cocaine-induced vasoconstriction when studied in the cardiac catheterization suite.[38]

Phentolamine

Phentolamine, a potent pure α-blocker, has a nitroglycerin-like ability to reverse cocaine-induced vasoconstriction.[39] Consider phentolamine as a second-line therapy.

Precautions

Though *labetalol* has been reported to be effective in case reports, use of this drug is controversial because it is a nonselective β-blocker.[40,41] Labetalol does not reverse coronary vasoconstriction.[42] *Propranolol* is contraindicated because it has been shown to worsen cocaine-induced vasoconstriction in patients studied in the cardiac catheterization suite.[43] *Esmolol,* despite being a selective β-blocker (β_1 but not β_2), can aggravate hypertension and induce hypotension.[44] Most toxicology experts consider not only propranolol but also esmolol, metoprolol, and labetalol to be contraindicated in the management of cocaine-induced ACS.[45]

Fibrinolytics

Acute coronary syndromes can result from cocaine use.[46] The management of ST-elevation myocardial infarction (STEMI) occurring as a result of cocaine use can be challenging. Although the initial mechanism reducing coronary flow involves spasm, thrombus evolves in the infarct-related coronary artery due to stasis. Although fibrinolytic therapy has been used in small numbers of reported patients, fibrinolytics are contraindicated if uncontrolled, severe drug-induced hypertension is present. It is important to be aware that patients presenting with ACS and STEMI may not initially acknowledge cocaine use. When percutaneous coronary intervention (PCI) is not available, fibrinolytic therapy may be appropriate if no contraindications are present and the risk-benefit ratio is favorable. Hollander et al[47] retrospectively evaluated the complications and reperfusion success of fibrinolytic therapy for cocaine-associated myocardial infarction, comparing patients who received such therapy (n = 25) with those who met electrocardiographic TIMI criteria but did not receive fibrinolytic therapy (n = 41). There were no major complications or deaths in patients who received fibrinolytic therapy (95% confidence interval, 0% to 12%). Minor complications occurred in only 2 patients. The presence or absence of clinical criteria for reperfusion was noted in the charts of 21 patients who received thrombolytic therapy: data suggested that reperfusion occurred in 67%. The investigators concluded that fibrinolytic therapy for cocaine-associated myocardial infarction appears to be safe, but whether it is an important therapeutic intervention for patients with cocaine-associated myocardial infarction

Table 3. Potentially Cardiotoxic Drugs: Cardiopulmonary Signs* of Toxicity and Therapy to Consider†

Potentially Toxic Drugs: by Type of Agent	Cardiopulmonary Signs* of Toxicity	Therapy to Consider†
Stimulants (sympathomimetics) • Amphetamines • Methamphetamines • Cocaine • Phencyclidine (PCP) • Ephedrine	• Tachycardia • Supraventricular arrhythmias • Ventricular arrhythmias • Impaired conduction • Hypertensive crises • Acute coronary syndromes • Shock • Cardiac arrest	• Benzodiazepines • Lidocaine • Sodium bicarbonate (for cocaine-related ventricular arrhythmias) • Nitroglycerin • Nitroprusside • Reperfusion strategy based on cardiac catheterization data • Phentolamine (α_1-adrenergic blocker) • β-Blockers relatively contraindicated (do not use propranolol for cocaine intoxication)
Calcium channel blockers • Verapamil • Nifedipine (and other dihydropyridines) • Diltiazem	• Bradycardia • Impaired conduction • Shock • Cardiac arrest	• NS boluses (0.5 to 1 L) • Epinephrine IV; or other α/β-agonists • Pacemakers • Circulatory assist devices? • Calcium infusions • Glucose/insulin infusion? • Glucagon
β-Adrenergic receptor antagonists • Propranolol • Atenolol • Sotalol • Metoprolol	• Bradycardia • Impaired conduction • Shock • Cardiac arrest	• NS boluses (0.5 to 1 L) • Epinephrine IV; or other α/β-agonists • Pacemakers • Circulatory assist devices? • Calcium infusions? • Glucose/insulin infusion? • Glucagon
Tricyclic antidepressants • Amitriptyline • Desipramine • Nortriptyline • Imipramine	• Tachycardia • Bradycardia • Ventricular arrhythmias • Impaired conduction • Shock • Cardiac arrest	• Sodium bicarbonate • Hyperventilation • NS boluses (0.5 to 1 L) • Magnesium sulfate • Lidocaine • Epinephrine IV; or other α/β-agonists
Cardiac glycosides • Digoxin • Digitoxin • Foxglove • Oleander	• Bradycardia • Supraventricular arrhythmias • Ventricular arrhythmias • Impaired conduction • Shock • Cardiac arrest	• Restore total body K^+, Mg^{++} • Restore intravascular volume • Digoxin-specific antibodies (Fab fragments: *Digibind* or *DigiFab*) • Atropine • Pacemakers (use caution and monitor for ventricular arrhythmias) • Lidocaine • Phenytoin?
Anticholinergics • Diphenhydramine • Doxylamine	• Tachycardia • Supraventricular arrhythmias • Ventricular arrhythmias • Impaired conduction • Shock, cardiac arrest	• Physostigmine

Potentially Toxic Drugs: by Type of Agent	Cardiopulmonary Signs* of Toxicity	Therapy to Consider†
Cholinergics • Carbamates • Nerve agents • Organophosphates	• Bradycardia • Ventricular arrhythmias • Impaired conduction, shock • Pulmonary edema • Bronchospasm • Cardiac arrest	• Atropine • Decontamination • Pralidoxime • Obidoxime
Opioids • Heroin • Fentanyl • Methadone • Morphine	• Hypoventilation (slow and shallow respirations, apnea) • Bradycardia • Hypotension • Miosis (pupil constriction)	• Assisted ventilation • Naloxone • Tracheal intubation • Nalmefene
Isoniazid	• Lactic acidosis with/without seizures • Tachycardia or bradycardia • Shock, cardiac arrest	• Pyridoxine (vitamin B_6) — large doses may be needed (ie, 1 g pyridoxine/per gram of ingested isoniazid)
Sodium channel blockers (Class I$_{VW}$ antiarrhythmics) • Procainamide • Disopyramide • Lidocaine • Propafenone • Flecainide	• Bradycardia • Ventricular arrhythmias • Impaired conduction • Seizures • Shock, cardiac arrest	• Sodium bicarbonate • Pacemakers • α- and β-agonist • Lidocaine (not for lidocaine overdose) • Hypertonic saline

*Unless stated otherwise, listed alterations of vital signs (bradycardia, tachycardia, tachypnea) are "hemodynamically significant."
†Specific *therapy to consider* should be based on specific indications. Therapies followed by "?" are *Class Indeterminate.*

remains unclear. Further prospective study of its efficacy is needed before routine use can be recommended.

Percutaneous coronary intervention is preferred by most experts for drug-induced ACS, especially when coronary atherosclerosis is known or may be present (older age, risk factors). If emergency cardiac catheterization reveals a thrombus without atherosclerotic disease, PCI with intracoronary antithrombin may be used. If a heavy thrombus load is present, antiplatelet therapy (eg, abciximab) may be needed.

Summary of Symptom-Based Therapy: Management of Cardiovascular Compromise Caused by Drugs or Toxins

In treatment of acute poison-induced shock and cardiac arrest, the standard ACLS protocols may not be effective.[48] Care of severely poisoned patients can be enhanced by urgent consultation with a medical toxicologist. The following alternative approaches may be needed for treatment of poisonings:

- The use of *higher doses* of drugs than usual
- The use of *drugs rarely given in cardiac arrest,* such as inamrinone, calcium, esmolol, glucagon, insulin, labetalol, phenylephrine, physostigmine, and sodium bicarbonate
- More frequent use of *heroic measures* such as prolonged CPR and circulatory assist devices
- *Earlier consideration of organ donation* when resuscitative efforts from a critical poisoning are unsuccessful and brain death is expected

When evaluating patients with cardiovascular emergencies, differentiate patients according to toxidromes, consider vital signs, and assess the 12-lead ECG. These steps will assist in the formulation of a differential diagnosis that can initially drive a therapy or treatment strategy while avoiding contraindicated drugs or interventions (Table 2). When a toxidrome is suspected, the cardiotoxicity of the specific drug or drug class can be evaluated and therapeutic recommendations considered (Table 3).

Management of Specific Poisonings

Table 4 summarizes potentially cardiotoxic drugs, the cardiovascular signs of toxicity they produce, and therapies to consider.

Calcium Channel Blocker and β-Blocker Toxicity

Both calcium channel blockers and β-blockers have negative inotropic (contractility) and negative chronotropic (heart rate) effects. Whereas calcium channel blockers possess varying degrees of direct vasodilatory properties,[49] β-blockers do not.[50]

Toxicity from calcium channel blockers and β-blockers can produce the following signs and symptoms:

- Hypotension
- Depression of myocardial contractility
- Bradycardias from depression of sinoatrial nodal, AV nodal, and intraventricular conduction; heart block
- Decreased level of consciousness, lethargy, or even coma
- Seizures (which may be the initial sign of serious toxicity), usually due to hypoperfusion of the central nervous system
- Hypoglycemia, hyperkalemia with β-blocker overdose
- Hyperglycemia associated with calcium channel blocker overdose
- Sudden decompensation to profound shock within minutes
- Cardiac arrest due to refractory AV block or pulseless electrical activity
- β-Blocker overdose may also cause a variety of arrhythmias, including torsades de pointes, VF, AV block, and in rare cases asystole

Time Course

Signs and symptoms of overdose from either calcium channel blockers or β-blockers typically develop within 2 to 4 hours of ingestion of *regular–release* preparations. Failure to develop symptomatology within 4 to 6 hours of regular-release ingestion indicates that moderate to severe toxicity is unlikely to occur. Toxic effects of controlled-release and long-acting preparations, however, may not be seen for up to 6 to 18 hours after ingestion.

Common Therapy for Calcium Channel and β-Blocker Overdoses

The optimal therapy for calcium channel and β-blocker overdoses has not been clearly defined. Evaluations of all available therapies have reported variable results. Initial therapies recommended by consensus include the following:

- Administer oxygen and monitor airway and ventilation (particularly if level of consciousness is depressed or seizures develop).
- Provide continuous ECG monitoring and be prepared to treat symptomatic or unstable arrhythmias.
- Perform careful assessment of blood pressure and hemodynamic status.
- Establish vascular access with 2 large-bore catheters.
- If hypotension is present, give a fluid challenge of 500 to 1000 mL of normal saline.[51,52] Monitor closely for signs of myocardial dysfunction and development of pulmonary edema.
- Determine the blood glucose concentration with a bedside rapid test.
- Consider activated charcoal for gastric decontamination in patients who are awake, alert, and present within 1 hour of ingestion with only mild hemodynamic effects.[53,54]
- Perform rapid sequence intubation followed by gastric lavage in patients who present within 1 hour of ingestion and have moderate to severe hemodynamic toxicity.
- Perform whole bowel irrigation when toxic quantities of controlled-release preparations have been consumed, medications are seen on the abdominal x-ray, and only if bowel sounds are still present.[53]
- Do not give syrup of ipecac. Ipecac has delayed onset and a propensity to worsen bradycardia through vomiting-induced increases in vagal tone. In addition, calcium blockers and β-blockers can cause rapid declines in hemodynamic stability, altered mental status, and seizures before ipecac can take effect.[55]

Specific Therapy for Calcium Channel Blocker Overdose

Immediate vascular access is established for the treatment of myocardial dysfunction and hypotension. The following treatment sequence for hypotension and hemodynamic instability can be individualized and requires continual assessment and reassessment.

Hypotension and Shock

- Give a *normal saline* fluid challenge, 1 to 2 boluses, 500 to 1000 mL each. Monitor for development of pulmonary edema. If hemodynamically significant signs and symptoms continue, add:

Rapid Response Interventions **1st Line Therapy: Calcium Infusions for Calcium Channel Blocker Toxicity**	The first-line drug therapy for calcium channel blocker–induced shock remains catecholamine-type vasopressors. • Calcium chloride infusions (1 to 3 g slow IV push) are recommended for calcium channel blocker–induced shock refractory to conventional catecholamine vasopressor therapy. • Additional calcium infusions (bolus or constant infusion) are warranted in patients who demonstrate a beneficial hemodynamic response to the initial calcium infusions. • Calcium infusions may be beneficial in other types of drug-induced shock. But they cannot be recommended because of limited supportive data (Class Indeterminate, level of evidence 6).

— *Epinephrine* infusion at 2 μg/min and titrate up to 100 μg/min. Catecholamine-like vasopressors (norepinephrine is another example) are the first-line drug therapy for hemodynamically significant hypotension or shock due to calcium channel blocker toxicity.[17,56]

• Consider *calcium chloride* 8 to 16 mg/kg (usually 5 to 10 mL or 0.5 to 1 g of a 10% solution from 10 mL vials with 100 mg/mL) if the shock fails to respond adequately to the fluid challenges and the epinephrine or norepinephrine infusion. Note that in case reports the effectiveness of this approach has varied greatly.

Additional IV calcium (slow IV push or continued infusion) to a total dose of 1 to 3 g IV is appropriate for patients who experience a positive hemodynamic response to the initial calcium infusion. Only limited supportive data exist for the use of calcium infusions in other types of drug-induced shock. Epinephrine and other α_1-agonists may sensitize the vasculature to the effects of calcium.

Bradycardia

Refractory hemodynamically significant bradycardia due to calcium channel blocker toxicity is treated with immediate transcutaneous pacing while preparations are made for transvenous access and pacing.

Additional Therapies to Consider

In specific cases and refractory patients, additional lifesaving measures and supportive therapy have been used. These therapies generally have been published as case reports or are supported only by animal data.

• *Glucose/insulin infusion:* Infusions of glucose and insulin have been used in the treatment of calcium channel blocker overdose; this intervention is supported by animal studies[57,58] and limited case series only.
• *Glucagon:* Myocardial toxicity due to calcium channel blockers has responded to glucagon in some animal studies and in case reports.[59] *Glucagon* is an inotropic agent that stimulates cyclic adenosine monophosphate in cardiac tissue via non-α, non-β receptors. Glucagon

has been administered in a dose of 1 to 5 mg IV. One method of administration is to give a 3 mg IV bolus and then initiate a continuous infusion at 3 mg/h, titrating as necessary.
• *Circulatory assist devices:* Devices such as the intra-aortic balloon pump or extracorporeal membrane oxygenation[60] should be considered if available for patients refractory to *maximal* medical therapy. Such support can maintain viability until the drug effects diminish below a lethal level, particularly for young, otherwise healthy, patients.
• There is reasonably good evidence that calcium salts may be beneficial in cases of mild to moderate calcium channel blocker poisoning. The efficacy of calcium salts in cases of more severe calcium channel blocker poisoning is more questionable. Stimulation of the α- and β-adrenergic receptors is believed to increase intracellular levels of calcium and to help reduce calcium channel blocker toxicity. Patients with severe, refractory calcium channel blocker–induced shock seem to have little to lose from modest doses of calcium salts. The safety and efficacy of high-dose calcium therapy have not been clearly established.

Specific Therapy for β-Blocker Overdose

General measures are the same as those for calcium channel blocker overdose. Assess and provide BLS Primary and ACLS Secondary measures for airway and ventilation as needed. Immediate vascular access is established as a priority for the treatment of myocardial dysfunction and hypotension. The following treatment sequence for hypotension and hemodynamic instability can be individualized and requires continual assessment and reassessment.

Hypotension and Shock

• Give a *normal saline* fluid challenge, 1 to 2 boluses, 500 to 1000 mL each. Monitor for development of pulmonary edema. If hemodynamically significant signs and symptoms continue, add:

- *Vasopressors:* If hemodynamically significant hypotension is present, treat with a vasopressor with moderate to high α-adrenergic activity, such as *epinephrine* infused at 2 to 10 µg/min. In case reports norepinephrine, dobutamine, isoproterenol, and dopamine have been associated with success.

- *Glucagon:* In animal models and some human case reports, glucagon showed promise as a valuable agent in *mild to moderate* β-blocker–induced shock. In reports of patients with more severe shock, however, consistent efficacy data is lacking. Glucagon in mild to moderate shock for patients unresponsive to vasopressors can be administered at a dose of 1 to 5 mg IV. One method of administration is to give a 3 mg IV bolus and then initiate a continuous infusion at 3 mg/h, titrating as necessary. Note that glucagon, like many inotropic agents, can further reduce SVR, so vasopressor adjuncts are often required.

- *Isoproterenol:* Isoproterenol can be used carefully as an adjunct with an epinephrine infusion or in combination with other agents, though significant improvement is rare. Do not use isoproterenol as a first-line agent.

- *Calcium:* Calcium infusions (8 to 16 mg/kg, usually 5 to 10 mL or 0.5 to 1 g of a 10% solution from 10 mL vials with 100 mg/mL) may be of benefit in β-blocker–induced shock that is unresponsive to glucagon and epinephrine. But calcium cannot be recommended specifically because the currently available evidence consists of limited animal data[61] and conflicting clinical case reports.[62,63]

Bradycardia

- *Refractory, hemodynamically significant bradycardia:* If hemodynamically significant bradycardia is present, add pacing (either transvenous or transcutaneous).
- *Additional therapies to consider:*
  - *Atropine:* While not harmful, atropine is rarely effective in β-blocker–induced bradycardia or in reversing symptomatic AV block.
  - *Circulatory assist devices:* As with calcium channel blocker overdose, circulatory assist devices or extracorporeal circulation may be effective for drug-induced shock that fails to respond to maximal medical therapy. But this approach must be started before irreversible end-organ damage has occurred.
  - *Glucose/insulin infusion:* Some success has been reported with glucose/insulin infusion in an animal model of treatment of shock caused by β-blocker overdose. This therapy may produce hypokalemia unless potassium is monitored and supplementation provided. The use of glucose and insulin for β-blocker toxicity remains a Class Indeterminate recommendation.

Cocaine Toxicity

Millions of people in the United States use cocaine. They inhale nasally or inject intravenously the crystalline form of the drug[64] or smoke the freebase form of the drug, commonly known as "crack."[65] Although arrhythmias and cardiac arrest from cocaine are relatively uncommon, cocaine use of any type by any route can cause disastrous complications.[64,65]

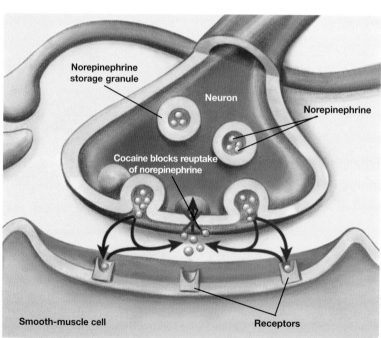

Figure 1. Mechanism of cocaine toxicity. Reprinted with permission from *The New England Journal of Medicine.* 2001;345:351-358.[10] Copyright 2001 Massachusetts Medical Society. All rights reserved. Published correction appears in *N Engl J Med.* 2001;345:1432.

Cocaine Toxicity

Cocaine first stimulates the release and then blocks the reuptake of norepinephrine, epinephrine, dopamine, and serotonin[64,66] (Figure 1). Cocaine abusers experience an elevation in blood pressure, tachycardia, and feelings of euphoria coupled with decreased fatigue. Cocaine toxicity is dose dependent. Numerous seizures, myocardial infarctions, and deaths have occurred in both new and long-term users who have taken only small quantities of the drug.[64,67,68]

Cardiac Toxicity

Serious cocaine-induced cardiac toxicity stems from the direct effect of cocaine on the heart. Cocaine also provokes the central nervous system to stimulate the cardiovascular system. The β-adrenergic effects of cocaine increase heart rate and myocardial contractility. The α-adrenergic effects of cocaine decrease coronary blood flow and may induce coronary artery spasm. Cocaine increases platelet adhesiveness, leading to increased risk of coronary thrombosis. These mechanisms lead to decreased coronary artery perfusion at a time of increased myocardial oxygen demand. Hypoxia from pulmonary edema and acidosis from cocaine-induced seizures may exacerbate the cardiotoxicity of cocaine.

Cocaine toxicity may cause thermoregulatory problems, including hyperpyrexia. A rise in the patient's body temperature can worsen existing tachycardia and neurologic symptoms. High ambient temperatures have also been associated with a significant increase in mortality in patients with cocaine toxicity.[10,67]

Treatment of Cocaine-Induced Arrhythmias

All patients with cocaine-induced CNS symptoms or cardiovascular complications require close observation. Treat fever and cool patients presenting with agitation, delirium, seizures, and elevated body temperature. If an arrhythmia or ACS is present, administer oxygen and provide continuous ECG monitoring.

Cocaine-Induced Supraventricular Arrhythmias

Cocaine-induced supraventricular arrhythmias include paroxysmal supraventricular tachycardia, rapid atrial fibrillation, and atrial flutter.[69] These arrhythmias are often short lived and seldom require therapy unless hemodynamic compromise is also present.[70-72]

Benzodiazepine

Treat persistent supraventricular arrhythmias in hemodynamically stable patients with a benzodiazepine, such as *diazepam* in a dose of 5 to 20 mg IV over 5 to 20 minutes. Benzodiazepines modulate the stimulatory effects of cocaine on the central nervous and cardiovascular systems, blunting the patient's hypersympathetic state.

Cocaine-Induced Stable Ventricular Tachycardia

Nonarrest ventricular arrhythmias due to cocaine include ventricular ectopy, episodes of nonsustained ventricular tachycardia, and stable monomorphic and polymorphic VT.[73,74]

Benzodiazepine

Like supraventricular arrhythmias, ventricular ectopy and tachycardia are often transient and may require only careful observation. Most experienced clinicians will administer a benzodiazepine in a titrated fashion (eg, diazepam 5 to 20 mg IV over 5 to 20 minutes).

Lidocaine

Many experts recommend lidocaine at the standard dose of 1 to 1.5 mg/kg for treatment of ventricular arrhythmias unresponsive to a titrated benzodiazepine. Cocaine, long established as a legitimate anesthetic agent, has properties of a sodium channel blocker (Class I_{vw} antiarrhythmic). Lidocaine, acting as a similar sodium channel blocker (Class I_{vw} antiarrhythmic), competes with cocaine at the sodium channel, thus decreasing cocaine's effects. The decision to use lidocaine must be carefully weighed against the increased risk of seizure due to the synergistic toxic effects of lidocaine in the presence of cocaine.[40,75]

Sodium Bicarbonate

Some experimental animal studies and human case reports[76,77] support the use of sodium bicarbonate (1 to 2 mEq/kg) in the treatment of cocaine-induced VF and VT.[78] Most toxicologists agree that sodium bicarbonate should be used *early* in the management of ventricular tachycardias resulting from the use of cocaine.[10,78,79]

Defibrillation

As a precaution have a defibrillator available at the bedside. Adhesive defibrillator pads can be preattached, and cardiac monitoring can be performed by conventional defibrillator/monitors.

Cocaine-Induced Ventricular Fibrillation

CPR and Defibrillation

The steps of the **BLS Primary and ACLS Secondary ABCD Surveys** apply to cocaine-induced VF arrest. These steps include CPR, defibrillation, airway control, and IV access.

Epinephrine

The initial medication given after unsuccessful shock(s) for VF arrest that is not associated with cocaine toxicity is an adrenergic agent, either *epinephrine* or *vasopressin*. Most experts agree that epinephrine is an appropriate vasoconstrictor to give in cocaine-induced VF arrest, even though the similar cardiovascular effects would argue otherwise. Little evidence exists to confirm either benefit or harm from an initial epinephrine dose of 1 mg. Clinicians should, however, increase the interval between subsequent doses of epinephrine to every 5 to 10 minutes and avoid high-dose epinephrine (>1 mg per dose) in patients with refractory VF.

Vasopressin

The ECC Guidelines 2000 experts added vasopressin 40 U IV push × 1 as an acceptable alternative to epinephrine for VF arrest. Extrapolation from pharmacologic principles suggests that vasopressin should offer considerable advantages over epinephrine for refractory, cocaine-induced VF arrest. Because of the current absence of data, this recommendation is a Class Indeterminate recommendation.

Lidocaine

For shock-refractory VF, give a lidocaine bolus of 1 to 1.5 mg/kg, and then reattempt defibrillation. Clinical evidence about the effect of lidocaine in cocaine toxicity is limited. The ECC Guidelines 2000 experts added amiodarone as an acceptable alternative to lidocaine for conventional management of shock-refractory VF. Whether this amiodarone recommendation applies to cocaine-induced persistent VF is unknown. In the absence of relevant data, omit amiodarone.

Sodium Bicarbonate

There is some evidence that supports the use of sodium bicarbonate (1 to 2 mEq/kg) in the treatment of cocaine-induced, stable VT and also may apply to cardiac arrest associated with VF.[76,77,80,81] Providers can consider a bolus of sodium bicarbonate after establishment of IV access and administration of a vasopressor and lidocaine.[10,78,79]

Summary: Treatment of Cocaine-Induced Arrhythmias

General Treatment

- Administer oxygen.
- Correct elevated body temperature.
- Perform continuous ECG monitoring.
- Monitor neurologic status.

Supraventricular Arrhythmias Requiring Therapy

- Diazepam 5 mg IV, escalating as needed to 20 mg.

Hemodynamically Stable Ventricular Tachycardia

- Diazepam 5 mg IV, escalating as needed to 20 mg.
- If persistent, lidocaine 1 to 1.5 mg/kg IV.
- Followed by sodium bicarbonate 1 to 2 mEq/kg IV.

Ventricular Fibrillation

Ventricular fibrillation should initially be treated in standard fashion:

- Attempt defibrillation with 1 shock per the ACLS protocol for a monophasic or biphasic defibrillator.
- If VF persists, follow with epinephrine 1 mg IV, limited to a single dose or repeated in 5 to 10 minutes, or vasopressin 40 U IV push × 1.
- If VF persists, follow with lidocaine 1 to 1.5 mg/kg IV bolus.
- If VF persists, follow with sodium bicarbonate 1 to 2 mEq/kg IV.

Treatment of Cocaine-Induced Hypertension and Pulmonary Edema

Cocaine-Induced Hypertension

Cocaine toxicity can produce hypertensive emergencies through effects on the central nervous system and peripheral α-agonist stimulation.

Benzodiazepine

Hypertensive patients should initially be treated with a benzodiazepine in an attempt to minimize the stimulatory effects of cocaine on the central nervous and cardiovascular systems.[40,82]

Nitroglycerin or Nitroprusside

Patients who require additional therapy should be treated with a vasodilator such as nitroglycerin or nitroprusside in a titrated dose. Nitroglycerin is preferable in patients with superimposed chest pain.

Precautions

Do not use β-blocking agents such as propranolol or esmolol.[44,83] Both have the potential to raise blood pressure by antagonizing cocaine-induced β-receptor stimulation and allowing unopposed cocaine-induced α-receptor stimulation. Labetalol, with both α-blocker and β-blocker effects, has shown inferior results compared with nitroglycerin or nitroprusside and should be avoided.[84,85] A pure α-blocker such as phentolamine (1 mg every 2 to 3 minutes; up to 10 mg) may be used, although it too is not well studied for treatment of cocaine toxicity.[86]

Cocaine-Induced Pulmonary Edema

The effects of cocaine on pulmonary dynamics may result in pulmonary edema. Pulmonary edema may also occur secondary to a subarachnoid hemorrhage, from a cocaine-induced myocardial infarction, or as a consequence of additional drugs of abuse, such as heroin.[66,87-89] Most patients respond to standard medical management. Positive-pressure ventilation with a continuous positive airway pressure mask or intubation supplemented by positive end-expiratory pressure will usually rapidly correct hypoxemia.

Treatment of Cocaine-Induced Chest Pain and ACS (See Also "ACS" on Page 269)

Cocaine-Induced Chest Pain

Chest pain is one of the most common complaints of cocaine users. The vast majority of patients have only transient chest pain with no evidence of acute ischemia on their ECG. Clinicians should be aware that abnormal but nondiagnostic ECGs are common in young adults who use cocaine.

See "FYI: Cardiovascular Complications of Cocaine Use" for a detailed discussion of this topic.

Cocaine-Induced ACS

Although rare, acute myocardial infarctions (AMIs) do occur in cocaine users. Most cocaine-related infarctions occur in patients who smoke cigarettes or who have other cardiac risk factors,[68,90,91] although some infarctions occur in active, healthy patients with no risk factors for ischemic heart disease.

Cocaine-related myocardial ischemia should be treated with *oxygen, aspirin, nitrates,* and a titrated dose of a

FYI **Cardiovascular Complications of Cocaine Use** **Cardiovascular Toxicity**	Cocaine causes myocardial ischemia through complex pathophysiologic mechanisms.[10] Acutely cocaine results in coronary artery vasoconstriction, tachycardia, systemic arterial hypertension, increased myocardial oxygen demand, platelet aggregation, and in situ thrombus formation. In long-term cocaine users, atherosclerosis and left ventricular hypertrophy develop at an accelerated pace. These conditions can further exacerbate the oxygen supply-demand mismatch. Myocardial ischemia and infarction may occur in patients with or without underlying atherosclerotic disease.
Cocaine-Associated ACS	The interval associated with the highest risk of myocardial ischemia and infarction after cocaine use has not been established. The risk of myocardial infarction is increased 24-fold in the first hour after cocaine use,[95] and most cocaine-associated myocardial infarctions occur within 24 hours of use.[91] Nonetheless spontaneous episodes of ST-segment elevation have been documented on ambulatory monitoring for up to 6 weeks after last use of cocaine.[96]
Evidence-Based Treatment?	The treatment of cocaine-associated ACS is methodologically difficult to study in randomized, controlled clinical trials. High-quality, prospective, multicenter cohort evaluations have provided valuable information.[97,98] Most consensus recommendations, however, are supported by evidence from case series; reasonable extrapolations from existing data; and rational conjecture (common sense) or common practices accepted before evidence-based guidelines. The basis for most current recommendations comes from a knowledge of successful therapies in patients with ACS unrelated to cocaine, animal investigations, and human volunteer studies, plus extrapolations from the known pathophysiologic mechanisms of cocaine-associated ACS.[10]
Treatment Differences: Cocaine-Related vs Cocaine-Unrelated ACS	*Benzodiazepines.* Benzodiazepines are recommended for patients with cocaine-associated ACS even though these agents are not routinely used in patients with ACS unrelated to cocaine.[10,48,71,99] In cocaine-induced ACS, benzodiazepines decrease central nervous system excitation and have a salutary effect on the centrally stimulated cardiovascular consequences of cocaine.[10] *β-Blockers.* Despite the success of β-blockers in AMI unrelated to cocaine, they are contraindicated for cocaine-associated ACS (see "The Evidence Against Use of β-Adrenergic Antagonists (β-Blockers) in Cocaine-Related AMI").[43,44,100] *Reperfusion Therapy.* Reperfusion therapy for patients with STEMI in the setting of cocaine use or toxicity has the same priority as reperfusion therapy in general. Coronary flow should be established as soon as possible to the ischemic region. In patients using cocaine the proximate cause of STEMI may be coronary spasm, which when combined with decreased coronary blood flow eventually causes intracoronary thrombus. Both the toxic effects of cocaine and thrombus formation require a thoughtful approach. Many cardiovascular experts prefer PCI to assess the status of the coronary artery involved and to guide therapy when this approach can be done in a timely manner.

Emergency Treatment of Cocaine-Induced ACS

Emergency treatment of patients with cocaine-associated myocardial ischemia targets the acute pathophysiologic effects of the process. Attempts to reduce or reverse the coronary vasoconstriction, hypertension, tachycardia, and predisposition to thrombus formation are the mainstays of treatment. The objective is to improve coronary artery perfusion and oxygen delivery while reducing myocardial oxygen demand.

Benzodiazepines

Multiple animal experiments, widespread anecdotal experience, and one randomized, controlled trial in humans support *diazepam* as the initial agent for treating all cocaine-intoxicated patients.[71,101] Benzodiazepines protect the central nervous system while decreasing sympathetic outflow, calming the patient and returning vital signs to the normal range. Additional direct effects on peripheral benzodiazepine receptors may counteract the vasoconstrictive properties of cocaine and its metabolite benzoylecgonine. The randomized, controlled trial showed that diazepam has the same effect as nitroglycerin on chest pain resolution and cardiac performance.[101]

Nitroglycerin

Specific anti-ischemic therapy begins with *nitroglycerin*. Neither reduction in infarct size nor mortality benefit has been assessed following nitroglycerin use in patients with cocaine-associated ACS. The *Class Indeterminate* recommendation for nitrates is based on experimental reversal of coronary vasoconstriction in humans and clinical relief of chest pain.[37,38,101]

Antiplatelet and Antithrombotic Agents

Attempts to decrease the acute coagulability of blood with *aspirin* or *heparin* are recommended with some support from clinical reports specific to cocaine users[102] (Class Indeterminate). The current understanding of the pharmacology of these agents suggests some value, as does the extensive clinical experience with ACS unrelated to cocaine.

Management of Refractory ACS

Patients with ischemia refractory to the above measures can be treated with either *phentolamine*, *calcium antagonists*, or *reperfusion therapy* depending on the clinical circumstances.[48]

Phentolamine

Phentolamine blocks the α-adrenergic effects of cocaine and reverses the coronary vasoconstrictive effects of cocaine.[39] One case report showed efficacy in a patient with cocaine-associated chest pain.[86] Because phentolamine may result in hypotension, use of small incremental doses (1 mg every 2 to 3 minutes) is recommended.

Calcium Antagonists

Calcium channel blockers do not have a clear role to play in patients with cocaine-induced vascular ischemia because data on the efficacy of these agents for the treatment of cocaine toxicity are contradictory.

- In a human cardiac catheterization model of cocaine toxicity, verapamil successfully reversed cocaine-induced coronary artery vasoconstriction.[103]
- In multicenter clinical trials in patients with ACS *not* associated with cocaine toxicity, researchers have found no benefit from calcium channel blockers on important outcomes such as survival.

Treatment Differences: Cocaine-Related vs Cocaine-Unrelated ACS *(continued)*	• In studies of cocaine-poisoned animals pretreated with calcium channel blockers, investigators have observed favorable results for a variety of end points, such as better survival, fewer seizures, and fewer cardiac arrhythmias. But in other studies investigators have found adverse effects. Positive results were reported only in animals that were *pretreated* with calcium channel blockers; *later* administration of calcium channel blockers showed no benefit.

The Evidence Against Use of β-Adrenergic Antagonists (β-Blockers) in Cocaine-Related AMI	Despite the success of β-blockers in patients with AMI unrelated to cocaine, β-blockers are contraindicated in recent cocaine users.[48] Clinicians should not administer β-blockers or mixed α-/β-blockers such as labetalol to patients who have recently used cocaine.
	
	• β-Blockers increase central nervous system toxicity and exacerbate coronary artery vasospasm in animal models of cocaine toxicity.
	• Human case series show that β-blockers do not reverse the hypertensive and tachycardic effects of cocaine.[44]
	• Studies in human volunteers show that β-blockers exacerbate cocaine-induced coronary artery vasoconstriction.[43]
	• Scientific agreement has not been established on the role, if any, of either pure β- or mixed α-/β-blockers in the treatment of cocaine intoxication. Labetalol, a mixed α-/β-antagonist, has attracted considerable attention from toxicologists. Labetalol does not appear to offer any advantages over pure β-antagonists even though it produced no adverse outcomes in some cases.[41,84,104] The evidence does not support the use of labetalol:
	   — It has more β-adrenergic antagonist effects than α-adrenergic antagonist effects.
	   — It leads to unopposed α effects with severe hypertension in patients with pheochromocytomas.
	   — It increases the risk of seizure and death in animal models of cocaine toxicity.
	   — It does not reverse coronary artery vasoconstriction in humans.[42]

benzodiazepine.[38,82] β-Blockers should *not* be used because of the possibility of α-mediated vasospasm.[43] Because of its antispasm effects and its beneficial role in myocardial infarction, *magnesium* can also be used for cocaine-related ischemia and infarction.[92,93] *Morphine* should be administered for continued pain.

STEMI and Reperfusion Therapy in Cocaine Toxicity

Perhaps half of all cocaine-related myocardial infarctions appear to be due to spasm, not plaque rupture. Additionally, patients with nonocclusive coronary disease may have abnormal vasomotor tone, predisposing them to the toxic effects of cocaine. Indications for fibrinolytic therapy must be reviewed in light of the fact that "false positive" ST-segment changes are common in cocaine users. These variant patterns include early repolarization and QRS complexes with elevated J points.[94] Before starting fibrinolytic therapy some clinicians require a diagnostic echocardiogram or evidence of infarction by a rapid assay technique of cardiac markers. These dilemmas have led many experts to prefer cardiac catheterization with coronary angiography so that the interventionalist can

select the appropriate reperfusion strategy (fibrinolytics vs percutaneous coronary interventions).

Tricyclic Antidepressants

When taken in excess the TCAs are among the most cardio-toxic agents in medicine. Although TCAs rarely cause cardiovascular side effects when taken in therapeutic amounts, they are the number one cause of death from overdose in patients who arrive at the hospital alive.[105]

The toxic side effects of TCAs are due to the interplay of their 4 major pharmacologic properties. Tricyclics

- Stimulate catecholamine release and then block reuptake at postganglionic synapses
- Have central and peripheral anticholinergic actions
- Inhibit potassium channels in myocardium and fast (voltage-dependent) sodium channels in brain and myocardium
- Have direct α-blocking actions

Major Signs of TCA Toxicity

As a toxic dose of a tricyclic begins to take effect, the following signs appear:

- Alterations in mental status, including agitation, irritability, confusion, delirium, hallucinations, hyper-activity, seizures, and hyperpyrexia
- Sinus tachycardia (especially in association with a rightward QRS axis); supraventricular tachycardia and hypertension may develop early after ingestion but are usually short lived because catecholamine depletion then develops
- Prolongation of the QT interval
- Anticholinergic effects, such as delirium, mydriasis, urinary retention, and gastric atony

More ominous signs that require immediate therapy are

- Coma
- Seizures
- QRS widening
- Wide-complex arrhythmias
- Ventricular arrhythmias
- Preterminal sinus bradycardia and AV block
- Hypotension
- Acidosis

The signs of significant TCA overdose may be recalled by the memory aid "Three C's and an A":

- **C**oma
- **C**onvulsions (seizures)
- **C**ardiac arrhythmias
- **A**cidosis

Serum levels usually are not readily available and are of little prognostic or therapeutic value in acute overdoses.

Time Course of TCA Toxicity

Most patients will manifest some sign of toxicity within 2 to 4 hours of ingestion of an excessive amount. Patients who are asymptomatic after 6 hours of continuous monitoring, with no QT prolongation on the 12-lead ECG, are at essentially no risk for toxicity.[106,107]

General Management of TCA Overdose

- Gastric decontamination with activated charcoal should be considered for all patients who present with an acute TCA overdose within 1 hour of ingestion.[54]
- Gastric lavage should be considered in all unconscious patients, particularly for patients who present within 1 to 2 hours of ingestion of a life-threatening quantity of a TCA.[108]
- Syrup of ipecac is unnecessary in the hospital care of patients, where superior gastric emptying techniques are readily available.[55]

Bicarbonate for TCA Overdose

Alkalinization With Sodium Bicarbonate

Alkalinization with sodium bicarbonate is the mainstay of therapy for severe TCA overdose.[106,109-111]

- Alkalinization decreases the free, non-protein-bound form of the tricyclic molecule and overrides the tricyclic-induced sodium channel blockade of phase 0 of the action potential.[107]
- Alkalinization is not required in patients who have only a mild resting tachycardia or mild prolongation of the QT interval.
- Alkalinization (raising serum pH to 7.50 to 7.55) is indicated for patients with
  - Prolongation of the QRS to >100 ms
  - Ventricular arrhythmias
  - Hypotension unresponsive to a saline bolus of 500 to 1000 mL

Alkalinization for the Unstable Patient With TCA Overdose

- Provide immediate hyperventilation to a pH of 7.50 to 7.55 for patients who present with seizures or inadequate respiratory function.[112]
- Give *sodium bicarbonate* 1 to 2 mEq/kg over 1 to 2 minutes.
- Follow with a *sodium bicarbonate* infusion of 3 ampules (150 mEq) plus KCl (30 mEq) mixed in 850 mL of D_5W, at an initial rate of 150 to 200 mL/h, titrated to keep pH at 7.50 to 7.55.
- The initial goal of therapy is to raise the pH to 7.50 to 7.55 and then to maintain that pH, confirming it by measurement of venous and arterial pH on a regular basis.
- Continue to infuse sodium bicarbonate until the patient's condition stabilizes (ie, QRS shortens to <100 ms, arrhythmias stop, and blood pressure returns to normal range).

Magnesium for TCA Overdose

Some patients may develop arrhythmias due to tricyclic actions on phase 2 of the action potential.

- The phase 2 effects are initially manifested by a prolongation of the QT interval. But they may result in the torsades de pointes variant of VT.[21,113-116]
- Magnesium sulfate is the drug of choice for this select group of patients.[21,114-116]
- The dose of magnesium is 1 to 2 g diluted in 10 mL D_5W IV push in unstable patients (a total of 5 to 10 g IV may be used). Give this dose more slowly (over 1 to 5 minutes) in hemodynamically stable patients.[21,114,117]

TCA-Induced Cardiac Arrest

TCA overdose usually causes profound myocardial depression. When cardiac arrest develops, it is often associated with pulseless electrical activity. The following recommendations apply to the treatment of TCA-induced cardiac arrest:

Rapid Response Interventions **ACLS Modification to Treatment of Cardiac Arrest**	The protocol for treating VF due to TCA overdose requires some modification of the standard ACLS Algorithm: • Attempt defibrillation with 1 shock. • Maintain airway and give a vasopressor. • Then *rapidly alkalinize the patient by administering sodium bicarbonate 1 to 2 mEq/kg IV push. If bicarbonate is not readily available, perform hyperventilation to create respiratory alkalosis.*

- Initiate the BLS Primary and ACLS Secondary ABCD Surveys.
- Start hyperventilation as soon as advanced control of the airway is achieved.
- Administer normal saline at 1000 mL/h when IV access is obtained.
- Slow push sodium bicarbonate 1 to 2 mEq/kg over 1 to 2 minutes.
- Follow with a sodium bicarbonate infusion of 3 ampules (150 mEq) with 30 mEq KCl mixed in 850 mL D_5W at 150 to 200 mL/h.
- Add epinephrine 1 mg IV every 3 to 5 minutes if the patient does not respond to alkalinization and the saline infusion.
- Load with lidocaine 1 to 1.5 mg/kg; follow with a maintenance infusion of 1 to 4 mg/min. Nonresponders at this point should be treated with magnesium sulfate 1 to 2 g diluted in 10 mL D_5W IV push.[117] Procainamide should not be used in TCA-induced arrhythmias because of its tricyclic-like pharmacologic properties.[110,118]

TCA-Induced Seizures and Hypotension

Seizures due to TCA overdose should be terminated immediately with benzodiazepines. Uncontrolled seizure activity results in hypoxia, acidosis, tachycardia, hypotension, and electrolyte fluxes. These responses increase morbidity and mortality from TCA overdose.

- Hypotension usually responds to infusions of 500 to 1000 mL of normal saline.
- Alkalinization with sodium bicarbonate is recommended for nonresponders.
- Patients with refractory hypotension may be treated with dopamine or norepinephrine.[24,119-121]

Digitalis Overdose and Cardiac Toxicity

Digitalis-induced cardiac toxicity may develop in long-term users of this widely prescribed medication. It may also be due to an acute overdose in a previously healthy patient.

Signs and Symptoms of Digitalis Toxicity

Many of the early symptoms of digitalis intoxication are nonspecific signs of central nervous system and gastrointestinal toxicity. Fatigue, visual symptoms, weakness, nausea, vomiting, and abdominal pain are common. Cardiac arrhythmias occur in the vast majority of patients with digitalis toxicity. The most common arrhythmias are ventricular ectopy and bradycardia, often in association with various degrees of AV block. The following rhythm disturbances should immediately suggest digitalis intoxication: atrial tachycardia with high-degree AV block, nonparoxysmal accelerated junctional tachycardia, multifocal VT, new onset bigeminy, and regularized atrial fibrillation.

Cardiac Toxicity of Digitalis

The cardiac toxicity of digitalis is due to the combination of its inhibitory effects on nodal conduction and its excitatory effects on individual atrial and ventricular fibers. Life-threatening digitalis toxicity most often is due to

- Bradyarrhythmias with resultant congestive heart failure
- Malignant ventricular arrhythmias
- Hyperkalemia resulting from digitalis poisoning of the sodium-potassium adenosine triphosphatase pump

General Approach to Treating Digitalis Toxicity

The treatment of arrhythmias due to digitalis toxicity is determined by the acuity of the overdose (ie, whether the overdose results from chronic therapy or acute ingestion) and the patient's hemodynamic function.

Management of Digitalis Toxicity Associated With Chronic Therapy

Digitalis intoxication in long-term users generally develops in association with hypokalemia, hypomagnesemia, dehydration, declining renal function, or loss of muscle mass. Patients who take non–potassium-sparing diuretics are especially prone to developing toxicity. Cardiotoxicity in these patients is initially treated by

- Replenishing total body potassium
- Replenishing total body magnesium stores[122]
- Replacing volume with normal saline

If the patient with digitalis toxicity is hypokalemic, assume that he is also hypomagnesemic until proven otherwise. Rapid replacement of potassium, magnesium, and volume will usually correct most arrhythmias in long-term digitalis users within a few hours. For severe toxicity consider use of digoxin-specific antibody (Fab fragments—see below).

General Management of Acute Digitalis Overdose

Gastric Decontamination With Activated Charcoal

Emergency physicians should consider decontamination with activated charcoal in all patients with an acute digitalis overdose who present within 1 hour of ingestion.[54,108] Syrup of ipecac is not useful in the hospital care of patients with digitalis overdose; other gastric emptying techniques are available.[55]

Life-Threatening Digitalis Overdose

In all *unconscious* patients perform rapid sequence intubation in preparation for orogastric lavage, administration of activated charcoal, or both. Some experts recommend gastric lavage for any patient seen within 1 to 2 hours of overdose with a life-threatening amount of digoxin whether the patient is conscious or unconscious.[108] Exercise caution if gastric lavage is selected, because it may induce a vagal response that can cause or exacerbate digitalis toxicity. Many experts recommend administration of 0.5 mg of atropine before gastric lavage to blunt this vagal response.

General Management Precautions

Patients with digitalis toxicity are more prone to pacemaker-induced ventricular rhythm disturbances. Use of trans-venous pacemakers should be highly selective.[119]

When arrhythmias develop, perform cardioversion or de-fibrillation when indicated. However, patients with digitalis toxicity may develop malignant ventricular arrhythmias or asystole after cardioversion. For this reason a lower initial cardioversion dose is used (see "Critical Concept: Synchronized Cardioversion in Unstable VT Associated With Digitalis Toxicity").

Patients with digitalis toxicity develop high levels of intracellular calcium, so do not give them additional calcium salts.[123] Hypokalemia and hypomagnesemia are risk factors for developing digitalis toxicity, although hyperkalemia may be present with acute severe toxicity (see below).

Management of Digitalis-Induced Symptomatic Bradycardias

Atropine

Patients with symptomatic bradycardia and AV block should initially receive atropine in doses starting at 0.5 mg IV. Because of the vagally mediated effects of digitalis, atropine may temporarily reverse digitalis intoxication.[122,124]

Digoxin-Specific Fab Fragment Therapy

The availability of digoxin-specific antibodies (Fab fragments) to treat severe chronic and acute toxicity has dramatically reduced morbidity and mortality from digitalis intoxication. Fab fragments bind to free digoxin, resulting in an inactive compound that is excreted in the urine. Use of Fab fragments results in lower levels of free serum digoxin; this concentration gradient pulls free digoxin from myocardial tissue. Effects begin in minutes; complete reversal of digitalis-mediated effects most often occurs within 30 minutes of administration.[125] The high cost per vial of Fab fragments must be weighed against the decreased need for prolonged and expensive intensive care therapy.

Dosing of Fab Fragments

The specific dose of Fab fragments is determined by the patient's weight and serum digoxin level (if known) or in the case of acute toxicity, by the estimated milligrams ingested. Each 40-mg vial of Fab fragments binds 0.6 mg of digoxin (Table 4). Serum digoxin levels rise dramatically after Fab fragment therapy; thus, the serum digoxin level should not be used to guide continuing therapy.

In general 3 to 5 vials are effective in patients with digitalis intoxication due to chronic use. Hemodynamically significant bradyarrhythmias and life-threatening AV block in acute overdose require much greater quantities of Fab fragments.

Table 4. Adult Dose Estimate of Digibind (Fab Fragments in Number of Vials) From Steady-State Serum Digoxin Concentration

Patient Weight (kg)	Serum Digoxin Concentration (ng/mL) (Vials)						
	1	2	4	8	12	16	20
40	0.5	1	2	3	5	7	8
60	0.5	1	3	5	7	10	12
70	1	2	3	5	9	11	14
80	1	2	3	7	10	13	16
100	1	2	3	8	12	15	20

Critical Concept **Synchronized Cardioversion in Unstable VT Associated With Digitalis Toxicity**	• If the patient is rapidly deteriorating and hemodynamically unstable, give an immediate shock using defibrillation doses. • Synchronized cardioversion attempts are preferable to unsynchronized shocks if the clinical situation allows the slightly longer time required to perform this procedure. • When performing immediate cardioversion, start at low energy levels of 25 to 50 J. The likelihood of postcountershock rhythm deterioration is increased in patients with digitalis toxicity. • If no response, immediately reattempt cardioversion using defibrillation doses. • When possible sedate the patient before shocks.

Use the dosing nomogram to determine the correct dose of antibody. Massive overdoses may require as many as 20 vials. There is no evidence to support attempts to totally correct elevated digoxin levels (ie, return the patient to a therapeutic level). Case reports suggest that this practice is frequently associated with undesirable outcomes.

Indications for Fab Fragment Therapy

The indications for Fab fragment therapy are digoxin toxicity in association with

- Life-threatening arrhythmias refractory to conventional therapy
- Shock or fulminant congestive heart failure
- Hyperkalemia (K^+ >5 mEq/L)
- Steady-state serum digoxin levels above 10 to 15 ng/mL in adults
- Cardiac arrest
- Acute ingestions greater than 10 mg in adults

Management of Digitalis-Induced Ventricular Arrhythmias

Potassium, Magnesium, and Normal Saline

Most episodes of digitalis toxicity–induced ventricular ectopy respond to simple administration of potassium, magnesium, and isotonic crystalloid.

Lidocaine

Lidocaine is the antiarrhythmic of choice if ventricular arrhythmias persist after administration of potassium, magnesium, and normal saline. Lidocaine acts rapidly and rarely causes acute toxicity when used in the recommended dose of 1 to 1.5 mg/kg.[122,124,126] Observe closely for early signs of lidocaine toxicity when placing elderly patients with congestive heart failure or renal impairment on a lidocaine maintenance infusion.

Phenytoin

In the past phenytoin was the preferred antiarrhythmic for digitalis-induced ventricular arrhythmias. The advantages of phenytoin were that it caused fewer central nervous system side effects than lidocaine and few adverse effects on AV conduction.

Magnesium

A number of reports suggest that magnesium may be the initial drug of choice for digitalis-induced ventricular tachyarrhythmias.[127,128] A dose of 1 to 2 g of magnesium sulfate diluted in 10 mL of D_5W and given IV push over 1 to 5 minutes may be used as first-line therapy. Some providers use magnesium only in patients with ventricular tachyarrhythmias unresponsive to lidocaine or phenytoin. A continuous magnesium infusion of 1 to 2 g (8 to 16 mEq) of magnesium diluted in 50 to 100 mL D_5W given over 1 hour and then 0.5 to 1 g per hour may be required for continued arrhythmia suppression.

Patients with arrhythmias refractory to pharmacologic therapy should be treated with Fab fragment antibodies.[129,130]

Management of Digitalis-Induced Stable VT

Fab Fragment Antibodies

When digitalis toxicity induces stable VT, Fab fragment antibodies combined with rapidly active antiarrhythmics are the treatment of choice.[122]

Lidocaine Infusion

A lidocaine bolus of 1 to 1.5 mg/kg is the best initial antiarrhythmic therapy. If the patient responds, begin a lidocaine infusion of 1 to 4 mg/min until the Fab fragment therapy is effective.

Magnesium Sulfate

Give magnesium sulfate 1 to 2 g (diluted in 10 mL D_5W) IV push over 1 to 2 minutes if there appears to be no response to the lidocaine. If a pharmacologic cardioversion occurs after the lidocaine and magnesium infusions, start a continuous magnesium infusion of 1 to 2 g (8 to 16 mEq) diluted in 50 to 100 mL D_5W for the next 30 to 60 minutes. This interval allows sufficient time for the Fab fragment to be administered and take effect. Patients with renal compromise may have developed digoxin toxicity on a renal basis, and magnesium administration poses a risk of iatrogenic arrhythmias for these patients.

FYI

Repeat Defibrillation After Fab Therapy

Attempt defibrillation approximately every 60 seconds until conversion is achieved or the arrest is terminated. Fab fragments take some time to bind to the digoxin in the body and bloodstream. When Fab fragments have been administered, more prolonged resuscitative efforts are indicated to allow time for the antibodies to be effective.

Management of Digitalis-Induced Unstable VT

Once digitalis-induced VT becomes clinically unstable, the treatment priorities are

- Synchronized cardioversion
- Immediate administration of Fab fragment antibodies
- Lidocaine
- Magnesium sulfate

Fab Fragment Antibodies

- Administer 10 to 20 vials of Fab fragments.

Lidocaine

- Give a loading dose of lidocaine of 1.5 mg/kg IV.
- If the patient responds to the lidocaine, begin a continuous infusion of 1 to 4 mg/min until the Fab fragment therapy takes effect.

Magnesium Sulfate

- Give magnesium sulfate 1 to 2 g diluted in 10 mL D$_5$W IV push over 1 to 2 minutes if there appears to be no response to the lidocaine. If there still appears to be no response to the lidocaine, give up to 5 to 10 g over the next 2 to 5 minutes.
- If pharmacologic cardioversion occurs after the lidocaine and magnesium infusions, start a continuous magnesium infusion of 1 to 2 g (8 to 16 mEq) diluted in 50 to 100 mL D$_5$W for the next 30 to 60 minutes. This interval allows sufficient time for the Fab fragments to be administered and take effect.

Management of Digitalis-Induced VF

Two Major Variations in Standard ACLS Protocols

Ventricular fibrillation due to digitalis overdose requires modifications to the standard ACLS guidelines. The Primary and Secondary ABCD Surveys should evolve in the standard pattern through the administration of epinephrine or vasopressin and shocks. Modify antiarrhythmic therapy and administer Fab fragments as indicated below:

- *Lidocaine* 1 to 1.5 mg/kg IV push
- Then administer *magnesium sulfate* 1 to 2 g diluted in 10 mL D$_5$W IV push
- *Fab fragment antibodies* 20 vials (or as many as available up to 20)

While awaiting response to Fab fragment therapy:

- *Magnesium sulfate* 1 to 2 g diluted in 10 mL D$_5$W IV push; repeat every minute up to a total of 5 to 10 g
- *Lidocaine* 0.5 mg/kg IV push; repeat every 8 to 10 minutes up to a total of 3 mg/kg

References

1. Mills CA, Flacke JW, Flacke WE, Bloor BC, Liu MD. Narcotic reversal in hypercapnic dogs: comparison of naloxone and nalbuphine. *Can J Anaesth*. 1990;37:238-244.

2. Kienbaum P, Scherbaum N, Thurauf N, Michel MC, Gastpar M, Peters J. Acute detoxification of opioid-addicted patients with naloxone during propofol or methohexital anesthesia: a comparison of withdrawal symptoms, neuroendocrine, metabolic, and cardiovascular patterns. *Crit Care Med*. 2000;28:969-976.

3. Gill AM, Cousins A, Nunn AJ, Choonara IA. Opiate-induced respiratory depression in pediatric patients. *Ann Pharmacother*. 1996;30:125-129.

4. Vilke GM, Buchanan J, Dunford JV, Chan TC. Are heroin overdose deaths related to patient release after prehospital treatment with naloxone? *Prehosp Emerg Care*. 1999;3:183-186.

5. Moss ST, Chan TC, Buchanan J, Dunford JV, Vilke GM. Outcome study of prehospital patients signed out against medical advice by field paramedics. *Ann Emerg Med*. 1998;31:247-250.

6. Bosse GM, Pope TM. Recurrent digoxin overdose and treatment with digoxin-specific Fab antibody fragments. *J Emerg Med*. 1994;12:179-185.

7. Eddleston M, Rajapakse S, Rajakanthan K, Jayalath S, Sjostrom L, Santharaj W, Thenabadu PN, Sheriff MH, Warrell DA. Anti-digoxin Fab fragments in cardiotoxicity induced by ingestion of yellow oleander: a randomised controlled trial. *Lancet*. 2000;355:967-972.

8. Dasgupta A, Szelei-Stevens KA. Neutralization of free digoxin-like immunoreactive components of oriental medicines Dan Shen and Lu-Shen-Wan by the Fab fragment of antidigoxin antibody (Digibind). *Am J Clin Pathol*. 2004;121:276-281.

9. Tracey JA, Cassidy N, Casey PB, Ali I. Bupropion (Zyban) toxicity. *Ir Med J*. 2002;95:23-24.

10. Lange RA, Hillis LD. Cardiovascular complications of cocaine use. *N Engl J Med*. 2001;345:351-358.

11. Lange RA, Willard JE. The cardiovascular effects of cocaine. *Heart Dis Stroke*. 1993;2:136-141.

12. Burns MJ, Linden CH, Graudins A, Brown RM, Fletcher KE. A comparison of physostigmine and benzodiazepines for the treatment of anticholinergic poisoning. *Ann Emerg Med*. 2000;35:374-381.

13. Brown TC. Tricyclic antidepressant overdosage: experimental studies on the management of circulatory complications. *Clin Toxicol*. 1976;9:255-272.

14. Brown TC, Barker GA, Dunlop ME, Loughnan PM. The use of sodium bicarbonate in the treatment of tricyclic antidepressant-induced arrhythmias. *Anaesth Intensive Care*. 1973;1:203-210.

15. Hoffman JR, McElroy CR. Bicarbonate therapy for dysrhythmia and hypotension in tricyclic antidepressant overdose. *West J Med*. 1981;134:60-64.

16. Bailey PM, Little M, Jelinek GA, Wilce JA. Jellyfish envenoming syndromes: unknown toxic mechanisms and unproven therapies. *Med J Aust*. 2003;178:34-37.

17. Proano L, Chiang WK, Wang RY. Calcium channel blocker overdose. *Am J Emerg Med*. 1995;13:444-450.

18. Mayron R, Ruiz E. Phenytoin: does it reverse tricyclic-antidepressant-induced cardiac conduction abnormalities? *Ann Emerg Med*. 1986;15:876-880.

19. Callaham M, Schumaker H, Pentel P. Phenytoin prophylaxis of cardiotoxicity in experimental amitriptyline poisoning. *J Pharmacol Exp Ther*. 1988;245:216-220.

20. Citak A, Soysal DD, Ucsel R, Karabocuoglu M, Uzel N. Efficacy of long duration resuscitation and magnesium sulphate treatment in amitriptyline poisoning. *Eur J Emerg Med*. 2002;9:63-66.

21. Knudsen K, Abrahamsson J. Effects of magnesium sulfate and lidocaine in the treatment of ventricular arrhythmias in experimental amitriptyline poisoning in the rat. *Crit Care Med*. 1994;22:494-498.

22. Shih RD, Hollander JE, Burstein JL, Nelson LS, Hoffman RS, Quick AM. Clinical safety of lidocaine in patients with cocaine-associated myocardial infarction. *Ann Emerg Med*. 1995;26:702-706.

23. Gowda RM, Khan IA, Wilbur SL, Vasavada BC, Sacchi TJ. Torsade de pointes: the clinical considerations. *Int J Cardiol*. 2004;96:1-6.

24. Vernon D, Banner W, Dean M. Dopamine and norepinephrine are equally effective for treatment of shock in amitriptyline intoxication. *Crit Care Med*. 1990;18:S239.

25. Vernon DD, Banner W Jr, Garrett JS, Dean JM. Efficacy of dopamine and norepinephrine for treatment of hemodynamic compromise in amitriptyline intoxication. *Crit Care Med*. 1991;19:544-549.

26. Wenzel V, Lindner KH. Employing vasopressin during cardiopulmonary resuscitation and vasodilatory shock as a lifesaving vasopressor. *Cardiovasc Res*. 2001;51:529-541.

27. Ramsay ID. Survival after imipramine poisoning. *Lancet*. 1967;2:1308-1309.

28. Southall DP, Kilpatrick SM. Imipramine poisoning: survival of a child after prolonged cardiac massage. *Br Med J*. 1974;4:508.

29. Kollef MH. Labetalol overdose successfully treated with amrinone and α-adrenergic receptor agonists. *Chest*. 1994;105:626-627.

30. Wolf LR, Spadafora MP, Otten EJ. Use of amrinone and glucagon in a case of calcium channel blocker overdose. *Ann Emerg Med*. 1993;22:1225-1228.

31. Love JN, Hanfling D, Howell JM. Hemodynamic effects of calcium chloride in a canine model of acute propranolol intoxication. *Ann Emerg Med*. 1996;28:1-6.

32. Love JN, Sachdeva DK, Bessman ES, Curtis LA, Howell JM. A potential role for glucagon in the treatment of drug-induced symptomatic bradycardia. *Chest*. 1998;114:323-326.

33. Burkhart KK. Intravenous propranolol reverses hypertension after sympathomimetic overdose: two case reports. *J Toxicol Clin Toxicol*. 1992;30:109-114.

34. Durward A, Guerguerian AM, Lefebvre M, Shemie SD. Massive diltiazem overdose treated with extracorporeal membrane oxygenation. *Pediatr Crit Care Med*. 2003;4:372-376.

35. Holzer M, Behringer W, Schorkhuber W, Zeiner A, Sterz F, Laggner AN, Frass M, Siostrozonek P, Ratheiser K, Kaff A. Mild hypothermia and outcome after CPR. Hypothermia for Cardiac Arrest (HACA) Study Group. *Acta Anaesthesiol Scand Suppl*. 1997;111:55-58.

36. Hebert MJ, Boucher A, Beaucage G, Girard R, Dandavino R. Transplantation of kidneys from a donor with carbon monoxide poisoning. *N Engl J Med*. 1992;326:1571.

37. Hollander JE, Hoffman RS, Gennis P, Fairweather P, DiSano MJ, Schumb DA, Feldman JA, Fish SS, Dyer S, Wax P, et al. Nitroglycerin in the treatment of cocaine associated chest pain—clinical safety and efficacy. *J Toxicol Clin Toxicol*. 1994;32:243-256.

38. Brogan WC III, Lange RA, Kim AS, Moliterno DJ, Hillis LD. Alleviation of cocaine-induced coronary vasoconstriction by nitroglycerin. *J Am Coll Cardiol*. 1991;18:581-586.

39. Lange RA, Cigarroa RG, Yancy CW Jr, Willard JE, Popma JJ, Sills MN, McBride W, Kim AS, Hillis LD. Cocaine-induced coronary-artery vasoconstriction. *N Engl J Med*. 1989;321:1557-1562.

40. Gay GR. Clinical management of acute and chronic cocaine poisoning. *Ann Emerg Med*. 1982;11:562-572.

41. Dusenberry SJ, Hicks MJ, Mariani PJ. Labetalol treatment of cocaine toxicity. *Ann Emerg Med*. 1987;16:235.

42. Boehrer JD, Moliterno DJ, Willard JE, Hillis LD, Lange RA. Influence of labetalol on cocaine-induced coronary vasoconstriction in humans. *Am J Med*. 1993;94:608-610.

43. Lange RA, Cigarroa RG, Flores ED, McBride W, Kim AS, Wells PJ, Bedotto JB, Danziger RS, Hillis LD. Potentiation of cocaine-induced coronary vasoconstriction by β-adrenergic blockade. *Ann Intern Med*. 1990;112:897-903.

44. Sand IC, Brody SL, Wrenn KD, Slovis CM. Experience with esmolol for the treatment of cocaine-associated cardiovascular complications. *Am J Emerg Med*. 1991;9:161-163.

45. Albertson TE, Dawson A, de Latorre F, Hoffman RS, Hollander JE, Jaeger A, Kerns WR II, Martin TG, Ross MP. TOX-ACLS: toxicologic-oriented advanced cardiac life support. *Ann Emerg Med*. 2001;37(4 suppl):S78-S90.

46. Hoffman RS, Hollander JE. Thrombolytic therapy and cocaine-induced myocardial infarction. *Am J Emerg Med*. 1996;14:693-695.

47. Hollander JE, Hoffman RS, Burstein JL, Shih RD, Thode HC Jr. Cocaine-associated myocardial infarction. Mortality and complications. Cocaine-Associated Myocardial Infarction Study Group. *Arch Intern Med*. 1995;155:1081-1086.

48. 2005 American Heart Association Guidelines for Cardiopulmonary Resuscitation and Emergency Cardiovascular Care. *Circulation*. 2005;112:IV1-IV203.

49. Pearigen PD, Benowitz NL. Poisoning due to calcium antagonists: experience with verapamil, diltiazem and nifedipine. *Drug Saf*. 1991;6:408-430.

50. Jackson CD, Fishbein L. A toxicological review of β-adrenergic blockers. *Fundam Appl Toxicol*. 1986;6:395-422.

51. Erickson FC, Ling LJ, Grande GA, Anderson DL. Diltiazem overdose: case report and review. *J Emerg Med*. 1991;9:357-366.

52. Weinstein RS. Recognition and management of poisoning with β-adrenergic blocking agents. *Ann Emerg Med*. 1984;13:1123-1131.

53. Kulig K, Bar-Or D, Cantrill SV, Rosen P, Rumack BH. Management of acutely poisoned patients without gastric emptying. *Ann Emerg Med*. 1985;14:562-567.

54. Park GD, Spector R, Goldberg MJ, Johnson GF. Expanded role of charcoal therapy in the poisoned and overdosed patient. *Arch Intern Med*. 1986;146:969-973.

55. Wrenn K, Rodewald L, Dockstader L. Potential misuse of ipecac. *Ann Emerg Med*. 1993;22:1408-1412.

56. Oe H, Taniura T, Ohgitani N. A case of severe verapamil overdose. *Jpn Circ J*. 1998;62:72-76.

57. Kline JA, Tomaszewski CA, Schroeder JD, Raymond RM. Insulin is a superior antidote for cardiovascular toxicity induced by verapamil in the anesthetized canine. *J Pharmacol Exp Ther*. 1993;267:744-750.

58. Yuan TH, Kerns WPI, Tomaszewski CA, Ford MD, Kline JA. Insulin-glucose as adjunctive therapy for severe calcium channel antagonist poisoning. *J Toxicol Clin Toxicol*. 1999;37:463-474.

59. Zaritsky AL, Horowitz M, Chernow B. Glucagon antagonism of calcium channel blocker–induced myocardial dysfunction. *Crit Care Med*. 1988;16:246-251.

60. Holzer M, Sterz F, Schoerkhuber W, Behringer W, Domanovits H, Weinmar D, Weinstabl C, Stimpfl T. Successful resuscitation of a verapamil-intoxicated patient with percutaneous cardiopulmonary bypass. *Crit Care Med*. 1999;27:2818-2823.

61. Waxman AB, White KP, Trawick DR. Electromechanical dissociation following verapamil and propranolol ingestion: a physiologic profile. *Cardiology*. 1997;88:478-481.

62. Snook CP, Sigvaldason K, Kristinsson J. Severe atenolol and diltiazem overdose. *J Toxicol Clin Toxicol*. 2000;38:661-665.

63. Pertoldi F, D'Orlando L, Mercante WP. Electromechanical dissociation 48 hours after atenolol overdose: usefulness of calcium chloride. *Ann Emerg Med*. 1998;31:777-781.

64. Cregler LL, Mark H. Medical complications of cocaine abuse. *N Engl J Med*. 1986;315:1495-1500.

65. Jekel JF, Allen DF, Podlewski H, Clarke N, Dean-Patterson S, Cartwright P. Epidemic free-base cocaine abuse. Case study from the Bahamas. *Lancet*. 1986;1:459-462.

66. Farrar HC, Kearns GL. Cocaine: clinical pharmacology and toxicology. *J Pediatr*. 1989;115(pt 1):665-675.

67. Lowenstein DH, Massa SM, Rowbotham MC, Collins SD, McKinney HE, Simon RP. Acute neurologic and psychiatric complications associated with cocaine abuse. *Am J Med*. 1987;83:841-846.

68. Gradman AH. Cardiac effects of cocaine: a review. *Yale J Biol Med*. 1988;61:137-147.

69. Barth CW III, Bray M, Roberts WC. Rupture of the ascending aorta during cocaine intoxication. *Am J Cardiol*. 1986;57:496.

70. Brody SL, Slovis CM, Wrenn KD. Cocaine-related medical problems: consecutive series of 233 patients. *Am J Med*. 1990;88:325-331.

71. Derlet RW, Albertson TE. Emergency department presentation of cocaine intoxication. *Ann Emerg Med*. 1989;18:182-186.

72. Rich JA, Singer DE. Cocaine-related symptoms in patients presenting to an urban emergency department. *Ann Emerg Med*. 1991;20:616-621.

73. Kloner RA, Hale S, Alker K, Rezkalla S. The effects of acute and chronic cocaine use on the heart. *Circulation*. 1992;85:407-419.

74. Isner JM, Estes NA III, Thompson PD, Costanzo-Nordin MR, Subramanian R, Miller G, Katsas G, Sweeney K, Sturner WQ. Acute cardiac events temporally related to cocaine abuse. *N Engl J Med*. 1986;315:1438-1443.

75. Derlet RW, Albertson TE, Tharratt RS. Lidocaine potentiation of cocaine toxicity. *Ann Emerg Med*. 1991;20:135-138.

76. Kerns W II, Garvey L, Owens J. Cocaine-induced wide complex dysrhythmia. *J Emerg Med*. 1997;15:321-329.

77. Wang RY. pH-dependent cocaine-induced cardiotoxicity. *Am J Emerg Med*. 1999;17:364-369.

78. Williams RG, Kavanagh KM, Teo KK. Pathophysiology and treatment of cocaine toxicity: implications for the heart and cardiovascular system. *Can J Cardiol*. 1996;12:1295-1301.

79. Noel B. Cardiovascular complications of cocaine use. *N Engl J Med*. 2001;345:1575, author reply 1576.

80. Beckman KJ, Parker RB, Hariman RJ, Gallastegui JL, Javaid JI, Bauman JL. Hemodynamic and electrophysiological actions of cocaine: effects of sodium bicarbonate as an antidote in dogs. *Circulation*. 1991;83:1799-1807.

81. Parker RB, Perry GY, Horan LG, Flowers NC. Comparative effects of sodium bicarbonate and sodium chloride on reversing cocaine-induced changes in the electrocardiogram. *J Cardiovasc Pharmacol*. 1999;34:864-869.

82. Silverstein W, Lewin NA, Goldfrank L. Management of the cocaine-intoxicated patient. *Ann Emerg Med*. 1987;16:234-235.

83. Ramoska E, Sacchetti AD. Propranolol-induced hypertension in treatment of cocaine intoxication. *Ann Emerg Med*. 1985;14:1112-1113.

84. Gay GR, Loper KA. The use of labetalol in the management of cocaine crisis. *Ann Emerg Med*. 1988;17:282-283.

85. Briggs RS, Birtwell AJ, Pohl JE. Hypertensive response to labetalol in phaeochromocytoma. *Lancet*. 1978;1:1045-1046.

86. Hollander JE, Carter WA, Hoffman RS. Use of phentolamine for cocaine-induced myocardial ischemia. *N Engl J Med*. 1992;327:361.

87. Mody CK, Miller BL, McIntyre HB, Cobb SK, Goldberg MA. Neurologic complications of cocaine abuse. *Neurology*. 1988;38:1189-1193.

88. Hoffman CK, Goodman PC. Pulmonary edema in cocaine smokers. *Radiology*. 1989;172:463-465.

89. Cucco RA, Yoo OH, Cregler L, Chang JC. Nonfatal pulmonary edema after "freebase" cocaine smoking. *Am Rev Respir Dis*. 1987;136:179-181.

90. Amin M, Gabelman G, Karpel J, Buttrick P. Acute myocardial infarction and chest pain syndromes after cocaine use. *Am J Cardiol*. 1990;66:1434-1437.

91. Hollander JE, Hoffman RS. Cocaine-induced myocardial infarction: an analysis and review of the literature. *J Emerg Med*. 1992;10:169-177.

92. Kimura T, Yasue H, Sakaino N, Rokutanda M, Jougasaki M, Araki H. Effects of magnesium on the tone of isolated human coronary arteries. Comparison with diltiazem and nitroglycerin. *Circulation*. 1989;79:1118-1124.

93. Woods KL, Fletcher S, Roffe C, Haider Y. Intravenous magnesium sulphate in suspected acute myocardial infarction: results of the second Leicester Intravenous Magnesium Intervention Trial (LIMIT-2). *Lancet*. 1992;339:1553-1558.

94. Gitter MJ, Goldsmith SR, Dunbar DN, Sharkey SW. Cocaine and chest pain: clinical features and outcome of patients hospitalized to rule out myocardial infarction. *Ann Intern Med*. 1991;115:277-282.

95. Mittleman MA, Mintzer D, Maclure M, Tofler GH, Sherwood JB, Muller JE. Triggering of myocardial infarction by cocaine. *Circulation*. 1999;99:2737-2741.

96. Nademanee K, Gorelick DA, Josephson MA, Ryan MA, Wilkins JN, Robertson HA, Mody FV, Intarachot V. Myocardial ischemia during cocaine withdrawal. *Ann Intern Med*. 1989;111:876-880.

97. Hollander JE, Hoffman RS, Gennis P, Fairweather P, DiSano MJ, Schumb DA, Feldman JA, Fish SS, Dyer S, Wax P, et al. Prospective multicenter evaluation of cocaine-associated chest pain. Cocaine Associated Chest Pain (COCHPA) Study Group. *Acad Emerg Med*. 1994;1:330-339.

98. Hollander JE, Shih RD, Hoffman RS, Harchelroad FP, Phillips S, Brent J, Kulig K, Thode HC Jr. Predictors of coronary artery disease in patients with cocaine-associated myocardial infarction. Cocaine-Associated Myocardial Infarction (CAMI) Study Group. *Am J Med*. 1997;102:158-163.

99. Hoffman RS, Hollander JE. Evaluation of patients with chest pain after cocaine use. *Crit Care Clin*. 1997;13:809-828.

100. Freemantle N, Cleland J, Young P, Mason J, Harrison J. β-Blockade after myocardial infarction: systematic review and meta regression analysis. *BMJ*. 1999;318:1730-1737.

101. Baumann BM, Perrone J, Hornig SE, Shofer FS, Hollander JE. Randomized, double-blind, placebo-controlled trial of diazepam, nitroglycerin, or both for treatment of patients with potential cocaine-associated acute coronary syndromes. *Acad Emerg Med*. 2000;7:878-885.

102. Heesch CM, Wilhelm CR, Ristich J, Adnane J, Bontempo FA, Wagner WR. Cocaine activates platelets and increases the formation of circulating platelet containing microaggregates in humans. *Heart*. 2000;83:688-695.

103. Negus BH, Willard JE, Hillis LD, Glamann DB, Landau C, Snyder RW, Lange RA. Alleviation of cocaine-induced coronary vasoconstriction with intravenous verapamil. *Am J Cardiol*. 1994;73:510-513.

104. Karch SB. Managing cocaine crisis. *Ann Emerg Med*. 1989;18:228-229.

105. Litovitz TL, Holm KC, Bailey KM, Schmitz BF. 1991 annual report of the American Association of Poison Control Centers National Data Collection System. *Am J Emerg Med*. 1992;10:452-505.

106. Frommer DA, Kulig KW, Marx JA, Rumack B. Tricyclic antidepressant overdose. A review. *JAMA*. 1987;257:521-526.

107. Callaham M, Kassel D. Epidemiology of fatal tricyclic antidepressant ingestion: implications for management. *Ann Emerg Med*. 1985;14:1-9.

108. Kulig K. Initial management of ingestions of toxic substances. *N Engl J Med*. 1992;326:1677-1681.

109. Braden NJ, Jackson JE, Walson PD. Tricyclic antidepressant overdose. *Pediatr Clin North Am*. 1986;33:287-297.

110. Marshall JB, Forker AD. Cardiovascular effects of tricyclic antidepressant drugs: therapeutic usage, overdose, and management of complications. *Am Heart J*. 1982;103:401-414.

111. Blackman K, Brown SG, Wilkes GJ. Plasma alkalinization for tricyclic antidepressant toxicity: a systematic review. *Emerg Med (Fremantle)*. 2001;13:204-210.

112. Bessen HA, Niemann JT. Improvement of cardiac conduction after hyperventilation in tricyclic antidepressant overdose. *J Toxicol Clin Toxicol*. 1985;23:537-546.

113. Liberatore MA, Robinson DS. Torsade de pointes: a mechanism for sudden death associated with neuroleptic drug therapy? *J Clin Psychopharmacol*. 1984;4:143-146.

114. Tzivoni D, Banai S, Schuger C, Benhorin J, Keren A, Gottlieb S, Stern S. Treatment of torsade de pointes with magnesium sulfate. *Circulation*. 1988;77:392-397.

115. Perticone F, Adinolfi L, Bonaduce D. Efficacy of magnesium sulfate in the treatment of torsade de pointes. *Am Heart J*. 1986;112:847-849.

116. Keren A, Tzivoni D, Gavish D, Levi J, Gottlieb S, Benhorin J, Stern S. Etiology, warning signs and therapy of torsade de pointes. A study of 10 patients. *Circulation*. 1981;64:1167-1174.

117. Iseri LT, Chung P, Tobis J. Magnesium therapy for intractable ventricular tachyarrhythmias in normomagnesemic patients. *West J Med*. 1983;138:823-828.

118. Glassman AH. Cardiovascular effects of tricyclic antidepressants. *Annu Rev Med*. 1984;35:503-511.

119. Teba L, Schiebel F, Dedhia HV, Lazzell VA. Beneficial effect of norepinephrine in the treatment of circulatory shock caused by tricyclic antidepressant overdose. *Am J Emerg Med*. 1988;6:566-568.

120. Tran TP, Panacek EA, Rhee KJ, Foulke GE. Response to dopamine vs norepinephrine in tricyclic antidepressant–induced hypotension. *Acad Emerg Med*. 1997;4:864-868.

121. Knudsen K, Abrahamsson J. Epinephrine and sodium bicarbonate independently and additively increase survival in experimental amitriptyline poisoning. *Crit Care Med*. 1997;25:669-674.

122. Dick M, Curwin J, Tepper D. Digitalis intoxication recognition and management. *J Clin Pharmacol*. 1991;31:444-447.

123. Davey M, Caldicott D. Calcium salts in management of hyperkalaemia. *Emerg Med J*. 2002;19:92-93.

124. Sharff JA, Bayer MJ. Acute and chronic digitalis toxicity: presentation and treatment. *Ann Emerg Med*. 1982;11:327-331.

125. Smith TW, Butler VP Jr, Haber E, Fozzard H, Marcus FI, Bremner WF, Schulman IC, Phillips A. Treatment of life-threatening digitalis intoxication with digoxin-specific Fab antibody fragments: experience in 26 cases. *N Engl J Med*. 1982;307:1357-1362.

126. Antman EM, Smith TW. Digitalis toxicity. *Annu Rev Med*. 1985;36:357-367.

127. Reisdorff EJ, Clark MR, Walters BL. Acute digitalis poisoning: the role of intravenous magnesium sulfate. *J Emerg Med*. 1986;4:463-469.

128. Cohen L, Kitzes R. Magnesium sulfate and digitalis-toxic arrhythmias. *JAMA*. 1983;249:2808-2810.

129. Antman EM, Wenger TL, Butler VP Jr, Haber E, Smith TW. Treatment of 150 cases of life-threatening digitalis intoxication with digoxin-specific Fab antibody fragments. Final report of a multicenter study. *Circulation*. 1990;81:1744-1752.

130. Woolf AD, Wenger T, Smith TW, Lovejoy FH Jr. The use of digoxin-specific Fab fragments for severe digitalis intoxication in children. *N Engl J Med*. 1992;326:1739-1744.

Chapter 14

Special Resuscitation Situations
Part 1: Hypothermia

Introduction

Unintentional hypothermia is a serious and preventable health problem. Severe hypothermia (body temperature <30°C [<86°F]) is associated with marked depression of critical body functions that may make the patient appear clinically dead during the initial assessment. But in some cases hypothermia may exert a protective effect on the brain and organs in cardiac arrest.[1] Intact neurologic recovery may be possible after hypothermic cardiac arrest, although those with nonasphyxial arrest have a better prognosis than those with asphyxia-associated hypothermic arrest.[2-4] With this in mind, rescuers should not withhold lifesaving procedures on the basis of clinical presentation. Patients should be transported as soon as possible to a center where monitored rewarming is possible.

Epidemiology

Unintentional hypothermia is defined as a decrease in core body temperature below 35°C or 36°C (95°F or 96.8°F). ACLS providers will most often encounter patients in cardiac arrest associated with unintentional hypothermia in 1 of 3 clinical settings:

- Cold stress or exposure (often subacute) in persons with thermoregulatory impairment
- Cold weather exposure
- Cold water immersion (with or without submersion)

Cold exposure in persons with impaired thermoregulatory function is surprisingly the most frequent cause of death from hypothermia.[3,5-15] *Impaired thermoregulatory function* may develop in many patient groups: the elderly, insulin-dependent diabetics, the malnourished, the alcohol-intoxicated or drug-intoxicated, the chronically ill, and the multiply medicated, medically disabled. These patients have decreased basal metabolism, dysfunctional shivering thermogenesis, and impaired vasoconstriction.

Patients with impaired thermoregulatory function who are impoverished, semistarved, or homeless and disabled are particularly at risk for cold exposure from lack of shelter, inadequate clothing, or improper residential heat.[11,12] Authors have applied the phrase "accidental urban hypothermia" to many of these patients.[16] This "at risk" population may develop hypothermia at ambient temperatures not usually considered "cold weather." Hypothermia is most likely to develop when these patients suffer cold exposure over long periods of time.[11,12]

Cold weather exposure can produce hypothermia in healthy people with normal thermogenesis when they experience long periods of adverse weather conditions. A number of predisposing factors play a role in the development of significant hypothermia in healthy people: severity of the cold weather, insulation properties of clothing or shelter, wind chill in a windy or exposed setting, exhaustion after heavy outdoor exercise, wet clothing, inadequate caloric intake, and associated injuries (such as frostbite or fractures) that interfere with self-protective actions.

Cold water immersion can also lead to significant hypothermia in healthy people. Sudden immersion in cold water (usually defined as water temperature <21°C or <70°F) most often occurs in association with boating or recreational aquatic mishaps.[17] Cooling occurs rapidly during cold water immersion because conductive heat loss is 25 to 35 times faster in water than in air. In water at 4.44°C (40°F), mortality approaches 50% after 1 hour. For perspective on water temperatures, note that the mean January water temperature is 21°C (70°F) off Miami, 24°C (75°F) off Honolulu, 11°C (52°F) off San Francisco, 14°C (57°F) off San Diego, and 3°C (37°F) off New York

City.[17] Victims of cold water immersion also face a high risk of *cold water submersion* with resultant aspiration, asphyxia, hypoxia, and even death. The protective value of hypothermia in cold water immersion with subsequent submersion is probably exaggerated. Recent experiments suggest that cold water immersion produces exhaustion (and subsequent submersion) faster than it produces a neurologically protective degree of core hypothermia.[18-20] Nearly all reports of successful resuscitation with full neurologic recovery describe prolonged cold water submersion in icy water (<5°C or <41°F).

Therapeutic hypothermia is intentional lowering of the patient's body temperature to reduce oxygen demand and metabolic rate. This therapy is undertaken to reduce complications of inadequate perfusion or reperfusion injury. New recommendations developed by the International Liaison Committee on Resuscitation and the American Heart Association advocate the use of therapeutic hypothermia as follows:

- When the initial rhythm was ventricular fibrillation (VF), unconscious adult patients with spontaneous circulation after out-of-hospital cardiac arrest should be cooled to 32°C to 34°C (89.6°F to 93.2°F) for 12 to 24 hours.
- For any other rhythm or for cardiac arrest in hospital, such cooling may also be beneficial.

Pathophysiology

Severe hypothermia (body temperature <30°C or <86°F) is associated with marked depression of cerebral blood flow and oxygen consumption, reduced cardiac output, and decreased arterial pressure.[21] Patients can appear to be clinically dead because of marked depression of brain function.[21-23]

Hypothermia may exert a protective effect on the brain and organs during cardiac arrest if the patient cools rapidly with no hypoxia before the cardiac arrest.[1,24] If the patient cools rapidly, oxygen consumption decreases and metabolism slows before the arrest, and this reduces organ ischemia during the arrest.[25]

This protective effect appears to account for the rare occurrence of resuscitation with intact neurologic recovery after hypothermic cardiac arrest.[4] The effects of hypothermia on cerebral oxygen consumption and metabolism are thought to be the mechanism for the therapeutic effects of induced hypothermia. Induced hypothermia for comatose survivors of out-of-hospital VF cardiac arrest has produced marked improvements in survival to hospital discharge,[26] 6-month mortality rate,[27] and neurologic outcomes.[27]

Severe unintentional hypothermia is a preventable health problem associated with significant morbidity and mortality, especially in urban areas. In inner cities hypothermia has a high association with mental illness, poverty, and use of drugs and alcohol.[28,29] In some rural areas more than 90% of deaths from hypothermia are associated with elevated blood alcohol levels.[30]

Hypothermia: Definitions, Signs, and Symptoms

The severity of hypothermia is determined from the patient's core body temperature. The Table presents the most commonly used definitions of hypothermia severity, based on a range of core body temperatures:

- **Mild hypothermia** (>34°C or >93.2°F): The clinical hallmark of mild hypothermia is the onset of shivering, which can become severe. Shivering represents a centrally mediated attempt at thermogenesis.[21] The onset of mental confusion and disorientation marks the symptomatic transition from mild to moderate hypothermia.
- **Moderate hypothermia** (30°C to 34°C or 86°F to 93.2°F): The hallmark of moderate hypothermia is progressive loss of higher cognitive functions with onset of marked confusion, disorientation, stupor, and loss of consciousness. With moderate hypothermia shivering diminishes and eventually disappears completely.
- **Severe hypothermia** (<30°C or <86°F): The hallmark of severe hypothermia is unconsciousness with immobility and the progressive loss of all signs of life. The vital functions disappear completely in roughly the following order as hypothermia becomes more and more severe:
  - Loss of consciousness and all voluntary movement
  - Loss of papillary light reflexes
  - Loss of deep tendon reflexes
  - Loss of spontaneous respirations
  - Loss of organized cardiac rhythm (onset of VF)
- **Profound hypothermia** (<20°C or <68°F): Profound hypothermia may be considered as a subcategory of severe hypothermia.[22,23] This category, however, has little clinical utility because it has no therapeutic implications. Profound hypothermia is managed the same way as severe hypothermia.

  - The hallmark of profound hypothermia is the total loss of any sign of life. Cardiac activity is completely lost, and the monitor displays only asystole. The electroencephalogram is totally silent with no detectable brain activity. No distinction can be made from death.

Table. Hypothermia: Definitions, Signs and Symptoms, and Recommended Therapy

Core Temperature*		Signs and Symptoms	Recommended Therapy		
°C	°F				
Mild hypothermia[31] >34°C or >93.2°F					
36°	96.8°	Muscle tone increases ("preshivering"). Metabolic rate and blood pressure increase to adjust for heat loss. Shivering begins.	Passive external rewarming	Active external rewarming: all areas	
35°	95°	Shivering continues and reaches maximum thermogenesis level. Victim is still mentally responsive.			
34°	93.2°	Extreme subjective coldness; some amnesia and dysarthria. Poor judgment and maladaptive behavior begin. Blood pressure is adequate; tachycardia and then progressive bradycardia occur.			
Moderate hypothermia 30°C to 34°C or 86°F to 93.2°F					
33°	91.4°	Mental confusion increases; ataxia; apathy; shivering decreases. Maximum respiratory stimulation with tachypnea, then progressive drop in minute volume.	Passive external rewarming	Active external rewarming: truncal areas only	
32°	89.6°	Consciousness is much more clouded; victim may become stuporous. Shivering almost stopped. Oxygen consumption <75% normal. Pupils may be dilated.			
31°	87.8°	Thermogenesis through shivering stops. Severe peripheral vasoconstriction; blood pressure is difficult to obtain.			
30°	86°	Muscles increasingly rigid; more loss of consciousness; risk of atrial fibrillation and other arrhythmias. Cardiac output drops to <67% of normal.			
Severe hypothermia <30°C or <86°F (purple shading = risk of VF with rough movements)					
29°	84.2°	Pulse and respirations slow perceptibly; cardiac arrhythmias become more frequent. Pupils usually dilated. Paradoxical undressing observed.	Passive external rewarming	Active external rewarming: truncal areas only	Active internal rewarming
28°	82.4°	**High risk of VF if heart is irritated from rough movements. Oxygen consumption <50% normal.**			
27°	80.6°	**Consciousness usually lost; all voluntary motion stops.**			

(Continued)

Core Temperature*		Signs and Symptoms	Recommended Therapy		
°C	°F		Passive external rewarming	Active external rewarming: truncal areas only	Active internal rewarming
26°	78.8°	Deep tendon and pupillary light reflexes usually absent. Victim can appear dead.			
25°	77°	VF can occur spontaneously even without irritation.			
24°	75.2°	Pulmonary edema, severe hypotension, and severe bradycardia may develop.			
23°	73.4°	VF risk very high; deathlike appearance; no corneal or oculocephalic reflexes.			
22°	71.6°	VF occurs spontaneously in majority of victims. Oxygen consumption <25% normal.			
21°	69.8°	VF amplitude diminishes.			
20°	68°	VF becomes very fine, more like "coarse asystole"; EEG signals flatten.			
Profound hypothermia (<20°C or <68°F)					
19°	66.2°	Either PEA or asystole; EEG almost flat.			
18°	64.4°	Almost invariably asystole.			
17°	62.6°	EEG totally silent.			
16°	60.8	Total irreversible cardiac and brain death (except in rare cases).			
15°	59°	Lowest recorded infant core temperature with intact neurologic recovery from accidental hypothermia.[63]			
13.7°	56.6°	Lowest recorded adult core temperature with full neurologic recovery from accidental hypothermia.[4]			
10°	50°	Oxygen consumption <8% normal.			
9°	48.2°	Lowest recorded core temperature for survival from therapeutic hypothermia.[23]			

*Adapted with permission from *ACLS Scenarios: Core Concepts for Case-Based Learning* by R.O. Cummins (Copyright 1996 Mosby, Inc.) with additional data from references 21-23.

— There have been rare case reports of successful resuscitation of patients with profound hypothermia using internal rewarming. Few of these patients have demonstrated complete neurologic recovery.[4]

The Hypothermia Algorithm (Figure) shows how the answers to these 2 questions determine the recommended actions for patients with unintentional hypothermia.

General Care of All Hypothermia Patients

The answers to 2 clinical questions shape the treatment of unintentional hypothermia:

- First, is the patient in cardiopulmonary arrest?
- Second, what is the core temperature?

When the patient is extremely cold but has maintained a perfusing rhythm, the provider should focus on interventions that prevent further heat loss and begin to rewarm the patient. If the hypothermic patient has not yet developed cardiac arrest, handle the patient gently for all procedures; physical manipulations have been reported to precipitate VF.[3,31] General care includes the following procedures:

- Prevent additional evaporative heat loss by removing wet garments and insulating the patient from further environmental exposure.
- Do not delay urgent procedures, such as intubation and insertion of vascular catheters, but perform them gently while closely monitoring cardiac rhythm. These patients are prone to develop VF.

Prearrest Interventions
Determine Core Body Temperature

The patient's core body temperature will determine subsequent treatment decisions. The core temperature is measured using a rectal or tympanic membrane thermometer. Standard mercury-filled glass thermometers are useful for mild hypothermia only because they do not register temperatures below 34°C (93.2°F). Lower-reading rectal probe thermometers with electronic-digital circuitry are readily available. They should be standard equipment in all emergency medical services vehicles, emergency departments (EDs), and first aid stations where hypothermic patients might require care.

Patients with a core temperature >34°C (>93.2°F) may be passively rewarmed with warm blankets and a warm environment. This form of rewarming will not be adequate for a patient with cardiopulmonary arrest or severe hypothermia.[10] For patients with moderate to severe hypothermia, therapy is determined by the presence or absence of a perfusing rhythm. General management of the patient with moderate to severe hypothermia and a perfusing rhythm is as follows:

- Moderate (30°C to 34°C [86°F to 93.2°F]): active external rewarming
- Severe (<30°C [86°F]): active internal rewarming; consider extracorporeal membrane oxygenation

Prehospital Interventions

In the prehospital setting, if the patient maintains a perfusing rhythm, providers focus on prevention of cardiac arrest. To prevent cardiac arrest, take the following steps:

- Prevent further heat loss
- Begin passive rewarming
- Begin clinical monitoring, particularly measurement of core temperature and monitoring of cardiac rhythm
- Provide rapid transport to definitive care

Prevent further conductive, convective, evaporative, and radiant heat losses by shielding the patient from wind, removing wet garments, and insulating the patient with blankets (especially reflective metallic-foil wraps), insulated sleeping bags and pads, dry clothing, or even newspapers or cardboard. Begin the process of passive rewarming with the insulating and shielding actions noted above.

Try to keep hypothermic patients in a horizontal position from the time of initial rescue and extrication (as feasible). Hypothermic patients are often volume depleted from "cold diuresis" with dysfunctional cardiovascular regulatory mechanisms. Avoid excess movement or rough activity. But do not delay urgently needed procedures such as rescue breathing, intubation, insertion of a vascular catheter, or even CPR chest compressions. Perform procedures gently, and monitor cardiac rhythm closely. An exaggerated fear of "precipitating VF" and other arrhythmias in hypothermic patients should not cause prehospital personnel to withhold essential interventions.

Spontaneous VF or VF secondary to jarring movements becomes a realistic risk only at severe levels of hypothermia (<30°C or <86°F).

Monitor Core Temperature and Rhythm

Monitor the cardiac rhythm. If the patient's skin is extremely cold, it may be impossible to record the cardiac rhythm using adhesive electrodes. In such cases you may use a sterile needle (1.5 inch, 22 gauge works well) to attach the electrodes to the skin. Use the needle as you would use a safety pin. Insert the needle through the electrode, through a small piece of skin, and back through the electrode.

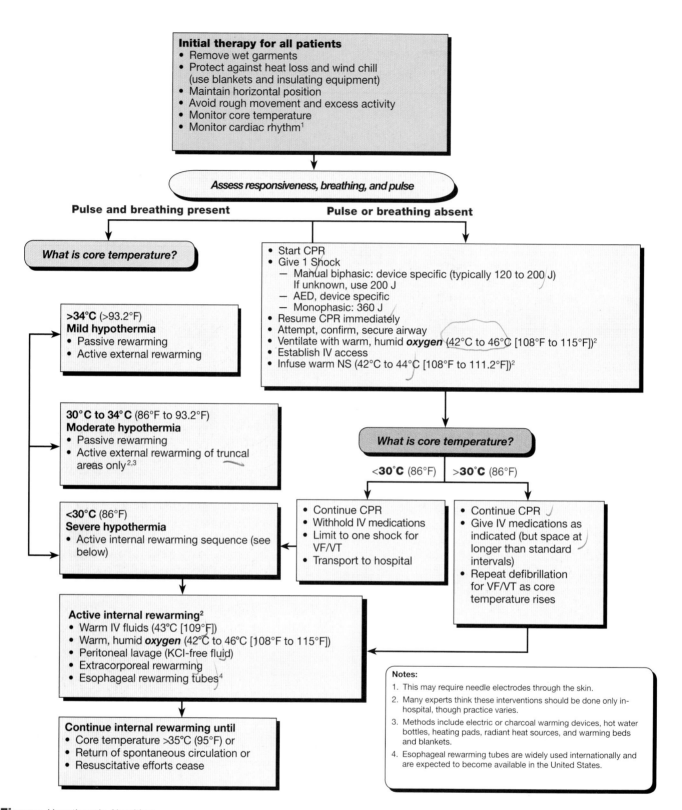

Figure. Hypothermia Algorithm.

Initial therapy for all patients
- Remove wet garments
- Protect against heat loss and wind chill (use blankets and insulating equipment)
- Maintain horizontal position
- Avoid rough movement and excess activity
- Monitor core temperature
- Monitor cardiac rhythm[1]

Assess responsiveness, breathing, and pulse

Pulse and breathing present

What is core temperature?

>34°C (>93.2°F)
Mild hypothermia
- Passive rewarming
- Active external rewarming

30°C to 34°C (86°F to 93.2°F)
Moderate hypothermia
- Passive rewarming
- Active external rewarming of truncal areas only[2,3]

<30°C (86°F)
Severe hypothermia
- Active internal rewarming sequence (see below)

Active internal rewarming[2]
- Warm IV fluids (43°C [109°F])
- Warm, humid *oxygen* (42°C to 46°C [108°F to 115°F])
- Peritoneal lavage (KCl-free fluid)
- Extracorporeal rewarming
- Esophageal rewarming tubes[4]

Continue internal rewarming until
- Core temperature >35°C (95°F) or
- Return of spontaneous circulation or
- Resuscitative efforts cease

Pulse or breathing absent
- Start CPR
- Give 1 Shock
  - Manual biphasic: device specific (typically 120 to 200 J) If unknown, use 200 J
  - AED, device specific
  - Monophasic: 360 J
- Resume CPR immediately
- Attempt, confirm, secure airway
- Ventilate with warm, humid *oxygen* (42°C to 46°C [108°F to 115°F])[2]
- Establish IV access
- Infuse warm NS (42°C to 44°C [108°F to 111.2°F])[2]

What is core temperature?

<30°C (86°F)
- Continue CPR
- Withhold IV medications
- Limit to one shock for VF/VT
- Transport to hospital

>30°C (86°F)
- Continue CPR
- Give IV medications as indicated (but space at longer than standard intervals)
- Repeat defibrillation for VF/VT as core temperature rises

Notes:
1. This may require needle electrodes through the skin.
2. Many experts think these interventions should be done only in-hospital, though practice varies.
3. Methods include electric or charcoal warming devices, hot water bottles, heating pads, radiant heat sources, and warming beds and blankets.
4. Esophageal rewarming tubes are widely used internationally and are expected to become available in the United States.

Rewarming Techniques

Management of the patient with hypothermia and a perfusing rhythm is determined by the core temperature.

Mild Hypothermia: >34°C (>93.2°F)

- Two methods are used to rewarm patients with mild hypothermia:
  - Passive rewarming (always)
  - Active external rewarming (when indicated; see below)

Passive Rewarming

As a general rule passive rewarming is the treatment of choice for hypothermia patients who can shiver (shivering thermogenesis stops at core temperatures below 32°C or 89.6°F). A wide variety of insulating materials are effective for passive rewarming. Blankets and reflective metallic-foil wraps are the most common. Passive rewarming occurs through internal heat generation by the patient. Rewarming rates are relatively slow, in the range of only 0.25°C to 0.5°C (0.45°F to 0.9°F) per hour.[32] In some studies, however, passive rewarming during out-of-hospital care was associated with a *fall* in core temperature.[33] Providers should also initiate and maintain passive rewarming for patients with moderate or severe hypothermia (see the Table). But passive rewarming alone will not effectively raise core body temperature for these patients or patients in cardiac arrest with any level of hypothermia.[25]

Active External Rewarming

Active external rewarming of all areas can be accomplished with a variety of *heating* and *heated* devices. Examples of heating devices are radiant heat, forced hot air, or warm bath water. Heating devices include warmed plastic bags of intravenous (IV) solutions, heated blankets, or chemical-reaction warm packs. In general do not place heated devices directly on the patient's skin. Both the patient and the device must be monitored. With all active external rewarming devices, especially chemical warm packs, verify that the temperature of the warming pack does not increase enough to cause skin burns. This is a particular risk for insensate patients with hypothermia. There are reports of chemical heating packs reaching hazardous temperatures.

In this form of passive rewarming, the entire body, including all 4 extremities and fingers and toes, are warmed. There is risk in external rewarming. As the arms and legs are rewarmed externally, rapid dilation of peripheral blood vessels occurs. As this cold blood returns to the central circulation, core body temperature may continue to fall—a phenomenon informally termed *afterdrop*. *Topical application of heated devices—especially to the fingers and toes—may result in tissue injury because peripheral tissues are often*

severely vasoconstricted. Apply heated devices like warm packs to truncal areas only (neck, armpits, or groin).

Moderate Hypothermia: 30°C to 34°C (86°F to <93.2°F)

The approach to patients with moderate hypothermia is also rewarming using 2 methods:

- Passive rewarming
- Active external rewarming: *truncal areas only*

Active external rewarming for moderate and severe hypothermia should specifically *exclude* rewarming of the arms and legs. The afterdrop phenomenon occurs much more frequently with moderate and severe hypothermia. In addition, *afterdrop acidosis* is more of a risk if the arms and legs are included in active external rewarming efforts. Active external rewarming of truncal areas can be accomplished in several ways.

Many of the innovative commercial rewarming techniques, such as forced hot air and warm water baths, cannot be used because these methods will not exclude the extremities. In wilderness medicine body-to-body contact inside an insulated bag has been used to increase core temperature at rates similar to spontaneous shivering.[34] The most convenient and least expensive device for truncal rewarming is the classic hot water bottle, disguised in most EDs as warmed plastic bags of IV fluids. (*Note:* Microwave warming of crystalloid fluids has been shown to be thermally safe.[35]) The addition of 1 or 2 standard electric heating pads under the patient's back and waist provides frugal yet respectable core temperature rewarming rates of about 1°C (1.8°F) per hour.[32] Forced-air warming blankets, with or without canopies,[36] are effective devices widely used for postoperative hypothermia.[37] They can produce rewarming rates of 1°C to 3°C (1.8°F to 5.4°F) per hour.[38] These devices have successfully rewarmed patients in hypothermic cardiac arrest; thus they may be useful in areas where cardiopulmonary bypass facilities are unavailable.[39] More elaborate and expensive techniques are available. These techniques include electric-powered warming vests; combustible-fueled warming belts and vests using charcoal, butane gas, or flammable liquids; and sophisticated truncal-centric heating mattresses.

Most heating devices should be applied first to the groin and axillary regions. Placement at these locations allows healthcare personnel unrestricted access to the patient's chest, neck, and arms for monitoring, diagnostic testing, and IV access. Active external rewarming of truncal areas can rewarm at a rate of about 1°C (1.8°F) per hour.[32] The number (and temperature) of heated devices applied to truncal areas determines the rewarming rate. Rewarming devices arrayed in the groin and axillae, around the neck, and next over the abdomen and then the chest can achieve even faster rewarming rates.

Severe Hypothermia: <30°C (<86°F)

The unique treatment for severe hypothermia is the addition of *active internal rewarming.* During active internal rewarming both passive rewarming and active external rewarming of truncal areas should continue (see the Table).

Healthcare personnel can accomplish active internal rewarming with several techniques. No randomized, controlled clinical trials comparing the efficacy of these methods have been reported.[25] Active internal rewarming should start with simple, inexpensive, and minimally invasive techniques, such as warm IV fluids and warm, humid oxygen. Active internal rewarming techniques also include more complex and invasive interventions. *Peritoneal lavage* is one example of "run-in/run-out heated lavage." These moderately invasive techniques include lavage of the stomach, colon, bladder, pleural cavity, and mediastinum.

- *Extracorporeal rewarming* includes full aortic-caval cannulation cardiopulmonary bypass[40] and a variety of femoral artery-vein (arterial-venous) and femoral vein-vein (veno-venous) bypass[41] methods.
- *Esophageal rewarming tubes* can be inserted.

During active internal rewarming of hypothermic patients in cardiac arrest, rescuers should remember the following:

- Use as many rewarming techniques simultaneously as possible while continuing CPR chest compressions and maintaining access to the patient.
- Start with the simple and minimally invasive techniques. Initiate more complex approaches as more resources and personnel become available.
- The following sequence may be used:

  — When the patient arrives in the ED, active external rewarming of truncal areas has already begun. The patient should be receiving warm, humid oxygen by tracheal tube and warm saline IV infusion.
  — ED staff place an electric heating pad under the trunk and abdomen and apply warm plastic bags of IV solution to the axillae and groin.
  — The emergency physician opens a dialysis tray before inserting a peritoneal dialysis catheter to begin peritoneal lavage. In the nearby operating room, technicians are preparing a cardiac bypass device to initiate extracorporeal rewarming as soon as the surgical team arrives to start the procedure.

Active Internal Rewarming

It is difficult to initiate an effective active internal rewarming strategy outside the hospital.[42] In fact, some experts think that active internal rewarming should be done only in hospital, though practice varies.[22,23]

Warm, Humid Oxygen (Administration Temperature: 42°C to 46°C or 108°F to 115°F)

Most experts recommend administration of warm, humid oxygen as a mainstay of active internal rewarming for patients with severe hypothermia but no cardiac arrest.[21-23,43,44] This method is particularly useful when other methods of internal rewarming are unavailable or delayed.[44] With the aerosol heated to 40°C (104°F), this technique rewarms at a rate of 1°C to 1.5°C (1.8°F to 2.7°F) per hour. Heated to 45°C (113°F), the rewarming rate increases to 1.5°C to 2°C (2.7°F to 3.6°F) per hour.[16,28,45]

Warm IV Fluids (42°C to 44°C or 108°F to 111°F)

Warm IV fluid is also infused centrally at a rate of approximately 150 to 200 mL/h IV. Avoid excessive fluid administration and provide sufficient fluid to maintain urinary output of 0.5 to 1 mL/kg per hour.

Peritoneal Lavage (KCl-Free Fluid, Warmed to 43°C or 109°F)

For peritoneal lavage, warm, potassium-free fluid can be administered 2 L at a time and then removed with zero dwell time using Y-connector tubing. Many experienced clinicians consider peritoneal lavage the preferred run-in/run-out heated lavage technique.[28] Peritoneal lavage has several advantages for emergency active internal rewarming. It is readily available in most hospitals and EDs. Equipment requirements are simple, and no special training or technical skills are needed. Other anatomic sites may be used for heated lavage, including the stomach, colon, bladder, chest (closed thoracic cavity lavage),[16,28] and heart (direct cardiac lavage can be performed after open thoracotomy and cardiac massage).[46]

Extracorporeal Rewarming (Cardiac Bypass)

Extracorporeal rewarming is the most effective technique for core rewarming of hypothermic patients in cardiac arrest.[47] When available this is the treatment of choice for these patients. Extracorporeal rewarming techniques have considerable advantages. They provide adequate support of oxygenation, ventilation, and perfusion, and they enable rapid core rewarming (up to 1°C or 1.8°F every 5 minutes).[47]

There are, however, significant disadvantages. These techniques require special equipment and highly trained personnel, which are unavailable in many hospitals. Long delays are imposed by the need to assemble the equipment and the specialized team and by the time needed to perform the procedures.

Other Active Internal Warming Techniques

Several other active internal rewarming techniques have resulted in neurologically intact survival from hypothermic cardiac arrest. These techniques include peritoneal lavage[48]; peritoneal lavage combined with warm water bags, warm IV fluids, and continuous CPR[49]; continuous, closed thoracostomy lavage using 2 chest tubes[50,51]; and forced, heated air[39,52] (an active external rewarming technique). The use of esophageal rewarming tubes in the United States has not been reported, but these tubes have been used extensively and successfully in Europe.[53]

Arrest Interventions

Patients in **hypothermic cardiac arrest** will require CPR with some modifications from conventional BLS and ACLS care and will require active internal rewarming.

- Moderate (30°C to 34°C [86°F to 93.2°F]): start CPR, attempt defibrillation, establish IV access, give IV medications spaced at longer intervals, provide active internal rewarming
- Severe (<30°C [<86°F]): start CPR, attempt defibrillation once, withhold medications until temperature is >30°C (>86°F), provide active internal rewarming

Patients with a core body temperature <30°C (<86°F) and cardiac arrest require active internal rewarming (ie, invasive techniques). With or without return of spontaneous circulation, these patients may benefit from prolonged CPR and internal warming (peritoneal lavage, esophageal rewarming tubes, cardiopulmonary bypass, extracorporeal circulation, etc).

Modifications to BLS for Hypothermia

In the field providers may withhold resuscitation if the patient has obvious lethal injuries or if the body is frozen so completely that chest compressions are impossible and the nose and mouth are blocked with ice.[28] Otherwise for patients in cardiac arrest, the general approach to BLS management should still target airway, breathing, and circulation but with some modifications in approach. When the victim is hypothermic, pulse and respiratory rates may be slow or difficult to detect. For these reasons the BLS healthcare provider should assess breathing and later assess the pulse for 30 to 45 seconds to confirm respiratory arrest, pulseless cardiac arrest, or bradycardia that is profound enough to require CPR.[54] If the patient is not breathing, start rescue breathing immediately. If possible, administer warm (42°C to 46°C [108°F to 115°F]), humid oxygen during bag-mask ventilation. If the patient is pulseless with no detectable signs of circulation, start chest compressions immediately. If there is any doubt about whether a pulse is present, begin compressions.

Clinical studies have not established the core body temperature at which defibrillation should first be attempted in hypothermic VF patients and how often it should be repeated. In general, providers should attempt defibrillation (1 shock) without regard to core body temperature. It is unacceptable to delay defibrillation attempts to assess core temperature.

But if ventricular tachycardia (VT) or VF is present, defibrillation should be attempted. Automated external defibrillators may be used for these patients. If VF is detected, it should be treated with 1 shock, then immediately followed by resumption of CPR. If the patient does not respond to 1 shock, further defibrillation attempts should be deferred, and the rescuer should focus on continuing CPR and rewarming the patient to a temperature of 32°C to 34°C (89.6°F to 93.2°F) before repeating the defibrillation attempt. If core temperature is <30°C (<86°F), successful conversion to normal sinus rhythm may not be possible until rewarming is accomplished.[55]

To prevent further core heat loss, remove wet garments and protect the victim from further environmental exposure. Insofar as possible this should be done while initial BLS therapies are provided. Beyond these critical initial steps the treatment of severe hypothermia (temperature <30°C [86°F]) in the field remains controversial. Many providers do not have the time or equipment to assess core body temperature or to institute aggressive rewarming techniques, although these methods should be initiated when available.[1,31,56,57]

Modifications to ACLS for Hypothermia

For unresponsive patients or those in arrest, endotracheal intubation is appropriate. Intubation serves 2 purposes in the management of hypothermia; it enables provision of effective ventilation with warm, humid oxygen, and it can isolate the airway to reduce the likelihood of aspiration.

ACLS management of cardiac arrest due to hypothermia focuses on more aggressive active core rewarming techniques as the primary therapeutic modality. The hypothermic heart may be unresponsive to cardiovascular drugs, pacemaker stimulation, and defibrillation.[31] In addition, drug metabolism is reduced. There is concern that in the severely hypothermic victim, cardioactive medications can accumulate to toxic levels in the peripheral circulation if given repeatedly. For these reasons IV drugs are often withheld if the patient's core body temperature is <30°C (<86°F). If the core body temperature is >30°C (>86°F), IV medications may be administered but at increased intervals between doses.

As noted previously, a defibrillation attempt is appropriate if VF/VT is present. If the patient fails to respond to the initial defibrillation attempt or initial drug therapy, defer subsequent defibrillation attempts or additional boluses of medication until the core temperature rises above 30°C (86°F).[31] Sinus bradycardia may be physiologic in severe hypothermia (ie, appropriate to maintain sufficient oxygen delivery when hypothermia is present), and cardiac pacing is usually not indicated.

In-hospital treatment of severely hypothermic (core temperature <30°C [86°F]) patients in cardiac arrest should be directed at rapid core rewarming. Techniques for in-hospital controlled rewarming include administration of warm, humid oxygen (42°C to 46°C [108°F to 115°F]), warm IV fluids (normal saline) at 42°C to 44°C (109°F), peritoneal lavage with warm fluids, pleural lavage with warm saline through chest tubes, extracorporeal blood warming with partial bypass,[31,56,58,59] and cardiopulmonary bypass.[60]

Because severe hypothermia is frequently preceded by other disorders (eg, drug overdose, alcohol use, or trauma), the clinician must look for and treat these underlying conditions while simultaneously treating the hypothermia.

Termination of Resuscitative Efforts

Prehospital providers should transport the hypothermic patient in persistent cardiac arrest to the nearest appropriate emergency facility. In-hospital personnel can initiate or continue active internal rewarming as clinically indicated. If drowning preceded hypothermia, successful resuscitation is unlikely. Some clinicians believe that patients who appear dead after prolonged exposure to cold temperatures should not be considered dead until they are warmed to near normal core temperature.[54,55] Hypothermia may exert a protective effect on the brain and organs if the hypothermia develops rapidly in cardiac arrest.

When a victim of hypothermia is discovered, however, it may be impossible to distinguish primary from secondary hypothermia. When it is clinically impossible to know whether the arrest or the hypothermia occurred first, rescuers should try to stabilize the patient with CPR. Basic maneuvers to limit heat loss and begin rewarming should be started. Complete rewarming is not indicated for all patients. Once in the hospital, physicians should use their clinical judgment to decide when resuscitative efforts should cease in a victim of hypothermic arrest.

Postcirculatory Arrest Management

If the patient regains spontaneous circulation, continue internal rewarming until the core temperature is >35°C (>95°F). During rewarming, patients who have been hypothermic for more than 45 to 60 minutes are likely to require volume administration because their vascular space expands with vasodilation. Healthcare providers must closely monitor heart rate, perfusion, and hemodynamics at this time. Routine administration of steroids, barbiturates, or antibiotics has not been documented to help increase survival or decrease postresuscitation damage.[61,62]

During rewarming there may be significant hyperkalemia. Extreme hyperkalemia has been reported in avalanche victims who sustain crushing injuries and hypothermia.[25] Severe hyperkalemia has also been reported among hypothermic patients who did not sustain crushing injuries.[28] In fact, the severity of hyperkalemia has been linked with mortality. Management of hyperkalemia should follow current ACLS guidelines. The recommendations include administration of calcium chloride, sodium bicarbonate, glucose plus insulin, and nebulized albuterol. More aggressive measures to reduce extremely high serum potassium levels may include dialysis or exchange transfusion.

Because severe hypothermia is frequently preceded by problems such as drug overdose, alcohol intoxication, or trauma, the clinician must look for and address these underlying conditions while treating the hypothermia. If the patient appears malnourished or has chronic alcoholism, administer thiamine (100 mg IV) early during rewarming. If submersion with asphyxiation preceded the patient's hypothermia, successful resuscitation is unlikely.

Differentiating Cardiac Arrest Due to Hypothermia From Normothermic Cardiac Arrest in a Cold Environment

Hypothermia may exert a protective effect on the brain and organs if core body temperature drops rapidly while the patient is still breathing and has a pulse. But when emergency personnel discover a patient with hypothermia in cardiac arrest, they may find it impossible to resolve a critical question: Did the patient suffer a normothermic cardiac arrest in a cold environment, or did the patient have spontaneous circulation but suffer progressive hypothermia ending in apnea and cardiac asystole? This question is important because the answer has important prognostic implications. If the patient cools rapidly before arrest, a decrease in oxygen consumption and metabolism can precede the arrest and reduce organ ischemia. If the arrest occurs while the patient is normothermic and then the patient later develops hypothermia, the hypothermia cannot exert any protective effect.

Emergency personnel and hospital providers are often unable to determine the precise sequence of events, but they may be able to speculate based on the circumstances of the arrest. For example, a normothermic person experiencing VF arrest while shoveling snow will develop hypothermia only *after* the arrest. A lone cross-country skier with a compound tibia-fibula fracture may experience a drop in core temperature over many hours before cardiac arrest occurs.

The hypothermic patient also may have sustained additional organ insults before the arrest, such as asphyxiation from submersion. In cold water immersion, for example, significant hypothermia occurs rapidly. But it may be hypothermia-induced exhaustion followed by submersion, aspiration, and hypoxia with eventual cardiac arrest. Successful resuscitation will be very unlikely in such circumstances. The recommended "default decision" is for providers to initiate full BLS and ACLS interventions when it is clinically impossible to determine whether the arrest or the hypothermia occurred first. Emergency care providers should modify these interventions as described in this chapter if significant hypothermia is documented.

Summary

Unintentional hypothermia is a special resuscitation situation in which prolonged and special resuscitative efforts can be beneficial and improve outcome. Careful management of the patient in the prearrest phase can prevent circulatory arrest and life-threatening arrhythmias. These patients require transport to specialized facilities with equipment and personnel knowledgeable in hypothermia care and rewarming. Many patients will also need integration of care with critical care specialists because multisystem complications are frequent. The Table defines the various degrees of hypothermia and correlates core temperature with symptoms and recommended therapy.

References

1. Holzer M, Behringer W, Schorkhuber W, Zeiner A, Sterz F, Laggner AN, Frass M, Siostrozonek P, Ratheiser K, Kaff A. Mild hypothermia and outcome after CPR. Hypothermia for Cardiac Arrest (HACA) Study Group. *Acta Anaesthesiol Scand Suppl.* 1997;111:55-58.

2. Farstad M, Andersen KS, Koller ME, Grong K, Segadal L, Husby P. Rewarming from accidental hypothermia by extra-corporeal circulation. A retrospective study. *Eur J Cardiothorac Surg.* 2001;20:58-64.

3. Schneider SM. Hypothermia: from recognition to rewarming. *Emerg Med Rep.* 1992;13:1-20.

4. Gilbert M, Busund R, Skagseth A, Nilsen PÅ, Solbø JP. Resuscitation from accidental hypothermia of 13.7°C with circulatory arrest. *Lancet.* 2000;355:375-376.

5. Exposure-related hypothermia deaths—District of Columbia, 1972-1982. *MMWR Morb Mortal Wkly Rep.* 1982;31:669-671.

6. Hypothermia-related deaths—Alaska, October 1998-April 1999, and trends in the United States, 1979-1996. *MMWR Morb Mortal Wkly Rep.* 2000;49:11-14.

7. Hypothermia-related deaths—Cook County, Illinois, November 1992-March 1993. *MMWR Morb Mortal Wkly Rep.* 1993;42:917-919.

8. Hypothermia-related deaths—Georgia, January 1996-December 1997, and United States, 1979-1995. *MMWR Morb Mortal Wkly Rep.* 1998;47:1037-1040.

9. Hypothermia-related deaths—New Mexico, October 1993-March 1994. *MMWR Morb Mortal Wkly Rep.* 1995;44:933-935.

10. Hypothermia-related deaths—North Carolina, November 1993-March 1994. *MMWR Morb Mortal Wkly Rep.* 1994;43:849, 855-856.

11. Hypothermia-related deaths—Suffolk County, New York, January 1999-March 2000, and United States, 1979-1998. *MMWR Morb Mortal Wkly Rep.* 2001;50:53-57.

12. Hypothermia-related deaths—Utah, 2000, and United States, 1979-1998. *MMWR Morb Mortal Wkly Rep.* 2002;51:76-78.

13. Hypothermia-related deaths—Vermont, October 1994-February 1996. *MMWR Morb Mortal Wkly Rep.* 1996;45:1093-1095.

14. Hypothermia-related deaths—Virginia, November 1996-April 1997. *MMWR Morb Mortal Wkly Rep.* 1997;46:1157-1159.

15. Hypothermia-associated deaths—United States, 1968-1980. *MMWR Morb Mortal Wkly Rep.* 1985;34:753-754.

16. Miller JW, Danzl DF, Thomas DM. Urban accidental hypothermia: 135 cases. *Ann Emerg Med.* 1980;9:456-461.

17. Steinman AM, Giesbrecht G. Immersion into cold water. In: Auerbach PS, ed. *Wilderness Medicine.* 4th ed. St Louis, Mo: Mosby; 2001:197-225.

18. Tipton M, Eglin C, Gennser M, Golden F. Immersion deaths and deterioration in swimming performance in cold water. *Lancet.* 1999;354:626-629.

19. Ryan JM. Immersion deaths and swim failure—implications for resuscitation and prevention. *Lancet.* 1999;354:613.

20. Teramoto S, Ouchi Y. Swimming in cold water. *Lancet.* 1999;354:1733.

21. Delaney K. Hypothermic sudden death. In: Paradis NA, Halperin HR, Nowak R, eds. *Cardiac Arrest: The Science and Practice of Resuscitation Medicine.* Baltimore, Md: Williams & Wilkins; 1996:745-760.

22. Danzl DF. Accidental hypothermia. In: Rosen P, Barkin R, eds. *Emergency Medicine: Concepts and Clinical Practice.* St Louis, Mo: Mosby; 1998:963-986.

23. Danzl DF. Accidental hypothermia. In: Auerbach PS, ed. *Wilderness Medicine.* 4th ed. St Louis, Mo: Mosby; 2001:135-177.

24. Sterz F, Behringer W, Berzanovich A. Active compression-decompression of thorax and abdomen (Lifestick CPR) in patients with cardiac arrest [abstract]. *Circulation.* 1996;94:I-9.

25. Larach MG. Accidental hypothermia. *Lancet.* 1995;345:493-498.

26. Bernard SA, Gray TW, Buist MD, Jones BM, Silvester W, Gutteridge G, Smith K. Treatment of comatose survivors of out-of-hospital cardiac arrest with induced hypothermia. *N Engl J Med.* 2002;346:557-563.

27. Hypothermia After Cardiac Arrest Study Group. Mild therapeutic hypothermia to improve the neurologic outcome after cardiac arrest. *N Engl J Med.* 2002;346:549-556.

28. Danzl DF, Pozos RS, Auerbach PS, Glazer S, Goetz W, Johnson E, Jui J, Lilja P, Marx JA, Miller J, et al. Multicenter hypothermia survey. *Ann Emerg Med.* 1987;16:1042-1055.

29. Woodhouse P, Keatinge WR, Coleshaw SR. Factors associated with hypothermia in patients admitted to a group of inner city hospitals. *Lancet.* 1989;2:1201-1205.

30. Gallaher MM, Fleming DW, Berger LR, Sewell CM. Pedestrian and hypothermia deaths among Native Americans in New Mexico: between bar and home [published correction appears in *JAMA.* 1992;268:2378]. *JAMA.* 1992;267:1345-1348.

31. Reuler JB. Hypothermia: pathophysiology, clinical settings, and management. *Ann Intern Med*. 1978;89:519-527.

32. Greif R, Rajek A, Laciny S, Bastanmehr H, Sessler DI. Resistive heating is more effective than metallic-foil insulation in an experimental model of accidental hypothermia: a randomized controlled trial. *Ann Emerg Med*. 2000;35:337-345.

33. Kober A, Scheck T, Fulesdi B, Lieba F, Vlach W, Friedman A, Sessler DI. Effectiveness of resistive heating compared with passive warming in treating hypothermia associated with minor trauma: a randomized trial. *Mayo Clin Proc*. 2001;76:369-375.

34. Giesbrecht GG, Sessler DI, Mekjavic IB, Schroeder M, Bristow GK. Treatment of mild immersion hypothermia by direct body-to-body contact. *J Appl Physiol*. 1994;76:2373-2379.

35. Lindhoff GA, Mac G, Palmer JH. An assessment of the thermal safety of microwave warming of crystalloid fluids. *Anaesthesia*. 2000;55:251-254.

36. Giesbrecht GG, Pachu P, Xu X. Design and evaluation of a portable rigid forced-air warming cover for prehospital transport of cold patients. *Aviat Space Environ Med*. 1998;69:1200-1203.

37. Giesbrecht GG, Ducharme MB, McGuire JP. Comparison of forced-air patient warming systems for perioperative use. *Anesthesiology*. 1994;80:671-679.

38. Giesbrecht GG, Schroeder M, Bristow GK. Treatment of mild immersion hypothermia by forced-air warming. *Aviat Space Environ Med*. 1994;65:803-808.

39. Koller R, Schnider TW, Neidhart P. Deep accidental hypothermia and cardiac arrest—rewarming with forced air. *Acta Anaesthesiol Scand*. 1997;41:1359-1364.

40. Dobson JAR, Burgess JJ. Resuscitation of severe hypothermia by extracorporeal rewarming in a child. *J Trauma*. 1996;40:483-485.

41. Waters DJ, Belz M, Lawse D, Ulstad D. Portable cardiopulmonary bypass: resuscitation from prolonged ice-water submersion and asystole. *Ann Thorac Surg*. 1994;57:1018-1019.

42. Sterba JA. Efficacy and safety of prehospital rewarming techniques to treat accidental hypothermia. *Ann Emerg Med*. 1991;20:896-901.

43. Giesbrecht GG, Paton B. Review article on inhalation rewarming. *Resuscitation*. 1998;38:59-60.

44. Weinberg AD. The role of inhalation rewarming in the early management of hypothermia. *Resuscitation*. 1998;36:101-104.

45. Hayward JS. Thermal protection performance of survival suits in ice-water. *Aviat Space Environ Med*. 1984;55:212-215.

46. Brunette DD, McVaney K. Hypothermic cardiac arrest: an 11 year review of ED management and outcome. *Am J Emerg Med*. 2000;18:418-422.

47. Walpoth BH, Walpoth-Aslan BN, Mattle HP, Radanov BP, Schroth G, Schaeffler L, Fischer AP, von Segesser L, Althaus U. Outcome of survivors of accidental deep hypothermia and circulatory arrest treated with extracorporeal blood warming. *N Engl J Med*. 1997;337:1500-1505.

48. Pickering BG, Bristow GK, Craig DB. Case history number 97: core rewarming by peritoneal irrigation in accidental hypothermia with cardiac arrest. *Anesth Analg*. 1977;56:574-577.

49. Lexow K. Severe accidental hypothermia: survival after 6 hours 30 minutes of cardiopulmonary resuscitation. *Arctic Med Res*. 1991;50(suppl 6):112-114.

50. Hall KN, Syverud SA. Closed thoracic cavity lavage in the treatment of severe hypothermia in human beings. *Ann Emerg Med*. 1990;19:204-206.

51. Iversen RJ, Atkin SH, Jaker MA, Quadrel MA, Tortella BJ, Odom JW. Successful CPR in a severely hypothermic patient using continuous thoracostomy lavage. *Ann Emerg Med*. 1990;19:1335-1337.

52. Kornberger E, Schwarz B, Lindner KH, Mair P. Forced air surface rewarming in patients with severe accidental hypothermia. *Resuscitation*. 1999;41:105-111.

53. Kristensen G, Drenck NE, Jordening H. Simple system for central rewarming of hypothermic patients. *Lancet*. 1986;2:1467-1468.

54. Steinman AM. Cardiopulmonary resuscitation and hypothermia. *Circulation*. 1986;74(pt 2):IV29-IV32.

55. Southwick FS, Dalglish PH Jr. Recovery after prolonged asystolic cardiac arrest in profound hypothermia: a case report and literature review. *JAMA*. 1980;243:1250-1253.

56. Weinberg AD, Hamlet MP, Paturas JL, White RD, McAninch GW. *Cold Weather Emergencies: Principles of Patient Management*. Branford, Conn: American Medical Publishing Co; 1990.

57. Romet TT. Mechanism of afterdrop after cold water immersion. *J Appl Physiol*. 1988;65:1535-1538.

58. Zell SC, Kurtz KJ. Severe exposure hypothermia: a resuscitation protocol. *Ann Emerg Med*. 1985;14:339-345.

59. Althaus U, Aeberhard P, Schupbach P, Nachbur BH, Muhlemann W. Management of profound accidental hypothermia with cardiorespiratory arrest. *Ann Surg*. 1982;195:492-495.

60. Silfvast T, Pettila V. Outcome from severe accidental hypothermia in Southern Finland—a 10-year review. *Resuscitation*. 2003;59:285-290.

61. Safar P. Cerebral resuscitation after cardiac arrest: research initiatives and future directions [published correction appears in *Ann Emerg Med*. 1993;22:759]. *Ann Emerg Med*. 1993;22:324-349.

62. Moss J. Accidental severe hypothermia. *Surg Gynecol Obstet*. 1986;162:501-513.

63. Nozaki R, Ishibashi K, Adachi N, Nishihara S, Adashi S. Accidental profound hypothermia [letter]. *N Engl J Med*. 1986;315:1680.

Chapter 14

Special Resuscitation Situations
Part 2: Drowning

This Chapter

- **The first and most important intervention for the drowning patient: immediate ventilation**
- **Removing water from the airway: Is it necessary? How should it be done?**
- **New evidence on routine stabilization of the cervical spine**
- **Whom to transport to the hospital**

Overview

Drownings are most common in children and young adults. These events can be traumatic for the relatives and loved ones of patients and for emergency providers.

Parents, baby-sitters, or guardians may experience grief and guilt for failing to protect the patient. They may also feel intense anger toward others who did not provide adequate supervision. Neighbors, friends, bystanders, and emergency personnel may feel guilty for participating in a rescue attempt that resulted in death or neurologic impairment.

Epidemiology

Drowning accounts for more than one half million deaths annually worldwide. This number is probably an underestimate because of underreporting. In highly developed countries the highest incidence of drowning is seen in children younger than 5 years of age and in persons 15 to 24 years of age.[1,2] In some countries drowning is the first or second leading cause of death in this age group.[3] Reports from many parts of the world emphasize that drowning is a leading cause of cardiopulmonary arrest in children and adolescents.[4-8]

Prevention

Many issues surrounding prevention of drownings are complex and controversial:

- Appropriate targets for prevention efforts.[9]
- Siblings bathing together without adult supervision. In a study from Utah every bathtub drowning occurred when siblings were bathing together without adult supervision.[10] Drowning occurred when one sibling stood or sat on another or held a sibling under the water.
- Pediatric "drowning proofing" is an unproven concept[11] that is specifically discouraged by the American Academy of Pediatrics.[12]
- Legal ordinances for swimming supervision and pool fencing vary widely.
- Legal ordinances regulating water sports, personal watercraft, boating, life vests, and flotation devices vary widely.
- Some drownings that involve homicide, manslaughter, and suicide are euphemistically termed "nonaccidental" or "intentional" drownings.

Many drowning incidents that result in death or neurologic impairment are preventable tragedies. Many are the result of poor judgment, alcohol consumption, or inadequate supervision of children. Despite the ACLS emphasis on immediate treatment, the definitive therapy for drowning is *prevention*. As in cardiac arrests associated with hypothermia (see Chapter 14, Part 1) or trauma (see Chapter 14, Part 5), the most effective way to reduce the number of deaths due to drowning is to prevent the initiating event or to provide immediate treatment to prevent a cardiac arrest. Once a drowning person deteriorates to a state of cardiac arrest, the chances for a successful outcome are minimal.

Rescue of drowning victims occurs on or near the water, exposing rescue teams to danger. Never forget the principle of provider safety: make sure the area is safe and avoid becoming a second victim.

Pathophysiology

The drowning process is a continuum that begins when a person's airway lies below the surface of liquid, usually water, at which time the person voluntarily holds his breath. Breathholding is usually followed by an involuntary period of laryngospasm secondary to the presence of liquid in the oropharynx or larynx.[13] During this period of breathholding and laryngospasm, the victim is unable to breathe gas. This results in oxygen being depleted and carbon dioxide not being eliminated. The victim then becomes hypercarbic, hypoxemic, and acidotic.[14] During this time the victim will frequently swallow large quantities of water.[15] The victim's respiratory movements may become very active, but there is no exchange of air because of the obstruction at the level of the larynx. As the victim's arterial oxygen tension drops further, laryngospasm abates, and the victim actively breathes liquid.[16] The amount of liquid inhaled varies considerably from victim to victim. Changes occur in the lungs, body fluids, blood-gas tensions, acid-base balance, and electrolyte concentrations, which are dependent on the composition and volume of the liquid aspirated and duration of submersion.[14,16,17] Surfactant washout, pulmonary hypertension, and shunting also contribute to development of hypoxemia.[18,19] Additional physiological derangements, such as the cold shock response, may occur in victims immersed in cold water. Water that is 10°C (50°F) or colder has pronounced cardiovascular effects, including increased blood pressure and ectopic tachyarrhythmias. The response may also trigger a gasp reflex followed by hyperventilation, which may occur while the victim is underwater.[20]

A victim can be rescued at any time during the drowning process. The victim may not require an intervention or may receive appropriate resuscitative measures. The victim may recover from the initial resuscitative efforts, with or without subsequent therapy to eliminate hypoxia, hypercarbia, and acidosis and restore normal organ function. If the victim is not ventilated soon enough, or does not start to breathe on his or her own, circulatory arrest will ensue, and in the absence of effective resuscitative efforts, multiple organ dysfunction and death will result, primarily because of tissue hypoxia. The heart and brain are the two organs at greatest risk for permanent, detrimental changes from relatively brief periods of hypoxia. The development of post-hypoxic encephalopathy with or without cerebral edema is the most common cause of death in hospitalized drowning patients.[21,22]

The duration of hypoxia is the critical determinant of drowning outcome. The duration of hypoxia can be reduced first by early rescue from the water, then by immediate provision of basic and advanced life support.

Providers should be prepared to treat trauma or hypothermia in drowning patients. Some patients may require cervical spine precautions. C-spine immobilization is recommended

---

Critical Concept

Prevention of Drowning

- Keep only a few inches of water in the bathtub when bathing young children. Never leave young children unsupervised in bathtubs.
- Never leave children alone in or near a pool even for a moment, regardless of safety precautions such as self-locking gate and pool alarms.
- Be sure adults and adolescents are trained in CPR so that they can rescue a child if necessary.
- Surround your pool on all 4 sides with a sturdy 5-foot fence. The house should not form one of the barriers to the pool if there is a doorway from the home to the pool area. Be sure that the gates self-close and self-latch at a height that children cannot reach.
- Keep rescue equipment—a shepherd's hook (a long pole with a hook on the end) and a life preserver—and a portable telephone near the pool.
- Avoid inflatable swimming aids such as "floaties." They are *not* a substitute for approved life vests and can give children a false sense of security.
- Generally children are not developmentally ready for swim lessons until after their fourth birthday.[12] Swim programs for children under 4 should not be seen as a way to decrease the risk of drowning.
- Whenever infants or toddlers are in or around water, an adult should be within arm's length, providing "touch supervision."

for patients whose drownings are associated with trauma, such as a dive or fall into water.[23] If you are unsure if trauma occurred, assume that C-spine immobilization is needed.

Primary or secondary hypothermia may develop in drowning patients. *Primary hypothermia* can develop when a drowning occurs in icy water (<5°C, <41°F). In icy water core body hypothermia may develop before significant hypoxia occurs. It is possible that such cold-water submersion may provide some protection from hypoxia and organ ischemia. The published studies reporting good outcomes from prolonged submersion describe young, small patients submerged in icy water. *Secondary hypothermia* occurs as a consequence of heat loss through evaporation after rescue from the water and during attempted resuscitation. Hypothermia in these patients offers no protective effects.

Drowning Outcomes: Research and Reporting
Uniform Definitions of Drowning

Physicians and other healthcare workers around the world deal with the consequences of drowning on a daily basis, yet there are few population-based surveillance studies on drowning incidents or prospective clinical studies of prognostic factors and outcomes of drowning. A long-standing problem of drowning research has been the lack of standardized definitions. Something as fundamental as the definition of drowning itself varies among reports, as do clinical characteristics of outcome measures. The lack of consistency makes assessment and analysis of studies difficult, both individually and as a whole.

To aid in the use of consistent terminology and the uniform reporting of drowning data, the American Heart Association recommends use of the Utstein definitions and style of data reporting[24,25]:

- *Drowning.* Drowning is a process resulting in primary respiratory impairment from submersion/immersion in a liquid medium. Implicit in this definition is that a liquid/air interface is present at the entrance of the victim's airway, preventing the victim from breathing air. The victim may live or die after this process, but whatever the outcome, he or she has been involved in a drowning incident.
- *Immersion.* Immersion is to be covered in water. For drowning to occur, usually at least the face and airway are immersed.
- *Submersion.* During submersion, the entire body, including the airway, is under water.
- The Utstein statement recommends that the following terms no longer be used:
  — Near-drowning
  — Wet and dry drowning
  — Active, passive, and silent drowning
  — Secondary drowning

The Utstein statement also de-emphasizes classification based on type of submersion fluid (salt water versus fresh water). Although theoretical differences have been reported in laboratory conditions, these have not been found to be clinically significant. The most important factors that determine outcome of drowning are the duration and severity of the hypoxia.

Rapid Response Intervention **Drowning**	• Rapid **A**irway and **B**reathing support play the major role in resuscitation from drowning. • This emphasis contrasts with the emphasis on rapid initiation of chest **C**ompressions and **D**efibrillation that is appropriate for most adults who have a sudden cardiac arrest.

FYI **Utstein Style** **Standard Definitions for Drowning Incidents**	• *Drowning.* A process resulting in primary respiratory impairment from submersion/immersion in a liquid medium. Implicit in this definition is that a liquid/air interface is present at the entrance of the victim's airway, preventing the victim from breathing air. The victim may live or die after this process, but whatever the outcome, he or she has been involved in a drowning incident. • *Immersion.* To be covered in water. For drowning to occur, usually at least the face and airway are immersed. • *Submersion.* The entire body, including the airway, is under water. • *Water rescue.* Occurs when a person is alert but experiences some distress while swimming. The patient may receive some help from others and displays minimal, transient symptoms such as coughing that clear quickly. In general the person does not require further evaluation.

Drowning Outcome Prediction

The Challenges

Emergency care providers face a number of difficult questions when attempting resuscitation of drowning patients:

- Should providers attempt resuscitation for a 60-year-old person pulled from a tropical vacation swimming pool cyanotic, cold, breathless, and pulseless after 10 minutes of submersion?
- What is the prognosis for a 5-year-old child who is cyanotic, cold, breathless, and pulseless when he is pulled from a frozen pond 30 minutes after falling through the ice and slipping underwater?
- Should emergency department (ED) personnel continue CPR and ACLS interventions for drowning patients who remain breathless and pulseless after 40 minutes of resuscitative efforts in the field? What if a family member or emergency responder risked his or her life in recovering the patient from the water?
- What is the value of restoring a heartbeat and spontaneous respirations to a child whose chance of meaningful neurologic recovery is virtually zero?

Such clinical and ethical challenges have stimulated considerable interest in outcome prediction for drowning patients. Accurate outcome prediction would assist providers in recognizing fatal drowning events for which resuscitative efforts should not be started and drowning events for which resuscitative efforts should be stopped in the field without "lights and siren" transport.

Accurate outcome prediction would also help prevent the tragedy of successful restoration of a beating heart and breathing lungs for patients with devastating and irreversible hypoxic neurologic insult.

Research in Outcome Prediction

Predictors of outcome have been generated on the basis of retrospective surveys and epidemiologic analyses rather than prospective studies. Retrospective analyses of a large observational database of drownings in children and adolescents (up to 20 years of age) from King County and Seattle, Washington, have contributed valuable insight into drowning outcomes.[26-29] This work confirmed duration of submersion as the most powerful predictor of outcome.[29] With increasing duration of submersion, the following associations with death or severe neurologic impairment were observed:

- 0 to <5 minutes: 10%
- 5 to <10 minutes: 56%
- 10 to <25 minutes: 88%
- ≥25 minutes, 100%

Note how 5 more minutes of submersion in the 5 to <10 minutes group increases mortality almost 6 times compared with the 0 to <5 minutes group.

The following factors have been associated with 100% mortality[28]:

- Submersion duration ≥25 minutes
- Resuscitation duration >25 minutes
- Pulseless cardiac arrest on arrival in the ED
- No return of consciousness (patient was comatose at the scene and on arrival at the hospital)

Slightly lower mortality rates were associated with the following factors[28]:

- VT/VF was observed on the initial field ECG: 93% mortality
- Pupils were dilated and unresponsive to light on arrival in the ED: 89% mortality
- Severe acidosis was documented in the ED: 89% mortality
- Respiratory arrest occurred after arrival in the ED: 87% mortality

Drowning patients who have spontaneous circulation and breathing in the field, before arrival at the ED, usually recover with good neurologic outcomes. In the King County database, no deaths occurred among patients who were responsive at the scene or in the ED.[26]

FYI

100% Mortality!

100% mortality is associated with the following factors[28]:

- Submersion duration ≥25 minutes
- Resuscitation duration >25 minutes
- Pulseless cardiac arrest on arrival in the ED
- No return of consciousness (patient was comatose at the scene and on arrival at the hospital)

Several classification systems have attempted to use clinical findings as predictors of outcome for drowning patients.[30,31] The most coherent and logical approach derives from a long-term analysis of 1831 drowning episodes from the beaches of Brazil.[30]

Unlike other researchers in this area, Szpilman and colleagues[30] did not start with an implicitly derived classification scheme and force each case into the scheme. Instead they derived the classification grades empirically after recognizing that the worse the cardiopulmonary compromise, the worse the mortality rate (Table 1). The Szpilman classification system is based on identification of cardiopulmonary compromise that is easily assessed by an on-scene physician using only 4 variables: coughing (yes or no), auscultation of the lungs, blood pressure, and heart rate.

Table 1. Severity Grades for Drowning Events Based on Clinical Findings With Associated Mortality Rates

Severity Grade	Clinical Findings	Mortality (%)[30]
1	Some coughing, normal auscultation	0
2	Coughing; with abnormal auscultation: rales in some lung fields on one side	0.6
3	Coughing; abnormal auscultation with acute pulmonary edema (bilateral rales); good cardiac function (no hypotension)	5.2
4	Coughing; abnormal auscultation with acute pulmonary edema (bilateral rales) with poor cardiac function (hypotension)	19.4
5	No spontaneous respirations, pulse is present	44
6	Cardiopulmonary arrest: no spontaneous breathing, no pulse	93

Uniform Reporting of Drowning Data: The Utstein Style

In addition to providing standardized definitions of drowning terms, the Utstein guidelines recommend core and supplemental data to collect on drownings (Table 2). Most resuscitations begin at the scene of the drowning and not at a hospital, making on-scene data extremely important. Furthermore, many, or possibly most, drowning patients have mild symptoms, recover at the scene, and may or may not be transported to a hospital. Thus, to have a complete understanding of drowning and to capture the full scope of this problem, it is crucial that data at the scene be included in drowning reports (Figure 1).

Precipitating Events

In each case of drowning, the precipitating event should be reported if known. Drowning is sometimes precipitated by an injury or a medical condition. Seizure is the most common initiating event in all age groups.[32] Loss of consciousness from any cause, however, such as hyperventilation before breathholding under water, concussion, stroke, or cardiac arrhythmia, may result in drowning. When assessing a drowning incident, it is important to recognize the role of intentional injury, suicide, homicide, and child abuse. Hypothermia, alcohol, and drugs may impair motor function and judgment. Moreover, alcohol may affect the cardiovascular response to submersion.[33,34] Several precipitating events, such as seizures, alcohol use, and hypothermia, are associated with an increased risk of death from drowning.[35,36] Thus, these precipitating events should be noted because they may be confounders in outcome. In some situations it may be difficult to identify the primary cause of death as drowning or another condition. For example, drowning in an older person may trigger a heart attack, whereas a heart attack may precipitate a drowning event.

Time Intervals and Time Points (Events)

The importance of time intervals in resuscitation science is exemplified by the duration of submersion. The number of minutes submersed is a measure of the period of hypoxic insult. Although this information is usually estimated by

---

Foundation Facts

Prognosis After Drowning Incident

- Drowning patients who have spontaneous circulation and breathing in the field, before arrival at the ED, usually recover with good neurologic outcomes.

- In the King County, Washington, database, no deaths occurred among patients who were responsive at the scene or in the ED.

bystanders and is inaccurate, it has been correlated with survival.[29,37-40]

Outcome

The primary outcome of a drowning episode should be categorized as either death or survival. *Survival* indicates that the patient remained alive after the acute event and any acute or subacute sequelae. For example, survival is the outcome of drowning patients who were successfully resuscitated from cardiac or respiratory arrest and were then discharged from the hospital or survived initially and subsequently died of other causes. A drowning in which the patient is successfully resuscitated at the scene but succumbs to a condition that is causally related to the drowning should be categorized as a *death due to drowning*.

Although differentiating death from survival is usually easy, judgment occasionally is required to determine whether

Table 2. Recommended Data to Report for Drownings: The Utstein Style[24,25]

	Core	Supplemental
Victim information	• Victim identifier • Gender • Age (estimate if necessary) • Date and time of day of incident • Precipitating event: known/unknown (if known, then specify)	• Race or ethnic category • Residence (city, county, state, country) • Preexisting illness: yes/no (If yes, then specify)
Scene information	• Witnessed (submersion is observed): yes/no • Body of water: bathtub, swimming pool, ocean, lake, river, or other bodies of water or containers • Unconscious when removed from water: yes/no • Resuscitation before EMS arrived: yes/no • EMS called: yes/no • Initial vital signs (spontaneous breathing, palpable pulse) • Time of first EMS resuscitation attempt • Neurologic status: ABC or other neurologic assessment • (AVPU, GCS)	• Water/liquid type: fresh, salt, chemical, other • Approximate water temperature: nonicy, icy • Time of submersion if known • Time of removal of victim from water if known • Cyanosis • If patient received resuscitation before EMS arrived, who gave CPR? Layperson, lifeguard, etc • Method of CPR: MTM, ventilation alone, MTM-CC, CC only, automated external defibrillation • EMS vehicle dispatched: yes/no • Time of first EMS assessment • Oxygen saturation, temperature, blood pressure, pupillary reaction (optional)
ED evaluation and treatment	• Vital signs: temperature, heart rate, respiratory rate, blood pressure • Oxygen hemoglobin saturation • Arterial blood gas analysis if unconscious or SaO_2 <95% on room air • Initial neurologic status (GCS, AVPU, or ABC) • Airway and ventilation requirements	• Pupillary reaction • Toxicology testing: blood alcohol level and other drugs
Hospital course	• Airway and ventilation requirements	• Serial neurologic function (admission, 6 hours, 24 hours, 72 hours, discharge) • Complicating illnesses

Disposition	• Alive or dead (if dead, report date, place, and time of death)
	• Date of hospital discharge
	• Neurologic outcome at hospital discharge
		• Quality of life (OPC, CPC, other)
		• Cause of death:
		  1. How was cause of death determined?
		  2. Autopsy: yes/no
		  3. Forensic information (suicide, homicide?)
		• Other injuries and morbidities

GCS indicates Glasgow Coma Scale; AVPU, Alert, responds to Verbal stimuli, responds to Painful stimuli, Unresponsive to all stimuli; and ABC, awake, blunted, comatose; MTM, mouth-to-mouth; CC, chest compression; OPC, overall performance category; CPC, cerebral performance category.

Patient ID

Gender = M ☐ F ☐ U*
Age = _____ or
Date of birth ___/___/___
                    DD/MM/YY

Date of event:
___/___/___
DD/MM/YY

Times:
Call received _____

EMS resus _____

Location of drowning:
bucket ☐   toilet ☐
bathtub ☐   lake ☐
ocean ☐   pool ☐
river/flowing water ☐   other ☐

Event witnessed? Yes ☐   No ☐
If yes: time of event = _____
         witnessed/monitored by
         layperson ☐   healthcare personnel ☐

At scene
Loss of consciousness   Yes ☐   No ☐
CPR before EMS   Yes ☐   No ☐
   by layperson ☐   healthcare personnel ☐
   techniques used: rescue breathing ☐
                       chest compression ☐

Precipitating event known?
No ☐   If yes: Intoxication ☐   Pre-existing medical
Yes ☐   Trauma ☐   List _____
                                           Drugs _____
                                           Other _____

EMS assessment/management:
Spont breathing   Yes ☐ No ☐ U* ☐   Initial neuro state: GCS: E __ V __ M __
Signs of circulation Yes ☐ No ☐ U* ☐   or   A ☐ V ☐ P ☐ U ☐
Airway interventions Yes ☐ No ☐ U* ☐   or   A ☐ B ☐ C ☐

EMS assessment/management:
Spont breathing   Yes ☐ No ☐ U* ☐   Initial neuro stage: GCS: E __ V __ M __
Palpable pulse   Yes ☐ No ☐ U* ☐   or   A ☐ V ☐ P ☐ U ☐
Tracheal tube/ventilation Yes ☐ No ☐ U* ☐   or   A ☐ B ☐ C ☐

Initial   temp _____   BP _____   RR _____   SpO$_2$ _____   FiO$_2$ _____

Outcome
ROSC: Survived to:
   Any   Yes ☐ No ☐ U* ☐   ICU/ED   Yes ☐ No ☐ U* ☐
   >20 min Yes ☐ No ☐ U* ☐   Hosp. admission   Yes ☐ No ☐ U* ☐
                                      Hosp. discharge   Yes ☐ No ☐ U* ☐
DNAR order Yes ☐ No ☐ U* ☐   If discharged alive: CPC _____   U* ☐
Date of discharge or death: ___/___/___
                            DD/MM/YY

Figure 1. Example of revised Utstein drowning data form. U* indicates unknown; ROSC, return of spontaneous circulation. Conn Drowning Coma Scale: A indicates alert; B, blunted; and C, comatose. GCS scale: E indicates eye opening; V, verbal response; and M, motor response. AVPU scale: A indicates alert or awake; V, response to voice; P, response to pain only; and U, unarousable. Reprinted with permission from Idris et al.[24,25]

FYI **Common Sequelae Leading to Drowning Deaths**	Following are examples of common sequelae leading to death from drowning. The most common cause of death in hospitalized drowning victims is posthypoxic encephalopathy. • Brain death attributable to severe hypoxic or ischemic brain injury • Acute respiratory distress syndrome • Multiorgan system dysfunction secondary to severe hypoxic or ischemic insult • Sepsis syndrome attributable to aspiration pneumonia or nosocomial infections

death after illnesses such as aspiration pneumonia or septic shock is causally related to the drowning episode. A death from such causes in the first few days or weeks after a drowning episode would generally be judged to be attributable to the drowning because the chain of causation is clear. Death from drowning would also be the ruling for a drowning patient who develops and dies from aspiration pneumonia after being stable with severe hypoxic encephalopathy for weeks to months. If that same patient died of acute myocardial infarction, however, it most likely would be classified as a death not related to drowning. Thus, there is no time limit between the drowning event and death from drowning if there is a clear chain of causality.

The survival category can be subclassified in terms of severity and type of morbidities, such as neurologic impairment or respiratory impairment (eg, ventilator dependence). Figure 1 is an example of an Utstein style drowning data form.

Proposed Approach to Grading Drowning Events

To stimulate international discussion of the shortcomings of submersion nomenclature and initiate preliminary solutions, participants in the Guidelines 2000 Consensus Conference developed an approach to grading drowning episodes (Figure 2). This algorithm can be used by epidemiologists to support a prospective database of drowning cases.

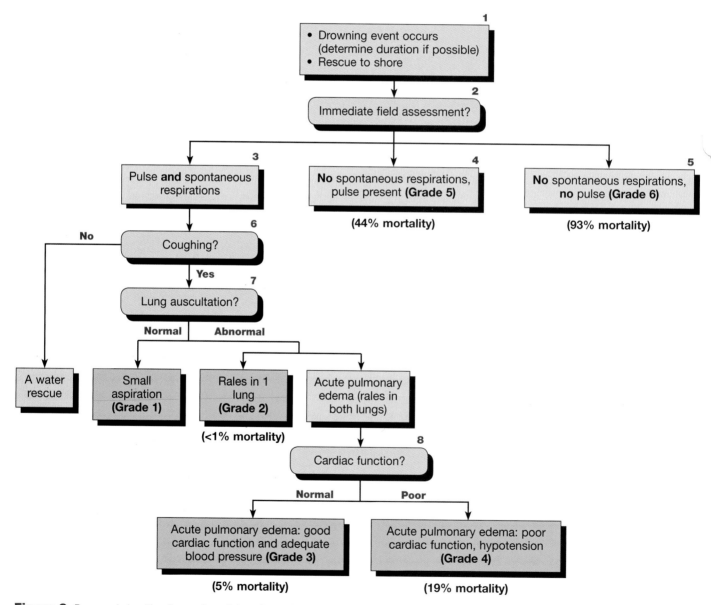

Figure 2. Proposed algorithm for grading of drowning episodes to facilitate uniform international reporting.

The algorithm is largely derived from the work of Szpilman and his Brazilian collaborators.[30] It has been validated retrospectively, demonstrating a relationship to outcomes (Table 1). Participants in the June 2002 Utstein consensus conference on drowning expressed agreement with the general principles of this algorithm and reviewed early drafts of the figure. The final version (Figure 2) reflects a number of modifications derived from this symposium. Continued use and evaluation of this algorithm could lead to future revisions and increased effectiveness.

The Proposed Drowning Episode Grading Algorithm: Underlying Concepts

The pathophysiology of drowning represents a continuum from the moment of submersion (head slips under the water), followed by some degree of aspiration, ineffective and then absent breathing, and then progressive hypoxia leading to irreversible apnea and then asystole (drowning death). An effective grading system needs to reflect the clinical signs demonstrated in patients rescued during the various stages of the drowning process.

- **Submersion:** The initial stage is an actual submersion. The head slips under water (or other liquid), there is no access to air, and some hypoxia develops with some aspiration of fluid into the hypopharynx, trachea, and lungs. Submersion is not really a problem until either hypoxia or aspiration occurs. Otherwise a person is simply swimming under water or voluntarily holding his or her breath.
- **Aspiration:** Experienced observers consider entrance of water into the respiratory passages with resultant stimulation of gag and cough reflexes as an essential stage in drowning events. *Coughing* is a critical dichotomous assessment point (Box 6). Coughing is an obvious physical sign with prognostic significance. If the patient is not coughing and has normal lung auscultation, the patient is classified as a *water rescue*. Although aspiration is assumed to occur during the stereotypical "struggle to keep the head above water," observers report many different scenarios. Modell[31] eloquently presents the range of submersion events that observers describe.
- **Apnea or breathlessness:** Absence of spontaneous breathing is an unambiguous physical sign that also relates to outcomes.

- **Spontaneous circulation:** If the period of hypoxia is prolonged, the heart stops beating. Hypoxia produces a well-established sequence of cardiac deterioration with tachycardia, then bradycardia, then a pulseless phase of ineffective cardiac contractions (PEA or VF/pulseless VT phase), followed by complete loss of cardiac rhythm and electrical activity (asystole). For this reason the absence of a pulse and other signs of circulation are easily assessed by providers, and their absence suggests that significant hypoxia has developed.

Algorithm for Drowning Episodes

Box 1

- A drowning event occurs. If possible determine the duration of submersion.
- If the provider can do so safely, the provider should open the patient's airway and check breathing and provide rescue breaths in the water if needed.
- Proceed with rescue to shore. Pay close attention to safety of both provider and patient. Take C-spine precautions (maintain cervical spine immobilization) *only* as indicated.

Box 2

- After the patient is rescued to shore (or another firm surface), immediately assess the ABCs of BLS: airway, breathing, and circulation.
- Immediately initiate all indicated BLS, ACLS, and pediatric resuscitation interventions based on the presence or absence of a patent airway, spontaneous respirations, and spontaneous pulse. These interventions include the following:
  - Send a second provider to phone 911. The lone provider should remain with the patient and provide 5 cycles of CPR (about 2 minutes) before leaving the patient to phone 911.
  - Provide basic life support, including all elements of the primary ABCs. When indicated provide ventilations and chest compressions. Continue until a defibrillator is available.
  - Once an AED or manual defibrillatoris available, check for the presence of VF/VT ("shockable rhythm") and deliver a defibrillatory shock if indicated.
  - Provide advanced adult and pediatric life support, including insertion of airway devices, establishment of IV access, and administration of IV medications.

Critical Concept

Lone Provider: When To Activate EMS

The lone provider should remain with the patient and provide 5 cycles of CPR (about 2 minutes) before leaving the patient to phone 911.

Box 3

- Drowning patients with spontaneous respirations and a sustained pulse are classified on the basis of 3 criteria:
  - Coughing (Box 6)
  - Lung auscultation (Box 7)
  - Cardiac function, eg, blood pressure (Box 8)

Box 4

- Drowning patients who have no spontaneous respirations but have a detectable pulse are classified as grade 5. On the warm-water beaches of Brazil with rapid BLS- and ACLS-level response teams, 56% of drowning patients with a severity of Grade 5 survive to hospital discharge.[30]
- If spontaneous respirations cannot be restored during resuscitative efforts and spontaneous cardiac activity ceases (asystole), treat as Grade 6 (Box 5).

Box 5

- Drowning patients who have no spontaneous respirations and no pulse on initial field assessment are classified as Grade 6. In Brazil only 7% of these nonbreathing, pulseless drowning patients survive to hospital discharge.[30]
- Patients who fail to respond to initial resuscitative efforts and fail to regain or sustain spontaneous respirations and pulse are classified as *deaths due to drowning*.

Box 6

- Assess whether the patient is coughing. Then auscultate the lungs.
- Coughing in drowning patients implies water aspiration.
- Drowning patients who are not coughing, have clear lungs on auscultation, and have maintained spontaneous circulation and respirations since rescue to shore are classified as water rescues.
- Drowning patients who are coughing repeatedly are further classified by the findings on lung auscultation.

Box 7

- The auscultation findings are used to further classify drowning patients with coughing:
  - Grade 1: Normal lung auscultation. Because these patients have been coughing, they are considered to have aspirated only a small amount of water.
  - Grade 2: Lung auscultation reveals some rales but in only one lung.
  - Grades 3 and 4: Lung auscultation reveals acute pulmonary edema (rales in both lungs). See Box 8 to separate Grade 3 from Grade 4.

Box 8

- In patients with acute pulmonary edema (rales in both lungs), cardiac function, and blood pressure, distinguish between Grades 3 and 4:

  - Grade 3: Good cardiac function and adequate blood pressure (5% mortality reported in Brazil[30])
  - Grade 4: Impaired cardiac function and hypotension (19% mortality reported in Brazil[30])

Drowning Outcome Prediction: Conclusions
Fate Factors but No System Factors for Drownings

The landmark work of Eisenberg et al[41] on out-of-hospital cardiac arrest identified what he termed *fate factors* and *system factors*.

- *Fate factors* are age, gender, initial arrest rhythm, location of arrest, and whether the arrest was witnessed. Although probability of survival is related to these factors, they cannot be changed or modified by providers.
- *System factors* include time to CPR, time to defibrillation, and time to and quality of early advanced care. These factors are amenable to effective organization and implementation of prehospital care. Community-based efforts to improve system factors and establish a strong Chain of Survival have revolutionized the approach to emergency medical services worldwide.

The epidemiologic studies of drowning events paint a pessimistic picture for improving outcomes. Multiple studies have established that outcome is determined largely by a single fate factor—*duration of submersion*.[28-30,37,42] The longer it takes to identify and rescue a drowning person, the worse the outcome.

The duration of hypoxia during submersion cannot be changed despite the best BLS and ACLS efforts. Immediate bystander CPR, however, can limit the duration of hypoxia to the time of submersion only. Delayed CPR results in a longer period of hypoxia.

Immediate provision of BLS and early ACLS contribute to the best outcome possible, given the duration of submersion. Nonetheless the relative contributions of these interventions are modest at best. Table 3 illustrates this problem. (Note that these are not published figures but rather data extrapolated from published sources.)

Table 3 shows that early BLS and ACLS significantly improve the chances of survival. But this data also shows the greater power that duration of submersion exerts over outcome. For example, patients rescued from the water within 5 minutes of submersion have a 70% chance of survival with late BLS and ACLS care and a 90% chance with immediate care. A person rescued from the water several minutes later, after 5 to <10 minutes of submersion, has markedly lower chances of survival regardless of

Table 3. Probability of Neurologically Intact Survival to Hospital Discharge Based on Duration of Submersion and Time to Basic and Advanced Life Support* (Extrapolated From Published Data[28-30,37,42])

Duration of Submersion (minutes)	Probability of Survival With Late BLS and Late ACLS	Probability of Survival With Early BLS and Late ACLS	Probability of Survival With Immediate BLS and ACLS
0 to <5	70%	80%	90%
5 to <10	30%	35%	44%
10 to <25	3%	5%	12%
≥25	0%	0%	0%

*Late is defined as BLS and ACLS personnel arriving >10 minutes after water rescue; early, BLS personnel arrive <10 minutes after water rescue; and immediate, BLS and ACLS personnel are present when patient is recovered from the water.

whether BLS and ACLS care is immediate (44%), early (35%), or late (30%).

Although survival from drowning episodes has increased in recent years, this increase does not appear to be attributable to improvements in medical treatment.[27]

"Do-Not-Start" and "When-to-Stop" Guidelines for Drowning Events

With the duration of submersion such a powerful determinant of outcome, one obvious guideline for emergency personnel would be not to initiate resuscitative efforts for a drowning patient with no respirations, no pulse, and a duration of submersion ≥25 minutes. But there are 2 critical problems with this guideline:

- It is often impossible to determine the precise duration of submersion.
- It is difficult for EMS systems to adopt specific do-not-start guidelines in the face of public perception that "miracle survivors" are commonplace.[43] This perception exists because of well-publicized anecdotes of successful resuscitations after prolonged submersions. But such media reports rarely (if ever) note that the survivors in these cases are almost exclusively young children submerged in icy cold water. Nor do they report that many of these "survivors" have severe neurologic impairment.

It seems reasonable to develop do-not-start and when-to-stop guidelines, based on objective information on the duration of submersion, for drowning patients who are in cardiopulmonary arrest upon rescue from the water (Grade 6 drowning). Very few of these patients are going to survive. For example, even in an excellent system like the one on Brazilian beaches, where physicians respond to drowning events, the survival rate for patients in cardiopulmonary arrest is only 7% regardless of the duration of submersion.[30]

- As a rule of thumb, about half of patients submerged for 5 to <10 minutes are pulseless upon water rescue.[28-30]
- Virtually all patients who ultimately survive from a Grade 6 drowning (not breathing, no pulse) will demonstrate a pulse in the field after a period of full BLS and ACLS interventions.
- King County data confirm this observation, noting that survival is unlikely if cardiac arrest persists despite resuscitation attempts for 25 minutes.[26,27] In studies from this EMS system, no one, not even pediatric patients, has survived to hospital discharge if spontaneous circulation did not return within 25 minutes of the start of resuscitative efforts.
  - Informal clinical guidelines in many EMS systems have evolved along the lines of "In normothermic patients, if pulse and respirations have not returned after 25 to 35 minutes of BLS and ALS support, they never will."

BLS Guidelines for Drowning Patients

Provider Safety

A cardinal rule of emergency medicine holds that the provider's primary obligation is to his or her personal safety. The provider must avoid creating "a second patient." The provider must always minimize danger to himself or herself. Providers should never attempt risky actions that are beyond the scope of their training and experience.

Recovery From the Water

When attempting to rescue a drowning person, the rescuer should get to the person as quickly as possible, preferably by some conveyance (boat, raft, surfboard, or flotation device). Recent evidence indicates that routine stabilization of the cervical spine is not necessary unless the circumstances leading to the drowning indicate that trauma is likely (see "Associated Trauma," below).

The Most Important Treatment for the Drowning Patient: Immediate Ventilation

The first and most important treatment for the drowning patient is the immediate provision of ventilation. Prompt initiation of rescue breathing increases the patient's chance of survival.[44] Rescue breathing is usually performed when the unresponsive victim is in shallow water or out of the water. If it is difficult for the rescuer to pinch the victim's nose, support the head, and open the airway in the water, mouth-to-nose ventilation may be used as an alternative to mouth-to-mouth ventilation. Untrained rescuers should not try to provide care while the victim is still in deep water.

- Flotation devices and some appliances can facilitate support of airway and breathing in the water if providers are trained in their use. Untrained providers should not attempt to use such adjuncts. Providers should not delay rescue breathing for lack of such equipment if they can otherwise provide it safely.

No Need to Drain Water From the Lungs

Management of the drowning patient's airway and breathing is similar to that recommended for any patient in cardiopulmonary arrest. There is no need to clear the airway of aspirated water. Only a modest amount of water is aspirated by the majority of drowning victims and it is rapidly absorbed into the central circulation, so it does not act as an obstruction in the trachea.[45,46] Some patients aspirate nothing because they develop laryngospasm or breathholding.[31,45] Most fluid obtained from attempts to drain the lungs comes from the stomach and not from the lungs.[46]

Attempts to remove water from the breathing passages by any means other than suction (eg, abdominal thrusts or the Heimlich maneuver) are unnecessary and potentially dangerous.[46] Reviews of this topic by the Institute of Medicine,[46] by the American Heart Association,[47] and in recognized textbooks in resuscitation[48] and emergency medicine[49,50] all conclude that there is no evidence to justify routine attempts to drain water from the lungs after submersion. Abdominal thrusts have been reported to cause regurgitation of gastric contents and subsequent

aspiration,[51-53] spinal cord injuries,[46] pharyngeal obstruction,[54] and rupture of the stomach.[55-60] Most important, provision of the Heimlich maneuver delays the initiation of ventilation that is critical to reverse hypoxia. The Heimlich maneuver for submersion patients should be reserved for patients with foreign-body airway obstruction or choking.[62,63] The routine use of abdominal thrusts or the Heimlich maneuver for drowning victims is not recommended.

Chest Compressions

As soon as the drowning patient is removed from the water, the rescuer should open the airway, check for breathing, and if there is no breathing, give 2 rescue breaths that make the chest rise (if this was not done in the water). After delivery of 2 effective breaths, the healthcare provider should check for a central pulse. The pulse may be difficult to appreciate in a drowning victim, particularly if the victim is cold. If the healthcare provider does not definitely feel a pulse within 10 seconds, the healthcare provider should start cycles of compressions and ventilations.

In general, providers should attempt chest compressions only on shore or on board a stable vessel or floating surface. External chest compressions can be performed in the water if rigid flotation devices are used or if the patient is extremely small and can be supported on the provider's forearm. Proper use of in-water resuscitation flotation devices requires device-specific training. Only trained rescuers should try to provide chest compressions in the water.

Vomiting During Resuscitation

Vomiting often occurs during chest compressions or rescue breathing, complicating efforts to maintain a patent airway. In a 10-year study in Australia, two thirds of patients who received rescue breathing and 86% of those who required compressions and ventilations vomited.[42] If vomiting occurs, turn the patient's mouth to the side and remove the vomitus using a finger, a cloth, or suction. If spinal cord injury is possible, log-roll the patient so that the head, neck, and torso are turned as a unit.

Defibrillation by BLS Providers

Although most drowning patients demonstrate asystole, some patients may demonstrate VF/pulseless VT. Once the patient is out of the water, if the patient is unresponsive and not breathing (and the healthcare provider does not feel a

Critical Concept *Abdominal Thrusts and the Heimlich Maneuver*	• Attempts to remove water from the airway by any means other than suction (eg, abdominal thrusts or the Heimlich maneuver) are unnecessary and potentially dangerous.
	• The routine use of abdominal thrusts or the Heimlich maneuver is not recommended.

pulse) after delivery of 2 rescue breaths, providers should attach an AED and attempt defibrillation if a shockable rhythm is identified.

You cannot safely attempt defibrillation in standing water. Patients must be moved out of standing water. Dry the patient's chest before attaching electrodes for monitoring or for defibrillation.

Deliver up to 5 cycles of CPR (about 2 minutes) and a shock. Then if you suspect hypothermia, evaluate the patient's core body temperature. If the patient's core body temperature is <30°C (<86°F) and VF persists, do not give further shocks until the patient's core body temperature rises above 30°C (86°F). Resume BLS and ACLS care until that time (see Chapter 14, Part 1: "Hypothermia").

Associated Trauma

Drowning events may be associated with trauma, and the issue of cervical spine immobilization is a difficult one. If the likelihood of head, neck, or spinal cord injury is significant, the provider should immobilize the head and neck and open the airway with a jaw thrust. But these maneuvers take time and may delay effective provision of rescue breathing.

- Providers should suspect spinal injuries in all drownings associated with diving; body, wind, or board surfing; falls from motorboats or sailboats; hang gliding; parasailing; falls from or crashes of personal watercraft; water slides; and in patients with signs of injury or alcohol intoxication.[23] Providers should immobilize the cervical spine for these patients.

- *Routine* cervical spine immobilization of *all* drowning patients is not recommended. In a retrospective survey of more than 2244 drownings, only 11 patients (<0.5%) had a C-spine injury, and all 11 had obvious trauma from diving, falling from height, or a motor vehicle crash.[23]

First-responding providers who suspect a spinal cord injury should

- Use their hands to stabilize the patient's neck in a neutral position (without flexion or extension).
- Open the airway using a jaw thrust without head tilt or chin lift. This method of airway opening is very difficult to perform in water, so the provider must weigh the

likelihood of cervical spine injury against the need for immediate rescue breathing in the water.

- Provide rescue breathing while maintaining the head in a neutral position. This method of rescue breathing is very difficult during in-water rescue.
- Float the patient, supine, onto a horizontal back-support device before removing the patient from the water.
- Align and support the head, neck, chest, and body if the patient must be turned.
- If you must move the patient, use a log-roll.

Associated Hypothermia (See Also Chapter 14, Part 1)

If the patient fails to respond to initial BLS, providers should evaluate the core temperature as soon as possible to rule out hypothermia. The provider should consider prolonging resuscitation attempts for a Grade 6 drowning patient if the patient's core temperature is <30°C (86°F). A core temperature at this level is an indication for active internal rewarming. To treat associated hypothermia, remove wet garments, dry the patient as soon as possible, and provide active rewarming when indicated (see Chapter 14, Part 1: "Hypothermia"). When hypothermia is present, use the following approach *without interrupting CPR:*

- Cover the patient with blankets or other materials to provide passive rewarming and to prevent further heat loss.
- Obtain rectal or tympanic (core body) temperature as soon as practical, and initiate hypothermia protocols as indicated in the Hypothermia Algorithm (Figure in Chapter 14, Part 1).
- If significant hypothermia is thought to be present, resuscitative efforts should continue until core temperature is measured to ensure that hypothermia is not contributing to ineffective resuscitative efforts.
- If the core temperature is >34°C (93.2°F), the hypothermia is insignificant and should not alter the duration of the resuscitation attempt.
- Between a core temperature of 30°C (86°F) and 34°C (93.2°F), clinical practice varies. Conservative protocols prolong the resuscitative effort until active external rewarming of truncal areas brings the core temperature up to >34°C (93.2°F). Little evidence supports this approach.

Foundation Facts **Respiration and Pulse Check in Suspected Hypothermia**	When a patient is hypothermic, respiration and pulse may be slow or difficult to detect. - Carefully assess breathing and confirm respiratory arrest. - Check the pulse for 30 to 45 seconds.

Consider the potential for hypothermia in all drowning events, especially when the initial immersion occurs in cold water. It is important to recognize that immersion in cold water is more likely to result in hypoxia than in development of protective central hypothermia.[64-66] This occurs because swimming in cold water typically produces a sequence of exhaustion, "swim failure" (inability to maintain horizontal swimming angle with body becoming more vertical relative to water surface), submersion, the beginning of the drowning process, and finally hypoxia.

This potentially terminal hypoxia occurs at relatively modest levels of central hypothermia that are insufficient to prevent organ ischemia. For example, Tipton et al[66] reported that competitive swimmers became exhausted after 60 to 90 minutes of swimming in 10°C (50°F) water. At that time of swim failure their rectal temperatures had dropped to only 35°C (94.5°F), a temperature that is too high to exert any protective effect.

ACLS Guidelines for Drowning Patients

Airway and Breathing

The submersion patient in cardiac arrest requires ACLS, including endotracheal intubation. Early endotracheal intubation is valuable for

- Improved oxygenation and ventilation
- Direct removal of foreign material from the tracheobronchial tree
- Application of continuous positive airway pressure (CPAP) or positive end-expiratory pressure (PEEP)

Circulation and Defibrillation

Patients in cardiac arrest may present with asystole (most common), pulseless electrical activity, or pulseless VF/VT. In children and adolescents VF/VT on the initial ECG is an extremely poor prognostic sign. Providers should follow ACLS guidelines for treatment of these rhythms. Treat drowning patients with severe hypothermia (core

body temperature <30°C or <86°F) according to the recommendations for hypothermia:

- Limit defibrillation attempts to one shock if hypothermia is severe and withhold further shocks, and then do not reattempt defibrillation until core body temp is 32°C to 34°C.
- If moderate hypothermia is present (core body temperature 30°C to 34°C or 86°F to 93.2°F), space intravenous medications at longer than standard intervals (see Chapter 14, Part 1: "Hypothermia").

Case reports document the use of surfactant for fresh water–induced respiratory distress, but further research is needed. The use of extracorporeal membrane oxygenation in young children with severe hypothermia after submersion is documented in case reports. There is insufficient evidence to support or refute the use of barbiturates, steroids, nitric oxide, therapeutic hypothermia after return of spontaneous circulation, or vasopressin.

Summary

- Prevention remains the most powerful therapeutic intervention for drowning.
- *Immediate provision of ventilations is the most important treatment for drowning.*
- The lack of an agreed-upon nomenclature has been a major obstacle to effective research in the epidemiology and treatment of drowning incidents. In 2003 international consensus guidelines for uniform definitions and reporting of data from studies of drowning incidents (the Utstein style) were published.[24,25] Use of these guidelines should improve the clarity of scientific communication and the comparability of scientific investigations related to drowning, as has occurred with use of the Utstein guidelines for reporting out-of-hospital cardiac arrest.
- Drowning events must be graded by severity. This grading is based on the clinical signs, ranging from simple aspiration with coughing to apnea with a beating heart to cardiopulmonary arrest (no breathing, no pulse).

Critical Concept **Consider Hypothermia**	Consider the potential for hypothermia in all drowning events. - Immersion in cold water is more likely to result in hypoxia than in development of protective central hypothermia. - Terminal hypoxia occurs at relatively modest levels of central hypothermia that are insufficient to prevent organ ischemia.

Critical Concept **Transport of Drowning Patients**	Every drowning patient, even one who requires only minimal resuscitation before recovery, requires monitored transport and evaluation at a medical facility.

- Do-not-start and when-to-stop guidelines are urgently needed to reduce danger to rescue personnel, poor use of resources, and the number of survivors with profound neurologic impairment.
  - Evidence supports the following "do-not-start resuscitation" guideline: *Do not start resuscitative efforts for drowning patients who were submerged for >25 minutes if there are no respirations and no heartbeat upon rescue from the water and if the patient is normothermic (core body temperature >34°C).* But no international consensus group has yet made such a recommendation.
  - Evidence now exists to support consideration of the following "when-to-stop resuscitation" guideline: *Stop resuscitative efforts if there has been no response (no respirations, no heartbeat) after >25 minutes of full BLS and ACLS interventions.* Again no international consensus group has yet made such a recommendation.
- When treating drowning patients, providers should consider the possibility of associated trauma and associated hypothermia.
  - A history or strong suspicion of trauma associated with a drowning event is the major indication for C-spine immobilization.
  - Routine C-spine immobilization for all drowning patients is not recommended at this time because it may compromise the delivery of rescue breathing.
  - The neuroprotective value of hypothermia for drowning patients in cardiac arrest is probably exaggerated. This effect is possible only when the hypothermia is severe (core body temperature <30°C or <86°F) and body cooling preceded the hypoxia that develops during submersion.
- ACLS personnel should strongly support effective prevention activities, which may at times require legislative and regulatory initiatives. Important prevention activities include
  - Unremitting, responsible, and mature adult supervision for all infants and children when near any source of the 1 to 2 inches of water necessary for a drowning death
  - Safe pool design with self-closing, self-locking gates and fencing that encloses the pool on all sides
  - Trained lifeguards at public pools and beaches

- Public swim areas fully equipped with rigid backboards, cervical collars, and BLS supplies, including AEDs
- Swimming and lifesaving classes
- Lay provider CPR-AED training
- Widespread availability and appropriate use of personal flotation devices

References

1. Peden MM, McGee K, Krug E, eds. *Injury: A Leading Cause of the Global Burden of Disease*, 2000. Geneva, Switzerland: World Health Organization; 2000.

2. Mulligan-Smith D, Pepe PE, Branche CM. A seven-year, statewide study of the epidemiology of pediatric drowning deaths. *Acad Emerg Med*. 2002;9:488-489.

3. Smith G. *Proceedings of the World Congress on Drowning*; 2002.

4. Weir E. Drowning in Canada. *CMAJ*. 2000;162:1867.

5. Steensberg J. Epidemiology of accidental drowning in Denmark 1989-1993. *Accid Anal Prev*. 1998;30:755-762.

6. Mackie IJ. Patterns of drowning in Australia, 1992-1997. *Med J Aust*. 1999;171:587-590.

7. Mizuta R, Fujita H, Osamura T, Kidowaki T, Kiyosawa N. Childhood drownings and near-drownings in Japan. *Acta Paediatr Jpn*. 1993;35:186-192.

8. Mogayzel C, Quan L, Graves JR, Tiedeman D, Fahrenbruch C, Herndon P. Out-of-hospital ventricular fibrillation in children and adolescents: causes and outcomes. *Ann Emerg Med*. 1995;25:484-491.

9. Quan L, Bennett E, Cummings P, Henderson P, Del Beccaro MA. Do parents value drowning prevention information at discharge from the emergency department? *Ann Emerg Med*. 2001;37:382-385.

10. Jensen LR, Williams SD, Thurman DJ, Keller PA. Submersion injuries in children younger than 5 years in urban Utah. *West J Med*. 1992;157:641-644.

11. Pitt WR, Cass DT. Preventing children drowning in Australia. *Med J Aust*. 2001;175:603-604.

12. Swimming programs for infants and toddlers. Committee on Sports Medicine and Fitness and Committee on Injury and Poison Prevention. American Academy of Pediatrics. *Pediatrics*. 2000;105(4 pt 1):868-870.

13. Miller RD, ed. *Anesthesia*. 5th ed. Philadelphia, Pa: Churchill Livingstone; 2000:1416-1417.

14. Modell JH, Gaub M, Moya F, Vestal B, Swarz H. Physiologic effects of near drowning with chlorinated fresh water, distilled water and isotonic saline. *Anesthesiology*. 1966;27:33-41.

15. Modell JH, Graves SA, Ketover A. Clinical course of 91 consecutive near-drowning victims. *Chest*. 1976;70:231-238.

16. Modell JH, Moya F. Effects of volume of aspirated fluid during chlorinated fresh water drowning. *Anesthesiology*. 1966;27:662-672.

17. Modell JH, Moya F, Newby EJ, Ruiz BC, Showers AV. The effects of fluid volume in seawater drowning. *Ann Intern Med*. 1967;67:68-80.

18. Halmagyi DF, Colebatch HJ. Ventilation and circulation after fluid aspiration. *J Appl Physiol*. 1961;16:35-40.

19. Giammona ST, Modell JH. Drowning by total immersion. Effects on pulmonary surfactant of distilled water, isotonic saline, and sea water. *Am J Dis Child*. 1967;114:612-616.

20. Tipton MJ. The initial responses to cold-water immersion in man. *Clin Sci (Lond)*. 1989;77:581-588.

21. Conn AW, Montes JE, Barker GA, Edmonds JF. Cerebral salvage in near-drowning following neurological classification by triage. *Can Anaesth Soc J*. 1980;27:201-210.

22. Eriksson R, Fredin H, Gerdman P, Thorson J. Sequelae of accidental near-drowning in childhood. *Scand J Soc Med*. 1973;1:3-6.

23. Watson RS, Cummings P, Quan L, Bratton S, Weiss NS. Cervical spine injuries among submersion victims. *J Trauma*. 2001;51:658-662.

24. Idris AH, Berg RA, Bierens J, Bossaert L, Branche CM, Gabrielli A, Graves SA, Handley AJ, Hoelle R, Morley PT, Papa L, Pepe PE, Quan L, Szpilman D, Wigginton JG, Modell JH. Recommended guidelines for uniform reporting of data from drowning: the "Utstein style." *Circulation*. 2003;108:2565-2574.

25. Idris AH, Berg RA, Bierens J, Bossaert L, Branche CM, Gabrielli A, Graves SA, Handley AJ, Hoelle R, Morley PT, Papa L, Pepe PE, Quan L, Szpilman D, Wigginton JG, Modell JH. Recommended guidelines for uniform reporting of data from drowning: the "Utstein style." *Resuscitation*. 2003;59:45-57.

26. Cummings P, Quan L. Trends in unintentional drowning: the role of alcohol and medical care. *JAMA*. 1999;281:2198-2202.

27. Quan L. Near-drowning. *Pediatr Rev*. 1999;20:255-259, quiz 260.

28. Quan L, Kinder D. Pediatric submersions: prehospital predictors of outcome. *Pediatrics*. 1992;90:909-913.

29. Quan L, Wentz KR, Gore EJ, Copass MK. Outcome and predictors of outcome in pediatric submersion victims receiving prehospital care in King County, Washington. *Pediatrics*. 1990;86:586-593.

30. Szpilman D. Near-drowning and drowning classification: a proposal to stratify mortality based on the analysis of 1,831 cases. *Chest*. 1997;112:660-665.

31. Modell JH. Drowning. *N Engl J Med*. 1993;328:253-256.

32. Quan L, Cummings P. Characteristics of drowning by different age groups. *Inj Prev*. 2003;9:163-168.

33. Plueckhahn VD. Alcohol and accidental drowning. A 25-year study. *Med J Aust*. 1984;141:22-25.

34. Plueckhahn VD. Alcohol consumption and death by drowning in adults; a 24-year epidemiological analysis. *J Stud Alcohol*. 1982;43:445-452.

35. Diekema DS, Quan L, Holt VL. Epilepsy as a risk factor for submersion injury in children. *Pediatrics*. 1993;91:612-616.

36. Smith GS, Keyl PM, Hadley JA, Bartley CL, Foss RD, Tolbert WG, McKnight J. Drinking and recreational boating fatalities: a population-based case-control study. *JAMA*. 2001;286:2974-2980.

37. Suominen P, Baillie C, Korpela R, Rautanen S, Ranta S, Olkkola KT. Impact of age, submersion time and water temperature on outcome in near-drowning. *Resuscitation*. 2002;52:247-254.

38. Nussbaum E. Prognostic variables in nearly drowned, comatose children. *Am J Dis Child*. 1985;139:1058-1059.

39. Peterson B. Morbidity of childhood near-drowning. *Pediatrics*. 1977;59:364-370.

40. Kruus S, Bergstrom L, Suutarinen T, Hyvonen R. The prognosis of near-drowned children. *Acta Paediatr Scand*. 1979;68: 315-322.

41. Eisenberg MS. Who shall live? Who shall die? In: Eisenberg MS, Bergner L, Hallstrom AP, eds. *Sudden Cardiac Death in the Community*. Philadelphia, Pa: Praeger Scientific; 1984:44-58.

42. Manolios N, Mackie I. Drowning and near-drowning on Australian beaches patrolled by life-savers: a 10-year study, 1973-1983. *Med J Aust*. 1988;148:165-167, 170-161.

43. Cummins RO. Personal communications regarding confidential medical reviews and consultations to medical-legal professionals. Seattle, Wash; 2002.

44. Kyriacou DN, Arcinue EL, Peek C, Kraus JF. Effect of immediate resuscitation on children with submersion injury. *Pediatrics*. 1994;94:137-142.

45. Modell JH, Davis JH. Electrolyte changes in human drowning victims. *Anesthesiology*. 1969;30:414-420.

46. Rosen P, Stoto M, Harley J. The use of the Heimlich maneuver in near drowning: Institute of Medicine report. *J Emerg Med*. 1995;13:397-405.

47. Quan L. Drowning issues in resuscitation. *Ann Emerg Med*. 1993;22:366-369.

48. Shaw KN, Lavelle JM. Drowned and near-drowned patients. In: Paradis NA, Halperin HR, Nowak RM, eds. *Cardiac Arrest: The Science and Practice of Resuscitation Medicine*. Baltimore, Md: Williams & Wilkins; 1997:820-829.

49. Feldhaus KM, Knopp RK. Near-drowning. In: Rosen P, Barkin R, eds. *Emergency Medicine: Concepts and Clinical Practice*. 4th ed. St Louis, Mo: Mosby; 1998:1061-1066.

50. Newman AB, Stewart RD. Submersion incidents. In: Auerbach PS, ed. *Wilderness Medicine: Management of Wilderness and Environmental Emergencies*. St Louis, Mo: Mosby; 2001.

51. Redding JS. The choking controversy: critique of evidence on the Heimlich maneuver. *Crit Care Med*. 1979;7:475-479.

52. Orlowski JP. Vomiting as a complication of the Heimlich maneuver. *JAMA*. 1987;258:512-513.

53. Fink JA, Klein RL. Complications of the Heimlich maneuver. *J Pediatr Surg*. 1989;24:486-487.

54. Anderson S, Buggy D. Prolonged pharyngeal obstruction after the Heimlich manoeuvre. *Anaesthesia*. 1999;54:308-309.

55. Visintine RE, Baick CH. Ruptured stomach after Heimlich maneuver. *JAMA*. 1975;234:415.

56. Cowan M, Bardole J, Dlesk A. Perforated stomach following the Heimlich maneuver. *Am J Emerg Med*. 1987;5:121-122.

57. van der Ham AC, Lange JF. Traumatic rupture of the stomach after Heimlich maneuver. *J Emerg Med*. 1990;8:713-715.

58. Dupre MW, Silva E, Brotman S. Traumatic rupture of the stomach secondary to Heimlich maneuver. *Am J Emerg Med*. 1993;11:611-612.

59. Bintz M, Cogbill TH. Gastric rupture after the Heimlich maneuver. *J Trauma*. 1996;40:159-160.

60. Majumdar A, Sedman PC. Gastric rupture secondary to successful Heimlich manoeuvre. *Postgrad Med J*. 1998;74:609-610.

61. Associated Press. Mom says 'thank you' to Heimlich; doctor's technique saved her son's life. *Cincinnati Post*. 1999.

62. Heimlich HJ. A life-saving maneuver to prevent food-choking. *JAMA*. 1975;234:398-401.

63. Patrick E. A case report: the Heimlich maneuver. *Emergency*. 1981;13:45-47.

64. Ryan JM. Immersion deaths and swim failure—implications for resuscitation and prevention. *Lancet*. 1999;354:613.

65. Teramoto S, Ouchi Y. Swimming in cold water. *Lancet*. 1999;354:1733.

66. Tipton M, Eglin C, Gennser M, Golden F. Immersion deaths and deterioration in swimming performance in cold water. *Lancet*. 1999;354:626-629.

Chapter 14

Special Resuscitation Situations
Part 3: Severe, Life-Threatening Asthma

Overview and Epidemiology

More than 22 million people in the US have asthma.[1] Asthma is responsible for more than 1.8 million emergency department (ED) visits per year, and approximately 10% to 25% of these visits results in a hospital admission.[2,3]

Severe asthma accounts for approximately 2% to 20% of admissions to intensive care units (ICUs), with up to one third of these patients requiring intubation and mechanical ventilation.[4] The CDC estimates approximately 4000 deaths annually due to asthma, many occurring in the prehospital setting. But this figure underestimates the total number of fatal asthma episodes. Experts think that more than 50% of asthma-related deaths are not recognized and attributed to other causes such as upper respiratory infection and influenza, especially in adult victims.[5] Most acute episodes resulting in death are related to severe underlying disease, inadequate baseline management, and acute exacerbations of inflammation. These potentially preventable deaths often strike the young, and they can be very painful for families, friends, and healthcare providers.

The *2005 American Heart Association Guidelines for Cardiopulmonary Resuscitation and Emergency Cardiovascular Care* do not discuss care for chronic asthma or typical exacerbations. But the guidelines do make recommendations for the management of *acute, severe, life-threatening asthma attacks*. These attacks have several labels and definitions. Near-fatal[10]; severe, life-threatening asthma[11]; and status asthmaticus are most common. Status asthmaticus refers to attacks that fail to respond to continuous, aggressive treatment after a specified amount of time (eg, 4 hours).

FYI

More Information on Asthma

Several consensus groups have developed excellent practice guidelines for the diagnosis and treatment of asthma. These groups include the National Asthma Education and Prevention Program of the National Institutes of Health,[6,7] the Global Initiative for Asthma,[8] and the Canadian Association of Emergency Physicians and the Canadian Thoracic Society.[9] The following websites are useful:

- National Asthma Education and Prevention Program: **http://www.nhlbi.nih.gov/about/naepp/**
- Global Initiative for Asthma: **http://www.ginasthma.com/**

Additional classifications for severity have been developed using more objective parameters. A 3-item asthma severity scale has been developed for the Global Initiative for Asthma.[12] This scale is based on history, current medication use, and forced expiratory volume in 1 second (FEV$_1$):

- **Severe hypoxemia:** for example, PaO$_2$ <65 mm Hg with 40% inspired oxygen, often with hypercarbia (PaCO$_2$ >40 mm Hg)
- **Severe airway obstruction:** defined by objective measures such as an FEV$_1$ or peak expiratory flow rate (PEFR or PEF) <40% of the predicted value
- **Speed of onset:** *rapid-onset asthma* develops in <2.5 hours; *slow-onset asthma* develops over several days[13]

Life-Threatening and Fatal Asthma
Pathophysiology

The pathophysiology of asthma consists of 3 key abnormalities:

- Bronchoconstriction
- Airway inflammation
- Mucous impaction

Severe exacerbations of asthma can lead rapidly to death. Cardiac arrest in patients with bronchial asthma has been linked to a variety of pathophysiologic mechanisms complicating exacerbations of asthma, but the most likely cause is thought to be bronchospasm with subsequent plugging of the narrowed airways by mucus (Figure 1).[14]

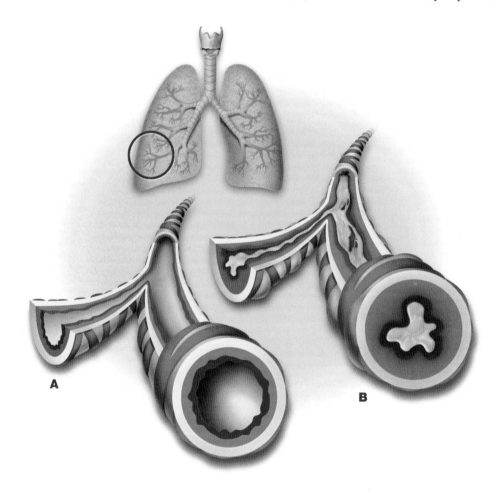

Figure 1. Asthma occurs in the setting of underlying inflammation. Diffuse bronchospasm occurs, causing air passages to constrict. Hypersecretion of mucous leads to mucous plugs, which block oxygenation and ventilation. **A,** Normal, healthy bronchiole. **B,** Bronchiole during an asthma attack.

FYI **Presentation of Severe, Life-Threatening Asthma**	Severe, life-threatening asthma (Table 1) will present to ACLS providers in 1 of 2 ways: • Clinical deterioration despite hours of therapy • Periarrest

Table 1. Asthma Severity Score: Classification of Mild, Moderate, and Severe Asthma*

Parameter†	Mild	Moderate	Severe	Subset: Respiratory Arrest Imminent
Breathless	While walking	While at rest (Infant—softer, shorter cry; difficulty feeding)	While at rest (Infant—stops feeding)	
	Can lie down	Prefers sitting	Sits upright	
Talks in	Sentences	Phrases	Words	
Alertness	May be agitated	Usually agitated	Usually agitated	Drowsy or confused
Respiratory rate	Increased	Increased	Often >30/min	
	Guide to rates of breathing in awake children: Age / Normal rate: <2 months <60/min; 2-12 months <50/min; 1-5 years <40/min; 6-8 years <30/min			
Use of accessory muscles; supra-sternal retractions	Usually not	Commonly	Usually	Paradoxical thoracoabdominal movement
Wheeze	Moderate, often only end expiratory	Loud; throughout exhalation	Usually loud; throughout inhalation and exhalation	Absence of wheeze
Pulse/minute	<100/min	100-120/min	>120/min	Bradycardia
	Guide to normal pulse rates in children: Age / Normal rate: 2-12 months <160/min; 1-2 years <120/min; 2-8 years <110/min			
Pulsus paradoxus	Absent <10 mm Hg	May be present 10 to 25 mm Hg	Often present >25 mm Hg (adult) 20-40 mm Hg (child)	Absence suggests respiratory muscle fatigue
PEF percent predicted or percent personal best	≥70%	Approx 40% to 69% or response lasts <2 hours	<40%	<25% Note: PEF testing may not be needed in very severe attacks
Pao₂ (on air)	Normal (test usually not necessary)	≥60 mm Hg (test not usually necessary)	<60 mm Hg: possible cyanosis	
and/or				
Pco₂‡	<42 mm Hg§ (test usually not necessary)	<42 mm Hg (test usually not necessary)	≥42 mm Hg: possible respiratory failure	
Sao₂ percent (on air) at sea level	>95% (test usually not necessary)	90-95% (test usually not necessary)	<90%	
	Hypercapnia (hypoventilation) develops more readily in young children than in adults and adolescents.			

Pao₂ indicates arterial oxygen pressure; Pco₂, partial pressure of carbon dioxide; PEF, peak expiratory flow; Sao₂, oxygen saturation.

*Reproduced from National Heart, Lung, and Blood Institute. Expert Panel Report: Guidelines for Diagnosis and Management of Asthma: Summary Report, 2007. US Department of Health and Human Services, Publication no. 08-0451.

†The presence of several parameters, but not necessarily all, indicates the general classification of the attack.

‡Kilopascals are used internationally; conversion would be appropriate in this regard.

§Hypercapnia (hyperventilation) develops more readily in young children than in adults and adolescents.

At autopsy these patients display marked mucous plugging, airway edema, exudation of plasma proteins, hypertrophy of airway smooth muscle, and cellular activation with increased production and activation of inflammatory mediators.[15-17] Some patients experience a sudden onset of severe bronchospasm that responds rapidly to inhaled β_2-agonists.[18] This observation suggests that marked bronchiolar smooth muscle spasm is the major component in some cases of fatal asthma.

Bronchoconstriction and airway obstruction from mucous plugging cause hyperinflation and increased airway resistance (Figure 1). As a consequence the work of breathing increases dramatically. For example, at an FEV_1 of 50% of predicted, the work of breathing increases to 10 times normal. At an FEV_1 of <25% of predicted, severe respiratory muscle fatigue can contribute to the development of respiratory arrest and death unless urgent treatment is provided. Some patients who receive mechanical ventilation develop auto-PEEP (positive end-expiratory pressure). A simple explanation of auto-PEEP is that the inspiratory tidal volume is greater than the expiratory tidal volume (see below). This net and ever increasing volume leads to an increase in intrathoracic pressure (the auto-PEEP), which decreases venous return to the heart. Hemodynamic compromise rapidly follows, largely as a result of inadequate cardiac output.

Severe asthma attacks are prone to be fatal when combined with one or more asthma-related complications. These complications include tension pneumothorax (often bilateral), pneumomediastinum, pneumonia, lobar atelectasis (from mucous plugging, often of larger airways), cardiac dysfunction, and pulmonary edema. Experts have long suspected that fatal cardiac arrhythmias occur from the use (or misuse) of β-adrenergic agonists.[16,17] In reviews of asthma-related deaths, however, several authors were unable to document an association between these drugs and fatal arrhythmias.[18-20] Recently data from registries of long QT pedigrees has confirmed that cohort members with asthma have more cardiac events than members without asthma. In these patients the β-adrenergic agonists cause increased prolongation of the QT interval.[21]

Signs and Symptoms

Fatal, near-fatal,[10] or life-threatening asthma[11] occurs more frequently in the following groups of asthma patients:

- Black men
- Inner-city residents
- Patients recently hospitalized for asthma[20]
- Patients who are steroid-dependent
- Patients recently intubated for asthma[20]
- Patients who delay seeking care for attacks and deteriorate at home

Asthma Triggers

Patient profiles and risk factors for asthma can be identified, as can triggers for attacks in many persons (Table 2). Some triggers are unavoidable, but they should

Table 2. Triggers of Fatal and Near-Fatal Asthma

1. Environment
   - Extremes of temperature
   - High humidity and dew points
   - Episodic contaminants (smoke, cigarette smoke)
2. Upper respiratory infections (viruses and bacteria)
3. Allergens (pollens and molds)
4. Exercise (cold-induced)
5. Other medical conditions (chronic obstructive pulmonary disease, gastroesophageal reflux)
6. Drugs (aspirin, β-blockers, non-steroidal anti-inflammatory medications)

Foundation Facts

Special Note for EMS and ED Personnel: Most deaths from asthma occur at home or during transport to an ED.

These patients are at higher risk for cardiac arrest!

The number of patients with severe asthma attacks who present to the ED at night is 10 times greater than the number presenting during the day; 2% of patients with acute asthma who present at night require intubation. The following patient groups are at increased risk for near-fatal and fatal asthma:

- Patients who fail to recognize the severity of their attack
- Patients who attempt to treat themselves during attacks without notifying their primary provider about exacerbations
- Patients with a high level of denial on psychological evaluation
- Patients who receive suboptimal treatment from their primary care provider
- Patients who are depressed or anxious
- Patients whose asthma was diagnosed when they were <5 years of age

be identified if possible. Others can be avoided in the future, or medical care can be sought early if patients and their families are aware of them. In some cases the trigger needs to be treated concomitantly with the asthma attack.

A somewhat stereotypical picture emerges of noncompliance, inadequate medication regimens, and denial. But a case-control study of fatal and near-fatal asthma events based on the experiences of more than 400 specialists noted that the stereotype was inaccurate for about half of life-threatening asthma events.[22] Nearly half of near-fatal and fatal attacks occurred suddenly and unexpectedly, outside the hospital, in stable, younger, atopic patients who were reportedly compliant with their medical plan of care and using inhaled corticosteroids daily.[22]

Signs and Symptoms: Assessing Severity

The patient's report of subjective symptoms is an inaccurate gauge of asthma severity.

- Reported severity correlates poorly with objective severity scores.
- Some patients with severe, life-threatening asthma have an impaired response to hypercapnia and hypoxia. Their perception of dyspnea appears to be blunted. These patients may present with severe abnormalities of oxygenation and respiratory acidosis.[23]

An asthmatic who is sitting upright to breathe, using accessory inspiratory muscles in the neck and chest, is at risk for sudden respiratory failure. Somnolence, mental confusion, and a moribund or exhausted appearance are ominous signs that respiratory arrest is imminent.

The key to assessing severity is to use asthma severity scores (Table 1). These scores are based on objective evaluation of clinical signs, airway obstruction and work of breathing, oxygenation (with oximetry) and ventilation, and either FEV_1 or PEF. Clinical severity scores are much more reliable than observations of healthcare providers.[25]

A peak flow meter provides a quick, accurate, and reproducible measure of PEF in cooperative adults that is not influenced by the person supervising the test.[26] Emergency departments should consider PEF as a vital sign for an asthmatic. A peak flow meter should be used in EDs and offices that might treat patients with acute asthma. A small box of disposable mouthpieces and a list of expected normal flow rates for men and women should be kept with the device.

Differential Diagnosis

When a patient presents with wheezing, the ACLS provider must determine if the patient has acute asthma. When a patient presents with extreme dyspnea, you may be unable to confirm a history of asthma.

Bronchospasm also may be caused by medications, such as β-blockers,[27] or by drugs such as cocaine and opiates.[28,29] Abrupt discontinuation of corticosteroids may lead to life-threatening asthma. Long-term corticosteroid use may produce a relative adrenal insufficiency because endogenous cortisol secretion is suppressed. If steroids are stopped abruptly, endogenous cortisol production may initially be inadequate, and this temporary adrenal insufficiency may precipitate a severe attack in these patients.

Prehospital Clinical Deterioration, Imminent Respiratory Arrest and Cardiopulmonary Arrest

ACLS providers will most often treat people with severe, life-threatening asthma attacks and those who are deteriorating despite therapy and may stop breathing within minutes. These patients are challenging for emergency providers. The immediate goal is to prevent deterioration to respiratory or cardiopulmonary arrest. The provider must make difficult

Foundation Facts **Wheezing and Asthma Severity— Don't Be Fooled!**	In severe asthma the severity of wheezing provides a poor indicator of airflow or adequacy of gas exchange. • A patient with severe bronchospasm and obstruction may not move air and may not wheeze at all.[24,25] • The silent asthmatic chest is an ominous sign. Treatment that results in the return of wheezes on auscultation is effective treatment.
Critical Concept **Oxygen Saturation Can Be Misleading**	Oxygen saturation (SaO_2) levels may not reflect progressive alveolar hypoventilation, particularly if O_2 is being administered. SaO_2 may initially fall during therapy because β-agonists produce both bronchodilation and vasodilation and may initially increase intrapulmonary shunting.

Other conditions may cause patients to wheeze and to be acutely short of breath. These conditions include

- Cardiac disease (congestive heart failure or myocarditis)
- Emphysema
- Pneumonia
- Upper airway obstruction (structural or psychogenic, due to vocal cord dysfunction)
- Acute allergic bronchospasm or anaphylaxis (aspirin, foods, or idiopathic)
- Pulmonary embolism

decisions about noninvasive ventilation, endotracheal intubation, and mechanical ventilation. With appropriate first-line asthma therapy, life-threatening asthma attacks should be infrequent.

Immediate Actions

If supplementary **oxygen** has not been initiated, start it at once; use a nonrebreathing mask with high-flow oxygen or a bag and mask. Immediately administer a **selective inhaled short-acting β2-agonist** by nebulizer or metered-dose inhaler (with spacer), whichever can be assembled more quickly. Administer every 20 minutes or continuously for 1 hour.

Combining several doses of ipratropium bromide (0.5 mg every 20 minutes for 3 doses, then as needed) to an inhaled selective β2-agonist improves bronchodilation and is recommended for severe exacerbation in the ED, but its use is not recommended after admission to the hospital.

Systemic corticosteroids are recommended for most patients with moderate or severe exacerbations or patients who don't respond completely to initial β2-agonist therapy.

Systemic **β2-agonists** can be administered SC or IV if inhaler therapy is not possible because the patient is unable to use the equipment effectively or if the inhaler equipment is not readily available. **Epinephrine** 0.3 to 0.5 mg or terbutaline 0.25 mg can be administer every 20 minutes up to 3 doses.

For severe exacerbations that do not respond to these initial therapies, consider magnesium sulfate or heliox as adjunct treatments (see discussion of Adjunct Treatments later in this chapter).

Evaluate Immediate Response

Evaluate how well the patient responds in the first 10 to 20 minutes to initial therapy. There should be unequivocal and significant objective improvement (eg, improvement in oxygenation and clinical appearance, a change in PEF from a severe degree of obstruction of <100 L/min to 150 to 200 L/min).

If the patient deteriorates, proceed immediately to rapid sequence intubation if resources and skilled personnel are available. Support ventilations with a bag-mask device while preparations are made.

Primary Therapy and Reassessment in the ED

Primary Therapy

Patients with severe, life-threatening asthma require urgent and aggressive treatment with simultaneous administration of oxygen, bronchodilators, and steroids. Healthcare providers must monitor these patients closely for deterioration. Although the pathophysiology of life-threatening asthma consists of bronchoconstriction, inflammation, and mucous impaction, only bronchoconstriction and inflammation are amenable to drug treatment. If the patient does not respond to therapy, early consultation or transfer to a pulmonologist or intensivist is appropriate.

Oxygen

- Start oxygen at 4 L/min for all patients with acute severe asthma. The immediate treatment goal is to achieve an arterial partial pressure of oxygen (PaO_2) of ≥92 mm Hg or oxyhemoglobin saturation ≥95%.
- Start supplementary oxygen before or simultaneously with initial inhaled β_2-agonists. Give oxygen to all asthmatic patients, including those with normal oxygen saturation.
  - Without administration of supplementary oxygen, a paradoxical worsening of hypoxemia could follow administration of inhaled bronchodilators.
  - β-Agonists may induce both pulmonary vasodilation and bronchodilation. This condition may produce a right-to-left shunt (shunting of systemic venous blood through the lungs so that it is desaturated when it returns to the left atrium), which will contribute to worsening of hypoxemia.
- Some patients may require high-flow oxygen by mask.

Inhaled β_2-Agonists

Albuterol and levalbuterol are equivalent β_2-selective β-agonists that act by relaxing bronchial smooth muscles. These drugs provide rapid, dose-dependent, short-acting reduction in bronchospasm with minimal adverse effects. Albuterol has gained almost universal acceptance as the therapeutic cornerstone for acute asthma. When first developed albuterol was given intravenously (IV). But inhaled albuterol, delivered through a nebulizer or a metered-dose inhaler (MDI), has proven much more effective than IV albuterol. Because the administered dose depends on lung volume and inspiratory flow rates, the same dose can be used in most adult patients regardless of age or size. Levalbuterol

has been shown to provide the same efficacy and safety as albuterol when administered at half the mg dose, but it has not been evaluated by continuous nebulization.

Metered-Dose Inhalers Versus Nebulizers

Although studies have shown no difference in the effects of continuous versus intermittent administration of nebulized albuterol, continuous administration was more effective in patients with severe exacerbations of asthma,[30,31] and it was more cost-effective in a pediatric trial.[32] A Cochrane meta-analysis showed no overall difference between the effects of albuterol delivered by MDI-spacer or nebulizer,[33] but MDI-spacer administration can be difficult in patients in severe distress. Delivery by nebulizer has become the most common ED treatment for acute asthma attacks. But a number of studies suggest that MDIs with spacers have several advantages over nebulizers,[34-37] although the technique of administration must be precise. MDI-spacer administration is less expensive, starting treatment is faster and easier, and there is more efficient use of staff time.

The recommended dose of albuterol by nebulizer is 2.5 or 5 mg every 20 minutes for 3 doses or continuous nebulization in a dose of 10 to 15 mg/h. Aggressive dosing for more severe cases calls for higher amounts of the agent at shorter intervals. The typical dose of albuterol by MDI-spacer (90 μg/puff) is 4 to 8 puffs every 20 minutes for up to 4 hours, then every 1 to 4 hours as needed.

Levalbuterol is the R-isomer of albuterol. Some studies have shown equivalent or slight improvement in bronchodilation with levalbuterol when compared with albuterol in the ED.[38-40] But the relative benefits of levalbuterol, which is more expensive than albuterol, have not been determined.[41]

Rapid Response Interventions
 	
Imminent Respiratory Arrest in Severe, Life-Threatening Asthma— Immediate Critical Interventions to Consider
	• Oxygen: high flow, nonrebreathing mask
	• β_2-agonists: by MDI and spacer or nebulizer
	• Epinephrine: 0.01 mg/kg *divided into 3 doses* or terbutaline 0.25 mg every 20 minutes for 3 doses SC
	• Noninvasive positive-pressure ventilation: if immediately available
	• Magnesium sulfate 1.2 to 2 g IV over 20 minutes or heliox
	• Inhaled ipratropium bromide 0.5 mg by nebulizer
	• Corticosteroids IV (eg, methylprednisolone 125 mg IV)
	• For severe refractory respiratory failure:
	  — Isoproterenol IV
	  — Extracorporeal membrane oxygenation

FYI **Administration of β_2-Selective β-Agonists**	There is no overall difference in effectiveness when albuterol is administered by continuous or intermittent dosing or by MDI-spacer or nebulizer. But • Continuous administration has been found more effective in patients with severe exacerbations of asthma • MDI-spacer administration can be difficult in patients in severe distress

Corticosteroids

Systemic corticosteroids are the only proven treatment for the inflammatory component of asthma, but the onset of their anti-inflammatory effects is 6 to 12 hours after administration. A comprehensive search of the literature by the Cochrane approach (including pediatric and adult patients) determined that early use of systemic steroids reduced rates of admission to the hospital.[42] In addition, reduction of inflammation and bronchial edema reduces length of hospital stay, in-hospital complications, readmissions, and return visits to the ED.[43,44]

Healthcare providers should administer steroids as early as possible to all patients with asthma but should not expect effects for several hours. Although there is no difference in clinical effects between oral and IV formulations of corticosteroids,[45] the IV route is preferable because patients with severe near-fatal asthma may vomit or be unable to swallow. A typical initial IV dose for mythylprednisolone is 125 mg. Then the dose for methylprednisolone, prednisone, and prednisolone is 40 to 80 mg/day in one or two divided doses until PEF is ≥70% of predicted value.

Other commonly accepted criteria[46] for immediately starting corticosteroids include slow response (>20 minutes) to inhaled β_2-agonists (moderate to severe attack), ED visit within the previous 7 days ("bounce-backs"), current use of oral corticosteroids ("steroid-dependent" patient), and recent tapering off corticosteroids ("steroid-dependent" patient).

Inhaled Steroids

Incorporation or substitution of inhaled steroids into this scheme remains controversial. A Cochrane meta-analysis of 7 randomized trials (4 adult and 3 pediatric) of inhaled corticosteroids concluded that steroids significantly reduced the likelihood of admission to the hospital, particularly in patients who were not receiving concomitant systemic steroids. But there was insufficient evidence to conclude that inhaled corticosteroids alone are as effective as systemic steroids.[43]

Adjunctive Therapy

Anticholinergics

Ipratropium bromide is an anticholinergic bronchodilator that is pharmacologically related to atropine. It can produce a clinically modest improvement in lung function compared with albuterol alone.[47,48] The nebulizer dose is 0.5 mg. It has a slow onset of action (approximately 20 minutes) with peak effectiveness at 60 to 90 minutes and no systemic side effects. It is typically given only once because of its prolonged onset of action, but some studies have shown clinical improvement only with repeated doses.[49] Given the few side effects, ipratropium should be considered an adjunct to albuterol. Tiotropium is a new, longer-acting anticholinergic that is currently undergoing clinical testing for use in acute asthma.[50]

Pharmacology

Ipratropium bromide (Atrovent) is an anticholinergic (parasympatholytic) bronchodilator that is pharmacologically related to atropine. Ipratropium inhibits vagally mediated constriction of bronchial smooth muscles. The result is local, site-specific bronchodilation. There are no systemic effects. Ipratropium bromide produces less bronchodilation than inhaled β_2-agonists,[48,51] and it has a slower onset (about 20 minutes longer).[52]

Use in Severe, Life-Threatening Asthma

There does appear to be a role for ipratropium bromide *in combination* with selective inhaled β-agonists for acute events. This beneficial effect appears to occur specifically in cases of severe, life-threatening asthma. Note that the only age groups with relevant studies are children and adolescents.[53] A systematic analysis of randomized, controlled trials in children and adolescents with moderately severe asthma (FEV_1 <55% of predicted)[54] noted that multiple doses of ipratropium added to inhaled β_2-agonists improved pulmonary function and reduced the rate of hospitalization by 30%. But this benefit was not observed when the asthma attacks were only mild or moderate. A meta-analysis of randomized, controlled trials limited to adult asthmatics observed a modest benefit from

Foundation Facts **Corticosteroids: Delayed Effect, Administer Early**	• Corticosteroids produce an objective effect only after 3 to 4 hours. • Improved airflow due to corticosteroids can be demonstrated only after 6 to 12 hours. • Early use of systemic steroids reduces hospital admissions.
FYI **NIH Expert Panel**	The National Institutes of Health Expert Panel on the Management of Asthma endorses the combination of β_2-agonists plus an inhaled anticholinergic agent for asthma patients with a PEF or FEV_1 <80% of the predicted normal value.[6]

ipratropium combined with β₂-agonists (7% improvement in FEV₁, 22% improvement in PEF).[55] Ipratropium bromide is not recommended for use after hospital admission.

Dose

Ipratropium bromide is usually mixed 0.5 mg in 2.5 mL of normal saline in a nebulizer with the first dose of albuterol and administered every 4 to 6 hours. Higher doses or dosing intervals less than 4 hours confer no added benefits.

Magnesium Sulfate

IV magnesium sulfate can modestly improve pulmonary function in patients with asthma when combined with nebulized β-adrenergic agents and corticosteroids.[56] Magnesium causes relaxation of bronchial smooth muscle independent of the serum magnesium level with only minor side effects (flushing, lightheadedness). A Cochrane meta-analysis of 7 studies concluded that IV magnesium sulfate improves pulmonary function and reduces hospital admissions, particularly for patients with the most severe exacerbations of asthma.[57]

Pharmacology

The exact mechanism of action of magnesium sulfate in asthma is unknown, but it may be similar to the tocolytic effects on smooth muscle. A number of clinical trials have reported that magnesium sulfate improves bronchodilation in patients persistently symptomatic after inhaled adrenergic agents and corticosteroids.[56-60]

Dose

The adult dose of magnesium sulfate 1.2 to 2 g IV given over 20 minutes when used with conventional therapy has been shown to reduce hospitalization rates for ED patients with severe exacerbations, but did not improve pulmonary function in patients whose initial FEV₁ was ≥25% of predicted.[1] When given with a β₂-agonist, nebulized magnesium sulfate improved pulmonary function during acute asthma but in contrast to the Cochrane meta-analysis, did not reduce the rate of hospitalization.[61]

Heliox

Heliox is a mixture of helium and oxygen (usually a 70:30 helium to oxygen ratio) that is less viscous than ambient air. Heliox has been shown to improve the delivery and deposition of nebulized albuterol and may decrease the likelihood of intubation.[1,62] Although a recent meta-analysis of 4 clinical trials did not support the use of heliox in the initial treatment of patients with acute asthma,[63] it may be useful for asthma that is refractory to conventional therapy.[64] The heliox mixture requires at least 70% helium for effect, so if the patient requires >30% oxygen, heliox cannot be used.

Parenteral Epinephrine or Terbutaline

Epinephrine and terbutaline are adrenergic agents that can be given subcutaneously to patients with acute severe asthma. Epinephrine is an effective bronchial smooth muscle dilator with rapid onset of action. The dose of subcutaneous epinephrine (concentration of 1:1000, 1 mg/mL) is divided into 3 doses of approximately 0.3 to 0.5 mg given at 20-minute intervals. The nonselective adrenergic properties of epinephrine may cause an increase in heart rate, myocardial irritability, and increased oxygen demand. But its use (even in patients >35 years of age) is well tolerated.[65] Terbutaline is given in a dose of 0.25 mg SC and can be repeated every 20 minutes for 3 doses. These drugs are more commonly administered to children with acute asthma. Although most studies have shown them to be equally efficacious, one study concluded that terbutaline was superior.[66]

Epinephrine

Pharmacology

Epinephrine is a nonselective β-agonist that requires parenteral (subcutaneous or IV) administration. The nonselective properties of epinephrine also produce tachycardia, acute blood pressure elevation, and myocardial irritability. Epinephrine will increase myocardial oxygen demand.

Indications

Adverse properties and side effects cause many experts to limit the use of epinephrine in acute asthma to patients under the age of 35 who are unable to use inhalers.[67] The exclusion of patients over age 35 is probably unjustified, particularly with subcutaneous epinephrine. Older prospective studies and reviews documented that subcutaneous epinephrine is well tolerated and effective for the treatment of older adults with asthma.

Use in Severe, Life-Threatening Asthma

Subcutaneous epinephrine can be administered to patients who are "too tight to wheeze" and cannot effectively inhale β₂-agonists through a metered-dose inhaler or nebulizer. As the patient deteriorates, the inspiratory flow rate decreases and compromises delivery of inhaled medications. There

Rapid Response Interventions **Epinephrine Prearrest**	Administer subcutaneous epinephrine to patients with severe acute asthma in prearrest. • At a concentration of 1:1000 the total dose is 0.01 mg/kg SC. It is usually divided into 3 doses of approximately 0.3 to 0.5 mg given at 20-minute intervals.

is little evidence to withhold epinephrine (even if it must be given IV) from patients with severe, life-threatening asthma solely because of their age.

Terbutaline

Pharmacology

Terbutaline is a selective β_2-agonist with pharmacologic and adverse effects similar to those of albuterol. Common trade names for terbutaline are Brethine and Bricanyl. Asthma patients use terbutaline in metered-dose inhalers, nebulized solution, or oral tablets. In the ED terbutaline is given by subcutaneous injection or IV infusion.

Use in Severe, Life-Threatening Asthma?

Compared with epinephrine, terbutaline has a slower onset of action (5 to 30 minutes), a longer time to peak effects (1 to 2 hours), and a much longer duration of action (3 to 6 hours). As an alternative to epinephrine, terbutaline has little role to play in adults with severe, life-threatening asthma because of the slow onset of action and longer time to peak effects. But in children at least one ED study has found terbutaline to be more efficacious than epinephrine for reversal of wheezing.

Dose

The dose of terbutaline is 0.25 mg SC. This dose can be administered every 20 minutes for 3 doses.

Other Agents

Ketamine

Ketamine is a parenteral dissociative anesthetic that has bronchodilatory properties. Ketamine may also have indirect effects in patients with asthma through its sedative properties. One case series[68] suggested substantial effectiveness, but the single randomized trial published to date[69] showed no benefit of ketamine when compared with standard care. Ketamine stimulates copious bronchial secretions. Sedation is not generally recommended because of the depressant effect on respiration.

Methylxanthines

Although previously a mainstay in the treatment of acute asthma, methylxanthines are infrequently used because of questionable efficacy, erratic pharmacokinetics, and known side effects and are no longer recommended for managing acute asthma exacerbations. A meta-analysis of 13 clinical trials concluded that the addition of aminophylline produced no increase in bronchodilation but an increase in adverse effects.[70] Side effects include nausea, vomiting, seizures, and cardiac arrhythmias. Theophylline is a substrate for the cytochrome p450 enzyme pathway. Theophylline levels are *increased* with concomitant administration of many drugs, such as cimetidine and verapamil. Theophylline levels are *decreased* with concomitant administration of isoproterenol, phenobarbital, phenytoin, and rifampin.

Leukotriene Receptor Antagonists

Leukotriene receptor antagonists (LTRAs) improve lung function and decrease the need for short-acting β-agonists during long-term asthma therapy, but their effectiveness during acute exacerbations of asthma is unproven. One study showed improvement in lung function with the addition of IV montelukast to standard therapy,[71] but further research is needed.

Inhaled Anesthetics

Case reports in adults[72] and children[73] suggest a benefit of inhalation anesthetics for patients with status asthmaticus unresponsive to maximal conventional therapy. These anesthetic agents may work directly as bronchodilators and may have indirect effects by enhancing patient-ventilator synchrony and reducing oxygen demand and carbon dioxide production. This therapy, however, requires an ICU setting, and there have been no randomized studies to evaluate its effectiveness.

Post-Treatment/Resuscitation Care

Response to Initial Treatment?

Clinical decision making for severe, life-threatening asthma is determined by the patient's response to initial treatment. This fact underscores the importance of asthma scoring systems that include evaluation of clinical appearance, work of breathing, pulse oximetry, and measurement of PEF or FEV_1. One study evaluated patients with severe asthma (pretreatment PEF <100 L/min) and noted the degree of improvement with initial therapy. Failure to achieve a PEF >300 L/min after first-line treatment was associated with a 92% admission rate.

To aid decision making, use the severity scoring system (Table 1). In addition, you can place patients into 1 of the following categories after first-line treatment:

- Clinical improvement and FEV_1 or PEF ≥70% of predicted after 1 to 3 hours of treatment: consider discharge home
- Some clinical improvement and FEV_1 or PEF 40% to 69% of predicted after 4 hours of intensive treatment: "incomplete responder"
- Inadequate clinical improvement and FEV_1 or PEF <40% of predicted after 4 hours of intensive treatment: hospital admission + noninvasive assisted ventilation
- No clinical improvement and FEV_1 or PEF <25% of predicted after 4 hours of intensive treatment: ICU admission + assisted ventilation

Clinical Improvement

FEV₁ or PEF ≥70% of Predicted After 1 to 3 Hours of Treatment: Consider Discharge Home

Most patients who improve clinically and are breathing room air with adequate oxygenation (oxyhemoglobin saturation of ≥95%) and FEV_1 or PEF ≥70% of predicted after 1 to 3 hours of inhaled short-acting β_2-agonists, anticholinergics, and oral corticosteroids can be discharged home. You may need to modify this disposition on the basis of the risk factors noted above and below.

- Observe these patients for at least 1 hour after they reach ≥70% of predicted FEV_1 or PEF to ensure their stability.
- Review the discharge medications closely. Studies confirm the value of continued inhaled or oral steroids and of inhaled β_2-agonists *after* an acute **exacerbation**. These medications significantly reduce the need for return ED visits and subsequent hospitalizations.

Some Clinical Improvement

FEV₁ or PEF 40% to 69% of Predicted After 4 Hours of Intensive Treatment: Incomplete Responders

Risk stratification for incomplete responders: Patients who achieve some clinical improvement but have persistent signs of moderate to severe asthma with improved oxygenation (oxyhemoglobin saturation of 90% to 95%) and FEV_1 or PEF 40% to 69% of predicted after 4 hours of intensive treatment are classified as *incomplete responders*. They require careful triage. To borrow from the nomenclature of acute coronary syndromes, the responsible clinician must "risk stratify" these patients. Concurrent comorbidity, such as insulin-dependent diabetes, coronary artery disease, cerebrovascular disease, chronic obstructive pulmonary disease, or acute pneumonia, adds to the risk.

Low-risk incomplete responders: Some incomplete responders are at low risk for continued deterioration and may be discharged conditionally. Appropriate discharge requires that patients have adequate discharge medications, home resources, access to follow-up care, and a detailed discharge care plan.

High-risk incomplete responders: Incomplete responders with 1 or more of the following risk factors should be hospitalized (with occasional individual exceptions):

- History of intubation and mechanical ventilation for acute, life-threatening asthma
- Recent (within 2 to 4 weeks) hospitalization for asthma
- Bounce-back ED visits (ie, patient was evaluated and treated in an ED in the previous 24 to 48 hours)
- Duration of attack is 1 week or longer

- Current use of oral steroids (steroid dependent); studies have not yet established whether patients currently using inhaled steroids should be stratified as high risk
- Inadequate home care resources
- Known or suspected poor compliance

Inadequate Clinical Improvement

FEV₁ or PEF 25% to 40% of Predicted After 4 Hours of Intensive Treatment: Hospital Admission + Noninvasive Assisted Ventilation

Emergency physicians should admit these patients to the hospital. Pulmonologists, emergency physicians, and other specialists are gaining considerable experience with noninvasive assisted ventilation techniques for these patients. Noninvasive positive-pressure ventilation (NIPPV) is rapidly emerging as an effective ED technique. These techniques, discussed in more detail below, are not initiated to prevent hospital admission. Their major clinical purpose is to prevent endotracheal intubation. These techniques are judged "effective" only if the patient avoids endotracheal intubation.

No Clinical Improvement

FEV₁ or PEF <25% of Predicted After 4 Hours of Intensive Treatment: ICU Admission + Assisted Ventilation

These patients need not only hospital admission but also intensive monitoring and care. They are seriously ill. Endotracheal intubation and mechanical ventilation may be necessary if the patient continues to be unresponsive to therapy.

Indications for ICU admission: In addition to an FEV_1 or PEF <25% of predicted, other objective signs and clinical symptoms indicate the need for ICU admission and probable intubation:

- Pao_2 <65 mm Hg with 40% inspired oxygen (oxyhemoglobin saturation <90%)
- $Paco_2$ >40 mm Hg (especially if rising during treatment in the ED)
- Altered level of consciousness
- Breathlessness that makes talking difficult
- Inability to lie supine
- Increasing fatigue and tiredness

Noninvasive Assisted Ventilation

Noninvasive positive-pressure ventilation may offer short-term support to patients with acute respiratory failure and may delay or eliminate the need for endotracheal intubation.[74] This therapy requires an alert patient with adequate spontaneous respiratory effort. Bilevel positive airway pressure (BiPAP), the most common way of delivering NIPPV, allows for separate control of inspiratory and expiratory pressures.

Description

The decision to intubate a patient with asthma is difficult. Noninvasive assisted ventilation techniques are emerging as an effective way for patients with severe, life-threatening asthma to avoid the need for intubation and mechanical ventilation.[76]

NIPPV uses a mechanical ventilation device to deliver positive-pressure ventilation through a mask to assist the patient's spontaneous respiratory efforts. The mask may cover a patient's face or nose or both. It must fit against the nose or face with a relatively tight seal.

Benefits

These devices are intended for patients suffering from severe, life-threatening asthma that is refractory to bronchodilators and steroids. In the past such compromised patients required endotracheal intubation and mechanical ventilation. By eliminating the need for intubation, these techniques convey numerous benefits.

NIPPV can enable support of ventilation without the need for and hazards of endotracheal tube placement. But the patient must have effective spontaneous respiratory effort and adequate airway protective mechanisms. Table 3 lists the initial steps and settings for NIPPV.

Requirements and Contraindications

Experienced clinicians often recommend NIPPV for patients who do not respond satisfactorily to aggressive first-line therapy. But 3 critical requirements remain. The patients must be

- Alert and able to protect the airway
- Cooperative
- Demonstrating effective spontaneous respirations

Contraindications: Noninvasive assisted ventilation techniques are contraindicated for patients who are

- Severely hypoxemic: PaO_2 <60 mm Hg or O_2 saturation <90% on rebreathing mask

- A rising $PaCO_2$ (>40 mm Hg) with a falling pH
- Deteriorating steadily or rapidly
- Confused, somnolent, moribund, or uncooperative
- Unable to protect the airway
- Hypotensive (BP <90 mm Hg)
- Known to have ischemic heart disease
- Having ventricular arrhythmias

Bilevel Positive Airway Pressure

Bilevel positive airway pressure (BiPAP) has proven to be the most effective type of NIPPV for life-threatening asthma. Intermittent assisted ventilation with a BiPAP ventilator may help to delay or eliminate the need for endotracheal intubation. The BiPAP ventilator is a variable-flow device that offers separate control of the inspiratory positive airway pressure and the expiratory positive airway pressure. Carefully selected settings allow this type of ventilator to counteract the effects of auto-PEEP. BiPAP devices reduce the work of breathing more than any other noninvasive respiratory support technique. They reduce the work of breathing by reducing the force required for exhalation and increasing the work of inspiration.

Most experts begin with an inspiratory positive airway pressure of 8 to 10 cm H_2O and an expiratory positive airway pressure of 3 to 5 cm H_2O.

Table 3. Initial Steps to Follow for NIPPV[75,76]

1. Secure a full face mask with head straps over the nose and mouth. Avoid a tight fit.

2. Connect the ventilator to the face mask. Use either a conventional mechanical ventilator or a ventilator specially made for NIPPV.

3. Start with continuous positive airway pressure (CPAP) set to 0 cm H_2O. Slowly increase CPAP to maintain positive end-expiratory pressure even during spontaneous inspiration.

4. Set positive-pressure support (inspiratory pressure) of ventilation at 10 cm H_2O. Adjust on the basis of arterial blood gases, but do not exceed 25 cm H_2O.

5. Set tidal volume at 500 mL (7 mL/kg).

6. Set ventilation rate at <25 breaths/min.

7. Continue to administer nebulized medications through the system.

Foundation Facts

When to Intubate in Severe Asthma

"The greatest challenge in intubating and managing the patient with asthma...is that the patient's clinical condition may worsen after intubation, when the patient may prove extremely difficult to ventilate and may be hemodynamically unstable. Thus the decision to intubate must be made carefully and the technique must be chosen to facilitate the best possible outcome."

—R.E. Schneider[75]

Endotracheal Intubation for Life-Threatening Asthma

"The patient's clinical condition may worsen after intubation.... The decision to intubate must be made carefully...."[75]

Endotracheal intubation does not solve the problem of small airway constriction in patients with severe asthma. In addition, intubation and positive-pressure ventilation can trigger further bronchoconstriction and complications such as breath stacking (auto-PEEP) and barotrauma. Although endotracheal intubation introduces risks, elective intubation should be performed if the asthmatic patient deteriorates despite aggressive management.

Rapid sequence intubation (RSI) is the technique of choice. The provider should use the largest endotracheal tube available (usually 8 or 9 mm) to decrease airway resistance. Immediately after intubation, confirm endotracheal tube placement by clinical examination and a device (eg, exhaled CO_2 detector) and obtain a chest radiograph.

Indications

The major indications for rapid endotracheal intubation in life-threatening asthma are

- Failure to improve after 4 hours of NIPPV.
- Continued deterioration despite aggressive first-line therapy.
- Association with anaphylaxis (see Chapter 14, Part 4 "Anaphylaxis").
- Deterioration with fatigue and exhaustion. With complete exhaustion the patient is simply too tired to maintain effective ventilation, and apnea and respiratory arrest are likely to develop.
- Onset of altered level of consciousness, confusion, or somnolence.
- A rising $PaCO_2$ (>40 mm Hg) with a falling pH. These values are particularly worrisome when associated with clinical signs of obtundation, somnolence, and poor muscle tone. These signs suggest the presence of exhaustion and respiratory failure. Note that isolated hypercarbia does not require immediate endotracheal intubation. *Treat the patient, not the numbers.*
- PaO_2 <50 mm Hg on a nonrebreathing mask, especially when associated with clinical signs of hypoxemia. These signs include severe agitation, confusion, and fighting against the oxygen mask.

Rapid Sequence Intubation (RSI)

Precautions

RSI is the technique of choice for endotracheal intubation in patients with severe, life-threatening asthma.[41,75] Other techniques, especially nasotracheal intubation, have a high rate of failure in these patients.

- Select the most experienced laryngoscopist to perform the procedure. In asthmatic patients the smallest amount of airway stimulation with a laryngoscope blade can provoke severe laryngospasm and reflex bronchoconstriction.
- It may be impossible to provide effective bag-mask ventilation when status asthmaticus is present. In patients with severe, life-threatening asthma, most air delivered with a bag and mask will divert away from the high-resistance airways and into the stomach. This can produce gastric distention, a further decrease in effective ventilation, regurgitation, and aspiration.
- Use the largest endotracheal tube (8 to 9 mm) possible. The larger the tube diameter, the less the airway resistance. Suctioning the airway secretions can be handled better with large-diameter tubes.

Premedications

The most critical of the **LOAD** premedications (lidocaine, opioids, atropine, defasciculating agent) is lidocaine.

- Give lidocaine 1.5 to 2 mg/kg IV 3 minutes before administration of opioids, sedatives, or paralytics. This dose will reduce bronchospasm induced by laryngoscopy and intubation.

Sedation and Anesthesia

Several anesthetics are powerful bronchodilators, especially halothane (not generally available) and other inhalational anesthetics (eg, isoflurane), ketamine, and propofol.[77,78] Only providers with extensive experience and knowledge of their side effects, precautions, and contraindications should use sedative and anesthetic agents for treating patients with severe life-threatening asthma.

Ketamine is an effective sedative, analgesic, and dissociative anesthetic. Many experts recommend ketamine as the IV anesthetic of choice for patients with status asthmaticus. Ketamine possesses strong bronchodilator properties.[69] Ketamine potentiates catecholamines and relaxes bronchiolar smooth muscle. Ketamine does not cause vasodilatation, circulatory collapse, or myocardial depression. A dose of 2 mg/kg IV (1 to 4 mg/kg pediatrics) induces anesthesia in 30 seconds and lasts 10 to 15 minutes. Because ketamine increases bronchial secretions, many experts also premedicate with **atropine** (0.01 mg/kg; minimum dose of 0.1 mg).

Propofol is another sedative with bronchodilator properties.[79] It is effective for both intubation and maintenance of sedation during mechanical ventilation. A dose of 2 to 2.5 mg/kg induces anesthesia in approximately 40 seconds and lasts 3 to 5 minutes. This drug may cause hypotension.

Etomidate is an acceptable hypnotic to use, though it lacks bronchodilator properties.[80] Etomidate is ultra short acting and has a safer hemodynamic profile than both ketamine and propofol. A dose of 0.2 to 0.6 mg/kg (0.2 to 0.4 mg/kg for pediatric patients) induces anesthesia in 60 seconds and lasts 3 to 5 minutes. This drug has no analgesic properties.

Inhaled volatile anesthetics: Physicians who care for patients with severe asthma should be aware of reports of the use of inhaled volatile anesthetics for patients with severe, life-threatening asthma. The volatile anesthetics are powerful bronchial smooth muscle relaxants. Enflurane and ether have been successful in the treatment of status asthmaticus refractory to all other treatments.[81] Use these agents with extreme caution because they are also vasodilators and myocardial depressants. Some of these anesthetics sensitize the myocardium to catecholamines, leading to life-threatening arrhythmias.

Paralysis

Two agents are commonly used for paralysis. **Succinylcholine,** at a dose of 1 to 2 mg/kg, is the clear paralytic agent of choice for RSI in patients with severe asthma and no contraindications to the drug. **Rocuronium,** at a dose of 0.6 to 1.2 mg/kg, is the second paralytic of choice. Its rapid onset of action is similar to that of succinylcholine, but it has a longer duration of action.

Immediately After Intubation

Airway Obstruction—A Persistent Problem

Endotracheal intubation enables use of external mechanical power to assist the patient's failing ventilation efforts. It does not solve the problem of airway obstruction. Patients with severe, life-threatening asthma may be extremely difficult to oxygenate before intubation, even with bag-mask ventilation. In addition, hypercarbia may create a respiratory acidosis. These problems with oxygenation and ventilation may persist even once the tube is in place.

- **Continue inhaled β_2-agonists:** Because breathing efforts may be inadequate, the patient may not have had adequate distribution of β_2-agonists before intubation. Immediately after intubation inject 2.5 to 5 mg of albuterol directly into the endotracheal tube.
- **Ventilate the patient slowly with 100% oxygen:** When severe asthma is present, significant obstruction to air flow persists even after intubation. In fact, if there is no significant obstruction to airflow immediately after intubation, you should reevaluate the diagnosis of acute asthma and consider the possibility that the resistance to airflow was present in the upper airway (eg, vocal cord dysfunction, tumor, or a foreign body).

Anyone performing manual ventilation for patients with severe asthma after intubation should *slowly* ventilate at a rate of only 6 to 10 breaths/min, allowing adequate time for exhalation between delivered breaths. This slow respiratory rate and adequate exhalation time can minimize the development of auto-PEEP and its serious consequence of severe hypotension and pneumothorax. Prevention of hyperventilation and auto-PEEP is preferable to treatment of the complications.

Acute asthma is occasionally confused with exacerbation of emphysema, especially in the elderly. Hyperventilation immediately after intubation can cause dire consequences in elderly patients with emphysema.

Table 4 summarizes the steps needed to insert an endotracheal tube and begin mechanical ventilatory support for patients with severe, life-threatening asthma.

Table 4. Summary of Steps to Initiate Mechanical Ventilatory Support for Severe Life-Threatening Asthma[75]

This sequence is one example. Variations are acceptable.

1. Place the patient in an upright position if comfortable.
2. Administer *lidocaine* 1.5 to 2 mg/kg three minutes before administration of anesthesia.
3. Administer *ketamine* 2 mg/kg.
4. *Immediately* follow with *succinylcholine* 1.5 mg/kg.
5. As the patient loses consciousness, apply *cricoid pressure.* Gently place the patient in the supine position.
6. Perform *laryngoscopy* and *endotracheal intubation.* Use an 8- to 9-mm tube if possible.
7. Perform primary and secondary confirmation of tube placement and begin mechanical ventilation support. Note that when patients have severe asthma, the esophageal detector device may reinflate rapidly, falsely suggesting endotracheal tube placement despite the presence of the tube in the esophagus. Providers should perform primary confirmation of tube placement and use exhaled CO_2 as a secondary confirmation device.
8. Begin maintenance sedation (*benzodiazepine or propofol*) and paralysis (*rocuronium*). Continue for 4 to 6 hours.
9. Adjust mechanical ventilation parameters as recommended in Table 5.
10. Provide additional *ketamine* as needed.
11. Administer inhalational agents via the endotracheal tube.
12. Monitor airway pressures to evaluate patient response to therapy.
13. Administer fluids (eg, normal saline) if needed to counteract the fall in blood pressure from auto-PEEP.

Mechanical Ventilation in Patients With Severe Asthma

Mechanical ventilation in patients with severe, life-threatening asthma is challenging and may produce several significant complications.

Troubleshooting Problems in the Intubated, Ventilator-Dependent Asthmatic

Auto-PEEP

Clinicians who provide mechanical ventilatory support for patients with severe asthma must understand the concept of auto-PEEP. Although asthmatics experience some obstruction of inspiration, they experience *marked* obstruction of expiration. As resistance to exhalation increases, the inevitable result will be air trapping and "breath stacking" (inspired air enters and then cannot exit).

With severe airway obstruction the duration of spontaneous expiration increases. But during mechanical ventilation, expiratory time is set. If expiratory time is inadequate, this can lead to "self-produced" or "auto-produced" PEEP. In this case end-expiratory pressure increases without addition of PEEP to the mechanical ventilatory circuit. Increased intrathoracic pressure from auto-PEEP can reduce venous return to the heart. This reduced venous return can lead to reduced cardiac output, hemodynamic compromise, and hypotension. Note that hyperinflation and increased intrathoracic pressure can also produce barotrauma, such as a tension pneumothorax.

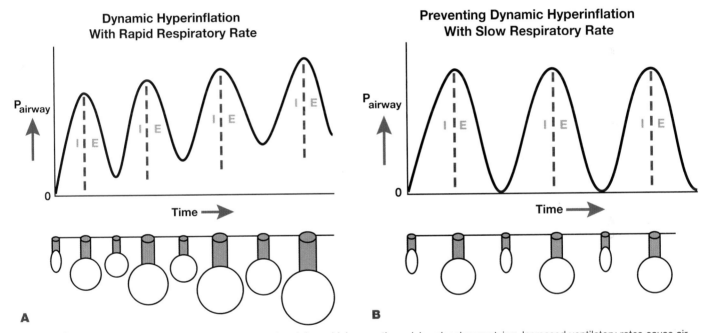

Figure 2. Dynamic hyperinflation. Bronchospasm and endobronchiole secretions delay alveolar emptying. Increased ventilatory rates cause air trapping (**A**) and increased alveolar volume, leading to decreased compliance or lung stiffness. Using a slower ventilation rate and lower volume (**B**) allows the alveolus more time to empty. I indicates inspiration; and E, expiration.

Critical Concept **Sudden Deterioration in a Ventilated Patient**	If the patient with asthma deteriorates or is difficult to ventilate, verify endotracheal tube position, eliminate tube obstruction (any mucous plugs and kinks), and rule out (or decompress) a pneumothorax. Only experienced providers should perform needle decompression or insertion of a chest tube for pneumothorax. Check the ventilator circuit for leaks or malfunction. High end-expiratory pressure can be quickly reduced by separating the patient from the ventilator circuit; this will allow PEEP to dissipate during passive exhalation. • To minimize auto-PEEP if present, decrease inhalation time (this increases exhalation time), decrease the respiratory rate by 2 breaths per minute, and reduce the tidal volume to 3 to 5 mL/kg. • Continue treatment with inhaled albuterol.

When severe bronchoconstriction is present, breath stacking (auto-PEEP) can develop during positive-pressure ventilation, leading to complications such as hyperinflation (Figure 2), tension pneumothorax, and hypotension. During manual or mechanical ventilation use a slower respiratory rate (6 to 10 breaths/min) with smaller tidal volumes (6 to 8 mL/kg),[41] shorter inspiratory time (adult inspiratory flow rate 80 to 100 mL/min), and longer expiratory time (inspiratory to expiratory ratio 1:4 or 1:5) than typical for nonasthmatic patients.

Ventilation With "Permissive Hypercapnia"

Adequate oxygenation is relatively easy to achieve with mechanical ventilation in patients with severe asthma. The problem is getting rid of the carbon dioxide—ventilation. Mild hypoventilation reduces the risk of barotrauma from significant levels of auto-PEEP and is typically well tolerated.[82] This concept of controlled hypoventilation, using ventilator settings that result in a mild elevation of $PaCO_2$, is referred to as *permissive hypercapnia or permissive hypercarbia.*

To prevent the development of significant levels of auto-PEEP, set the mechanical ventilator to low tidal volume, low respiratory rate, and long expiratory time. These settings will lead to a mild increase in $PaCO_2$, but because ventilatory support is controlled, hypercapnia develops gradually ($PaCO_2$ levels may rise to 70 to 90 mm Hg over 3 to 4 hours). Acidemia also develops, with pH values in the range of 7.2 to 7.3, but the level is controlled by controlling the rise in $PaCO_2$. Within 24 to 48 hours the patient's serum pH will be restored to a near-normal level because the kidneys will reabsorb bicarbonate to compensate for the respiratory acidosis.

In addition to setting the ventilator for reduced tidal volume and slower respiratory rates, you should increase the inspiratory flow rate to 80 to 120 L/min. To tolerate such settings patients usually require complete paralysis and heavy sedation. Closely monitor patient tolerance of the respiratory acidosis, particularly during the first 24 to 48 hours of therapy, before renal compensation has occurred. In some patients arrhythmias may develop when acidosis is present, and this may limit the level of permissive hypercapnia used. It may be necessary to allow the $PaCO_2$ to rise in smaller increments over a longer period of time. Table 5 provides an example of initial settings for mechanical ventilation after endotracheal intubation.

Patient Is Difficult to Ventilate

When ventilation is difficult or inadequate, clinical assessment and evaluation may be difficult and elusive in patients with severe refractory asthma. Auscultatory clues may be missing because the chest is often silent. This lack of audible breath sounds comes from poor airflow and hyperinflation of the chest wall.

Table 5. Example of Initial Settings for Ventilation After Endotracheal Intubation[75]

1. Calculate the patient's **ideal body weight.**
2. **Tidal volume:** Set to 6 to 8 mL/kg.
3. **Respiratory rate:** Set to 8 to 10 breaths/min.
4. **Inspiratory flow rate:** Set to 80 to 100 L/min. The objective is to achieve a ratio of inspired to expired air (I:E) of 1:4 to 1:5.
5. **Positive inspiratory pressure:** Start at 10 cm H_2O. Do not set at >25 cm H_2O. Keep the **peak inspiratory pressure (PIP)** under 40 cm H_2O. This level will reduce the occurrence of barotrauma and hemodynamic compromise. Sudden increases in the inspiratory pressures may indicate a pneumothorax, obstructed endotracheal tube, or mucous plugging. Conversely a precipitous fall in PIP may indicate extubation. Investigate any sudden change in PIP.
6. **Permissive hypercarbia:** Titrate tidal volume and respiratory rate to allow the gradual development of hypercarbia. It often will occur if inspiratory pressure is maintained at <25 cm H_2O.
7. **Continue sedation:** Maintain continuous sedation with propofol or a benzodiazepine.
8. **Maintain paralysis:** Maintain continuous paralysis with a longer-acting, nondepolarizing muscle relaxant, such as *rocuronium.*
9. **Administer inhalational medications:** Continue to provide (as indicated) the first-line asthma therapies (inhaled β_2-agonists, anticholinergics, and corticosteroids) by nebulizer delivery of drugs through the ventilator and endotracheal tube.

Foundation Facts

D-O-P-E: Causes of Difficult Ventilation

Four common causes of acute deterioration in any intubated patient are recalled by the mnemonic DOPE:

1. **D**isplacement (tube)
2. **O**bstruction (tube)
3. **P**neumothorax
4. **E**quipment failure

If the patient is extremely "tight" (with airway constriction) and difficult to ventilate, perform the following procedures *in order* until ventilation is adequate:

1. Ensure that the patient is adequately sedated and paralyzed so that there is a passive patient-ventilator interaction.
2. Check the endotracheal tube for patency. Look for obstruction from kinking, mucous plugging, or biting. Suction the tube.
3. Change to a *square-wave pattern* of airflow. You may need to increase the time for exhalation, shorten the time for inhalation, and markedly increase the limit of peak inspiratory pressure to ensure that the patient is receiving the set tidal volume.
4. Reduce the respiratory rate to 6 to 8 breaths/min to reduce auto-PEEP to ≤15 mm Hg.
5. Reduce the tidal volume to 3 to 5 mL/kg to reduce auto-PEEP to ≤15 mm Hg.
6. Increase peak flow to >60 L/min (90 to 120 L/min is commonly used) to further shorten inspiratory time and increase exhalation time.

Hypoxia or Hypotension Occurs After Intubation

There are 4 common causes of significant hypoxia or hypotension immediately after intubation: incorrect placement of the endotracheal tube, obstruction of the endotracheal tube, significant auto-PEEP buildup, and tension pneumothorax.

Incorrect Placement of the Endotracheal Tube

With any drop in oxygen saturation or exhaled CO_2, reconfirm tube position immediately. Do this even if correct tube position was verified by primary and secondary confirmation. Check that the endotracheal tube has not been inserted too far. It may be in either the right (most likely) or left main bronchus. The tube should be inserted to 21 cm (measure at the incisors) in most men and to 20 cm in most women. Use lengths slightly shorter (eg, 19 to 20 cm) in smaller adults. If you suspect incorrect placement of the endotracheal tube, evaluate tube placement *immediately using primary and secondary confirmation techniques.* Do not take time to obtain a chest radiograph. It is appropriate to obtain a chest radiograph after intubation, but it may not confirm tube misplacement. Spontaneous extubation or tube migration into a main bronchus is always a respiratory emergency. This is particularly true if the patient has severe, life-threatening asthma. The patient cannot tolerate the delay that would occur with a confirmatory radiograph.

Note that patients with status asthmaticus can demonstrate false-negative results with the esophageal detector device. When the endotracheal tube is in the esophagus of a patient with severe asthma, the detector bulb may re-expand immediately, suggesting endotracheal tube placement. Providers must be aware that severe asthma may cause erroneous results with the esophageal detector device; use exhaled CO_2 detectors as another secondary confirmation device.

Obstruction of the Endotracheal Tube

If the patient is difficult to ventilate manually, check for patency of the tube. If the tube is patent, attempt to suction the tube and check for tube obstructions from kinking, mucous plugging, or biting.

Massive Auto-PEEP Buildup

The most common cause of profound hypotension after intubation is a massive buildup of auto-PEEP. If auto-PEEP is suspected, first stop ventilating the patient for a brief time (20 to 40 seconds). This pause allows the auto-PEEP to dissipate. Monitor the patient's oxygenation and resume ventilation after auto-PEEP dissipates or if the patient develops significant hypoxemia or clinical signs of further deterioration.

Tension Pneumothorax

Evidence of a tension pneumothorax includes decreased chest expansion and decreased breath sounds on the side of the pneumothorax, shifting of the trachea away from the side of the pneumothorax, or the development of subcutaneous emphysema. The immediate lifesaving treatment is *needle decompression* to release air from the pleural space. This procedure is often followed by placement of a chest tube. Slowly insert a 16-gauge cannula (over-the-needle catheter) in the second intercostal space along the midclavicular line. Be careful to avoid direct puncture of the lung. Hearing or feeling the venting of compressed air is diagnostic. Several commercial products, based on the 1-way valve principle, are available. You can use these devices after relief of a

---

Critical Concept

Needle Decompression: Use Extreme Caution!

An attempt at needle decompression or insertion of a chest tube in a patient with severe, refractory asthma without a pneumothorax can be a life-threatening error.

- The visceral pleura of the hyperinflated lung can be punctured, producing an iatrogenic pneumothorax.
- Air would be released through the needle catheter or thoracostomy tube, just as occurs with relief of a tension pneumothorax.
- The high pressures in the contralateral, mechanically ventilated lung plus the coexisting auto-PEEP could generate a contralateral tension pneumothorax.

tension pneumothorax to prevent further buildup of pneumatic tension. Nonetheless patients often require a chest tube.

Final Interventions to Consider

ACLS providers may encounter a patient with severe asthma and progressive hypoxia and hypercapnia refractory to the therapy described above. At that time, if at all possible, a pulmonologist or critical care specialist should be consulted. The following "interventions of desperation" have occasionally met with some success, at least as recounted in case reports and anecdotes.

Empiric Bilateral Needle Decompression for Bilateral Pneumothoraxes

Evidence from anecdotal case reports and surveys of chest radiographs suggests that unrecognized bilateral tension pneumothoraxes may underlie some cases of fatal asthma. There is insufficient published data to support a recommendation for empiric attempts at bilateral needle decompression in all severely compromised asthma patients. The critical point is *to consider* whether unrecognized pneumothoraxes may have precipitated an asthmatic cardiac arrest.

Intravenous β-Agonist (Isoproterenol)

Isoproterenol given by IV infusion over 60 to 90 minutes has been effective for severely ill patients unable to tolerate inhalational therapy. Start with 0.1 µg/kg per minute; increase to a maximum of 6 µg/kg per minute. Titrate according to heart rate.

Extracorporeal Membrane Oxygenation

There are increasing reports of success with this technique in mechanically ventilated patients who could not be adequately oxygenated.[83] Additional therapies such as so-called "lung massage" have been reported to benefit some patients in status asthmaticus. But positive reports from animal studies were not verified in humans, and such techniques should not be attempted.[84,85]

References

1. Expert Panel Report 3 (EPR-3): Guidelines for the Diagnosis and Management of Asthma—Summary Report 2007. *J Allergy Clin Immunol*. 2007;120:S94-138.

2. Pollack CV Jr, Pollack ES, Baren JM, Smith SR, Woodruff PG, Clark S, Camargo CA. A prospective multicenter study of patient factors associated with hospital admission from the emergency department among children with acute asthma. *Arch Pediatr Adolesc Med*. 2002;156:934-940.

3. Weber EJ, Silverman RA, Callaham ML, Pollack CV, Woodruff PG, Clark S, Camargo CA Jr. A prospective multicenter study of factors associated with hospital admission among adults with acute asthma. *Am J Med*. 2002;113:371-378.

4. Division of Data Services. New asthma estimates: tracking prevalence, health care, and mortality. In: Hyattsville, MD: National Center for Health Statistics; 2001.

5. McCoy L, Redelings M, Sorvillo F, Simon P. A multiple cause-of-death analysis of asthma mortality in the United States, 1990-2001. *J Asthma*. 2005;42:757-763.

6. Keahey L, Bulloch B, Becker AB, Pollack CV Jr, Clark S, Camargo CA Jr. Initial oxygen saturation as a predictor of admission in children presenting to the emergency department with acute asthma. *Ann Emerg Med*. 2002;40:300-307.

7. Emond SD, Camargo CA Jr, Nowak RM. 1997 National Asthma Education and Prevention Program guidelines: a practical summary for emergency physicians. *Ann Emerg Med*. 1998; 31:579-589.

8. Alvey Smaha D. Asthma emergency care: national guidelines summary. *Heart Lung*. 2001;30:472-474.

9. Beveridge RC, Grunfeld AF, Hodder RV, Verbeek PR. Guidelines for the emergency management of asthma in adults. CAEP/CTS Asthma Advisory Committee. Canadian Association of Emergency Physicians and the Canadian Thoracic Society. *CMAJ*. 1996;155:25-37.

10. Mitchell I, Tough SC, Semple LK, Green FH, Hessel PA. Near-fatal asthma: a population-based study of risk factors. *Chest*. 2002;121:1407-1413.

11. Kolbe J, Fergusson W, Vamos M, Garrett J. Case-control study of severe life threatening asthma (SLTA) in adults: psychological factors. *Thorax*. 2002;57:317-322.

12. Liard R, Leynaert B, Zureik M, Beguin FX, Neukirch F. Using Global Initiative for Asthma guidelines to assess asthma severity in populations. *Eur Respir J*. 2000;16:615-620.

13. Wasserfallen JB, Schaller MD, Feihl F, Perret CH. Sudden asphyxic asthma: a distinct entity? *Am Rev Respir Dis*. 1990; 142:108-111.

14. Molfino NA, Nannini LJ, Martelli AN, Slutsky AS. Respiratory arrest in near-fatal asthma. *N Engl J Med*. 1991;324:285-288.

15. Reid LM. The presence or absence of bronchial mucus in fatal asthma. *J Allergy Clin Immunol*. 1987;80:415-416.

16. Robin ED, McCauley R. Sudden cardiac death in bronchial asthma, and inhaled β-adrenergic agonists. *Chest*. 1992; 101:1699-1702.

17. Robin ED, Lewiston N. Unexpected, unexplained sudden death in young asthmatic subjects. *Chest*. 1989;96:790-793.

18. Kallenbach JM, Frankel AH, Lapinsky SE, Thornton AS, Blott JA, Smith C, Feldman C, Zwi S. Determinants of near fatality in acute severe asthma. *Am J Med*. 1993;95:265-272.

19. Abramson MJ, Bailey MJ, Couper FJ, Driver JS, Drummer OH, Forbes AB, McNeil JJ, Haydn Walters E. Are asthma medications and management related to deaths from asthma? *Am J Respir Crit Care Med*. 2001;163:12-18.

20. McFadden ER Jr, Warren EL. Observations on asthma mortality. *Ann Intern Med*. 1997;127:142-147.

21. Rosero SZ, Zareba W, Moss AJ, Robinson JL, Hajj Ali RH, Locati EH, Benhorin J, Andrews ML. Asthma and the risk of cardiac events in the long QT syndrome. Long QT Syndrome Investigative Group. *Am J Cardiol*. 1999;84:1406-1411.

22. Hannaway PJ. Demographic characteristics of patients experiencing near-fatal and fatal asthma: results of a regional survey of 400 asthma specialists. *Ann Allergy Asthma Immunol*. 2000;84:587-593.

23. Kikuchi Y, Okabe S, Tamura G, Hida W, Homma M, Shirato K, Takishima T. Chemosensitivity and perception of dyspnea in patients with a history of near-fatal asthma. *N Engl J Med*. 1994;330:1329-1334.

24. Nowak RM, Pensler MI, Sarkar DD, Anderson JA, Kvale PA, Ortiz AE, Tomlanovich MC. Comparison of peak expiratory flow and FEV₁ admission criteria for acute bronchial asthma. *Ann Emerg Med*. 1982;11:64-69.

25. Shim CS, Williams MH Jr. Evaluation of the severity of asthma: patients versus physicians. *Am J Med*. 1980;68:11-13.

26. Levin E, Gold MI. The mini-Wright expiratory peak flow meter. *Can Anaesth Soc J*. 1981;28:285-287.

27. Odeh M, Oliven A, Bassan H. Timolol eyedrop-induced fatal bronchospasm in an asthmatic patient. *J Fam Pract*. 1991; 32:97-98.

28. Weitzman JB, Kanarek NF, Smialek JE. Medical examiner asthma death autopsies: a distinct subgroup of asthma deaths with implications for public health preventive strategies. *Arch Pathol Lab Med*. 1998;122:691-699.

29. Levenson T, Greenberger PA, Donoghue ER, Lifschultz BD. Asthma deaths confounded by substance abuse: an assessment of fatal asthma. *Chest*. 1996;110:604-610.

30. Lin RY, Sauter D, Newman T, Sirleaf J, Walters J, Tavakol M. Continuous versus intermittent albuterol nebulization in the treatment of acute asthma. *Ann Emerg Med*. 1993;22:1847-1853.

31. Rudnitsky GS, Eberlein RS, Schoffstall JM, Mazur JE, Spivey WH. Comparison of intermittent and continuously nebulized albuterol for treatment of asthma in an urban emergency department. *Ann Emerg Med*. 1993;22:1842-1846.

32. Khine H, Fuchs SM, Saville AL. Continuous vs intermittent nebulized albuterol for emergency management of asthma. *Acad Emerg Med*. 1996;3:1019-1024.

33. Newman KB, Milne S, Hamilton C, Hall K. A comparison of albuterol administered by metered-dose inhaler and spacer with albuterol by nebulizer in adults presenting to an urban emergency department with acute asthma. *Chest*. 2002;121:1036-1041.

34. Bowton DL. Metered-dose inhalers versus hand-held nebulizers: some answers and new questions. *Chest*. 1992;101:298-299.

35. Bowton DL, Goldsmith WM, Haponik EF. Substitution of metered-dose inhalers for hand-held nebulizers: success and cost savings in a large, acute-care hospital. *Chest*. 1992;101:305-308.

36. Colacone A, Afilalo M, Wolkove N, Kreisman H. A comparison of albuterol administered by metered dose inhaler (and holding chamber) or wet nebulizer in acute asthma. *Chest*. 1993;104:835-841.

37. Idris AH, McDermott MF, Raucci JC, Morrabel A, McGorray S, Hendeles L. Emergency department treatment of severe asthma: metered-dose inhaler plus holding chamber is equivalent in effectiveness to nebulizer. *Chest*. 1993;103:665-672.

38. Gawchik SM, Saccar CL, Noonan M, Reasner DS, DeGraw SS. The safety and efficacy of nebulized levalbuterol compared with racemic albuterol and placebo in the treatment of asthma in pediatric patients. *J Allergy Clin Immunol*. 1999;103:615-621.

39. Nelson HS, Bensch G, Pleskow WW, DiSantostefano R, DeGraw S, Reasner DS, Rollins TE, Rubin PD. Improved bronchodilation with levalbuterol compared with racemic albuterol in patients with asthma. *J Allergy Clin Immunol*. 1998;102:943-952.

40. Nelson HS. Clinical experience with levalbuterol. *J Allergy Clin Immunol*. 1999;104(2 pt 2):S77-S84.

41. Marik PE, Varon J, Fromm R Jr. The management of acute severe asthma. *J Emerg Med*. 2002;23:257-268.

42. Gibbs MA, Camargo CA Jr, Rowe BH, Silverman RA. State of the art: therapeutic controversies in severe acute asthma. *Acad Emerg Med*. 2000;7:800-815.

43. Rowe BH, Spooner CH, Ducharme FM, Bretzlaff JA, Bota GW. Early emergency department treatment of acute asthma with systemic corticosteroids. *Cochrane Database Syst Rev*. 2000: CD002178.

44. Rowe BH, Keller JL, Oxman AD. Effectiveness of steroid therapy in acute exacerbations of asthma: a meta-analysis. *Am J Emerg Med*. 1992;10:301-310.

45. Ratto D, Alfaro C, Sipsey J, Glovsky MM, Sharma OP. Are intravenous corticosteroids required in status asthmaticus? *JAMA*. 1988;260:527-529.

46. Mengert TJ. Asthma. In: Copass MK, ed. *Emergency Medical Therapy*. 4th ed. Philadelphia, Pa: WB Saunders; 1996:300-316.

47. Aaron SD. The use of ipratropium bromide for the management of acute asthma exacerbation in adults and children: a systematic review. *J Asthma*. 2001;38:521-530.

48. Rodrigo G, Rodrigo C. Ipratropium bromide in acute asthma: small beneficial effects? [letter]. *Chest*. 1999;115:1482.

49. Plotnick LH, Ducharme FM. Acute asthma in children and adolescents: should inhaled anticholinergics be added to beta(2)-agonists? *Am J Respir Med*. 2003;2:109-115.

50. Keam SJ, Keating GM. Tiotropium bromide. A review of its use as maintenance therapy in patients with COPD. *Treat Respir Med*. 2004;3:247-268.

51. Rodrigo G, Rodrigo C, Burschtin O. A meta-analysis of the effects of ipratropium bromide in adults with acute asthma. *Am J Med*. 1999;107:363-370.

52. Karpel JP, Schacter EN, Fanta C, Levey D, Spiro P, Aldrich T, Menjoge SS, Witek TJ. A comparison of ipratropium and albuterol vs albuterol alone for the treatment of acute asthma. *Chest*. 1996;110:611-616.

53. Qureshi F, Zaritsky A, Lakkis H. Efficacy of nebulized ipratropium in severely asthmatic children. *Ann Emerg Med*. 1997; 29:205-211.

54. Plotnick LH, Ducharme FM. Combined inhaled anticholinergic agents and β₂-agonists for initial treatment of acute asthma in children. *Cochrane Database Syst Rev*. 2000:CD000060.

55. Stoodley RG, Aaron SD, Dales RE. The role of ipratropium bromide in the emergency management of acute asthma exacerbation: a metaanalysis of randomized clinical trials. *Ann Emerg Med*. 1999;34:8-18.

56. Silverman RA, Osborn H, Runge J, Gallagher EJ, Chiang W, Feldman J, Gaeta T, Freeman K, Levin B, Mancherje N, Scharf S. IV magnesium sulfate in the treatment of acute severe asthma: a multicenter randomized controlled trial. *Chest*. 2002;122:489-497.

57. Rowe BH, Bretzlaff JA, Bourdon C, Bota GW, Camargo CA Jr. Magnesium sulfate for treating exacerbations of acute asthma in the emergency department. *Cochrane Database Syst Rev*. 2000:CD001490.

58. Schiermeyer RP, Finkelstein JA. Rapid infusion of magnesium sulfate obviates need for intubation in status asthmaticus. *Am J Emerg Med*. 1994;12:164-166.

59. Rowe BH, Bretzlaff JA, Bourdon C, Bota GW, Camargo CA. Systematic review of magnesium sulfate in the treatment of acute asthma. *Cochrane Database Syst Rev*. 1998;4.

60. Rowe BH, Edmonds ML, Spooner CH, Camargo CA. Evidence-based treatments for acute asthma. *Respir Care*. 2001;46:1380-1390; discussion 1390-1391.

61. Blitz M, Blitz S, Beasely R, Diner BM, Hughes R, Knopp JA, Rowe BH. Inhaled magnesium sulfate in the treatment of acute asthma. *Cochrane Database Syst Rev*. 2005:CD003898.

62. Hess DR, Acosta FL, Ritz RH, Kacmarek RM, Camargo CA Jr. The effect of heliox on nebulizer function using a beta-agonist bronchodilator. *Chest*. 1999;115:184-189.

63. Rodrigo GJ, Rodrigo C, Pollack CV, Rowe B. Use of helium-oxygen mixtures in the treatment of acute asthma: a systematic review. *Chest*. 2003;123:891-896.

64. Reuben AD, Harris AR. Heliox for asthma in the emergency department: a review of the literature. *Emerg Med J*. 2004;21:131-135.

65. Cydulka R, Davison R, Grammer L, Parker M, Mathews J. The use of epinephrine in the treatment of older adult asthmatics. *Ann Emerg Med*. 1988;17:322-326.

66. Victoria MS, Battista CJ, Nangia BS. Comparison between epinephrine and terbutaline injections in the acute management of asthma. *J Asthma*. 1989;26:287-290.

67. Safdar B, Cone DC, Pham KT. Subcutaneous epinephrine in the prehospital setting. *Prehosp Emerg Care*. 2001;5:200-207.

68. Petrillo TM, Fortenberry JD, Linzer JF, Simon HK. Emergency department use of ketamine in pediatric status asthmaticus. *J Asthma*. 2001;38:657-664.

69. Howton JC, Rose J, Duffy S, Zoltanski T, Levitt MA. Randomized, double-blind, placebo-controlled trial of intravenous ketamine in acute asthma. *Ann Emerg Med*. 1996;27:170-175.

70. Parameswaran K, Belda J, Rowe BH. Addition of intravenous aminophylline to β_2-agonists in adults with acute asthma. *Cochrane Database Syst Rev*. 2000:CD002742.

71. Camargo CA Jr, Smithline HA, Malice MP, Green SA, Reiss TF. A randomized controlled trial of intravenous montelukast in acute asthma. *Am J Respir Crit Care Med*. 2003;167:528-533.

72. Schultz TE. Sevoflurane administration in status asthmaticus: a case report. *AANA J*. 2005;73:35-36.

73. Wheeler DS, Clapp CR, Ponaman ML, Bsn HM, Poss WB. Isoflurane therapy for status asthmaticus in children: a case series and protocol. *Pediatr Crit Care Med*. 2000;1:55-59.

74. Soroksky A, Stav D, Shpirer I. A pilot prospective, randomized, placebo-controlled trial of bilevel positive airway pressure in acute asthmatic attack. *Chest*. 2003;123:1018-1025.

75. Schneider R. Asthma and COPD. In: Walls RM, Luten RC, Murphy MF, Schneider RE, eds. *Manual of Emergency Airway Management*. Philadelphia, Pa: Lippincott Williams & Wilkins; 2000:164-168.

76. Meduri GU, Cook TR, Turner RE, Cohen M, Leeper KV. Noninvasive positive pressure ventilation in status asthmaticus. *Chest*. 1996;110:767-774.

77. Maltais F, Sovilj M, Goldberg P, Gottfried SB. Respiratory mechanics in status asthmaticus: effects of inhalational anesthesia. *Chest*. 1994;106:1401-1406.

78. Rooke GA, Choi JH, Bishop MJ. The effect of isoflurane, halothane, sevoflurane, and thiopental/nitrous oxide on respiratory system resistance after tracheal intubation. *Anesthesiology*. 1997;86:1294-1299.

79. Eames WO, Rooke GA, Wu RS, Bishop MJ. Comparison of the effects of etomidate, propofol, and thiopental on respiratory resistance after tracheal intubation. *Anesthesiology*. 1996;84:1307-1311.

80. Bergen JM, Smith DC. A review of etomidate for rapid sequence intubation in the emergency department. *J Emerg Med*. 1997; 15:221-230.

81. Saulnier FF, Durocher AV, Deturck RA, Lefebvre MC, Wattel FE. Respiratory and hemodynamic effects of halothane in status asthmaticus. *Intensive Care Med*. 1990;16:104-107.

82. Mazzeo AT, Spada A, Pratico C, Lucanto T, Santamaria LB. Hypercapnia: what is the limit in paediatric patients? A case of near-fatal asthma successfully treated by multipharmacological approach. *Paediatr Anaesth*. 2004;14:596-603.

83. Shapiro MB, Kleaveland AC, Bartlett RH. Extracorporeal life support for status asthmaticus. *Chest*. 1993;103:1651-1654.

84. Van der Touw T, Tully A, Amis TC, Brancatisano A, Rynn M, Mudaliar Y, Engel LA. Cardiorespiratory consequences of expiratory chest wall compression during mechanical ventilation and severe hyperinflation. *Crit Care Med*. 1993;21:1908-1914.

85. Van der Touw T, Mudaliar Y, Nayyar V. Cardiorespiratory effects of manually compressing the rib cage during tidal expiration in mechanically ventilated patients recovering from acute severe asthma. *Crit Care Med*. 1998;26:1361-1367.

Special Resuscitation Situations
Part 4: Anaphylaxis

This Chapter

- *Emergency differential diagnosis of anaphylaxis*
- *Dosing and use of epinephrine in life-threatening anaphylaxis*
- *Priorities for airway management in angioedema*
- *Special attention for volume status for cardiovascular instability*

Definitions

Anaphylaxis is a severe, systemic allergic reaction characterized by multisystem involvement, including the skin, airway, vascular system, and gastrointestinal tract. Severe cases may result in complete obstruction of the airway, cardiovascular collapse, and death.

Immunologic Definitions

The term *classic anaphylaxis* refers to hypersensitivity reactions mediated by the subclass of antibodies immunoglobulins IgE and IgG. Prior sensitization to an allergen has occurred, producing antigen-specific immunoglobulins. Subsequent reexposure to the allergen provokes the anaphylactic reaction. Many anaphylactic reactions, however, occur without a documented prior exposure.

Anaphylactoid reactions are similar to anaphylactic reactions, but they are triggered by materials such as radiocontrast material and certain parenteral medications and are not mediated by an IgE antibody response. The clinical presentation and management of anaphylactic and anaphylactoid reactions are similar, so it is unnecessary to distinguish between them when determining treatment for an acute attack.

Clinical Definitions

Some authors define *anaphylaxis* as a generalized, rapid-onset allergic reaction (including urticaria) with laryngeal edema, angioedema, or bronchospasm from increased bronchial smooth muscle tone, which causes shortness of breath.[1] Anaphylaxis is graded as severe if loss of consciousness (syncope) or hypotension occurs. These effects are produced by the release of mediators, including histamine, leukotriene C_4, prostaglandin D_2, and tryptase.

Incidence

Although prior exposure is essential for development of true anaphylaxis, reactions occur even when no documented prior exposure exists. Thus patients may appear to react to their initial exposure to an antibiotic or insect sting. As we age we all are exposed to potential allergens that can create

Foundation Facts	Anaphylactoid or pseudoanaphylactic reactions display a similar clinical syndrome, but they are not immune-mediated. Treatment for the two conditions is similar. Some anaphylactic reactions may be mediated by complement (eg, allergic reactions to blood products). Generally signs of an anaphylactic reaction develop after reexposure to a sensitizing antigen.
Anaphylactoid Reactions	

sensitivity. For this reason children are at lowest risk and the elderly are at the greatest risk of developing anaphylaxis.

The annual incidence of anaphylaxis is unknown. Researchers do not use national or international standards for either *numerators* (case definitions) or *denominators* (source of cases). A population-based study from the state of Minnesota estimated the annual rate of *occurrence* of anaphylaxis to be 30 per 100 000 person-years (95% CI). Because some people had more than one episode of anaphylaxis, the average annual rate of *incidence* of anaphylaxis was lower, at 21 per 100 000 person-years (95% CI, 17 to 25).[2] Clinicians identified a suspect allergen in 68% of cases of anaphylaxis. The most commonly identified allergens were food, medication, and insect sting. Seven percent of persons with anaphylaxis required hospitalization.

In the United Kingdom investigators reported an annual incidence rate using the number of patients evaluated at the accident and emergency department (ED) of a single hospital as the denominator.[1] Anaphylaxis, defined as a generalized allergic reaction that caused shortness of breath, occurred in 1 of 2300 ED patients. Severe anaphylaxis, with loss of consciousness, occurred in 1 of 6000 ED patients. The annual incidence of severe anaphylactic reactions in 3 European countries has been estimated at 154 per 1 million hospitalized patients, with 4 deaths per 1 million hospitalized patients.[3]

Etiology

Insect stings, drugs, contrast media, and some foods (eg, milk, eggs, and fish in children and shellfish in adults) are the most common causes of anaphylaxis. Any antigen capable of activating IgE can be a trigger for anaphylaxis. In terms of etiology, researchers generally list the following categories of causes: pharmacologic agents, latex, stinging insects, and foods. In up to 5% of cases the antigenic agent cannot be identified.

Other causes are diverse, and frequently precipitating antigens cannot be identified. Exercise-induced anaphylaxis (especially after ingestion of certain foods) has been reported. Some allergens such as dust, pollen, and dander are inhaled. Anaphylaxis may even be idiopathic. Without a known allergen, these patients must be managed with long-term oral steroid therapy. β-Blockers may increase the severity of anaphylaxis, blocking the response to endogenous catecholamines and exogenous epinephrine.

Pharmacologic Agents

Antibiotics (especially parenteral penicillins and other β-lactams), aspirin and nonsteroidal anti-inflammatory drugs, and intravenous (IV) contrast agents are the medications most frequently associated with life-threatening anaphylaxis.

Latex

Much attention has focused on latex-induced anaphylaxis, but it is actually quite rare.[4,5] A decade-long registry of anaphylactic deaths in England has not registered any latex-associated deaths.[6,7]

Stinging Insects

Fatal anaphylaxis has long been associated with stings from Hymenoptera (membrane-winged insects), including ants, bees, hornets, wasps, and yellow jackets. When a person with IgE antibodies induced by a previous sting is stung again, a fatal reaction can occur within 10 to 15 minutes. Cardiovascular collapse is the most common mechanism.[6-8] The issue of hypersensitivity to Hymenoptera stings has become complex and controversial because of medical, economic, and legal issues related to the poor performance of venom skin testing as a diagnostic test[9,10] and the absence of appropriate indications for Hymenoptera desensitization. In one recent study of people who had been stung once *and* who had a reaction to that sting, subjects were given a challenge sting at rest. Of these subjects, 35% to 60% experienced anaphylaxis from the challenge sting.[11]

Foods

Peanuts, tree-grown nuts, seafood, and wheat are the foods most frequently associated with life-threatening anaphylaxis.[12] Bronchospasm and asphyxia are the most frequent mechanisms.[6-8] Allergies to peanuts and tree nuts (Brazil, almond, hazel, and macadamia nuts) have recently been recognized as particularly dangerous.[13]

Pathophysiology

The manifestations of anaphylaxis are related to release of chemical mediators from mast cells. These mediators are released when antigens (allergens) bind to antigen-specific IgE attached to previously sensitized basophils and mast cells. In an anaphylactoid reaction, exposure to an antigen causes direct release of mediators, a process that is not mediated by IgE.

The most important mediators of anaphylaxis are histamines, leukotrienes, prostaglandins, thromboxanes, and bradykinins. These mediators contribute to vasodilation, increased capillary permeability, and airway constriction and produce the clinical signs of hypotension, angioedema, and bronchospasm. The sooner the reaction occurs after exposure, the more likely it is to be severe.

The location and concentration of the mast cells determine which organs are affected. The signs and symptoms are determined by the body system involved.

Signs and Symptoms

Signs and symptoms can be cutaneous, cardiovascular, respiratory, and gastrointestinal. Consider anaphylaxis when responses from 2 or more body systems (cutaneous, respiratory, cardiovascular, neurologic, or gastrointestinal) are noted; the cardiovascular and respiratory systems may not be involved. The shorter the interval between exposure and reaction, the more likely the reaction is to be severe. Signs and symptoms include the following:

Respiratory

Serious upper airway (laryngeal) edema, lower airway edema (asthma), or both may develop, causing stridor and wheezing. Rhinitis is often an early sign of respiratory involvement.

Cardiovascular

Cardiovascular collapse is the most common periarrest manifestation. Vasodilation produces a relative hypovolemia. Increased capillary permeability contributes to further intravascular volume loss. The patient may be agitated or anxious and may appear either flushed or pale. Additional cardiac dysfunction may result from underlying disease or the development of myocardial ischemia from administration of epinephrine.[6-8]

Gastrointestinal

Gastrointestinal signs and symptoms of anaphylaxis include abdominal pain, vomiting, and diarrhea. These signs may be particularly prominent in children.

Cutaneous

These symptoms may include diffuse urticaria and conjunctivitis. The patient may appear either flushed or pale.

Differential Diagnosis

Patients with anaphylaxis can present with a wide variety of signs and symptoms. No single finding is pathognomonic. Many conditions can produce clinical signs that are similar to anaphylaxis but that require different treatments. To provide optimal therapy and avoid inappropriate treatment,[14] providers must differentiate between anaphylaxis and other diseases. The ACLS provider must recognize the following frequently encountered anaphylaxis "look-alikes":

- **Urticaria** is characterized by distinctive small skin eruptions *(hives)* with well-defined borders and pale centers surrounded by patches of red skin *(wheal-and-flare reaction)*. Typically these red areas are intensely itchy *(pruritus)*.

- **Angioedema** and urticaria are variable manifestations of the same pathologic process. This response is mediated by vasoactive substances, which cause the arterioles to dilate. Capillary fluid leak and edema develop in both conditions. Angioedema involves vessels in the subdermal skin layers. Urticaria is localized in skin layers superficial to the dermis. Angioedema results in areas of well-demarcated, localized, nonpitting edema. Although angioedema may be caused by anaphylaxis, the provider must consider other potential causes of angioedema and urticaria.

- **Hereditary angioedema** (in which there is a family history of angioedema) does not cause urticaria but does cause gastrointestinal edema, which can lead to severe abdominal pain, or respiratory mucosal edema, which can lead to airway compromise. This form of angioedema is treated with fresh frozen plasma. Angioedema is treated with C1 esterase inhibitor replacement concentrate if available. Otherwise fresh frozen plasma may be used.

- **Severe, life-threatening asthma.** Although bronchospasm is often a component of anaphylaxis, asthma and anaphylaxis are two distinct entities that require very different treatment. Failure to identify and treat either anaphylaxis or asthma could be fatal for the patient.[14]

- **Functional vocal cord dysfunction.** Change in voice or loss of voice can lead to a suspicion of the angioedema in the pharynx that occurs with allergic/anaphylactic reactions.

Foundation Facts

Both Absolute and Relative Hypovolemia Often Contribute to Hemodynamic Instability

- Vasodilation produces a relative hypovolemia.

- Increased capillary permeability contributes to further intravascular volume loss.

- Correction of the hypovolemia may require significant volume replacement and is critical to resuscitation.

- **Scombroid poisoning.** This food-related illness often develops within 30 minutes of eating spoiled tuna, mackerel, or dolphin (mahi-mahi). Ingestion typically causes urticaria, nausea, vomiting, diarrhea, and headache. These symptoms are caused by histamine produced by bacteria on the fish. Histamine levels can be higher than 20 to 50 mg/100 g of toxic fish. Antihistamines (H_1 and $_2$ blockers) are safe and are often effective in reducing or eliminating these symptoms.
- **Angiotensin-converting enzyme (ACE) inhibitors** are associated with a reactive angioedema predominantly of the upper airway. This reaction can develop as late as days or years after ACE inhibitors are first used. The best medical treatment for this form of angioedema is unclear. ACLS providers must focus on aggressive early airway management.[15]
- **Panic disorder and panic attacks.** In some forms of panic attacks, functional stridor develops from forced adduction of the vocal cords. Panic attacks are not associated with urticaria, angioedema, or hypotension.
- **Vasovagal reactions.** Patients with classic "fainting" may appear to be either flushed or pale when they collapse or lose consciousness.

Treatment of Anaphylaxis

The treatment of anaphylaxis has not been standardized, and recommendations to prevent cardiopulmonary arrest are difficult to standardize because etiology, clinical presentation (including severity and course), and organ involvement vary widely.[17] Few randomized trials of treatment approaches have been reported. Providers must be aware that the patient can deteriorate quickly and that urgent support of airway, breathing, and circulation is essential.

Interventions to Prevent Cardiac Arrest

The following therapies are commonly used and widely accepted but are based more on consensus than evidence.

Oxygen: Administer at High Flow Rates

Administer oxygen to all patients, and administer a high concentration of oxygen to patients with respiratory distress. Titrate oxygen administration based on pulse oximetry evaluation of oxyhemoglobin saturation. Be prepared to intubate the patient and provide mechanical ventilatory support if laryngeal edema produces severe upper airway obstruction or if bronchospasm causes severe respiratory distress (see "Special Considerations in Anaphylaxis Management," below).

Epinephrine

Absorption and subsequent achievement of maximum plasma concentration after subcutaneous administration are slower and may be significantly delayed with shock.[18,19] Thus, intramuscular (IM) administration is favored. Close monitoring is critical because fatal overdose of epinephrine has been reported.[6,20]

- Administer epinephrine by IM injection early to all patients with signs of a systemic reaction, especially hypotension, airway swelling, or definite difficulty breathing.
- Use an IM dose of 0.3 to 0.5 mg (1 mL of 1:1000) repeated every 15 to 20 minutes if there is no clinical improvement.

IV Epinephrine

Administer IV epinephrine if anaphylaxis appears to be severe with immediate life-threatening manifestations.[22]

- Use epinephrine (10 mL of 1:10 000) 0.1 mg IV slowly over 5 minutes. Epinephrine may be diluted to a 1:10 000 solution before infusion.
- An IV infusion at rates of 1 to 4 µg/min may prevent the need to repeat epinephrine injections frequently.[23]

Critical Concept **Exclude Anaphylaxis First**	A number of disease processes produce some of the signs and symptoms of anaphylaxis. • Only after the clinician eliminates anaphylaxis as a diagnosis should the other conditions be considered, because failure to identify and appropriately treat anaphylaxis can be fatal.[14,16]

Rapid Response Interventions **Patients Taking β-Blockers**	Patients who are taking β-blockers have increased incidence and severity of anaphylaxis and can develop a paradoxical response to epinephrine.[21] • Consider glucagon as well as ipratropium for these patients.

Critical Concept **Administration of Epinephrine** **IM > IV ≠ SC**	The preferred route for administration of epinephrine is IM. • Administer IV epinephrine if anaphylaxis appears to be severe with immediate life-threatening manifestations.[22] • Do not give epinephrine *subcutaneously* because absorption and achievement of maximum plasma concentration are delayed when systemic perfusion is poor.

Aggressive Fluid Resuscitation

Give isotonic crystalloid (eg, normal saline) if hypotension is present and does not respond rapidly to epinephrine. A rapid infusion of 1 to 2 L or even 4 L may be needed initially. Monitor for the development of pulmonary edema and be prepared to support oxygenation and ventilation.

Antihistamines

Administer antihistamines slowly IV or IM (eg, 25 to 50 mg of diphenhydramine).

H₂ Blockers

Administer H_2 blockers such as cimetidine (300 mg orally, IM, or IV).[24]

Inhaled β-Adrenergic Agents

Provide inhaled albuterol if bronchospasm is a major feature. Inhaled ipratropium may be especially useful for treatment of bronchospasm in patients on β-blockers. Note that some patients treated for near-fatal asthma actually had anaphylaxis, so they received repeated doses of conventional bronchodilators rather than epinephrine.[25]

Corticosteroids

Infuse high-dose IV corticosteroids early in the course of therapy. Beneficial effects are delayed at least 4 to 6 hours.

Potential Therapies

Potential additional therapies based on limited case reports or pathophysiologic mechanisms include vasopressin, atropine, and glucagon.

• **Vasopressin.** There are case reports that vasopressin may benefit severely hypotensive patients.[27,28]
• **Atropine.** Case reports also suggest that when relative or severe bradycardia is present, there may be a role for administration of atropine.[16]

• **Glucagon.** For patients who are unresponsive to epinephrine, especially those receiving β-blockers, glucagon may be effective. This agent is short-acting (1 to 2 mg every 5 minutes IM or IV). Nausea, vomiting, and hyperglycemia are common side effects.

Post-Treatment Management

Patients who respond to therapy require observation, but there is no evidence to suggest the length of observation time needed. Symptoms may recur in some patients (up to 20%) within 1 to 8 hours (biphasic response) despite an intervening asymptomatic period. Biphasic responses have been reported to occur up to 36 hours after the initial reaction.[2,21,24,29-31] A patient who remains symptom-free for 4 hours after treatment may be discharged.[32] Severe reactions or other problems, however, may necessitate longer periods of observation.

Cardiac Arrest

Cardiac arrest from anaphylaxis may be associated with profound vasodilation, total cardiovascular collapse, tissue hypoxia, and asystole. There is no research data to guide specific modifications in resuscitation procedures. Providers may find it difficult to achieve adequate volume replacement and ventilation. Consensus recommendations have been made following experience with nonfatal cases.

Death from anaphylaxis is usually due to cardiovascular collapse with massive vasodilation, cardiac pump failure, and progressive shock. The major clinical challenge is providing adequate volume replacement into a cardiovascular "tank" undergoing a life-threatening, but unknown, increase in capacity and capillary leak.

FAQ **Should you remove the venom sac?** **How?**	In rare cases insect envenomation by bees, but not wasps, leaves a venom sac attached to the victim's skin. • At some point during initial assessment, look at the sting site. If you see a stinger, immediately scrape it or any insect parts at the site of the sting using the dull edge of a knife.[26] • Avoid compressing or squeezing any insect parts near the skin because squeezing may increase envenomation.

If cardiac arrest develops, CPR, volume administration, and adrenergic drugs are the cornerstones of therapy. Initial therapy should be reviewed for completeness and titration. Critical therapies are as follows:

- **Aggressive volume expansion.** Near-fatal anaphylaxis produces profound vasodilation that significantly increases intravascular capacity. Massive volume replacement is needed. Use at least 2 large-bore IVs with pressure bags to administer large volumes (typically totals between 4 and 8 L) of isotonic crystalloid as quickly as possible.
- **High-dose epinephrine IV.** Use a rapid progression to high dose without hesitation in patients in full cardiac arrest. A commonly used sequence is 1 to 3 mg IV (3 minutes), 3 to 5 mg IV (3 minutes), then 4 to 10 µg/min infusion.
- **Antihistamine IV.** There is little data about the value of antihistamines in anaphylactic cardiac arrest, but it is reasonable to assume that little additional harm could result.[24]
- **Steroid therapy.** Steroids given during a cardiac arrest will have little effect, but they may have value in the early hours of any postresuscitation period.
- **Asystole/Pulseless Electrical Activity (PEA) Algorithms.** The arrest rhythm in anaphylaxis is often PEA or asystole. See the Pulseless Arrest Algorithm in Part 1, Chapter 6, "Asystole/PEA."

Special Considerations in Anaphylaxis Management

Treatment of Severe Airway Obstruction

Monitor the patient's airway and breathing closely during therapy (see above). Perform early *elective* intubation if the patient develops hoarseness, lingual edema, posterior or oropharyngeal swelling, or severe bronchospasm. Be prepared to perform *semi-elective* (awake, sedated) endotracheal intubation without paralytic agents when signs of distress develop and before respiratory arrest is imminent.

Early Endotracheal Intubation: Some Precautions

If intubation is delayed, patients can deteriorate relatively quickly (within ½ to 3 hours) with development of progressive stridor, laryngeal edema, massive lingual swelling, facial and neck swelling, and hypoxemia. At this point both endotracheal intubation and cricothyrotomy may be difficult or impossible. Attempts at endotracheal intubation may only further increase laryngeal edema or compromise the airway with bleeding into the oropharynx and narrow glottic opening.

Hypoxia may lead to agitation and combativeness during administration of oxygen. Initiation of paralysis before an endotracheal intubation attempt may prove lethal in these patients. The glottic opening is narrow and difficult to visualize when lingual and oropharyngeal edema are present. Once paralyzing agents are administered, the patient will be unable to contribute to ventilation.

If endotracheal intubation is unsuccessful, it may be impossible to provide effective bag-mask ventilation. Laryngeal edema prevents air entry. Facial edema prevents creation of an effective seal between the face and the bag-mask device. Pharmacologic paralysis at this point may deprive the patient of his/her only mechanism for ventilation, ie, spontaneous breathing attempts.

Airway, Oxygenation, and Ventilation in Cardiac Arrest

Cardiac arrest may result from angioedema and upper or lower airway obstruction. Bag-mask ventilation and endotracheal intubation may be impossible. Cricothyrotomy may not be possible because landmarks are obliterated by severe swelling.

Rapid sequence or crash intubation, similar to that done for severe, life-threatening asthma, should be initiated early rather than late. Note the precaution above about administration of paralyzing agents.

FYI **Prolonged CPR May Be Indicated**	Patients with anaphylaxis are often young with healthy hearts and cardiovascular systems, and they may respond to rapid correction of vasodilation and low blood volume. Effective CPR may maintain sufficient oxygen delivery until the catastrophic effects of the anaphylactic reaction resolve.
Rapid Response Interventions ***Pay Special Attention to Patients With Angioedema***	Early, elective intubation is recommended for patients who develop hoarseness, lingual edema, stridor, or oropharyngeal swelling. • Patients with angioedema pose a particularly worrisome problem because they are at high risk for rapid deterioration.

In these desperate circumstances, consider the following airway techniques:

- Fiberoptic endotracheal intubation
- Digital endotracheal intubation, in which the fingers guide insertion of a small (<7.0 mm) endotracheal tube
- Needle cricothyrotomy followed by trans-endotracheal oxygenation (ventilation will not be very effective unless a larger airway can be inserted)
- Cricothyrotomy as described for patients with massive neck swelling[33]

References

1. Stewart AG, Ewan PW. The incidence, aetiology and management of anaphylaxis presenting to an accident and emergency department. *Q J Med*. 1996;89:859-864.

2. Yocum MW, Butterfield JH, Klein JS, Volcheck GW, Schroeder DR, Silverstein MD. Epidemiology of anaphylaxis in Olmsted County: a population-based study. *J Allergy Clin Immunol*. 1999;104(pt 1):452-456.

3. An epidemiologic study of severe anaphylactic and anaphylactoid reactions among hospital patients: methods and overall risks. The International Collaborative Study of Severe Anaphylaxis. *Epidemiology*. 1998;9:141-146.

4. Dreyfus DH, Fraser B, Randolph CC. Anaphylaxis to latex in patients without identified risk factors for latex allergy. *Conn Med*. 2004;68:217-222.

5. Ownby DR. A history of latex allergy. *J Allergy Clin Immunol*. 2002;110:S27-S32.

6. Pumphrey RS. Lessons for management of anaphylaxis from a study of fatal reactions. *Clin Exp Allergy*. 2000;30:1144-1150.

7. Pumphrey RS. Fatal anaphylaxis in the UK, 1992-2001. *Novartis Found Symp*. 2004;257:116-128; discussion 128-132, 157-160, 276-285.

8. Pumphrey RS, Roberts IS. Postmortem findings after fatal anaphylactic reactions. *J Clin Pathol*. 2000;53:273-276.

9. Golden DBK, Kagey-Sobotka A, Norman PS, Hamilton RG, Lichtenstein LM. Insect sting allergy with negative venom skin test responses. *J Allergy Clin Immunol*. 2001;107:897-901.

10. Reisman RE. Insect sting allergy: the dilemma of the negative skin test reactor. *J Allergy Clin Immunol*. 2001;107:781-782.

11. Hauk P, Friedl K, Kaufmehl K, Urbanek R, Forster J. Subsequent insect stings in children with hypersensitivity to Hymenoptera. *J Pediatr*. 1995;126:185-190.

12. Mullins RJ. Anaphylaxis: risk factors for recurrence. *Clin Exp Allergy*. 2003;33:1033-1040.

13. Ewan PW. Clinical study of peanut and nut allergy in 62 consecutive patients: new features and associations. *BMJ*. 1996;312:1074-1078.

14. Brown AF. Anaphylaxis: quintessence, quarrels, and quandaries. *Emerg Med J*. 2001;18:328.

15. Ishoo E, Shah UK, Grillone GA, Stram JR, Fuleihan NS. Predicting airway risk in angioedema: staging system based on presentation. *Otolaryngol Head Neck Surg*. 1999;121:263-268.

16. Brown AF. Anaphylaxis gets the adrenaline going. *Emerg Med J*. 2004;21:128-129.

17. Gavalas M, Walford C, Sadana A, O'Donnell C. Medical treatment of anaphylaxis. *J Accid Emerg Med*. 2000;17:152; author reply 152-153.

18. Simons FE, Gu X, Simons KJ. Epinephrine absorption in adults: intramuscular versus subcutaneous injection. *J Allergy Clin Immunol*. 2001;108:871-873.

19. Simons FER, Chan ES, Gu X, Simons KJ. Epinephrine for the out-of-hospital (first-aid) treatment of anaphylaxis in infants: is the ampule/syringe/needle method practical? *J Allergy Clin Immunol*. 2001;108:1040-1044.

20. Pumphrey R. Anaphylaxis: can we tell who is at risk of a fatal reaction? *Curr Opin Allergy Clin Immunol*. 2004;4:285-290.

21. Ellis AK, Day JH. Diagnosis and management of anaphylaxis. *CMAJ*. 2003;169:307-311.

22. Brown SG, Blackman KE, Stenlake V, Heddle RJ. Insect sting anaphylaxis: prospective evaluation of treatment with intravenous adrenaline and volume resuscitation. *Emerg Med J*. 2004;21:149-154.

23. Barach EM, Nowak RM, Lee TG, Tomlanovich MC. Epinephrine for treatment of anaphylactic shock. *JAMA*. 1984;251:2118-2122.

24. Winbery SL, Lieberman PL. Histamine and antihistamines in anaphylaxis. *Clin Allergy Immunol*. 2002;17:287-317.

25. Rainbow J, Browne GJ. Fatal asthma or anaphylaxis? *Emerg Med J*. 2002;19:415-417.

26. Visscher PK, Vetter RS, Camazine S. Removing bee stings. *Lancet*. 1996;348:301-302.

27. Kill C, Wranze E, Wulf H. Successful treatment of severe anaphylactic shock with vasopressin. Two case reports. *Int Arch Allergy Immunol*. 2004;134:260-261.

28. Williams SR, Denault AY, Pellerin M, Martineau R. Vasopressin for treatment of shock following aprotinin administration. *Can J Anaesth*. 2004;51:169-172.

29. Smith PL, Kagey-Sobotka A, Bleecker ER, Traystman R, Kaplan AP, Gralnick H, Valentine MD, Permutt S, Lichtenstein LM. Physiologic manifestations of human anaphylaxis. *J Clin Invest*. 1980;66:1072-1080.

30. Stark BJ, Sullivan TJ. Biphasic and protracted anaphylaxis. *J Allergy Clin Immunol*. 1986;78:76-83.

31. Brazil E, MacNamara AF. "Not so immediate" hypersensitivity: the danger of biphasic anaphylactic reactions. *J Accid Emerg Med*. 1998;15:252-253.

32. Brady WJ Jr, Luber S, Carter CT, Guertler A, Lindbeck G. Multiphasic anaphylaxis: an uncommon event in the emergency department. *Acad Emerg Med*. 1997;4:193-197.

33. Simon R, Brenner B. Airway procedures. In: *Emergency Procedures and Techniques*. Baltimore, Md: Williams & Wilkins; 1994:79.

Special Resuscitation Situations
Part 5: Impending Cardiac Arrest and Resucitation Due to Trauma

---

This Chapter

- *Rapid scene survey and provider safety first*
- *How to rapidly assess a deteriorating patient to prevent arrest*
- *Emergency thoracotomy and penetrating chest trauma*
- *Poor survival guidelines: when to withhold or terminate resuscitation*

Overview and Epidemiology

In industrialized nations trauma is the leading cause of death from the age of 6 months through young adulthood.[1,2] When anyone is severely injured, resuscitation must begin as soon as possible, preferably at the scene.[3] Early and effective support of airway, ventilation, oxygenation, and perfusion is vital because survival from out-of-hospital cardiac arrest secondary to blunt trauma is uniformly low in children and adults.[4-6] In some out-of-hospital and emergency department settings, resuscitative efforts are withheld when patients with blunt trauma are found in asystole or agonal electrical cardiac activity. Survival after cardiac arrest resulting from penetrating trauma is only slightly better. Following penetrating trauma, rapid transport to a trauma center is associated with better outcomes than prolonged resuscitative attempts in the field.[7]

Despite a rapid and effective out-of-hospital and trauma center response, patients with out-of-hospital cardiac arrest due to trauma rarely survive.[8-11] Those patients with the best outcome from trauma arrest generally are young, have treatable penetrating injuries, have received early (out-of-hospital) endotracheal intubation, and undergo prompt

---

FYI

Trauma Terminology

- *Scene survey:* Quick assessment to determine the safety of the scene.
- *Primary survey (ATLS) or initial assessment (NHTSA):* Rapid evaluation and stabilization of airway, breathing, circulation, disability (neurologic function), and exposure.
- *Secondary survey (ATLS) or focused history and detailed physical examination (NHTSA):* A complete head-to-toe physical examination. The detailed physical examination of the NHTSA course includes a *focused history*. Use the AMPLE mnemonic to identify important aspects of the patient's history and presenting complaint:

  - **A**llergies
  - **M**edications
  - **P**ast medical history
  - **L**ast meal
  - **E**vents leading up to the scenario

transport (typically ≤10 minutes) to a trauma care facility.[10-13] Cardiac arrest in the field due to blunt trauma is fatal in all age groups.[4-6]

BLS and ALS for the trauma patient are fundamentally the same as the care for a patient with a primary cardiac or respiratory arrest. In trauma resuscitation providers perform a "Primary Survey" to rapidly identify and immediately treat life-threatening conditions that will interfere with establishing an effective airway, oxygenation, ventilation, and circulation.[3] After completion of the Primary Survey, the provider should perform a more detailed Secondary Survey (also called the Focused History and Detailed Physical Examination). The terminology used to describe these assessments is presented in the Critical Concepts box. Cardiopulmonary deterioration associated with trauma has several possible causes. The management plan may vary for each.

Initial Evaluation and Triage

Extricate and Evaluate

Specially trained providers should rapidly extricate the patient while immobilizing the cervical spine. Provide immediate BLS and ALS interventions to ensure adequate airway, oxygenation, ventilation, and circulation. Prepare the patient for rapid transport to a facility that provides definitive trauma care. Use lateral neck supports, strapping, and backboards throughout transport to minimize exacerbation of an occult neck or spinal cord injury.

For years there has been a debate over whether ACLS providers should deploy a full armamentarium of interventions when treating patients of severe trauma at the scene. A number of studies have questioned the clinical effectiveness of on-site advanced airway management via endotracheal intubation as well as circulatory support with rapid intravenous (IV) infusions. The case against these

interventions centers on two arguments: whether they are truly safe and effective and whether they adversely delay transport to, and definitive management at, a hospital or emergency department (ED).

There is considerable evidence that out-of-hospital endotracheal intubation is either harmful or at best ineffective for most EMS patients.[14-17] Researchers and emergency medical services (EMS) leaders have also questioned the safety and effectiveness of aggressive out-of-hospital IV fluid resuscitation in an urban environment.[7,18-20] In addition, field ACLS interventions unquestionably prolong time at the scene, delay transport to the ED or trauma center, and thereby delay essential interventions such as surgical control of life-threatening bleeding.[20-23]

With the above discussion in mind, the focus of prehospital resuscitation should be to safely extricate and attempt to stabilize the patient and to minimize interventions that will delay transport to definitive care. Strict attention should be paid to stabilizing the spine during care. Patients suspected of having severe traumatic injuries should be transported or receive early transfer to a facility that can provide definitive trauma care. Attempts to stabilize the patient are typically performed during transport to avoid delay.

Multicasualty Triage

When multiple patients have serious injuries, emergency personnel must establish priorities for care. When the number of patients with critical injuries exceeds the capability of the EMS providers at the scene, patients without a pulse are the lowest priority for care. Most EMS systems have guidelines that permit out-of-hospital pronouncement of death or withholding of cardiac resuscitative efforts when there are multiple patients with critical injuries or when patients have injuries incompatible with life. EMS personnel should work within such guidelines when available.

| **Rapid Response Interventions**

Consider These Causes and Intervene Before Cardiac Arrest | Potential causes of cardiopulmonary deterioration and arrest include the following:

• Severe central neurologic injury with secondary cardiovascular collapse
• Hypoxia secondary to respiratory insufficiency, resulting from neurologic injury, airway obstruction, large open pneumothorax, or severe tracheobronchial laceration or crush
• Direct and severe injury to vital structures such as the heart, aorta, or pulmonary arteries
• Underlying medical problems or other conditions that led to the injury, such as sudden cardiac arrest or stroke in the driver of a motor vehicle
• Severely diminished cardiac output from tension pneumothorax or pericardial tamponade
• Exsanguination leading to hypovolemia and severely diminished oxygen delivery
• Injuries in a cold environment (eg, fractured leg) complicated by secondary severe hypothermia |

ATLS and NHTSA Terminology

Primary Survey = initial assessment
Secondary Survey = focused history and detailed physical examination

The National Highway Traffic Safety Administration (NHTSA) EMS National Standard Curricula uses some terms for the initial assessment and stabilization of the injured patient that differ slightly from those used in the Advanced Trauma Life Support Course (ATLS) offered by the American College of Surgeons. The ACLS provider should be familiar with the terms used by the two courses to describe the same provider actions and should be able to apply both sets of terms to the care of the injured patient.

In cases of cardiac arrest associated with uncontrolled internal hemorrhage or pericardial tamponade, the best outcomes are associated with rapid transport of the patient to an emergency facility with immediate operative capabilities.

Despite rapid and effective out-of-hospital and trauma center response, survival is poor in patients with out-of-hospital cardiopulmonary arrest due to blunt trauma. Patients who do survive out-of-hospital cardiopulmonary arrest associated with trauma generally are young, have penetrating injuries, receive early (out-of-hospital) endotracheal intubation, and receive prompt transport by highly skilled paramedics to a definitive care facility.

Trauma care should be provided within a planned system that promotes excellence in prehospital, in-hospital, and rehabilitative care. Such a system includes protocols for management of common complications of injury, early consultation with a surgeon when indicated, and an ongoing program of quality improvement. Detailed presentation of trauma management is beyond the scope of this textbook. Advanced courses are taught by several organizations, including the American College of Surgeons (Advanced Trauma Life Support Course) and the National Association of Emergency Medical Technicians (Pre-Hospital Trauma Life Support Course). Whenever possible, recommendations in this chapter were made consistent with the recommendations taught in those courses.

Withholding or Terminating Resuscitation in Prehospital Traumatic Cardiopulmonary Arrest

In January 2003 the National Association of EMS Physicians and the American College of Surgeons Committee on Trauma published a position statement on withholding or terminating resuscitation in prehospital traumatic cardiopulmonary arrest.[24-26] These valuable guidelines are summarized in Table 1. In addition, in 2001 the American College of Surgeons Committee on Advanced Trauma Life Support published their seventh edition of recommendations for Advanced Trauma Life Support.[3]

Modifications to BLS for Cardiac Arrest Associated With Trauma

Establish Unresponsiveness

Head trauma, shock, or respiratory arrest may produce loss of consciousness. If spinal cord injury is present, the patient may be conscious but unable to move. Throughout initial assessment and stabilization, the provider should monitor the patient's responsiveness. Deterioration could indicate either neurologic compromise or cardiorespiratory failure.

Airway

Cervical Spine Precautions

When head or neck injury or multisystem trauma is present, providers must immobilize the cervical spine throughout BLS maneuvers. Use a jaw thrust without head extension instead of a head tilt–chin lift to open the airway. If at all possible a second provider should be responsible for immobilizing the head and neck until spinal immobilization equipment is applied.

After opening the airway manually, clear the mouth of blood, vomitus, and other secretions. Remove this material with a (gloved) finger sweep, or use gauze or a towel to wipe the mouth. You may also use suction.

Breathing and Ventilation

Once a patent airway is established, assess for breathing. If breathing is absent, agonal, or slow and extremely shallow, manual ventilation is needed. When ventilation is provided with a barrier device, a pocket mask, or a bag-mask device, the rescuer must still maintain cervical spine stabilization. Deliver breaths slowly to reduce risk of gastric inflation. If the chest does not expand during ventilation despite the presence of an adequate and patent airway, rule out tension pneumothorax or hemothorax. If there is a risk of cervical spine injury, immobilize the spine while providing rescue breathing. Maintain immobilization throughout the rescue attempt.

Table 1. Guidelines for Withholding or Terminating of Resuscitation in Prehospital Traumatic Cardiopulmonary Arrest

A. Specific Criteria and Recommendations by Type of Trauma

Patient in Cardiac Arrest Associated With Trauma Upon Arrival of EMS Personnel		
Type of Trauma	**Specific Criteria**	**Recommendations**
Blunt	• Thorough primary assessment finds patient to be apneic, pulseless, with no organized ECG activity	• DO NOT START resuscitative efforts
Penetrating	• Further assessment finds **POSITIVE** secondary signs of life (eg, pupillary reflexes, spontaneous movement, agonal respirations, organized ECG activity)	• START resuscitative efforts • TRANSPORT to nearest ED or trauma center
	• Further assessment finds **NO** secondary signs of life (eg, pupillary reflexes, spontaneous movement, agonal respirations, organized ECG activity)	• DO NOT START resuscitative efforts
Blunt or Penetrating	• Injuries are obviously incompatible with life (eg, decapitation, hemicorporectomy)	• DO NOT START resuscitative efforts
	• Evidence of death (eg, dependent lividity, rigor mortis, decomposition)	
	• Possible nontraumatic cardiac arrest: mechanism of injury does not correlate with clinical condition	• START resuscitative efforts • TRANSPORT to nearest ED or trauma center
	• No response, or no sustained response, to 15 minutes of resuscitation and CPR if EMS personnel witnessed arrest → nonsalvageable	• STOP resuscitative efforts
	• More than 15 minutes transport time to nearest ED or trauma center → nonsalvageable	

B. Guideline Elements and Recommendations

Guideline Element	**Recommendations**
System factors to consider	• Average transport time within EMS system • Definitive care capabilities (trauma centers) within EMS system • Transport time based on accomplishment of IV access and airway management during transport
Special resuscitation situations	• Give special consideration (following specific protocols) to victims of drowning, lightning strike, and significant hypothermia
Training	• EMS providers must be thoroughly familiar with all guidelines and protocols for decisions to withhold or stop resuscitative efforts
Medical direction	• EMS medical director should develop and implement all protocols • Online medical control should be available to help determine the appropriateness of withholding or stopping resuscitation
Notification policies and protocols	• Procedures must include notification of appropriate law enforcement agencies, including medical examiners or coroners, about final disposition of the body
Survivor and provider support	• The family of the deceased should have access to resources (eg, clergy, social workers, counseling personnel) as needed • EMS providers should have access to resources for debriefing and counseling as needed
Quality review	• Polices and protocols for termination or withholding of resuscitation should be monitored through a quality review system

Modified from Hopson et al.[25,26]

Circulation

The provider should stop any visible hemorrhage using direct compression and appropriate dressings. After opening the airway and delivering 2 effective rescue breaths, the healthcare provider should attempt to feel a carotid pulse. If the healthcare provider does not definitely feel a pulse within 10 seconds, the provider should begin chest compressions and provide cycles of compressions and ventilations. During CPR rescuers should provide compressions of adequate number and depth (push hard and fast), allow full chest recoil after each compression, and minimize interruptions in chest compressions.

When CPR is provided for a patient with an advanced airway in place, 2 rescuers no longer deliver cycles of compressions interrupted with pauses for ventilation. Instead, the compressing rescuer should deliver 100 compressions per minute continuously, without pauses for ventilation. The rescuer delivering the ventilations should give 8 to 10 breaths per minute and should be careful to avoid delivering an excessive number of ventilations. The 2 rescuers should change compressor and ventilator roles approximately every 2 minutes to prevent compressor fatigue and deterioration in quality and rate of chest compressions. When multiple rescuers are present, they should rotate the compressor role about every 2 minutes.

Defibrillation

Sudden cardiac arrest associated with VF/pulseless VT may cause trauma. If the patient develops VF/pulseless VT, the patient will lose consciousness, and this can lead to falls and car crashes.

If an automated external defibrillator (AED) is available, turn it on and attach it. The AED will evaluate the patient's cardiac rhythm and advise delivery of a shock if appropriate. If VF is present, note that the VF may have been the cause rather than the consequence of the trauma (eg, an automobile driver develops VF sudden cardiac arrest and when he loses consciousness he crashes the car). The patient may require further cardiac evaluation after resuscitation.

Disability

Throughout all interventions assess the patient's level of consciousness and general neurologic status. Monitor closely for signs of neurologic deterioration during BLS care. The Glasgow Coma Scale is useful and can be calculated in seconds (see Chapter 9: "Stroke").

Exposure

The patient may lose heat to the environment through conduction, convection, and evaporation. Such heat loss will be exacerbated when the patient's clothes are removed or if the patient is covered in blood or water. Take all practical actions to maintain the patient's temperature.

Modifications to ACLS for Cardiac Arrest Associated With Trauma

ACLS includes continued assessment and support of the airway, oxygenation and ventilation (breathing), and circulation. Some of these procedures may be performed only after the patient has arrived at the hospital.

Airway

Indications for intubation in the injured patient include

- Respiratory arrest or apnea
- Respiratory failure, including severe hypoventilation, hypoxemia despite oxygen therapy, or respiratory acidosis
- Shock
- Severe head injury
- Inability to protect the upper airway (eg, loss of gag reflex, depressed level of consciousness, coma)
- Thoracic injuries (eg, flail chest, pulmonary contusion, penetrating trauma)
- Signs of airway obstruction
- Injuries associated with potential airway obstruction (eg, crushing facial or neck injuries)
- Anticipated need for mechanical ventilatory support

Perform endotracheal intubation with cervical spine immobilization. Orotracheal intubation is the preferred method. You should avoid nasotracheal intubation, especially if you suspect cervical spine injury, because nasotracheal intubation is more likely than orotracheal intubation to require excessive manipulation of the cervical spine. Also avoid nasotracheal intubation if you suspect maxillofacial injury or basilar skull fracture. If the maxillofacial injury is associated with a dural tear, a nasogastric or endotracheal tube placed through the nose may migrate intracranially.[27] Nasotracheal intubation also may result in the introduction of bacteria through the dura. ACLS providers should confirm proper endotracheal tube placement by both clinical assessment and a device.

Maintain proper tube placement by use of commercial endotracheal tube holders. Continuously confirm proper tube position by use of pulse oximetry and exhaled CO_2 monitoring during transport and after any transfer of the patient (eg, from ambulance to hospital gurney). In the prehospital setting, immobilization of the cervical spine with a collar or backboard or both can serve as an additional aid to prevent tube dislodgement, although the use and effect of these immobilizers on tube placement has not been reported.

The inability to intubate the trachea of the patient with massive facial injury and edema is an indication for a surgical airway. An emergent cricothyrotomy will provide an immediate, secure airway that supports oxygenation, although ventilation will be suboptimal. Commercial cricothyrotomy kits and transtracheal catheters are now widely available for use by prehospital and ED ACLS providers.

Complications

If CPR is needed after endotracheal intubation, provision of simultaneous ventilations and compressions may cause a tension pneumothorax. The patient may require needle decompression and insertion of a 1-way valve. There is a high risk for the development of a tension pneumothorax if lung injury has occurred, especially if the patient has fractured ribs or a fractured sternum.

Stomach Decompression

Insert a gastric tube to decompress the stomach. Insert an orogastric rather than a nasogastric tube in patients with severe head or maxillofacial injuries. If the dura is torn, a nasogastric tube can migrate into sinuses or even into the brain.[27] Always confirm proper orogastric or nasogastric tube placement into the stomach by auscultation over the gastric region while injecting air through a syringe.

Ventilation

Provide high concentrations of oxygen even if the patient's oxygenation appears to be adequate. Once you ensure a patent airway, assess breath sounds and chest expansion.

Complications

Signs of a pneumothorax are a unilateral decrease in breath sounds and inadequate chest expansion during positive-pressure ventilation. Assume that these signs are caused by a *tension pneumothorax* until that complication is either confirmed or ruled out. Perform needle decompression of the pneumothorax immediately and then insert a chest tube. Surgical exploration is indicated if thoracic decompression does not produce immediate hemodynamic improvement or if the patient has a penetrating thoracic wound.[12]

Providers should look for and seal any significant *open pneumothorax*. Tension pneumothorax may develop after sealing of an open pneumothorax, so decompression may be needed.[8] A traumatic *hemothorax* also may interfere with ventilation and chest expansion. Treat significant hemothorax with blood replacement and chest tube insertion. If the hemorrhage is severe and continues, the patient may require surgical exploration.

If the patient has a significant *flail chest,* spontaneous ventilation likely will be inadequate to maintain oxygenation. Flail chest results from multiple fractures of adjacent ribs. These fractures cause instability of a portion of the chest wall. This instability may cause respiratory failure, particularly if the patient is breathing spontaneously. Treat flail chest with positive-pressure ventilation.

Circulation

Once airway, oxygenation, and ventilation are addressed, evaluate and manage circulation. In the setting of trauma and pulseless arrest, the outcome will be poor unless a reversible cause can be immediately identified and treated (eg, tension pneumothorax).

Control external bleeding with pressure. This control is particularly important in the prehospital setting when surgical intervention is not possible. If hypovolemic shock is present, establish vascular access with the largest bore catheter possible and administer boluses of isotonic crystalloids (see "Volume Resuscitation," below). Note that volume resuscitation is no substitute for manual or surgical control of hemorrhage.[3]

Volume Resuscitation

Volume resuscitation is an important but controversial part of trauma resuscitation. ACLS providers should establish large-bore IV access while en route to the ED or trauma center, limiting attempts to two. Isotonic crystalloid is the resuscitation fluid of choice because research has not clearly established any specific type of solution as superior.[28] When replacement of blood loss is required in the hospital, it is accomplished with a combination of packed red blood cells and isotonic crystalloid.

Aggressive fluid resuscitation is not required for trauma patients who have no evidence of hemodynamic compromise. Recommendations for volume resuscitation in trauma patients with signs of hypovolemic shock are determined by the type of trauma (penetrating vs blunt) and the setting (urban vs rural). A high rate of volume infusion with the therapeutic goal of a systolic blood pressure ≥100 mm Hg is now recommended only for patients with isolated head or extremity trauma, either blunt or penetrating. In the urban setting, aggressive prehospital volume resuscitation for penetrating trauma is no longer recommended because it is likely to increase blood pressure and consequently accelerate the rate of blood loss, delay arrival at the trauma center, and delay surgical interventions to repair or ligate bleeding vessels.[7,11,29] Such delay cannot be justified when the patient can be delivered to a trauma center within a few minutes. In rural settings, transport times to trauma centers will be longer, so volume resuscitation for blunt or penetrating trauma is provided during transport to maintain a systolic blood pressure of 90 mm Hg.

Arrest Rhythms

The most common terminal cardiac rhythms observed in trauma patients are pulseless electrical activity (PEA) and bradyasystolic rhythms. Occasionally VF/VT occurs.

Treatment of PEA requires identification and treatment of reversible causes, such as severe hypovolemia, hypothermia, cardiac tamponade, or tension pneumothorax.[12] Development of bradyasystolic rhythms often indicates the presence of severe hypovolemia, severe hypoxemia, or cardiorespiratory failure. Treat VF/VT with defibrillation. Although epinephrine is typically administered during ACLS treatment of these arrhythmias, it may be ineffective in the presence of severe hypovolemia.

Emergency Thoracotomy

Since publication of the *ECC Guidelines 2000* several centers have reported their retrospective observations about resuscitative thoracotomies for patients in traumatic cardiac arrest.[30-33] For example, one series reported 49 patients with *penetrating* chest trauma who underwent resuscitative thoracotomy in the ED.[33] None of the patients in cardiac arrest or without signs of life before thoracotomy survived to hospital discharge.

In a 2002 report of resuscitative thoracotomies for trauma patients in the ED,[30] the 3 survivors of 10 patients with penetrating trauma all had signs of life and vital signs on arrival at the ED. In contrast, all 19 patients with blunt trauma died, despite the fact that 14 of the 19 "had vital signs" at the time of the thoracotomy. In a database of 959 resuscitative thoracotomies,[32] 22 victims of penetrating trauma and 4 victims of blunt trauma survived to hospital discharge after receiving prehospital CPR (overall survival rate of 3%).

In 2001 the Committee on Trauma of the American College of Surgeons published a systematic review of 42 studies of ED thoracotomies involving nearly 7000 patients, published from 1966 to 1999.[34] In this database, survival was 11% (500 of 4482) for patients with penetrating trauma and 1.6% (35 of 2193) for patients with blunt trauma.

These studies suggest that there may be a role for open thoracotomy in specific patients or situations. Table 2 describes conditions under which an open thoracotomy may be considered. Open thoracotomy does not improve outcome from out-of-hospital blunt trauma arrest, but it can be lifesaving for patients with penetrating chest trauma if the patient has an arrest immediately before arrival at the ED or while in the ED. During concurrent volume resuscitation for penetrating trauma, prompt emergency thoracotomy will permit direct massage of the heart, relief of cardiac tamponade, control of thoracic and extrathoracic

Table 2. Suggested Indications for Resuscitative Thoracotomy: Patients With Traumatic Cardiac Arrest

Type of Injury	Assessment
Blunt trauma	• Patient arrives at ED or trauma center with pulse, blood pressure, and spontaneous respirations, *and* • then experiences witnessed cardiac arrest
Penetrating cardiac trauma	• Patient experiences a witnessed cardiac arrest in ED or trauma center *or* • Patient arrives in ED or trauma center after <5 minutes of out-of-hospital CPR and with positive secondary signs of life (eg, pupillary reflexes, spontaneous movement, organized ECG activity)
Penetrating thoracic (noncardiac) trauma	• Patient experiences a witnessed cardiac arrest in ED or trauma center *or* • Patient arrives in ED or trauma center after <15 minutes of out-of-hospital CPR and with positive secondary signs of life (eg, pupillary reflexes, spontaneous movement, organized ECG activity)
Exsanguinating abdominal vascular trauma	• Patient experiences a witnessed cardiac arrest in ED or trauma center *or* • Patient arrives in ED or trauma center with positive secondary signs of life (eg, pupillary reflexes, spontaneous movement, organized ECG activity) *plus* • Resources available for definitive repair of abdominal-vascular injuries

hemorrhage, and aortic cross-clamping.[9,11] This procedure should be performed only by experienced providers.

Penetrating Cardiac Injury

Providers should suspect penetrating cardiac injury with any penetrating trauma to the left chest, particularly when the penetrating injury is associated with low cardiac output or signs of tamponade (eg, distended neck veins, hypotension, and decreased heart tones). Remember that bullet and stab wounds may cause thoracic and cardiac injury even when the entrance site is in the right chest, back, or abdomen.

The **F**ocused **A**ssessment **S**onogram in **T**rauma (FAST) is a rapid and accurate method of imaging the heart and the pericardium that can be performed in the emergency department. When used by an experienced operator, the FAST is up to 90% accurate for the diagnosis of pericardial fluid.[3] FAST, however, is not available in all hospitals.

Pericardiocentesis can be useful for both diagnosis and treatment of cardiac tamponade. In general, efforts to relieve pericardial tamponade due to penetrating injury should occur in the hospital. Pericardiocentesis can be used to stabilize the patient until exploration, pericardiotomy, and repair of the injury can be accomplished in the operating room.[3]

Cardiac Contusions

Cardiac contusions causing significant arrhythmias or impairing cardiac function are present in approximately 10% to 20% of adult patients with severe blunt chest trauma.[35] You should suspect myocardial contusion if the trauma patient has extreme tachycardia, arrhythmias, and ST-segment T-wave changes.

The myocardial band fraction of creatine kinase (CK-MB) is frequently elevated in patients with blunt chest injuries, but the elevation has little diagnostic or prognostic significance. Patients with an elevated level are just as likely as others to do well, and patients with a normal level may still have significant cardiac dysfunction. An MB fraction >5% has been used historically to diagnose cardiac contusion, but this isoenzyme is not a sensitive indicator of myocardial contusion.[36] Although cardiac troponins may signal the presence of cardiac injury, they do not provide more information than a 12-lead ECG.[3] Confirm the diagnosis of myocardial contusion by echocardiography or radionuclide angiography.

Indications for Surgical Exploration

Resuscitation may be impossible in the presence of severe, uncontrolled hemorrhage or in the presence of significant cardiac, thoracic, or abdominal injuries. Patients with such injuries require surgical intervention. The following conditions are generally thought to be indications for urgent surgical exploration.[3]

- Hemodynamic instability despite volume resuscitation.
- Thoracic injury associated with
  - Excessive chest tube drainage (1.5 to 2 L or more total, or >300 mL/h for 3 or more hours).
  - Significant hemothorax on chest x-ray.
  - Suspected cardiac or aortic injury. The helical, contrast-enhanced computed tomography of the chest is extremely accurate for diagnosis of aortic injury.[3]
- Gunshot wounds thought to traverse the peritoneal cavity or visceral/vascular retroperitoneum (note that the path of the bullet may be unpredictable).
- Penetrating torso trauma, particularly if associated with
  - Peritoneal perforation or hypotension.
  - Bleeding from the stomach, rectum, or genitourinary tract.
- Blunt abdominal trauma with the following:
  - Hypotension and clinical evidence of intraperitoneal bleeding.
  - Positive diagnostic peritoneal lavage or ultrasound.
- Significant solid-organ, diaphragm, or bowel injury or peritonitis.
  - Contrast-enhanced CT indicates a ruptured gastrointestinal tract, intraperitoneal bladder injury, renal pedicle injury, or severe visceral parenchymal injury after blunt or penetrating injury.
  - Peritonitis (on presentation or as a later complication).
  - Free air, retroperitoneal air, or rupture of the hemidiaphragm after blunt trauma.

Transfer

If a patient arrives at a facility with limited trauma capability, hospital staff should treat identifiable and reversible injuries to their capability. The patient should then be rapidly transferred to a facility that can provide definitive trauma care.

References

1. *World Health Statistical Annual, 1994*. Geneva, Switzerland: World Health Organization; 1994.

2. Anderson RN. Deaths: leading causes for 2000. *Natl Vital Stat Rep*. 2002;50:1-85.

3. Parks SN, ATLS Subcommittee, American College of Surgeons Committee on Trauma. *Advanced Trauma Life Support, Overview of Changes for 7th Edition*. Chicago, Ill: American College of Surgeons; 2001.

4. Rosemurgy AS, Norris PA, Olson SM, Hurst JM, Albrink MH. Prehospital traumatic cardiac arrest: the cost of futility. *J Trauma*. 1993;35:468-473.

5. Hazinski MF, Chahine AA, Holcomb GW III, Morris JA Jr. Outcome of cardiovascular collapse in pediatric blunt trauma. *Ann Emerg Med*. 1994;23:1229-1235.

6. Bouillon B, Walther T, Kramer M, Neugebauer E. Trauma and circulatory arrest: 224 preclinical resuscitations in Cologne in 1987-1990 [in German]. *Anaesthesist*. 1994;43:786-790.

7. Bickell WH, Wall MJ Jr, Pepe PE, Martin RR, Ginger VF, Allen MK, Mattox KL. Immediate versus delayed fluid resuscitation for hypotensive patients with penetrating torso injuries. *N Engl J Med*. 1994;331:1105-1109.

8. Pepe PE. Emergency medical services systems and prehospital management of patients requiring critical care. Philadelphia, Pa: WB Saunders Co; 1993:9-24.

9. Rozycki G, Adams C, Champion H, Kihn R. Resuscitative thoracotomy—trends in outcome. *Ann Emerg Med*. 1990;19:462.

10. Copass MK, Oreskovich MR, Bladergroen MR, Carrico CJ. Prehospital cardiopulmonary resuscitation of the critically injured patient. *Am J Surg*. 1984;148:20-26.

11. Durham LA III, Richardson RJ, Wall MJ Jr, Pepe PE, Mattox KL. Emergency center thoracotomy: impact of prehospital resuscitation. *J Trauma*. 1992;32:775-779.

12. Kloeck W. Prehospital advanced CPR in the trauma patient. *Trauma Emerg Med*. 1993;10:772-776.

13. Schmidt U, Frame SB, Nerlich ML, Rowe DW, Enderson BL, Maull KI, Tscherne H. On-scene helicopter transport of patients with multiple injuries—comparison of a German and an American system. *J Trauma*. 1992;33:548-553.

14. Cummins RO, Hazinski MF. Guidelines based on the principle 'First, do no harm'. New guidelines on tracheal tube confirmation and prevention of dislodgment. *Resuscitation*. 2000;46:443-447.

15. Katz SH, Falk JL. Misplaced endotracheal tubes by paramedics in an urban emergency medical services system. *Ann Emerg Med*. 2001;37:32-37.

16. Gausche M, Lewis RJ, Stratton SJ, Haynes BE, Gunter CS, Goodrich SM, Poore PD, McCollough MD, Henderson DP, Pratt FD, Seidel JS. Effect of out-of-hospital pediatric endotracheal intubation on survival and neurological outcome: a controlled clinical trial. *JAMA*. 2000;283:783-790.

17. Dutton RP, Mackenzie CF, Scalea TM. Hypotensive resuscitation during active hemorrhage: impact on in-hospital mortality. *J Trauma*. 2002;52:1141-1146.

18. Dretzke J, Sandercock J, Bayliss S, Burls A. Clinical effectiveness and cost-effectiveness of prehospital intravenous fluids in trauma patients. *Health Technol Assess*. 2004;8:iii, 1-103.

19. Dula DJ, Wood GC, Rejmer AR, Starr M, Leicht M. Use of prehospital fluids in hypotensive blunt trauma patients. *Prehosp Emerg Care*. 2002;6:417-420.

20. Greaves I, Porter KM, Revell MP. Fluid resuscitation in prehospital trauma care: a consensus view. *J R Coll Surg Edinb*. 2002;47:451-457.

21. Koenig KL. Quo vadis: "scoop and run," "stay and treat," or "treat and street"? *Acad Emerg Med*. 1995;2:477-479.

22. Deakin CD, Soreide E. Pre-hospital trauma care. *Curr Opin Anaesthesiol*. 2001;14:191-195.

23. Nolan J. Advanced life support training. *Resuscitation*. 2001;50:9-11.

24. Hopson LR, Hirsh E, Delgado J, Domeier RM, Krohmer J, McSwain NE Jr, Weldon C, Friel M, Hoyt DB. Guidelines for withholding or termination of resuscitation in prehospital traumatic cardiopulmonary arrest. *J Am Coll Surg*. 2003;196:475-481.

25. Hopson LR, Hirsh E, Delgado J, Domeier RM, McSwain NE Jr, Krohmer J. Guidelines for withholding or termination of resuscitation in prehospital traumatic cardiopulmonary arrest: a joint position paper from the National Association of EMS Physicians Standards and Clinical Practice Committee and the American College of Surgeons Committee on Trauma. *Prehosp Emerg Care*. 2003;7:141-146.

26. Hopson LR, Hirsh E, Delgado J, Domeier RM, McSwain NE, Krohmer J. Guidelines for withholding or termination of resuscitation in prehospital traumatic cardiopulmonary arrest: joint position statement of the National Association of EMS Physicians and the American College of Surgeons Committee on Trauma. *J Am Coll Surg*. 2003;196:106-112.

27. Baskaya MK. Inadvertent intracranial placement of a nasogastric tube in patients with head injuries. *Surg Neurol*. 1999;52:426-427.

28. Moore FA, McKinley BA, Moore EE. The next generation in shock resuscitation. *Lancet*. 2004;363:1988-1996.

29. Solomonov E, Hirsh M, Yahiya A, Krausz MM. The effect of vigorous fluid resuscitation in uncontrolled hemorrhagic shock after massive splenic injury. *Crit Care Med*. 2000;28:749-754.

30. Grove CA, Lemmon G, Anderson G, McCarthy M. Emergency thoracotomy: appropriate use in the resuscitation of trauma patients. *Am Surg*. 2002;68:313-316; discussion 316-317.

31. Ladd AP, Gomez GA, Jacobson LE, Broadie TA, Scherer LR III, Solotkin KC. Emergency room thoracotomy: updated guidelines for a level I trauma center. *Am Surg*. 2002;68:421-424.

32. Powell DW, Moore EE, Cothren CC, Ciesla DJ, Burch JM, Moore JB, Johnson JL. Is emergency department resuscitative thoracotomy futile care for the critically injured patient requiring prehospital cardiopulmonary resuscitation? *J Am Coll Surg*. 2004;199:211-215.

33. Aihara R, Millham FH, Blansfield J, Hirsch EF. Emergency room thoracotomy for penetrating chest injury: effect of an institutional protocol. *J Trauma*. 2001;50:1027-1030.

34. Practice management guidelines for emergency department thoracotomy. Working Group, Ad Hoc Subcommittee on Outcomes, American College of Surgeons–Committee on Trauma. *J Am Coll Surg*. 2001;193:303-309.

35. McLean RF, Devitt JH, Dubbin J, McLellan BA. Incidence of abnormal RNA studies and dysrhythmias in patients with blunt chest trauma. *J Trauma*. 1991;31:968-970.

36. Paone RF, Peacock JB, Smith DL. Diagnosis of myocardial contusion. *South Med J*. 1993;86:867-870.

Chapter 14

Special Resuscitation Situations
Part 6: Cardiac Arrest During Pregnancy

Background

During attempted resuscitation of a pregnant woman, providers have 2 potential patients, the mother and the fetus. The best hope for fetal survival is maternal survival. For the critically ill patient who is pregnant, rescuers must provide appropriate resuscitation with consideration of the physiologic changes due to pregnancy.

Essential Facts

Pregnancy stimulates a variety of physiologic changes that make the pregnant woman more vulnerable to cardiovascular insult. These changes can complicate attempted resuscitation during cardiac arrest (see "Critical Concepts: Physiologic Changes of Pregnancy That May Affect Resuscitation"). The ACLS provider should be aware of the unique physiology of pregnancy and be able to adapt resuscitation techniques to support the mother and the child.

Frequency

Cardiovascular emergencies in pregnant women are uncommon. Death related to pregnancy itself is rare, occurring at an estimated rate of 3.3 pregnancy-related deaths for every 100 000 live births.[1-4] But when non–pregnancy-related deaths are included, the rate increases to 9.2 deaths of pregnant women per 100 000 live births.

In the United States the 3 leading causes of death in pregnant women are homicide, suicide, and motor vehicle crashes.[5,6] In areas as disparate as North Carolina[6] and New York City,[5] homicide is the most common cause of death in pregnant women, exceeding any single pregnancy-related cause, preexisting medical condition, or obstetric complication.[7] The major subcategory for homicide is "domestic violence."

Pregnant women suffer the same problems of motor vehicle crashes, falls, assault, attempted suicide, and penetrating trauma (eg, stabbings and gunshot wounds) as the rest of modern society. These injuries often require heroic interventions. Our response has been to craft harsh phrases to guide emergency care, such as "postmortem C-section," "perimortem delivery," "sacrifice mother or child," or "save mother or child," and "harvest the fetus." We walk a thin line between aiding our memory and demeaning our patients. These guidelines will avoid such phrases as much as possible.

Much of the literature on cardiac arrest associated with pregnancy comes from the specialties of emergency medicine and trauma rather than obstetrics and anesthesiology. The ACLS Course for Experienced Providers includes a teaching scenario dealing with attempted resuscitation of a pregnant woman with traumatic cardiac arrest.

Critical Concept

Physiologic Changes of Pregnancy That May Affect Resuscitation

Airway and Pulmonary Function
- The larynx is displaced anteriorly, with increased edema and blood flow.
- Oxygen consumption increases 20%.
- Elevation of the diaphragm causes decreased functional residual capacity and functional residual volume, which predispose to rapid desaturation during hypoxia.
- Tidal volume and minute ventilation are increased to support increased cardiac output and oxygen demand during pregnancy.
- The normal maternal arterial blood gases reflect a respiratory alkalosis with a mild compensatory metabolic acidosis. Mild maternal hypocarbia ($PaCO_2$ 28 to 32 mm Hg) is needed to create a gradient in the placenta to facilitate removal of fetal CO_2. Because respiratory alkalosis is already present, the mother's ability to compensate for any new acid load is limited.

Circulation
- During most of the pregnancy there is a 40% increase in cardiac output and plasma volume; late in the third trimester, cardiac output decreases, particularly when the mother is supine.
- Physiologic anemia may reduce arterial oxygen content even if oxyhemoglobin saturation and PaO_2 are satisfactory.
- Systemic and pulmonary vascular resistance decrease.
- Beyond 20 weeks' gestation the uterus compresses the inferior vena cava and aorta, compromising systemic venous return and systemic blood flow.

Gastrointestinal Function
- Hormonal changes contribute to an incompetent gastroesophageal sphincter even under normal conditions.
- An incompetent gastroesophageal sphincter predisposes the mother to regurgitation and the risk of aspiration with loss of consciousness.

—*Contributed by Carolyn M. Zelop, MD, St. Francis Hospital and Medical Center, Hartford, CT*

The Second Patient

A cardiovascular emergency in a pregnant woman creates a special situation for the ACLS provider. This emergency involves 2 potential patients, the mother and the fetus. You must always consider the fetus when an adverse cardiovascular event occurs in a pregnant woman. At a gestational age of approximately ≥20 weeks, the size of the uterus begins to adversely affect the attempted resuscitation. At a gestational age of approximately 24 to 25 weeks, the fetus may survive outside the womb.

Decisions About Cesarean Delivery

The decision of whether to perform an emergency cesarean delivery must be made quickly when the mother is in cardiac arrest. Emergency cesarean delivery—also known as hysterotomy—may improve the outcome for both mother and child.

Causes of Maternal Cardiopulmonary Arrest

The many causes of cardiac arrest in pregnant women can be grouped into several defining categories (see Table 1 for a detailed list):

- Injury/trauma
- Obstetric complications at the time of delivery
- Iatrogenic complications
- Medical conditions related to pregnancy
- Preexisting medical conditions

Changes in Maternal and Fetal Physiology: Relation to Cardiac Arrest

Uterine-Placental Blood Flow

During pregnancy the mother's cardiac output and plasma volume increase by 40%, and one third of maternal cardiac output flows through the uteroplacental unit. During pregnancy the uterus and placenta form a passive, low-resistance system. Maternal perfusion pressure is the sole determinant of uteroplacental and fetal blood flow. Consequently any cardiovascular compromise in the mother

Table 1. Potential Causes of Maternal Cardiopulmonary Arrest[7,8]

Injury/trauma
• Homicide • Suicide • Motor vehicle crash • Illicit drug use, unintentional overdose
Obstetric complications at the time of delivery

• Amniotic fluid embolism
• Hemorrhagic events:
  — Placenta previa, accreta, increta, or percreta
  — Placental abruption
  — Uterine atony
  — Disseminated intravascular coagulopathy
• Pregnancy-induced malignant hypertension
• Idiopathic peripartum cardiomyopathy

Iatrogenic complications
• Intubation errors • Pulmonary aspiration • Anesthetic overdose (intrathecal, intravascular) • Medication-related errors (overdose, allergies) • Hypermagnesemia
Medical conditions related to pregnancy (increased risk during pregnancy)
• Pulmonary embolism from thrombus, air, or fat (most common nontraumatic cause) • Infection or sepsis
Preexisting medical conditions

• Asthma
• Cerebral hemorrhage
• Cerebral aneurysm
• Cerebral thrombosis
• Malignant hyperthermia
• Cardiac pathology:
  — Acute coronary syndromes
  — Arrhythmias
  — Congenital or vascular heart disease

can severely impair blood flow to the uterus, placenta, and fetus. Restoration and support of maternal systemic perfusion is essential for the mother and the fetus.

Effect of the Enlarging Uterus

By the 20th week of pregnancy the gravid uterus is large enough to significantly compress the inferior vena cava and the aorta. Compression of the inferior vena cava reduces venous return to the heart, and compression of the aorta compromises forward flow. These factors can compromise cardiac output even in a normal pregnancy, particularly when the mother is supine.

If cardiac arrest develops, the gravid uterus can compromise the effectiveness of resuscitation. Because there is obstruction of venous return, you should not administer resuscitation medications through a subdiaphragmatic vein. During cardiac arrest these medications may not reach the mother's heart unless or until the fetus is delivered.

Maternal Physiology

A number of factors can compromise maternal oxygen delivery and ability to compensate for hypoxia and acidosis. If the mother is anemic, arterial oxygen content will be reduced even when oxyhemoglobin saturation and PaO_2 are adequate. By the third trimester the gravid uterus pushes the diaphragm up enough to significantly reduce the functional residual capacity and functional residual volume.

Relevant Research

In a study published in 1969, Uleland and colleagues[9] performed serial cardiovascular studies in 11 pregnant patients. They studied normal hemodynamics and the effects of changes in patient position and exercise during the course of normal pregnancy. This is still considered the definitive study of the hemodynamics of pregnancy. Uleland and colleagues noted the effects of the gravid uterus on normal maternal cardiac output and the importance of the lateral decubitus position:

> In this study it became apparent that cardiac output was elevated early in pregnancy and was maintained at a high level for a considerable length of time. Late in gestation cardiac output declines toward nonpregnant levels, regardless of maternal position.... "The increasing influence of the enlarging uterus as pregnancy advances is apparent from our data; a change in position from the supine to lying on the side produced a... rise of 8 percent... at 20 to 24 weeks' gestation, 13.6 percent at 28 to 32 weeks' gestation, and 28.5 percent ($P < 0.01$) at term."

The decrease in these lung volumes coupled with the high oxygen consumption that exists during pregnancy can predispose the mother to rapid arterial oxygen desaturation if hypoxia develops. If the mother is supine during cardiac arrest, this reduction in functional residual capacity limits the effectiveness of efforts to oxygenate and ventilate the patient.

Because the pregnant woman maintains a respiratory alkalosis with mild compensatory acidosis, the mother will have limited ability to buffer an acid load. The high level of progesterone during pregnancy reduces the tone of the lower esophageal sphincter. Incompetence of this sphincter increases the risk that positive-pressure ventilation during CPR will cause regurgitation and aspiration of gastric contents. For this reason the ACLS provider should establish a protected airway early in resuscitation. Maternal laryngeal edema may make intubation more difficult and may require use of a smaller tracheal tube. Increased laryngeal blood flow increases the risk of bleeding when any tube (orogastric, nasogastric, nasopharyngeal, endotracheal) is inserted into the oropharynx or nasopharynx.

Fetal Physiology

Fetal physiology may offer the fetus some protection during the first minutes of maternal hypoxia or cardiac arrest. Fetal hemoglobin differs from "adult" hemoglobin in that it binds more readily with oxygen. For this reason it is better saturated at lower arterial oxygen tension. As a result fetal arterial oxygen content is higher at a given PaO_2. Fetal cardiac output is higher per kilogram of body weight than newborn cardiac output.

There has been a single case report of intact newborn survival after 20 minutes of maternal cardiac arrest (but not more than 25 minutes).[10] In this case the mother received uninterrupted CPR during the emergency cesarean delivery and for several minutes afterward.

The effects of maternal CPR on fetal blood flow have not been studied in humans. Decades-old laboratory research showed that primate fetuses can survive up to 7 minutes of in utero asphyxiation without evidence of neurologic damage after birth. But this laboratory experience contradicts anecdotal reports of human perimortem cesarean delivery. For the human fetus the window of reversible damage appears to be no wider than 4 to 5 minutes.[11]

Resuscitation of the Pregnant Woman in Cardiac Arrest

Basic Life Support

Several modifications to standard BLS approaches are appropriate for the pregnant woman in cardiac arrest (Table 2). At a gestational age of 20 weeks and beyond, the pregnant uterus can press against the inferior vena cava and the aorta, impeding venous return and cardiac output. Uterine obstruction of venous return can produce prearrest hypotension or shock and in the critically ill patient may precipitate arrest.[12,13]

Shifting the Gravid Uterus

In cardiac arrest the compromise in venous return and cardiac output by the gravid uterus limits the effectiveness of chest compressions. The gravid uterus may be shifted away from the inferior vena cava and the aorta by placing the patient 15° to 30° back from the left lateral position (Class IIa) or by pulling the gravid uterus to the side.[14] This may be accomplished manually or by placement of a rolled blanket or other object under the right hip and lumbar area.

Manual Displacement

Relieve compression of the inferior vena cava and the aorta by shifting the gravid uterus to the left:

- Stand on the left side of the patient, level with the top of the uterus.
- Reach across the midline with both hands and pull the gravid uterus toward your abdomen.
- Pull until the patient's right hip/buttock begins to rise from the surface where the woman is lying.

Mechanical Techniques

The Cardiff wedge is a firm, wedge-shaped cushion that is available commercially. Such firm, wedge-shaped supports not only shift the uterus to the left but also provide a wide, firm, angled surface to support the tilted torso during chest compressions. In emergency circumstances such single-purpose equipment is often unavailable.

Alternative means of support are the angled backs of 2 or 3 chairs or the angled thighs of several providers. Overturn a 4-legged chair so that the top of the chair back touches the floor. Align 1 or 2 more overturned chairs on either side of the first so that all are tilted in the same manner. Place

Rapid Response Interventions **To Prevent Cardiac Arrest in Pregnancy**	To treat the critically ill pregnant patient: • Place the patient in the left lateral position (Figure). • Give 100% oxygen. • Establish IV access and give a fluid bolus. • Consider reversible causes of cardiac arrest and identify any preexisting medical conditions that may be complicating the resuscitation.

Table 2. Primary and Secondary ABCD Surveys: Modifications for Pregnant Women

ACLS Approach	Modifications to BLS and ACLS Guidelines

Primary ABCD Survey	**Airway**
	• No modifications.
	
	Breathing
	• No modifications.
	
	Circulation
	• Place the woman on her left side with her back angled 15° to 30° from the left lateral position. Then start chest compressions.
	    or
	• Place a wedge under the woman's right side (so that she tilts toward her left side).
	    or
	• Have one rescuer kneel next to the woman's left side and pull the gravid uterus laterally. This maneuver will relieve pressure on the inferior vena cava.
	
	Defibrillation
	• No modifications in dose or pad position.
	• Defibrillation shocks transfer no significant current to the fetus.
	• Remove any fetal or uterine monitors before shock delivery.

Secondary ABCD Survey	**Airway**
	• Insert an advanced the airway early in resuscitation to reduce the risk of regurgitation and aspiration.
	• Airway edema and swelling may reduce the diameter of the trachea. Be prepared to use an endotracheal tube that is slightly smaller than the one you would use for a nonpregnant woman of similar size.
	• Monitor for excessive bleeding following insertion of any tube into the oropharynx or nasopharynx.
	• No modifications to intubation techniques. A provider experienced in intubation should insert the endotracheal tube.
	• Effective preoxygenation is critical because hypoxia can develop quickly.
	• Rapid sequence intubation with continuous cricoid pressure is the preferred technique.
	• Agents for anesthesia or deep sedation should be selected to minimize hypotension.
	
	Breathing
	• No modifications of confirmation of tube placement. Note that the esophageal detector device may suggest esophageal placement despite correct endotracheal tube placement.
	• The gravid uterus elevates the diaphragm:
	  — Patients can develop hypoxemia if either oxygen demand or pulmonary function is compromised. They have less reserve because functional residual capacity and functional residual volume are decreased. Minute ventilation and tidal volume are increased.
	  — Tailor ventilatory support to produce effective oxygenation and ventilation.
	
	Circulation
	• Follow standard ACLS recommendations for administration of all resuscitation medications.
	• Do not use the femoral vein or other lower extremity sites for venous access. Drugs administered through these sites may not reach the maternal heart unless or until the fetus is delivered.
	
	Differential Diagnosis and Decisions
	• Decide whether to perform emergency hysterotomy.
	• Identify and treat reversible causes of the arrest. Consider causes related to pregnancy and causes considered for all ACLS patients (see Table 1 in this chapter and Table 1 in Chapter 11).

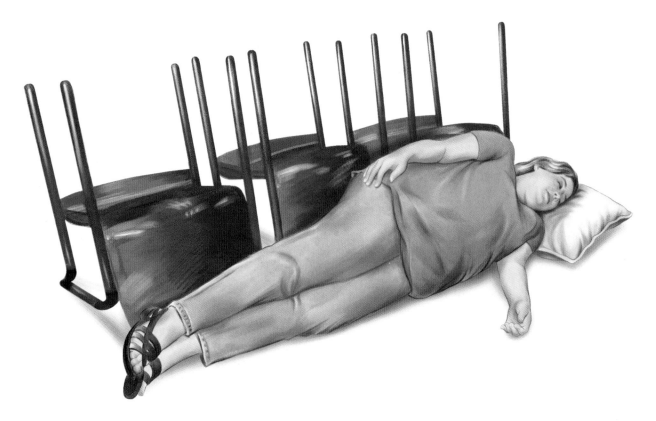

Figure. Left lateral position for pregnant woman. The gravid uterus may be shifted away from the inferior vena cava and the aorta by placing the patient 15° to 30° back from the left lateral position (Class IIa) or by pulling the gravid uterus to the side.

the woman on her left side, align her torso parallel with the chair backs, and begin chest compressions (see Figure).

Airway and Breathing

Hormonal changes promote insufficiency of the gastroesophageal sphincter, increasing the risk of regurgitation. Apply continuous cricoid pressure during positive-pressure ventilation for any unconscious pregnant woman.

Chest Compressions

Perform chest compressions higher on the sternum. This shift in hand placement will adjust for the elevation of the diaphragm and abdominal contents by the gravid uterus. We lack clear guidelines on how far the compression point should be shifted. Use the pulse check during chest compressions to adjust the sternal compression point.

Defibrillation

If the pregnant woman has ventricular fibrillation, administer defibrillation shocks at the doses recommended in the ACLS guidelines. There is no evidence that shocks from a direct-current defibrillator have adverse effects on the heart of the fetus. If fetal or uterine monitors are in place, remove them before you deliver shocks.

Complications of CPR in the Pregnant Woman

The physical changes associated with pregnancy and the challenges of performing modified chest compressions increase the risk of several CPR complications, including liver lacerations, uterine rupture, hemothorax, and hemopericardium.

Advanced Cardiac Life Support

The treatments listed in the standard ACLS Pulseless Arrest Algorithm, including recommendations and doses for defibrillation, medications, and intubation apply to cardiac arrest in the pregnant woman (Table 2). There are important considerations to keep in mind, however, about airway, breathing, circulation, and the differential diagnosis.

Airway

Secure the airway early in resuscitation. Hormonal changes promote insufficiency of the gastroesophageal sphincter and increase the risk of regurgitation. Intubation of a pregnant woman during attempted resuscitation can be difficult.

- A provider experienced in intubation should perform the procedure.

- Edema and swelling may narrow the woman's airway. It may be necessary to use an endotracheal tube that is slightly smaller (0.5 to 1 mm smaller ID) than the one used for a nonpregnant woman of similar size. The provider must be aware that a smaller tube will increase resistance to air flow and work of breathing during spontaneous ventilation.
- Effective preoxygenation before each intubation attempt is especially important because the decrease in functional residual capacity and functional residual volume predispose to rapid development of hypoxia.
- Rapid sequence intubation with continuous cricoid pressure is the preferred technique. Etomidate or thiopental is preferred for anesthesia or deep sedation.
- Blood flow to the larynx increases during pregnancy. Watch for excessive bleeding in the airway following insertion of any tube into the oropharynx or nasopharynx.

Breathing

Verify correct endotracheal tube placement using primary and secondary confirmation techniques. Note that in late pregnancy the esophageal detector device may suggest esophageal placement (the aspirating bulb does not re-inflate after compression) when the tube is actually in the trachea. This false-positive result could lead the provider to remove a properly placed endotracheal tube.

Pregnancy decreases functional residual capacity and functional residual volume, but the tidal volume and minute ventilation are increased. As a result, you must tailor ventilatory support based on evaluation of oxygenation and ventilation.

Circulation

Follow the ACLS guidelines for choice of resuscitation medications. Vasopressor agents such as epinephrine, vasopressin, and dopamine will significantly decrease blood flow to the uterus. But there are no alternatives to using all indicated medications in recommended doses. You must resuscitate the mother or the chance of resuscitating the fetus vanishes. Recall the time-honored clinical aphorism that maternal resuscitation is the best method for fetal resuscitation.

Differential Diagnosis

The same reversible causes of cardiac arrest that occur in nonpregnant women can occur during pregnancy. But providers should be familiar with pregnancy-specific diseases and procedural complications (Table 1). Providers should try to identify these common and reversible causes of cardiac arrest in pregnancy during resuscitation attempts. The use of abdominal ultrasound by a skilled operator should be considered in detecting pregnancy and possible causes of the cardiac arrest, but this should not delay other treatments.

- **Excess magnesium sulfate.** Iatrogenic overdose is possible in women with eclampsia who receive magnesium sulfate, particularly if the woman becomes oliguric. Administration of calcium gluconate (1 ampule or 1 g) is the treatment of choice for magnesium toxicity. Empiric calcium administration may be lifesaving.[15,16]
- **Acute coronary syndromes.** Pregnant women may experience acute coronary syndromes, typically in association with other medical conditions. Because fibrinolytics are relatively contraindicated in pregnancy, percutaneous coronary intervention is the reperfusion strategy of choice for ST-elevation myocardial infarction.[11] But there are reports of successful use of fibrinolytics for massive, life-threatening pulmonary embolism in pregnant women.[17]
- **Pre-eclampsia/eclampsia.** Pre-eclampsia/eclampsia develops after the 20th week of gestation and can produce severe hypertension and ultimate diffuse organ system failure. If untreated it may result in maternal and fetal morbidity and mortality.
- **Aortic dissection.** Pregnant women are at increased risk for spontaneous aortic dissection.
- **Life-threatening pulmonary embolism and stroke.** Successful use of fibrinolytics for a massive, life-threatening pulmonary embolism[18-20] and ischemic stroke[21] have been reported in pregnant women.
- **Amniotic fluid embolism.** Clinicians have reported successful use of cardiopulmonary bypass for women with a life-threatening amniotic fluid embolism during labor and delivery.[22]

Critical Concept *Use of Sodium Bicarbonate in Prolonged Resuscitation*	The ACLS guidelines do not recommend routine use of sodium bicarbonate. The use of sodium bicarbonate creates particular problems in attempted resuscitation during pregnancy. It is unlikely to buffer the fetal pH but may temporarily buffer maternal pH, so it may mask the severity of the fetal acidosis.

- **Trauma and drug overdose.** Pregnant women are not exempt from the accidents and mental illnesses that afflict much of society. Domestic violence also increases during pregnancy; in fact, homicide and suicide are leading causes of mortality during pregnancy.[8]

Emergency Hysterotomy (Cesarean Delivery) for the Pregnant Woman in Cardiac Arrest

Maternal Cardiac Arrest Persists/Not Immediately Reversed by BLS and ACLS

Clinicians treating a pregnant woman in cardiac arrest must never forget the second patient, the unborn child. With the mother in cardiac arrest, the blood supply to the fetus becomes hypoxic and acidotic. This will prove fatal to the fetus without rapid restoration of the mother's spontaneous circulation. *The key to resuscitation of the infant is resuscitation of the mother.* After approximately 20 to 23 gestational weeks, however, the *key to resuscitation of the mother is removal of the fetus from the gravid uterus.* After 20 to 23 weeks the gravid uterus obstructs the inferior vena cava, preventing venous return to the heart, and compresses the aorta, threatening arterial blood flow to critical organs.

The emergency ("crash") hysterotomy or cesarean delivery has gained general acceptance as a way of resuscitating a pregnant woman who remains in cardiac arrest after the initial few minutes of BLS and ACLS. Although the crash hysterotomy also offers the best chance of resuscitating the gestationally advanced fetus, cesarean delivery mandates sacrifice of a fetus below the gestational age of 20 to 23 weeks. The ECC guidelines first recommended the crash hysterotomy in 1992. The evidence for this recommendation consisted of a small number of case reports. With candid acknowledgement of the lack of definitive evidence from large-scale studies, the crash hysterotomy, as detailed below, has become widely cited, and the updated 2005 guidelines retained this recommendation. Candor, however, requires acknowledging that the published evidence leaves the crash hysterotomy as a generally accepted *intervention of desperation* for both the mother and the fetus. Designating the crash hysterotomy the "standard of care" for all emergency settings must await further published evidence.

Recommendations Based on Gestational Age

Hysterotomy allows access to the infant so that newborn resuscitation can begin. It also leads to immediate correction of much of the abnormal physiology of the full-term mother. The critical point to remember is that *both mother and infant will die if you cannot restore blood flow to the mother's heart.*

Once the fetus is delivered, the uterus is decompressed and the abdominal incision may enable direct massage of the mother's heart through the diaphragm. Internal cardiac compression through a thoracotomy may also be attempted. Evidence to support these interventions is lacking.

The gravid uterus reaches a size that will begin to compromise aortocaval blood flow at approximately 20 weeks' gestation for the single fetus. Fetal viability is estimated to begin at approximately 24 to 25 weeks. Consequently there is general acceptance of the following recommendations:

- **Attempt to determine gestational age from history and examination:** As a rule the uterus is palpable at the maternal umbilicus at approximately 20 weeks' gestation. For every centimeter above the umbilicus that the uterus is palpable, add 1 week to the estimated gestational age. Note that this estimate applies only to the single fetus. The uterus will be larger earlier in gestation if there is more than one fetus in the uterus.
- **Gestational age <20 weeks:** Resuscitation protocols should focus on the mother. If there is a single fetus, there is no need to consider urgent hysterotomy. The size of the uterus is unlikely to significantly compromise maternal venous return and cardiac output. But if there is more than one fetus, the uterus may compromise maternal blood flow, and emergency hysterotomy may be advisable.
- **Gestational age approximately 20 to 23 weeks:** Perform emergency hysterotomy and deliver the fetus to save the life of the mother. If the mother remains in cardiac arrest, unresponsive to BLS and ACLS for more than 5 minutes, delivery of the fetus will relieve the obstruction on the inferior vena cava and the aorta and may enable successful resuscitation of the mother. Survival of the newborn infant is unlikely.

- **Gestational age approximately >24 to 25 weeks:** After consideration of the factors listed in Table 3, perform emergency hysterotomy to save the life of both the mother and the fetus.
- **Consider infant factors that influence infant survival:** The factors that influence the newborn's chance of survival are gestational age, birth weight, and lung maturity. Survival is unlikely for the infant born at a gestational age less than 24 to 25 weeks and a birth weight less than 500 g.
- **Several factors related to the survival of a cardiac arrest infant:** The following arrest conditions have been linked with increased infant survival:
  — Short interval between the mother's arrest and delivery of the infant:
    - <5 minutes: Excellent probability of survival
    - 5 to <10 minutes: Good survival
    - 10 to <15 minutes: Fair survival
    - 15 to <20 minutes: Poor survival
    - 20 minutes: Only 1 case report[23]
  — Mother's cardiac arrest is not associated with sustained prearrest hypoxia
  — No or minimal signs of fetal distress at the time of the mother's cardiac arrest
  — Mother's resuscitation is conducted effectively and aggressively
  — Hysterotomy occurs in a medical center with a neonatal intensive care unit

Factors to Consider

Table 3 lists the many factors to consider in a very short time during a maternal cardiac arrest and attempted resuscitation.

Every emergency department should rehearse its plan of action for this type of event, including location of supplies, sources of extra equipment, and best methods for obtaining subspecialty assistance. All planning should be done in collaboration with obstetrical and neonatal or pediatric specialists.

Avoid chaos. Cardiac arrest in the pregnant woman, especially if it occurs outside the operating room or labor and delivery suites, can become a chaotic event. The following quotation describes an all too common reality:

> Resuscitation of a pregnant patient can become a chaotic event. Particularly in major centers, there may be other specialists involved, including pediatricians, neonatologists, anesthesiologists, obstetricians, and possibly others. These specialists have unique skills and experience that will help in the resuscitation. However, many of the specialists are poorly versed in emergency medicine and advanced cardiac life support protocols. It is particularly important that the team leader of the resuscitation take strict control of the events and the order in which they occur. The other specialists involved should not be allowed to deviate from the proper process.... The emergency physician must be the director of the resuscitation and take firm control.
>
> *—From Datner and Promes, "Resuscitation Issues in Pregnancy."*[7]

Table 3. The Emergency Hysterotomy (Cesarean Delivery) Decision: Factors to Consider Upon Maternal Arrest

Factors to Consider	Comments

Arrest Factors
 	
• If the mother fails to respond to initial resuscitative efforts and the gestational age is >20 weeks, ask that personnel and equipment be assembled for emergency hysterotomy. This will allow simultaneous continuation of resuscitative efforts and preparation for the cesarean delivery.
• Is the mother receiving appropriate BLS and ACLS care, including
   — CPR with compressions performed with the mother angled to the left?
   — Early intubation with verification of proper placement of the endotracheal tube?
   — Administration of indicated IV medications to a venous site above the diaphragm?
• Has the mother responded to arrest interventions?
• Are there any potentially reversible causes of arrest?
	Arrest Factors
	
	• Survival probabilities for the mother and fetus decrease as the interval from maternal arrest increases.
	• Aim for an interval of 5 minutes or less from maternal arrest to delivery of the fetus. This goal requires efficient assembly of personnel and equipment.
	• Do not wait until 5 minutes of unsuccessful resuscitation have passed before you begin to consider the need to deliver the fetus emergently. You should consider the need for hysterotomy within minutes to enable assembly of personnel and equipment.
	• Ensure that the mother has received superior resuscitative efforts. She cannot be declared "refractory" to CPR and ACLS unless all interventions have been implemented and implemented well.

Mother-Infant Factors • Is the fetus old enough to survive? • Has too much time passed for the mother to survive? • Is the mother's cardiac arrest due to a chronic hypoxic state? • What is the status of the fetus at the time of the mother's cardiac arrest?	**Mother-Infant Factors** • This question recognizes the critical importance of gestational age. Survival is unlikely for the infant born at a gestational age less than approximately 24 to 25 weeks and a birth weight less than 500 g. • Do not lose site of the goal of this dramatic event: a live, neurologically intact infant and mother. • Carefully consider the future before pushing the margins of survivability. • Even if the fetus is unlikely to survive (gestational age of 20 to 23 weeks), the mother may benefit from emergency hysterotomy.
Setting and Personnel • Are appropriate equipment and supplies available? • Is hysterotomy within the rescuer's skill "comfort zone"? • Are skilled neonatal or pediatric support personnel available to care for the infant, especially if it is not at full term? • Are obstetric personnel immediately available to support the mother after delivery? • In both in-hospital and out-of-hospital settings, is there adequate staff and equipment support? In out-of-hospital settings, is bystander support available?	
Differential Diagnosis • Consider whether persistent arrest is due to an immediately reversible problem (eg, excess anesthesia, reaction to analgesia, or severe bronchospasm). If it is, correct the problem and there may be no need for hysterotomy. • Consider whether persistent arrest is due to a fatal, untreatable problem (eg, massive amniotic fluid embolism). If it is, an immediate hysterotomy may save the fetus.	

References

1. Berg CJ, Atrash HK, Koonin LM, Tucker M. Pregnancy-related mortality in the United States, 1987-1990. *Obstet Gynecol*. 1996;88:161-167.

2. Beasley JW, Byrd JE, Damos JR, Roberts RG, Koller WS. Advanced life support in obstetrics course. *Am Fam Physician*. 1993;47:579-580.

3. Beasley JW, Damos JR, Roberts RG, Nesbitt TS. The advanced life support in obstetrics course: a national program to enhance obstetric emergency skills and to support maternity care practice. *Arch Fam Med*. 1994;3:1037-1041.

4. Wolcomir M. *Advanced Life Support for Obstetrics*. Kansas City, Mo: American Academy of Family Physicians; 1996.

5. Dannenberg AL, Carter DM, Lawson HW, Ashton DM, Dorfman SF, Graham EH. Homicide and other injuries as causes of maternal death in New York City, 1987 through 1991. *Am J Obstet Gynecol*. 1995;172:1557-1564.

6. Harper M, Parsons L. Maternal deaths due to homicide and other injuries in North Carolina: 1992-1994. *Obstet Gynecol*. 1997;90:920-923.

7. Datner EM, Promes SB. Resuscitation issues in pregnancy. In: Rosen P, Barkin R, eds. *Emergency Medicine: Concepts and Clinical Practice*. 4th ed. St Louis, Mo: Mosby; 1998:71-76.

8. Johnson MD, Luppi CJ, Over DC. Cardiopulmonary resuscitation. In: Gambling DR, Douglas MJ, eds. *Obstetric Anesthesia and Uncommon Disorders*. Philadelphia, Pa: WB Saunders; 1998:51-74.

9. Uleland K. Maternal cardiovascular dynamics: the influence of gestational age. *Am J Obstet Gynecol*. 1969;104:856-864.

10. Oates S, Williams GL, Rees GA. Cardiopulmonary resuscitation in late pregnancy. *BMJ*. 1988;297:404-405.

11. Doan-Wiggins L. Resuscitation of the pregnant patient suffering sudden death. In: Paradis NA, Halperin HR, Nowak RM, eds. *Cardiac Arrest: The Science and Practice of Resuscitation Medicine*. Baltimore, Md: Williams & Wilkins; 1997:812-819.

12. Page-Rodriguez A, Gonzalez-Sanchez JA. Perimortem cesarean section of twin pregnancy: case report and review of the literature. *Acad Emerg Med*. 1999;6:1072-1074.

13. Cardosi RJ, Porter KB. Cesarean delivery of twins during maternal cardiopulmonary arrest. *Obstet Gynecol*. 1998;92:695-697.

14. Goodwin AP, Pearce AJ. The human wedge. A manoeuvre to relieve aortocaval compression during resuscitation in late pregnancy. *Anaesthesia*. 1992;47:433-434.

15. Poole JH, Long J. Maternal mortality--a review of current trends. *Crit Care Nurs Clin North Am*. 2004;16:227-230.

16. Munro PT. Management of eclampsia in the accident and emergency department. *J Accid Emerg Med*. 2000;17:7-11.

17. Strong THJ, Lowe RA. Perimortem cesarean section. *Am J Emerg Med*. 1989;7:489-494.

18. Turrentine MA, Braems G, Ramirez MM. Use of thrombolytics for the treatment of thromboembolic disease during pregnancy. *Obstet Gynecol Surv*. 1995;50:534-541.

19. Thabut G, Thabut D, Myers RP, Bernard-Chabert B, Marrash-Chahla R, Mal H, Fournier M. Thrombolytic therapy of pulmonary embolism: a meta-analysis. *J Am Coll Cardiol*. 2002;40:1660-1667.

20. Patel RK, Fasan O, Arya R. Thrombolysis in pregnancy. *Thromb Haemost*. 2003;90:1216-1217.

21. Dapprich M, Boessenecker W. Fibrinolysis with alteplase in a pregnant woman with stroke. *Cerebrovasc Dis*. 2002;13:290.

22. Stanten RD, Iverson LI, Daugharty TM, Lovett SM, Terry C, Blumenstock E. Amniotic fluid embolism causing catastrophic pulmonary vasoconstriction: diagnosis by transesophageal echocardiogram and treatment by cardiopulmonary bypass. *Obstet Gynecol*. 2003;102:496-498.

23. Windle WF. Brain damage at birth: functional and structural modifications with time. *JAMA*. 1968;206:1967-1972.

Special Resuscitation Situations
Part 7: Electric Current and Lightning Injuries

This Chapter

- **Groups most at risk for electric current and lightning injuries**
- **Prevention of electric current and lightning injuries**
- **Considerations for early subspecialty involvement**
- **Critical BLS and ACLS interventions**
- **Postarrest management**

Introduction

Electric current can be a great force for good in the community. Our society has become dependent on electric power for heating and cooling, cooking and food preservation, and motive force, as well as the multitude of electronic gadgets that make our lives easier, more enjoyable, and more productive. Electric current offers many therapeutic opportunities in modern medicine. Defibrillation can control and possibly restore cardiac action. Electrical stimulation can facilitate bone growth. Physical therapies rely on many means of electrical stimulation. Even in psychiatry, electroconvulsive therapy has support.

Nonetheless uncontrolled electric current can cause severe injuries when it enters the body accidentally. There are 2 major means by which this occurs: technical electric current and lightning current.

Technical Electric Current

Technical electric current can cause massive deep injury and not infrequently death. Devastating internal burning may be seen, and some victims experience tetanic skeletal muscle contractions and "lock" to the source of current, prolonging exposure and multiplying the injury. (This "no-let-go" phenomenon has also been linked to the development of posttraumatic stress disorder.[1]) Current impinging on the heart can induce physical injury (such as burning, bruising, and physical disruption) and arrhythmias, including ventricular fibrillation (VF) and asystole. It may also cause fatal pump impairment and electromechanical dissociation. Even low-voltage sources, such as those involved in bathtub incidents, can cause cardiac arrest. There is often little external evidence in these cases because skin resistance has been lowered to such an extent that no skin burns occur, but the current affects the heart maximally.

Lightning Current

Lightning current presents a unique injury constellation of its own. Burns are of minimal concern, but cardiac injury is significant, and central nervous system and autonomic nervous system injury can be marked.

Blunt trauma and blunt head injury may occur with both types of current because of muscle contraction or falls, a blast effect from arcing or circuit box explosion, or the concussive effects of being close to a lightning strike point. Long-term neurocognitive damage with chronic pain, sometimes termed *post–electric shock syndrome,* has been consistently identified. This syndrome contributes to marked long-term disability and dysfunction.

The ACLS provider who treats cardiac arrest caused by electric shock or lightning strike must provide CPR

FYI

Injuries From Technical Electric Current and Lightning Current

Technical electric current:
- Physical injuries such as burning and bruising
- Arrhythmias, including VF and asystole
- Fatal pump impairment
- Electromechanical dissociation

Lightning current:
- Significant cardiac injury
- Marked central nervous system and autonomic nervous system injury
- Burns are of minimal concern

Both types of current:
- Blunt trauma
- Blunt head injury
- Long-term neurocognitive damage with chronic pain (*post–electric shock syndrome*)

and trauma and burn care. In general more prolonged resuscitative efforts and more aggressive fluid resuscitation are indicated for these patients than for other patients in cardiac arrest.

Epidemiology

Electric shock injuries cause approximately 500 deaths annually in the United States,[2] and lightning injuries cause approximately 40 to 60 deaths in the United States per year. Historically, up to 150 to 300 deaths per year occurred.[3] Although these are not common causes of traumatic death (Table 1), they are responsible for an estimated 52 000 trauma admissions per year and 4% to 7% of burn center admissions.[3] Many people who survive electric shock or lightning strike have permanent sequelae.

Electric Shock

Various groups are at particular risk for electrical injury. In perhaps the most comprehensive epidemiological analysis of deaths due to electric shock, Lindstrom et al[5] identified patterns of injury using data from 285 electricity-related deaths in Sweden from 1975 to 2000. The investigators defined "electrocution" as a *cause of death* that included death from electric shock, from burns caused by arcs, and from falls from a height. The vast majority of victims were male (94%); 132 incidents (46%) were related to work activities and 151 (53%) to recreational or leisure activities (2 cases unknown). Thirty-six deaths (13%) occurred in adolescents. Approximately 20% of cases involved alcohol. Over the total period, occupational and recreational deaths tended to parallel each other in a decreasing trend.

Similarly deaths due to high-voltage current (>1000 V) and to low-voltage current (<1000 V) decreased, the former by a larger percentage.

Forty-six percent of the 132 work-related electrocutions occurred in electrical workers, 14% occurred in agricultural

Table 1. Estimated Lifetime Risk of Death (by Age 70) From Various Causes

Cause of Death	Lifetime Risk* (numerator/denominator) Interpretation: a total of (numerator) people will die from (cause of death) before reaching age 70 in a population of (denominator)
Measles	1.5/1 000 000
Smallpox vaccination	5/1 000 000
Lightning strike	3/100 000
Electrocution	3/10 000
Drowning	2.5/1000
Falls	6/1000
Motor vehicle crash	1.5/100

*These estimates are based on actuarial data and represent "best estimates" of risk rather than "upper bounds" of risk. Lifetime risks are derived by multiplying annual deaths by 70 years, then dividing the product by the total US population.[4]

workers, and 11% occurred in construction workers.[5] Neglect of proper use of protective devices and procedures was considered to be a significant contributor to electrocution in 65% of those cases.

The most dangerous situation remains accidental contact with aerial power lines, and these deaths are roughly equally distributed between recreational and occupational deaths. Such incidents accounted for 40% of the total. Of these, the most dangerous location was railway lines (61 of 113, 54%), followed by forest and field lines (23 of 113,

FYI ***Electrocution vs Electric Current or Electric Shock Injury***	Loose terminology might refer to any electric shock as an "electrocution." But this term specifically refers to *death* from electric current. Otherwise the victim suffers an "electric current injury" or "electric shock injury."

20%), and public road lines (7 of 113, 6%). The remaining 22 deaths (19%) due to contact with power lines occurred in substations, farms, over watercourses, and at other minor locations.[5]

Carelessness, including lifting ladders, media truck satellite probes, and other long metal apparatus into overhead lines, is common in this injury. Nor can one ignore foolhardy and often illegal activities such as entering power substations or railway property; in the Swedish study, 20 of the 36 adolescents who died were electrocuted while climbing on railway carriages and touching overhead lines. In leisure activities alcohol was a significant factor in 35% of the cases.

Lindstrom et al[5] identified several significantly dangerous activities: performing unauthorized repairs, using alcohol, overlooking overhead power lines, or simply using poor judgment. These findings emphasize the importance of staying clear of fallen lines and of keeping domestic electric apparatus in good repair.

Although aerial power lines pose the greatest risk of electric shock, these injuries can occur in nearly all areas in which we move, including indoor residential properties and even gardens (Table 2). Electric injuries in the home account for nearly half of the annual deaths from electric shock.[3] They result from failure to properly ground tools or appliances or

Table 2. Common Locations for Electrocution

Location	Occupational	Leisure
Railway site	23/64	41/64
Residential	6/55	49/55
Substation	25/30	5/30
Farmhouse	19/25	6/25
Garden	0/21	21/21
Workshop	15/18	3/18
Construction site	15/16	1/16
Power pole	12/15	3/15
Water area	1/11	10/11
Other	16/28	12/28
TOTAL	132/283	151/283

Data from Lindstrom et al.[5]

Critical Concept ***Disability, Not Death, Is the Issue***	Although accidental death is an undoubted tragedy, survivors of electrical injury demonstrate tremendous ongoing disability,[7] which is important both personally and for society.

FYI ***Risk Groups for Electrocution***	Various groups are at particular risk for electrocution[5]: • Males • Adolescents • Utility, agricultural, and construction workers The following activities are significantly dangerous: • Performing unauthorized repairs • Using alcohol • Overlooking overhead power lines • Employing poor judgment Neglect of proper use of protective devices and procedures is a significant contributor to the electrocution in work-related cases.

from using electric appliances near water. Pediatric electric shock injuries typically occur around the home—when the child bites an electrical wire, places an object in an electrical socket, contacts an exposed low-voltage wire or appliance, or touches a high-voltage wire outdoors.[6]

Although accidental death is an undoubted tragedy, survivors of electrical injury demonstrate tremendous ongoing disability,[7] which is important both personally and for society. Prevention of electrical accidents will reduce not only deaths but also chronic and severe disability.

Lightning Strike

Lightning strike is a leading environmental cause of cardiac arrest. It exposes the victim to a potentially very large current for a very short time. Victims may be injured by a direct strike or through a side flash or splash (Figure 1), or from shock waves created in the surrounding air. In many cases of apparent direct strike, victims who receive immediate resuscitation can survive because much of the lightning current "flashes over" the victim and only a small amount enters the body. Figures 2A and 2B show the unique "ferning" pattern that can be produced on the skin by this flashover phenomenon.

Lightning strikes kill hundreds of people internationally every year and injure many times that number. Approximately 30% of victims of lightning strike die, and up to 70% of survivors sustain significant and permanent sequelae.[8-10]

Cloud-to-ground lightning strikes the surface of the United States about 25 million times a year. The largest number of cloud-to-ground flashes per area is located in central Florida between Tampa and Orlando.[11,12] Other regions of Florida and across the Gulf Coast also have high flash densities due to the warm humid air at the surface and coastal sea breezes, which fuel thunderstorm growth on most afternoons during a 6-month storm season. Regions in the western United States with mountains and large slopes in terrain also have high flash densities.[13]

During many recent years lightning has been second only to floods and flash floods in terms of US storm deaths. Florida leads the nation in the number of lightning deaths, and Colorado is second. When population is taken into account, the highest death rates are clustered in the southeast and Rocky Mountain states. The mountain west maximum is attributed to more people being outside at the same time of year and day when thunderstorms occur as well as the

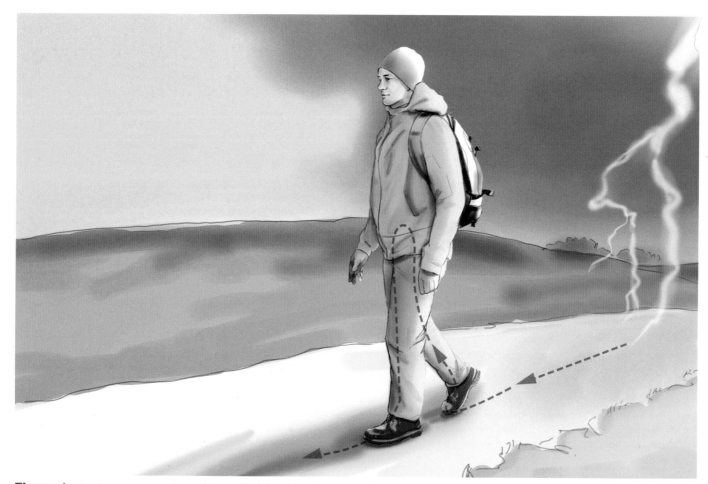

Figure 1. Side flash or splash. Current from a lightning strike is conducted to a nearby victim through the ground. The victim's legs conduct the current through his lower body.

less intense rain associated with lightning, which gives the impression of a less dangerous situation than is the case.

Two thirds of lightning casualties occur between noon and 6 PM in the summer months. Males are much more often victims of lightning than females.[14] This fact is attributed to the larger amount of time males spend outdoors in work and recreational activities, a tendency to underestimate the dangers of lightning, and perhaps to greater risk-taking behavior as well as aversion to changing activities already begun.

Lightning deaths are tracked more carefully than injuries because fatalities are reported more completely.[15] One reason for the difficulty in reporting lightning casualties is that about 90% of all deaths and injuries occur to one person at a time. For many reasons these may never be recorded in hospital admission data, coroner reports, or newspaper accounts, all sources of data for assessing the impact of lightning strikes. Nonfatal injuries are notoriously underreported because a significant number of the injured do not seek immediate medical care or do not need to be admitted for care. Nonetheless a ratio of 10 injuries per

death is considered to be the most reasonable estimate of injuries over the long term.[16]

The number of lightning deaths is determined from *Storm Data,* a monthly publication of the National Weather Service. The current fatality total in the United States is 40 to 60 per year. The fatality rate in the United States has dropped by more than an order of magnitude in recent decades, from 6 per 1 million population during the early 20th century to below 0.5 per million in recent years. A similar drop has been documented in other developed countries. This reduced fatality rate is attributed to the large decrease in the percentage of the population working and living in rural areas and the higher quality of building construction. Most people in developed regions live and work in large, enclosed buildings that are safe from lightning because of the "Faraday cage effect" of wiring and plumbing. Other factors include better awareness of weather, better medical care and communications, and the availability of metal-topped, fully enclosed vehicles for traveling. In parts of the world where people work in labor-intensive agriculture and live in unsafe structures, it has been estimated that 24 000 deaths and 240 000 injuries occur annually.[17]

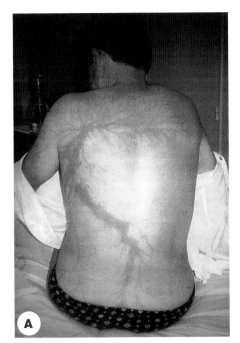
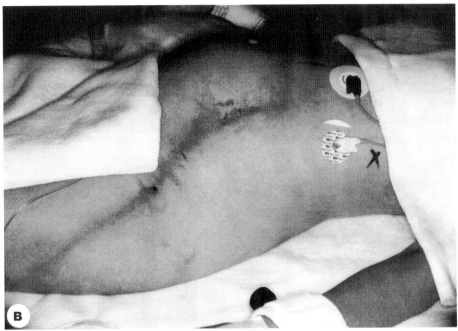

Figure 2. A. A 54-year-old man struck by lightning with initial stupor but rapid return of consciousness and eventual full recovery. His back displays an erythematous, fern-leaf pattern that was painless. This pattern has been referred to as "Lichtenberg figures." No blistering occurred and the marks disappeared completely within 48 hours. Reprinted with permission from *The New England Journal of Medicine.* 2000;343:1536. © 2000 Massachusetts Medical Society. All rights reserved. **B.** A 24-year-old woman, in her 26th week of pregnancy, struck by lightning while standing under a tree during a thunderstorm. The lightning entered her body through a necklace on the right side of her neck. As the lightning traveled to the ground it encountered the baby's head and was deflected to the left. An erythematous fern-leaf "print" of the lightning marks her skin. Although the woman survived, the baby died. Reprinted with permission from *The New England Journal of Medicine.* 1994;330:1492. © 1994 Massachusetts Medical Society. All rights reserved.

A century ago indoor fatalities were the most frequent, but today only 2% of lightning deaths occur inside houses. Outdoor incidents are the most frequent, and victims often are standing under trees.[18] A high percentage of lightning deaths occur during recreation, especially in beach, water, and camping settings. In addition, incidents during sports activities such as soccer, baseball and softball, golf, and hiking have become more common in recent years.[19,20] Rural casualties are now half as frequent as urban cases.

Prevention

Identification of risk groups, the most common settings for electric shocks and lightning strikes, and epidemiologic trends enables us to introduce measures to prevent many of these injuries and deaths.

Electric Current Injury Prevention

Several useful strategies have been developed to help prevent technical electrical injuries. These include building construction techniques and codes to require insulation of conductors in overhead cable swings so that they are insulated where contact might likely occur.

The adoption of standards for safe equipment manufacture has led to the development of circuit breaker closure and reclosure apparatus, semi-insulated cable plugs, and molded integrated plugs and sockets to prevent tampering and unauthorized repair. A significant advance is development of *residual current devices*. These devices compare the current flowing to and from a device, which should be equal. If the device detects an imbalance, it is assumed that the imbalance is caused by diversion of current through a person and the power is disconnected.

Many companies have adopted workplace codes, safe procedures, and specific protocols for responding to accidents. Although adoption of such codes and procedures necessitates a significant amount of employee training, it also provides a pool of skilled workers more attuned to safety. Companies are encouraged to frequently reinforce use of protective devices.

Lightning Injury Prevention

Lightning safety is not convenient, but then neither are other forms of safety. Lightning injury prevention for the most part is an individual responsibility unless large venues such as summer camps or sports stadiums are involved.

Prevention requires familiarity with lightning safety guidelines:

1. Know the weather forecast before starting an activity.
2. If bad weather is predicted, make alternate plans.
3. Know the weather patterns in the area where you are planning to be. Be off of mountains, golf courses, and other lightning-prone areas before the time of maximum lightning exposure, generally the afternoon hours.
4. Have a "weather eye"—watch the sky for signs of a storm.
5. At the first sound of thunder, which rarely can be heard more than 10 miles away (and often a lot less), you are already in danger and should be in safer shelter, such as a substantial (habitable) building with plumbing and wiring or a fully enclosed metal vehicle with all the windows closed.
6. Do not resume outdoor activities until at least 30 minutes after the last thunder is heard or lightning is seen.

Information about lightning safety for larger venues is available from the National Weather Service (www.lightningsafety.noaa.gov).

Major Effects of Electric Shock and Lightning Strike

Fatal Arrhythmias

The greatest danger for death from electric shock or lightning strike is the induction of arrhythmias. In the Lindstrom et al[5] study, the most common mechanism of fatal injury by far was fatal cardiac arrhythmia (79%). In the US study of Jones et al,[21] 85% of deaths were due to arrhythmias. The arrhythmias of most importance are those that give rise to cardiac arrest, namely asystole, which is thought to occur more commonly in lightning strike, and VF, thought to occur in "lesser" technical electric shocks. Because VF deteriorates to asystole, these observations may be related more to the timing of discovery or rescue of the victim than real.

Most other arrhythmias, including atrial tachycardia and fibrillation, ventricular tachycardia, and atrial and ventricular ectopia, are inducible with electric shock. But these arrhythmias do not necessarily lead to immediate death. Some clinicians have observed a delayed induction of arrhythmias within the first few days to 1 to 2 weeks after recovery from electric shock. There is little discussion of this phenomenon in the literature, although eventually it may become understood.

A current of around 20 µA applied directly to the heart is sufficient to induce an asystolic state or VF. Conversely this level of current can act as a defibrillating current when directly applied.

Other abnormalities in the myocardium have been reported. Other injuries caused by electric shock are neural dysfunction and tissue damage from burns.

Neural Dysfunction

Common sense reasoning assumes that because nervous tissue is by nature electrical in function, it must be susceptible to electric damage. This view assumes that neural membranes are immediately available to the passage of current. But nerve trunks are enclosed in a protective sheath of highly fatty and relatively resistive tissue, so electric current may not have the immediately deleterious effects on nerve function as might seem likely at first. This view also ignores electrical field, electroporation, and thermal effects.

Myocardial Tissue Damage by Burn Injury

Tissue, including myocardial tissue, may be damaged by burns. Burn damage produces a focal area of damaged myocardium not unlike that seen in infarction, and this area can become a site of myocardial rupture. Electric current most often travels hand to foot, so burn damage usually occurs inferiorly and may be reflected on the ECG in inferior leads II, III, and aVF.

Several authors have reported this type of damage and ECG pattern typical of infarction immediately after electric injury. Romero et al[22] reported severe antero-apical myocardial necrosis in a healthy 22-year-old man who sustained an electric current injury. Homma et al[23] reported persistent ventricular dysfunction, evident on the echocardiogram, in 2 patients. They proposed that the 2 mechanisms of cardiac damage in electrical injury are heat-induced myocardial tissue burn and arrhythmia-induced hypotension, the latter being most important in their patients. Xenopoulos et al[24] described a patient with rapid resolution of ECG changes but profound and ongoing echocardiographic dysfunction that continued until cardiac arrest occurred and the patient died. The myocardium at autopsy showed dramatic hemorrhage but normal patent coronary circulation. Many histologic signs of failure and inotropic therapy (eg, contraction bands) were evident on

microscopic examination. These changes led to a marked heterogeneity of viable and nonviable muscle.

The ECG in Electrical Injury

Conventional wisdom has been that once a patient survives an acute electric shock, the ECG changes and myocardial damage resolve and myocardial function returns. But resolution of ECG changes and abnormal cardiac marker levels are insufficient to indicate recovery of the myocardium, as the cases above illustrate. For this reason it may be necessary to conduct additional studies (eg, echocardiography, SPECT) to assess the extent and severity of myocardial damage. Also important is consideration of the effects of catecholamine excess and hypertension, which can develop from inotropic and vascular changes, on the damaged heart. Chandra et al[25] report that the best clinical predictors of myocardial damage are the extent of surface burns and a pathway of current involving the heart, which they define as one where the entry and exit points are superior and inferior to the heart, respectively. The current-time profile is another parameter to consider.

A valuable overview of these issues is given by Fish,[26] although the comments regarding preferential susceptibility of nervous tissue may not reflect the true pathophysiology. The mechanisms of induction of arrhythmias have also been well outlined by Bridges et al[27] and Geddes et al.[28]

Lightning injury seems more straightforward. It is commonly agreed, and appears supported, that even though many different ECG patterns may be seen acutely, full resolution of signs and complete recovery of function is the norm.

Pathophysiology
Electric Current Injuries

Electric shock injuries result from the direct effects of current on cell membranes and vascular smooth muscle. Injuries also occur with the conversion of electric energy into thermal energy as current passes through body tissues.

| **Critical Concept**

Assessing Myocardial Damage in Patients With Electrical Injury | Conventional wisdom has been that once a patient survives an acute electric shock, the ECG changes and myocardial damage resolve and myocardial function returns. But resolution of ECG changes and abnormal enzyme levels alone does not indicate recovery of the myocardium. If clinically indicated, the clinician should also consider

• Findings on additional studies (eg, echocardiography, SPECT)
• Effects of catecholamine excess and hypertension on the damaged heart
• Current-time profile

Perhaps the best clinical predictors of myocardial damage are the extent of surface burns and a pathway of current involving the heart (ie, one where the entry and exit points are superior and inferior to the heart, respectively).[25] |

Life-threatening arrhythmias, including ventricular tachycardia or ventricular ectopy, may result from either low-intensity or high-intensity electric current, and cardiopulmonary arrest may result. Low-voltage alternating current typically causes VF, while high-intensity current can cause asystole. In addition to arrhythmias, the current may create a brief but substantial inotropic stimulus, widespread muscle contraction and probable muscle cell rupture, myocardial cell damage, coronary artery spasm, and decreased coronary artery perfusion. These factors can contribute to cardiopulmonary arrest, postshock arrhythmias, and persistent myocardial dysfunction.

Respiratory arrest can be caused by the passage of electric current through the brain, by contraction of the diaphragm and chest wall muscles, from prolonged paralysis of the respiratory muscles, and by cessation of brain perfusion secondary to cardiac arrest. The respiratory arrest may persist even after circulation is restored.

Metabolic and systemic complications of electric injury include organ, muscle, and joint injuries and burns. Fractures of long bones and joint dislocations following electric shock can be caused by severe muscle contractions or falls. Many patients demonstrate hypovolemia and metabolic acidosis from fluid loss through skin damage and tissue destruction. Rhabdomyolysis may result from muscle injury and may lead to renal failure.

Vascular complications may compromise perfusion to extremities, and neurologic injuries can range from coma or altered level of consciousness to peripheral nerve damage.

Little is known about how electric current affects individual cells, but some understanding and data are available based on our knowledge of *electroporation,* a technique used in molecular biology. In this technique electric current is applied to a cell plasma membrane (or other living surface, such as skin) to increase its electrical conductivity and permeability. With exposure to current, pores will form in the membrane, allowing introduction of a substance such as a drug or coding DNA. If the voltage and duration of exposure are appropriate, these pores will reseal in a short time with no long-term damage to the cell. But if the voltage is too high or exposure too long, the cell will become unstable and progress to lysis. This same process is thought to occur in victims of electric shock.

Lightning Injury

The most common cause of death in lightning strike is cardiac arrest. The arrest may be associated with primary VF or asystole.

Lightning acts as an instantaneous, massive, direct-current shock that depolarizes the entire myocardium at once. In the 70% of lightning strike victims who survive, cardiac

---

FYI

Mechanisms of Electric Current Effects in Lightning Strike

There are 5 mechanisms by which electric current in a lightning strike may affect a person[34,35]:

1. Direct strike—self-explanatory and not nearly as common as it appears in the press: <10% of injuries.
2. Side flash or splash—when a person is standing next to a struck object and a portion of current jumps to the person: 25% to 40% of injuries.
3. Contact potential—when a person is touching a struck object and a portion of the current is diverted through the person: 3% to 10% of injuries.
4. Ground potential (step voltage, stride potential)—when lightning hits an object on the ground at a distance from the person, current is injected into the ground and flows radially from the struck object; injury to a person occurs as the current travels through the ground or as it arcs across an irregular surface through which it is traveling: 30% to 60% of injuries.
5. Upward streamer—the electrical field in a thundercloud induces opposite charges and "upward streamers" that may pass through anything in the field, including people. Even when the streamer fails to contact the lightning channel to complete the stroke, the current can be significant enough to cause serious injury or death: 10% to 25% of injuries.

Each of these mechanisms has a range of severity of injury and likelihood of cardiac arrest. Although it is "common sense" that the direct strike is more likely to cause fatalities, this has never been substantiated by clinical or laboratory studies. The physics of lightning is incredibly complex; lightning is a current phenomenon, not the voltage phenomenon of generated electricity with which we are more familiar.

automaticity resumes spontaneously. Organized cardiac activity and a perfusing rhythm soon follow.

Victims of lightning strike frequently suffer acute respiratory arrest. If apnea continues for more than 1 to 4 minutes, secondary hypoxic cardiac arrest will occur. This cessation of breathing may be caused by a variety of mechanisms, such as electric current passing through the brain and stopping further respiratory center activity in the medulla, tetanic contraction of the diaphragm and chest wall musculature during exposure to the current, and prolonged paralysis of respiratory muscles, which may continue for minutes after the electric shock ends.

Respiratory arrest due to thoracic muscle spasm or suppression of the respiratory center may persist after return of spontaneous circulation. Unless ventilatory assistance is provided, a secondary hypoxic cardiac arrest may occur.

Lightning strikes have widespread effects on the cardiovascular system. The strikes produce extensive catecholamine release, stimulating the autonomic nervous system. If cardiac arrest does not occur, the victim may develop hypertension, tachycardia, and nonspecific ECG changes (including prolongation of the QT interval and transient T-wave inversion). Myocardial necrosis with release of creatine kinase-MB may occur. Right and left ventricular ejection fractions may also be depressed, but this effect appears to be reversible.

Lightning can produce a wide spectrum of neurologic injuries. Injuries may be primary, resulting from effects on the brain, or secondary, developing as complications of cardiac arrest and hypoxia. The current can produce brain hemorrhage, edema, and small-vessel and neuronal injury. Hypoxic encephalopathy can result from cardiac arrest. A lightning strike can also damage myelin of peripheral nerves.

The etiology of respiratory and cardiac arrest following lightning injury has not been well studied, but these events may result from injury to the central nervous system; the autonomic nervous system; or the sinoatrial node, atrioventricular node, or other conducting pathways as current traverses through or around the outside of the body ("flashover"). Autonomic injury has been reported both clinically and in laboratory studies.[29-32] An animal study has shown that a portion of the current may enter the body at various cranial ports of entry (eye, mouth, nose, ears). Once diverted internally, the pathway is short to deep structures, including the brainstem and hypothalamus. The same study showed preferential damage to the brainstem respiratory centers.

Lightning injury is not scalable—one cannot use experience with generated electricity to predict findings or outcomes in a victim of lightning strike. For example, lightning injury rarely includes deep burns despite the tremendous energy involved. Part of the reason for this is that lightning is so short-lived that it may not be around long enough to heat up the skin to cause a burn.[33] In addition, although a small portion of lightning energy may go "through" a victim, the vast majority from a direct strike (and perhaps some of the other mechanisms) flashes around the person (flashover). There are 5 mechanisms by which electric current in a lightning strike may affect a person (FYI: "Mechanisms of Electric Current Effects in Lightning Strike").[34,35] It is not known how much current goes through or around a person in any of these mechanisms, although numbers can be modeled. Electromagnetic field effects are probably negligible.[36,37]

As noted above, although inherent automaticity may restart the myocardium, ventilation does not always recommence and a secondary hypoxic cardiac arrest may follow. Whether ventilation and oxygenation at this point may be restorative or whether the respiratory arrest signifies a more severe, and perhaps irrecoverable, injury has not been studied. But this sequence of events highlights the importance of CPR and airway management as interventions.

Out-of-Hospital Management
Electrical Injury

Out-of-hospital management is essentially standard BLS and ACLS management with minor modifications and extra precaution on-site. With electric shock the most important consideration is to not convert a situation with one victim into a situation with multiple victims.

The first task is extrication of the victim. It is most important to know—and this is entirely different from lightning-injured persons—that *a victim remaining in contact with electric current is dangerous to touch.* A rescuer who touches a victim before the source of current is turned off may be shocked. In addition, any material can conduct high-voltage current, and current can flow through the ground surrounding the victim. For these reasons the rescuer should not even approach the victim until the power source is turned off.

The first step is to break the connection between the person and the current source. For incidents involving a utility worker atop a pole, the specific protocols for pole-top rescue must be followed, and all workers should be well trained in these procedures. *Only rescuers specifically trained to break a live connection should attempt this intervention.*

For incidents occurring during recreational activities, the following process can be used:

1. Safely switch off the power to the apparatus or line that is thought to be the source of the shock, either at the switch or by pulling the plug. This must be done safely—with *no contact with any conductor.* A wise policy is to do this with one hand only and no other environmental body contact.
2. If immediate disconnection is not possible, switch off a circuit breaker or pull the appropriate fuse at the switchboard.
3. Alternatively, turn off the whole installation at the main switch.

Alternative methods of removing a victim from the source have been proposed. These methods include dragging the victim away with insulated hands and using a dry pole as a lever to move the victim. These methods should be used with extreme caution.

Once the power supply is off, the victim is safe to touch. Waiting until the power supply is off may mean that the victim has prolonged contact with current and dies. Although this scenario is highly distressing for rescuers, the loss of multiple lives is a worse consequence.

Lightning Injury

As with electric current injury, the top priority in lightning injury is safety. Victims of lightning strike will not be connected to the source of electricity when rescuers arrive, but if weather conditions are still inclement, the scene is still dangerous. Rescuers should remove the victim from the lightning-prone area to a safe shelter or EMS vehicle as soon as possible and provide BLS and ACLS as described below.

Basic Life Support for Electric Current and Lightning Injury

If immediate resuscitation is provided, survival from cardiac arrest caused by lightning strike is higher than that reported following cardiac arrest from other non-VF causes. Aggressive and persistent resuscitative efforts (20 to 30 minutes) are justified even when the interval between collapse and the start of resuscitation is prolonged or when cardiac arrest persists despite initial efforts. The goal is to oxygenate the heart and brain adequately until

cardiac activity resumes. Victims in respiratory arrest may require only ventilation and oxygenation to avoid secondary hypoxic cardiac arrest.

Once the victim is separated from the source of current and the scene is safe, determine cardiorespiratory status. Immediately after electrocution, respiration or circulation or both may fail. If spontaneous respiration or circulation is absent, immediately initiate BLS, including activation of the emergency medical services (EMS) system, prompt provision of CPR, and use of an automated external defibrillator (AED) when available. Immediate provision of ventilation and compressions (if needed) is essential. Use the AED to identify and treat ventricular tachycardia or VF.

Maintain spinal stabilization throughout extrication and treatment if there is a likelihood of head or neck trauma. Both lightning and electrical trauma often cause multiple trauma, including injury to the spine and muscular strains, internal injuries from being thrown, and fractures caused by the tetanic response of skeletal muscles. Remove smoldering clothing, shoes, and belts to prevent further thermal damage.

Vigorous resuscitative measures are indicated even for those who appear dead on initial evaluation. Because many victims are young, without preexisting cardiopulmonary disease, they have a good chance of survival if immediate support of cardiopulmonary function is provided.

The Concept of Reverse Triage for Lightning Injury

In multiple-casualty emergencies, especially from traumatic events, victims in cardiac arrest are given the lowest priority (see "Cardiac Arrest Associated With Trauma"). The harsh but evidence-based principle is that these victims have a very low probability of survival even with aggressive resuscitative efforts. Emergency personnel, especially if they are limited in numbers, will save more lives if they support victims who are not in cardiac arrest.

But in a multicasualty lightning strike event, the victim who develops immediate cardiac arrest has a high probability of survival and recovery *if BLS is provided without delay.* When multiple victims suffer simultaneous lightning strike, rescuers should give highest priority to victims who are in

Critical Concept

"Reverse Triage" for Multiple Victims of Lightning Strike

In a multicasualty lightning strike event, the victim who develops immediate cardiac arrest has a high probability of survival and recovery *if BLS is provided without delay.* When multiple victims suffer simultaneous lightning strike, give highest priority to victims who are in respiratory or cardiac arrest. Victims of lightning strike who do not suffer immediate cardiopulmonary arrest are unlikely to do so. They have an excellent chance of recovery with little additional treatment.

respiratory or cardiac arrest. Victims of lightning strike who do not suffer immediate cardiopulmonary arrest are unlikely to do so. They have an excellent chance of recovery with little additional treatment. Survival is high when victims with cardiac or respiratory arrest receive immediate resuscitation. This is true even when the presenting rhythm is asystole or when prolonged efforts are required.

Advanced Cardiovascular Life Support for Electric Current and Lightning Injury

When treating electric current and lightning injury, rescuers must first be sure that the scene is safe. Patients who are unresponsive after an electrical injury may be in either respiratory or cardiac arrest. Airway control, prompt CPR, and attempts at defibrillation (if indicated) are critically important. Treat VF, asystole, and other serious arrhythmias with the ACLS techniques outlined in this text. Quickly start CPR and attempt defibrillation at the scene if needed. Then take steps to manage the airway, including early placement of an advanced airway (eg, endotracheal intubation). Establishing an airway may be difficult for patients with electric burns of the face, mouth, or anterior neck. But extensive soft-tissue swelling may develop rapidly, complicating airway control measures. For this reason early intubation should be performed for patients with evidence of extensive burns even if the patient has begun to breathe spontaneously. ACLS providers should be prepared to provide respiratory support in case respiratory arrest persists even after return of spontaneous circulation.

Initial support of cardiovascular function requires treatment of arrest rhythms and then treatment of any life-threatening arrhythmias. Once spontaneous perfusion is restored, the victim may require fluid therapy and inotropic or vasopressor support. Victims with electric injuries have greater fluid requirements than those with thermal burns and will require rapid intravascular fluid administration to replace ongoing fluid losses and prevent hemodynamic compromise. For victims with hypovolemic shock or significant tissue destruction, rapid intravenous fluid administration is indicated to counteract shock and correct ongoing fluid losses due to third spacing. Fluid administration should be adequate to maintain a brisk diuresis. Fluid replacement will facilitate renal excretion of myoglobin, potassium, and other byproducts of tissue destruction (this is particularly true for patients with electrical injury).

Early Subspecialty Involvement and Transfer

As significant as the external injuries may appear after electrothermal shock, the underlying tissue damage is far more extensive, and survivors may have permanent neurologic and cardiac sequelae. Early consultation with or transfer to a physician and a facility (eg, burn center) familiar with treatment of these injuries is critical.

ED Management
The Medical Emergency Team

The management of cardiac arrest from electrical injury is similar to the management of cardiac arrest from other traumatic mechanisms. Most victims are young with little cardiac risk. For patients struck by lightning, management varies tremendously but is supportive and guided by the injuries. Management of cardiac arrest due to electric or lightning current generally involves ventilatory support, monitoring, cardiac compression, and standard drugs. There is no research to suggest that some drugs are more effective for these patients.

However, these patients may have other severe injuries, including trauma from a fall, deep burns, and even injuries due to exposure. A multidisciplinary medical emergency team (MET) with subspecialists from critical care, trauma, neurology, surgery, and cardiology can be very beneficial for these patients and should be activated early.

Differential Diagnosis

Increased capillary permeability will occur in association with tissue injury. Expect the development of local tissue edema at the site of injury.

Compartment syndromes can rapidly develop in any extremity, especially if circumferential burns are present. This severe tissue edema can produce local areas of vascular compromise and tissue necrosis.

Electrothermal burns and underlying tissue injury may require surgical attention for debridement or fasciotomies. Seek early consultation with a physician skilled in treatment of electrical injuries.

Postarrest Management

An important question is how long a patient should be monitored after an electrical injury. A well person with no signs of cardiac dysfunction, no abnormal cardiac markers, and a normal ECG can generally be discharged within 6 hours of the shock. A middle course is to monitor the patient for 24 hours and if all remains well, then to discharge. Any abnormality that develops should be treated as appropriate before discharge.

But as noted above, many patients with electrical injury have permanent neurologic, cardiac, or physical sequelae. These patients will require rehabilitation and long-term follow-up care.

References

1. Kelley KM, Tkachenko TA, Pliskin NH, Fink JW, Lee RC. Life after electrical injury. Risk factors for psychiatric sequelae. *Ann N Y Acad Sci*. 1999;888:356-363.

2. National Safety Council. *1999 Injury Facts*. Itasca, IL: National Safety Council; 1999.

3. Fontanarosa PB. Electrical shock and lightning strike. *Ann Emerg Med*. 1993;22:378-387.

4. Klaassen C, Eaton E. Principles of toxicology. In: Klaassen C, ed. *Casarett and Doull's Toxicology: The Basic Science of Poisons*. 4th ed. New York, NY: McGraw-Hill; 1993:12-49.

5. Lindstrom R, Bylund PO, Eriksson A. Accidental deaths caused by electricity in Sweden, 1975-2000. *J Forensic Sci*. 2006;51:1383-1388.

6. Kobernick M. Electrical injuries: pathophysiology and emergency management. *Ann Emerg Med*. 1982;11:633-638.

7. Cooper MA, Andrews CJ. Disability, not death, is the issue in lightning injury. Presented at: International Conference on Lightning and Static Electricity; Seattle, WA; 2005.

8. Cooper MA. Lightning injuries: prognostic signs for death. *Ann Emerg Med*. 1980;9:134-138.

9. Kleinschmidt-DeMasters BK. Neuropathology of lightning-strike injuries. *Semin Neurol*. 1995;15:323-328.

10. Stewart CE. When lightning strikes. *Emerg Med Serv*. 2000;29:57-67; quiz 103.

11. Huffines GR, Orville RE. Lightning ground flash density and thunderstorm duration in the contiguous United States: 1989-1996. *J Appl Meteorol*. 1999;38:1013.

12. Orville RE, Huffines GR, Burrows WR, Holle RL, Cummins KL. The North American Lightning Detection Network (NALDN)—first results: 1998-2000. *Mon Wea Rev*. 2002;130:2098.

13. López RE, et al. Spatial and temporal distributions of lightning over Arizona from a power utility perspective. *J Appl Meteorol*. 1997;36:825.

14. Curran EB, Holle RL, López RE. Lightning fatalities, injuries, and damage reports in the United States from 1959–1994. Silver Spring, Md: National Oceanic and Atmospheric Administration; 1997. Technical memo NWS SR-193.

15. López RE. The underreporting of lightning injuries and deaths in Colorado. *Bull Am Meteorol Soc*. 1993;74:2171.

16. Cherington M, et al. Closing the gap on the actual numbers of lightning casualties and deaths. Presented at: 11th Conference on Applied Climatology; Dallas, Tex; January 10-15, 1999.

17. Holle RL, López RE. A comparison of current lightning death rates in the U.S. with other locations and times. Presented at: International Conference on Lightning and Static Electricity; Blackpool, UK; September 16-18, 2003.

18. Holle RL, López RE, Navarro BC. Deaths, injuries, and damages from lightning in the United States in the 1890s in comparison with the 1990s. *J Appl Meteorol*. 2005;44:1563-1573.

19. Holle RL. Activities and locations of recreation deaths and injuries from lightning. Presented at: International Conference on Lightning and Static Electricity; Blackpool, UK; September 16-18, 2003.

20. Holle RL. Lightning-caused deaths and injuries during hiking and mountain climbing. Presented at: International Conference on Lightning and Static Electricity; Seattle, WA; September 20-22, 2005.

21. Jones JE, Armstrong CW, Woolard CD, Miller GB Jr. Fatal occupational electrical injuries in Virginia. *J Occup Med*. 1991;33:57-63.

22. Romero B, Candell-Riera J, Gracia RM, Fernandez MA, Aguade S, Peracaula R, Soler-Soler J. Myocardial necrosis by electrocution: evaluation of noninvasive methods. *J Nucl Med*. 1997;38:250-251.

23. Homma S, Gillam LD, Weyman AE. Echocardiographic observations in survivors of acute electrical injury. *Chest*. 1990;97:103-105.

24. Xenopoulos N, Movahed A, Hudson P, Reeves WC. Myocardial injury in electrocution. *Am Heart J*. 1991;122:1481-1484.

25. Chandra NC, Siu CO, Munster AM. Clinical predictors of myocardial damage after high voltage electrical injury. *Crit Care Med*. 1990;18:293-297.

26. Fish R. Electric shock, part II: nature and mechanisms of injury. *J Emerg Med*. 1993;11:457-462.

27. Bridges JE, et al, eds. *Electrical Shock Safety Criteria: Proceedings of the First International Symposium on Electrical Shock Safety Criteria*. New York, NY: Pergamon Press; 1985.

28. Geddes LA, Bourland JD, Ford G. The mechanism underlying sudden death from electric shock. *Med Instrum*. 1986; 20:303-315.

29. Grubb BP, Karabin B. New onset postural tachycardia syndrome following lightning injury. *Pacing Clin Electrophysiol*. 2007;30:1036-1038.

30. Weeramanthri TS, Puddey IB, Beilin LJ. Lightning strike and autonomic failure—coincidence or causally related? *J R Soc Med*. 1991;84:687-688.

31. Cooper MA, Kotsos T, Gandhi MV, Neideen T. Acute autonomic and cardiac effects of simulated lightning strike in rodents. Presented at: International Bioengineering Symposium; Chicago, Ill; July 2000.

32. Cooper MA. The acute effects of simulated lightning strike on the cardiac and autonomic nervous system in an animal model. Presented at: International Conference on Lightning and Static Electricity; Blackpool, UK; September 15-19, 2003.

33. Cooper MA. Lightning burns are usually minor, superficial, and less common than expected. Presented at: International Lightning Detection Conference; Tucson, Ariz; April 24-25, 2006.

34. Cooper MA. A fifth mechanism of lightning injury. *Acad Emerg Med*. 2002;9:172-174.

35. Cooper MA, Andrews CJ, Holle RL. Distribution of lightning injury mechanisms. Presented at: International Lightning Detection Conference; Tucson, Ariz; April 24-25, 2006.

36. Cherington M, Wachtel H, Yarnell PR. Could lightning injury be magnetically induced? *Lancet*. 1998;351:1788.

37. Andrews CJ, Cooper MA, Kotsos T, Kitigawa N, Mackerras D. Magnetic effects of lightning strokes. *Electronic J Lightning Res*. 2007.

Life-Threatening Electrolyte and Acid-Base Abnormalities

This Chapter

- **Most common causes of electrolyte imbalances**
- **Early recognition of symptoms of electrolyte and acid-base disorders**
- **Diagnostic and therapeutic equations for treating electrolyte abnormalities**
- **Rapid response interventions for life-threatening electrolyte imbalances**
- **Diagnosing acid-base imbalances**
- **Diabetic ketoacidosis in patients without insulin-dependent diabetes?**
- **The importance of potassium in diabetic ketoacidosis**
- **Classic findings of nonketotic hyperosmolar syndrome**

Introduction

Electrolyte and acid-base abnormalities are commonly associated with cardiovascular emergencies. Identified abnormalities probably represent only the tip of the iceberg—the numerator of a much larger, unrecognized denominator. The true frequency of a causative role of electrolyte and acid-base abnormalities in periarrest emergencies remains unknown.

When faced with an unexplained cardiovascular emergency, healthcare professionals should consider that the origin lies in electrolyte and acid-base problems. When patients with underlying conditions develop unexpected cardiovascular deterioration, the astute clinician should remember to search for the explanation in the original condition. Conditions that can frequently cause electrolyte and acid-base abnormalities are listed in Table 1.

If you identify predisposing conditions, you may be able to provide *anticipatory therapy* to prevent development of

Table 1. Conditions Frequently Associated With Life-Threatening Electrolyte or Acid-Base Abnormalities

Possible Presenting Signs and Symptoms	
• Vomiting	• Confusion, lethargy, irritability
• Diarrhea, constipation	• Weakness, fatigue

Acute Conditions	
• Anorexia	• Poor oral intake
• Use of multiple medications	• Recent seizures
• Alcohol abuse, acute	• Recent surgery
• Pancreatitis	• Peritonitis

Chronic Medical Problems	
• Renal failure	• Older age (>65 years)
• Renal dialysis	• Insulin-dependent diabetes
• Drug abuse	• Hypertension
• Metastatic cancer	• Cirrhosis
• Immobilization	• Congestive heart failure
• Alcohol abuse, chronic	• Weight loss, chronic
• Hyperalimentation	
• Malnutrition, chronic	
• Nephrotic syndrome	

Table 2. A, Normal Values of Electrolytes. **B,** Diagnostic and Therapeutic Equations

Table 2A. Normal Values			
Parameter (Symbol)	**Reference Range (Normal)**	**Parameter (Symbol)**	**Reference Range (Normal)**
Sodium (Na^+)	135 to 145 mEq/L	**Arterial Blood Gases (Room Air)**	
Potassium (K^+)	3.5 to 5 mEq/L	pH	7.35 to 7.45
Chloride (Cl^-)	98 to 108 mEq/L	PCO_2	35 to 45 mm Hg
Carbon dioxide (HCO_3^-)	7 ± 4 mEq/L	Base excess	> + 2 = Metabolic alkalosis
Anion gap	10 to 15 mEq/L	Base deficit	< − 2 = Metabolic acidosis
Glucose	62 to 125 mg/dL	Calculated vs measured pH	See below
Urea nitrogen (BUN)	8 to 21 mg/dL		
Creatinine	0.3 to 1.2 mg/dL		
Calcium, total (Ca^{2+})	8.5 to 10.5 mg/dL		
Calcium, ionized	4.2 to 4.8 mg/dL		
Magnesium (Mg^{2+})	1.3 to 2.2 mEq/L		
Urine specific gravity	1.005 to 1.030 mg/mL		
Albumin	3.5 to 5.2 g/dL		
Protein, total	6 to 8.2 g/dL		
Osmolality, serum	275 to 295 mOsm/L		

Table 2B. Useful Calculations and Formulae*		
Calculation	**Formula**	**Comments**
Anion gap (serum concentration in mEq/L)	$[Na^+] - ([Cl^-] + [HCO_3^-])$	Normal range: 10 to 15 mEq/L. A gap >15 suggests metabolic acidosis.
Osmolal gap	$Osmolality_{measured} - Osmolality_{calculated}$ Normal = <10	Osmolal gap normally <10. If osmolal gap is >10, suspect unknown osmotically active substances.
Calculated osmolality (in mOsm/L)	$(2 \times [Na^+]) + ([Glucose] \div 18) + ([BUN] \div 2.8)$	Simplified to give *effective* osmolality. Normal = 272 to 300 mOsm/L
Total free water deficit (in L)	$\frac{([Na^+]_{measured} - 140) \times TBW}{140}$ $TBW_{in L} = (0.6_{men}\ or\ 0.5_{women}) \times Weight_{in kg}$	Use to calculate quantity of water needed to correct water deficit in hypernatremia.
Sodium deficit (in total mEq)	$([Na^+]_{desired} - [Na^+]_{measured}) \times TBW_{in L}$ $TBW_{in L} = (0.6_{men}\ or\ 0.5_{women}) \times Weight_{in kg}$	Use to calculate sodium deficit to replace with 3% saline in severe hyponatremia (3% saline contains 513 mEq sodium per liter).
Determination of predicted pH	$(40 - PCO_2) \times 0.008 =$ $\pm\Delta$ in pH from 7.4	For every 1 mm Hg change in PCO_2 from 40, pH will change by 0.008. Measured pH less than calculated pH: metabolic acidosis is present. Measured pH greater than predicted pH: metabolic alkalosis is present.

*See text for details. Concentration units are the same as listed above. TBW indicates total body water.

life-threatening electrolyte and acid-base disorders. You may need to start empiric treatment on the basis of history, physical examination, and objective signs before laboratory results become available.

This chapter refers to electrolyte values that are above or below the normal range. For ease of reference Table 2 presents the normal range for a number of relevant clinical parameters. Table 2 also contains the various diagnostic and therapeutic equations presented throughout the chapter. But be sure to check the reference ranges for your laboratory because there may be slight variations based on patient demographics and test variability.

Potassium

The magnitude of the potassium gradient across cell membranes determines excitability of nerve and muscle cells, including the myocardium. Rapid or significant changes in the serum potassium concentration can have life-threatening consequences. Potassium is a positive ion that is present in much higher concentration inside cells than in the extracellular space that includes the serum. The difference in potassium concentration between the inside and outside of cells is called the *potassium gradient*. Maintaining the potassium gradient across cell membranes is critical for muscular and neurologic function. Minor changes in the serum potassium concentration can have major effects on the excitability of the heart and conduction within it. Of all significant electrolyte abnormalities, rapid changes in serum potassium are the most likely to be life-threatening.

Hyperkalemia

Normal potassium range: 3.5 to 5 mEq/L
The normal potassium range in serum is 3.5 to 5 mEq/L, but it may vary slightly between laboratories. Under physiologic conditions serum potassium is tightly regulated within this range.

Causes

There are multiple causes of hyperkalemia; Table 3 lists the most common ones. Hyperkalemia generally is caused by either increased K^+ release from cells or impaired excretion by the kidneys. Evaluation of serum potassium must consider the effects of changes in serum pH. When serum pH falls, serum potassium rises because potassium shifts from the cellular to the vascular space. When serum pH rises, serum potassium falls because potassium shifts from the vascular space into the cells. A good way to remember the relationship between pH and serum potassium is that *serum potassium changes in a direction opposite serum pH*. Effects of pH changes on serum potassium should be anticipated during therapy for hyperkalemia or hypokalemia and during any therapy that may cause changes in serum pH (eg, treatment of diabetic ketoacidosis).

Early recognition of conditions that cause hyperkalemia may prevent or minimize hyperkalemic cardiac arrhythmias.[1-3] The most common cause of severe, life-threatening hyperkalemia is kidney failure—classically in a dialysis patient who misses scheduled dialysis appointments and presents with severe weakness.[4] These patients can experience good outcomes if the hyperkalemia is recognized and resuscitation includes concomitant hemodialysis.[5]

Medications are the most frequent *exogenous* cause of hyperkalemia.

- Potassium supplements prescribed to prevent *hypo*kalemia are the most frequent cause of hyperkalemia in hospitalized patients.

Rapid Response Interventions for the MET (Medical Emergency Team) or RRT (Rapid Response Team)
 	
 Emergency Treatment of Acute Moderate and Severe Hyperkalemia
	Although hyperkalemia is defined as a serum potassium concentration >5 mEq/L, it is moderate (6 to 7 mEq/L) and severe (>7 mEq/L) hyperkalemia that are life-threatening and require immediate therapy.
	
	 • For *mild* elevation (5 to 6 mEq/L), remove potassium from the body with
	   — Diuretics: Furosemide 40 to 80 mg IV
	   — Resins: Kayexalate 15 to 30 g in 50 to 100 mL of 20% sorbitol, either orally or by retention enema
	 • For *moderate* elevation (6 to 7 mEq/L), shift potassium intracellularly with
	   — Glucose plus insulin: Mix 25 g (50 mL of D_{50}) glucose and 10 U regular insulin and give IV over 15 to 30 minutes
	   — Sodium bicarbonate: 50 mEq IV over 5 minutes (sodium bicarbonate alone is less effective than glucose plus insulin or nebulized albuterol, particularly for treatment of patients with renal failure; it is best used in conjunction with these medications)
	   — Nebulized albuterol: 10 to 20 mg nebulized over 15 minutes

- Potassium-sparing diuretics, such as spironolactone, triamterene, and amiloride, are another well-recognized cause of hyperkalemia.
- Use of angiotensin-converting enzyme (ACE) inhibitors (eg, captopril) can also lead to elevation of serum potassium, particularly when combined with oral potassium supplements.
- Nonsteroidal anti-inflammatory agents (eg, ibuprofen) can cause hyperkalemia through direct effects on the kidney.

Diagnosis

The most common symptoms of hyperkalemia are non-specific: *weakness, hypotension, and paresthesias.* As serum potassium rises an *ascending paralysis* may develop.

The physical examination, the 12-lead ECG, and serum potassium concentration provide important (though indirect) information about the significance of the hyperkalemia. These evaluations must be performed promptly for critically ill patients. As the hyperkalemia worsens, the ECG becomes abnormal. Table 4 lists these ECG changes in roughly the sequence in which they occur, and Figure 1 illustrates their appearance. The development of widened QRS complexes heralds significant cardiac dysfunction. If untreated at this point, progressive hyperkalemia leads to sine-wave-like complexes, unstable and symptomatic arrhythmias, and finally asystole and death.

Treatment

The first critical action in treating hyperkalemia is to reduce potassium intake as much as possible:

- Stop any potassium supplementation.
- Identify and discontinue any prescribed or over-the-counter drugs that can cause hyperkalemia. If necessary call the patient's pharmacist to determine which medications may be involved.

Further treatment of hyperkalemia varies by the level of serum potassium and the severity of the patient's clinical status. Therapeutic interventions involve treatments that antagonize or inhibit the action of potassium on cell membranes (calcium), induce a transcellular shift of potassium (insulin/dextrose, albuterol, sodium bicarbonate), and enhance clearance (resins, loop diuretics, hemodialysis).

Table 3. Common Causes of Hyperkalemia

Endogenous Causes
• Chronic renal failure
• Metabolic acidosis (eg, diabetic ketoacidosis)
• Pseudohypoaldosteronism type II (also known as Gordon's syndrome; familial hyperkalemia and hypertension)
• Chemotherapy causing tumor lysis
• Muscle breakdown (rhabdomyolysis)
• Renal tubular acidosis
• Hemolysis
• Hypoaldosteronism (Addison's disease, hyporeninemia)
• Hyperkalemic periodic paralysis

Exogenous Causes
• Medications: K^+-sparing diuretics, ACE inhibitors, nonsteroidal anti-inflammatory drugs, potassium supplements, penicillin derivatives, succinylcholine (in paralyzed patients), β-blockers
• Blood administration (particularly with older "bank" blood)
• Diet (rarely the sole cause), salt substitutes
• Pseudohyperkalemia (due to blood sampling or hemolysis, high white blood cell count, high platelets, tumor lysis syndrome)

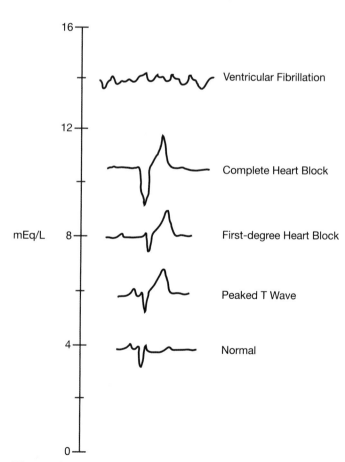

Figure 1. ECG changes associated with progressive hyperkalemia. Adapted with permission from Burch and Winsor.[6]

- **Mild hyperkalemia (5 to 6 mEq/L):** Remove potassium from the body by one or more of the following therapies:
  - Diuretics: Furosemide 1 mg/kg slow IV
  - Resins: Kayexalate 15 to 30 g in 50 to 100 mL of 20% sorbitol, either orally or by retention enema
  - Dialysis: For patients with chronic renal failure receiving peritoneal or hemodialysis
- **Moderate elevation (6 to 7 mEq/L):** Initiate a temporary intracellular shift of potassium using the following agents:
  - Sodium bicarbonate: 50 mEq IV or up to 1 mEq/kg over 5 minutes
  - Glucose/insulin: Mix 10 U regular insulin and 25 g (50 mL of D_{50}) glucose, and give IV over 15 to 30 minutes
  - Nebulized albuterol: 5 to 20 mg over 15 minutes

The Periarrest Hyperkalemic Patient

Hyperkalemic patients in periarrest usually have renal failure. Often they are patients on renal dialysis who have missed one or more treatments. Hyperkalemia can also complicate systemic acidosis, so therapy must also be directed at reversing the cause of the acidosis. Patients with severe potassium elevation (>7 mEq/L), especially those with widened QRS complexes, require urgent care.

- **Severe elevation (>7 mEq/L with potassium-induced ECG changes):**
  - First and most urgent, give 5 to 10 mL of 10% calcium chloride IV over 2 to 5 minutes. Calcium chloride will antagonize the toxic effects of potassium at the myocardial cell membrane, lowering the risk of ventricular fibrillation (VF).
  - Second, initiate a rapid shift of K^+ into cells with sodium bicarbonate, glucose plus insulin, and nebulized albuterol (as for moderate hyperkalemia; see Table 5).

  - Third, begin removal of K^+ from the body with diuretics, resins, or dialysis as described for mild hyperkalemia. Dialysis is the treatment of choice for patients with renal failure.

The clinical case illustrates the critical actions necessary for severe hyperkalemia. Table 5 summarizes the emergency treatments and treatment sequence recommended for hyperkalemia.

Hypokalemia

Normal potassium range: 3.5 to 5 mEq/L

Hypokalemia is defined as a serum potassium level <3.5 mEq/L. The major consequences of severe hypokalemia result from its effects on nerves and muscles (including the heart). The myocardium is extremely sensitive to the effects of hypokalemia, particularly if the patient has coronary artery disease or is taking a digitalis derivative. Symptoms of mild hypokalemia are weakness, fatigue, paralysis, respiratory difficulty, constipation, paralytic ileus, and leg cramps; more severe hypokalemia will alter cardiac tissue excitability and conduction. Hypokalemia can produce ECG changes such as U waves, T-wave flattening, and arrhythmias, especially if the patient is taking digoxin and particularly ventricular arrhythmias. Pulseless electrical activity or asystole may develop.

Causes

The most common causes of low serum potassium are gastrointestinal (GI) loss (diarrhea, laxatives), renal loss (hyperaldosteronism, severe hyperglycemia, potassium-depleting diuretics, carbenicillin, sodium penicillin, amphotericin B), intracellular shift (alkalosis or a rise in pH), and malnutrition. Table 6 lists the most common causes of low serum potassium.

Table 4. Increasing Serum Potassium Levels and Most Frequently Associated ECG Findings

Serum Potassium Range (mEq/L)	Frequent ECG Findings
5.5 to <6	• Peaking (tenting) of T waves (most prominent early ECG change)
6 to <6.5	• Increasing PR and QT intervals
6.5 to <7	• Flattened P waves and ST segments
7 to <7.5	• Widened QRS complexes
7.5 to <8	• Deepening S waves; merging of S and T waves
8 to <10	• Sine-wave-shaped complexes begin; idioventricular complexes and rhythms; VT-like appearance
≥10	• PEA (often with a "sine wave" appearance), VF/VT, asystole

Table 5. Emergency Treatments and Treatment Sequence for Hyperkalemia

Therapy	Dose	Effect Mechanism	Onset of Effect	Duration of Effect
Calcium chloride	• 5 to 10 mL IV 10% solution (500 to 1000 mg)	• Antagonism of toxic effects of hyperkalemia at cell membrane	• 1 to 3 min	• 30 to 60 min
Sodium bicarbonate	• Begin with 1 ampule; give up to 1 mEq/kg Repeat in 15 min • Then give 2 ampules (100 mEq) in 1 L D_5W IV PRN over next 1 to 2 hours	• Redistribution: intracellular shift	• 5 to 10 min	• 1 to 2 h
Insulin plus glucose (use 1 U insulin per 5 g glucose)	• 10 U regular insulin IV plus 1 ampule (50 mL) D_{50} (25 g) • Then give 10 to 20 U regular insulin and 500 mL $D_{10}W$ IV over 1 hr PRN	• Redistribution: intracellular shift	• 30 min	• 4 to 6 h
Nebulized albuterol	• 10 to 20 mg over 15 min • May repeat	• Redistribution: intracellular shift	• 15 min	• 15 to 90 min
Diuresis with furosemide	• 40 to 80 mg IV bolus	• Removal from body	• At start of diuresis	• Until end of diuresis
Cation-exchange resin (Kayexalate)	• 15 to 50 g PO or PR plus sorbitol	• Removal from body	• 1 to 2 h	• 4 to 6 h
Peritoneal or hemodialysis	• Per institutional protocol	• Removal from body	• At start of dialysis	• Until end of dialysis

Clinical Case Example: Hyperkalemia in Patients With End-Stage Renal Failure

A 24-year-old man with type I diabetes mellitus and dialysis-dependent kidney failure presents to the ED. The patient reports severe weakness, shortness of breath, nausea, vomiting, and dizziness. He missed his last two scheduled dialysis sessions while out of town on vacation. On examination the patient looks ill and uncomfortable. Vital signs are as follows: temperature 35.3°C, pulse 108/min, BP 175/110 mm Hg, RR 32/min and labored, and oxyhemoglobin saturation per pulse oximetry is 93% on room air. Auscultation reveals bibasilar rales and an S_3 gallop.

Findings of the initial exam are consistent with volume overload. *Initiate O₂–IV–monitor.*

A 12-lead ECG shows wide-complex sinus tachycardia. STAT laboratory studies (including serum K^+) are pending.

In view of the wide QRS complexes, the situation is critical. *Immediate therapy for hyperkalemia is warranted,* so do not delay treatment while waiting for lab results.

- Administer IV calcium chloride 10% solution (500 to 1000 mg) over 2 to 5 minutes to antagonize the effects of potassium at the cell membrane.
- Next give medications that shift K^+ into the cells.
  In end-stage renal disease, sodium bicarbonate has little effect. Moreover, the Na^+ load associated with use of bicarbonate can worsen existing volume overload.
  — In this case 10 U of regular insulin IV plus 50 mL of D_{50} glucose should shift K^+ intracellularly.
  — Nebulized albuterol (10 to 20 mg over 15 minutes) also shifts K^+ intracellularly through the mechanism of adrenergic stimulation, an effect known for nearly 3 decades. Albuterol inhalation is particularly effective in patients with renal failure. It also helps prevent the hypoglycemia associated with use of glucose/insulin.
- Finally, initiate agents and methods to remove K^+ from the body, such as diuresis with furosemide (though it may not work in end-stage renal disease), Kayexalate, and urgent dialysis.

Table 6. Common Causes of Hypokalemia

Decreased Intake
• Poor dietary intake
• Malnutrition

Gastrointestinal and Sweat Losses
• Vomiting (including eating disorders)
• Nasogastric suction
• Diarrhea (including laxative or enema abuse)
• Malabsorption syndromes
• Enteric fistula
• Ureterosigmoidostomy
• Loss through sweating (heavy exercise, heatstroke, febrile illnesses)

Increased Renal Losses
• Diuretic use
• Renal tubular acidosis
• Primary aldosteronism
• Secondary aldosteronism (renal artery stenosis, CHF, cirrhosis plus ascites, excess of ACTH or glucocorticosteroids)
• Licorice ingestion
• Chewing tobacco
• Rare causes of renal loss:
— Bartter's syndrome: Disorder of renal tubules causing high aldosterone, low potassium, and metabolic alkalosis
— Liddle's syndrome: Autosomal dominant condition of renal tubules causing increased potassium secretion

Medications
• Aminoglycosides
• Penicillins (eg, Carbenicillin)
• Cisplatin, amphotericin B
• L-Dopa
• Lithium
• Thallium
• Theophylline

Redistribution: Extracellular to Intracellular Potassium Shifts
• Redistribution with pH changes:
— Acidosis (or fall in pH) raises serum K^+
— Alkalosis (or rise in pH) lowers serum K^+
• Treatment of diabetic ketoacidosis
• Insulin administration
• Hypomagnesemia
• β_2-Adrenergic agents (eg, albuterol)
• Hypokalemic periodic paralysis (congenital disorder causing intermittent episodes of muscle weakness due to low serum potassium)

Diagnosis

In one survey severe hypokalemia (potassium <3.0 mEq/L) was present in 2.6% of hospitalized patients and was associated with a 21% mortality rate.[7] Hypokalemia in patients hospitalized with acute myocardial infarction is an independent risk factor for VF.[8] Hypokalemia may exist for several reasons. Patients with cardiovascular disease may be taking potassium-wasting diuretics. In addition, stress hormones such as catecholamines can cause a transcellular shift of potassium into cells, causing or aggravating hypokalemia. Patients with cardiac ischemia, heart failure, or ventricular hypertrophy have an increased risk of cardiac arrhythmias even with mild to moderate hypokalemia.[9]

Signs and symptoms of hypokalemia correlate with both the level of serum potassium and the speed of the fall in serum potassium[10]:

- **Mild (3 to 3.5 mEq/L):** Often no symptoms
- **Moderate (2.5 to <3.0 mEq/L):** Generalized weakness, fatigue, lassitude, constipation, leg cramps
- **Severe (2.0 to <2.5 mEq/L):** Muscle breakdown (rhabdomyolysis), paralytic ileus, bowel obstruction
- **Life-threatening (<2.0 mEq/L):** Development of ascending paralysis, impairment of respiratory function, unstable cardiac arrhythmias

Hypokalemia is suggested by changes in the ECG (see Table 7).

Treatment

The treatment of hypokalemia consists of minimizing further potassium loss and providing potassium replacement. Intravenous (IV) administration of potassium is indicated when arrhythmias are present or hypokalemia is severe (potassium level of <2.5 mEq/L). Gradual correction of hypokalemia is preferable to rapid correction unless the patient is clinically unstable.

Table 7. Decreasing Potassium Levels and Most Frequently Associated ECG Findings

Serum Potassium Range (mEq/L)	Frequent ECG Findings
2.5 to 3	• U waves begin, flattened T waves, low QRS voltage, prominent P waves
2 to <2.5	• More prominent U waves, more ST-segment changes
<2	• Widened QRS complexes, arrhythmias, PEA, asystole

The Periarrest Hypokalemic Patient

To treat malignant ventricular arrhythmias in patients with severe hypokalemia:

- Give an initial infusion of KCl, 2 mEq/min IV over 10 minutes (20 mEq total).
- Follow with 1 mEq/min over the next 10 minutes (10 mEq total).
- Document in the chart that the rapid infusion is intentional to treat life-threatening hypokalemia.
- As the patient improves and stabilizes, reduce the KCl infusion rate.

Mild and Moderate Hypokalemia

Whereas critical hypokalemia is treated empirically, calculated potassium replacement for mild and moderate hypokalemia should be based on an estimate of the total body potassium deficit:

- As a rule of thumb, for every 1 mEq/L decrease in serum potassium, the total body deficit is 150 to 400 mEq.
- Total body potassium and estimated deficit is based on age, sex, and body size. For example, the 150 mEq estimated deficit is appropriate for an elderly woman with low muscle mass. But for a young, muscular man, an estimated deficit of 400 mEq for every 1 mEq/L decrease in serum K^+ is more appropriate.
- Because changes in pH affect serum potassium, another rule of thumb has evolved: serum K^+ decreases by about 0.3 mEq/L for every 0.1 unit increase in pH above normal. Consequently a patient with alkalosis (pH >7.45) will have a lower serum potassium than expected on the basis of total body potassium.

The astute clinician will decrease the amount of replacement potassium for an alkalotic patient with hypokalemia if the alkalosis is also corrected.

- Base decisions about route (oral vs IV) and speed (fast vs slow) of potassium replacement on the clinical condition of the patient. In general, oral potassium replacement is preferable. Rapid correction is appropriate only for clinically unstable patients.
- Stable patients: Limit the potassium replacement dose to approximately 10 to 20 mEq/h.
  - Maximum concentration: Approximately 40 mEq in 1 L of normal saline. Peripheral IV sites are preferable. Use a central line for concentrations greater than 20 mEq/L.
  - Maximum rate: Approximately 40 mEq in 1 hour. A 40 mEq infusion will acutely raise the serum potassium concentration by approximately 0.5 mEq/L.
  - Monitor the ECG continuously during IV potassium infusion. If potassium is infused through a central line, the tip of the catheter should not be in the right atrium. Potassium infusion into the coronary sinus is thought to contribute to life-threatening arrhythmias.

Sodium

Sodium is the major intravascular ion that influences serum osmolality. An acute increase in serum sodium will produce an acute increase in serum osmolality; an acute decrease in serum sodium will produce an acute fall in serum osmolality. Sodium concentration and osmolality in the intravascular and interstitial spaces equilibrate across the vascular membrane.

Rapid Response Interventions for the MET (Medical Emergency Team) or RRT (Rapid Response Team)	Administration of potassium may be empirical and emergent in potentially life-threatening conditions. Intravenous potassium replacement can cause life-threatening hyperkalemia, so this route of replacement is usually reserved for the following situations:
Emergency Treatment of Severe Hypokalemia	<ul><li>The patient cannot tolerate oral K^+</li><li>Severe, life-threatening hypokalemia (K^+ <2.5 mEq/L)</li><li>Imminent cardiac arrest or extenuating emergency conditions (eg, digitalis intoxication with recurrent life-threatening arrhythmias)</li></ul>The maximum amount of IV potassium replacement should not exceed 10 to 20 mEq/h. *Continuous* ECG monitoring during infusion is required.<ul><li>If cardiac arrest from hypokalemia is imminent (ie, malignant ventricular arrhythmias are present), rapid replacement of potassium is required. Give an initial infusion of 10 mEq IV over 5 minutes; repeat once if needed. A more concentrated solution of potassium may be infused if a central line is used, but the tip of the catheter used for the infusion should not extend into the right atrium.</li><li>Document in the patient's chart that rapid infusion is intentional in response to life-threatening hypokalemia.</li></ul>

FYI

ECG Changes in Hypokalemia

For more information see Weaver and Burchell's classic article on ECG changes in

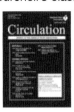

Weaver WF, Burchell HB. Serum Potassium and the Electrocardiogram in Hypokalemia. *Circulation*, April 1960, volume 21.

Acute changes in serum sodium will produce free water shifts into and out of the vascular space until osmolality equilibrates in these compartments. An acute fall in serum sodium will produce an acute shift of free water from the vascular into the interstitial space and may cause cerebral edema.[11-13] An acute rise in serum sodium will produce an acute shift of free water from the interstitial to the vascular space. Rapid correction of hyponatremia has been associated with development of rhabdomyolysis,[14,15] pontine myelinolysis,[16,17] and cerebral bleeding.[14,16,17] For these reasons monitor neurologic function closely in the patient with hypernatremia or hyponatremia, particularly during correction of these conditions. Whenever possible, correct serum sodium slowly, carefully controlling the total change in serum sodium over 48 hours and avoiding overcorrection.[18,19]

Under normal conditions the serum sodium concentration and serum osmolality are controlled through the *renin-angiotensin-aldosterone system* and with the *antidiuretic hormone* (ADH, also known as arginine vasopressin or AVP). Sodium, the most abundant positive ion in the extracellular space, determines the size of the extracellular fluid (ECF) volume. Abnormalities in sodium concentration generally reflect abnormalities of total body water.

Sodium is an extracellular ion. It is present in relatively small concentrations intracellularly and relatively large concentrations extracellularly (in the interstitial space). When the body's total sodium content increases, ECF will increase, resulting in volume overload. Sodium retention and ECF volume overload occur frequently with congestive heart failure (CHF), congestive cirrhosis of the liver, and the nephrotic syndrome. When the total sodium content decreases, ECF volume also decreases (volume depletion). This causes signs of poor skin turgor, tachycardia, and orthostatic hypotension.

Remember these general rules:

1. High serum sodium concentration generally indicates free water depletion; low serum sodium concentration indicates free water overload.

2. Abnormally high or low serum sodium concentration usually indicates volume-related problems.

3. Clinical problems related to inappropriate intravascular volume (eg, CHF, edema, orthostatic syncope) often reflect problems in sodium concentration.

Hypernatremia

Normal sodium range: 135 to 145 mEq/L

Hypernatremia is defined as a serum sodium concentration >145 to 150 mEq/L. It may be caused by a primary gain in Na^+ or excess loss of water. Hypernatremia may cause neurologic symptoms such as altered mental status, weakness, irritability, focal neurologic deficits, and even coma or seizures. The severity of symptoms is determined by the speed and magnitude of the change in serum sodium concentration.

Causes

Gains in sodium can result from hyperaldosteronism (excess mineralocorticoid), Cushing's syndrome (excess glucocorticoid), or excessive hypertonic saline or sodium bicarbonate administration. Loss of free water can result from GI losses or renal excretion (eg, osmotic diuresis or diabetes insipidus).

Hypernatremia is generally caused by 1 of 3 mechanisms:

1. Insufficient water intake, resulting most often in *normovolemic hypernatremia*

2. Loss of water and sodium (but water loss in excess of sodium loss), resulting most often in *hypovolemic hypernatremia*

3. Gain of water and sodium (but sodium gain exceeds water gain), resulting most often in *hypervolemic hypernatremia*

The most frequent clinical scenario is loss of both water and sodium, but more water relative to sodium (hypovolemic hypernatremia). Most hypernatremic patients in periarrest are hypovolemic. Somewhat counterintuitive, patients with hypernatremia usually have an absolute reduction in total body sodium. As serum sodium is lowered to a safe level, these patients will require administration of normal saline to replenish total body stores. Table 8 lists the most common causes of hypernatremia according to these 3 mechanisms. This method of classification helps identify the cause of the hypernatremia and provides guidance for therapy.

Diagnosis

Hypernatremia causes water to shift from the interstitial space into the vascular space. Significant hypernatremia can cause a shift of free water from the cellular space, causing intracellular dehydration. The severity of symptoms depends on the acuteness and severity of the rise in serum sodium. If the sodium concentration rises quickly or substantially, the signs and symptoms will be more severe.

Table 8. Common Causes of Hypernatremia

Reduced Intake of Free Water: Normovolemic or Hypovolemic Hypernatremia
• Mild free water loss, such as increased insensible water losses • Conditions that lead to inability to obtain free water: — Infancy — Coma, dementia — Bed confinement, intubation — Injuries — Environmental emergencies (wilderness travel, castaways)
Significant Loss of Free Water (With Moderate Loss of Sodium): Hypovolemic Hypernatremia
• Gastrointestinal losses: vomiting, diarrhea, nasogastric suctioning, fistulas • Renal losses: — Osmotic diuresis such as mannitol administration — Diabetes insipidus with loss of concentrating ability: central (no vasopressin from pituitary gland) or nephrogenic (no renal response to vasopressin) — Postobstructive state • Dermal losses: sweating, burns
Significant Gain of Sodium (With Moderate Gain of Free Water): Hypervolemic Hypernatremia
• Excessive sodium bicarbonate administration • Hypertonic saline administration, salt tablets, errors in formula preparation • Seawater ingestion • Excess mineralocorticoid (primary aldosteronism) • Excess glucocorticoid (Cushing's disease, exogenous, ectopic ACTH syndromes)

- **Neurologic symptoms:** An acute free water shift from the interstitial to the vascular space can cause nausea and vomiting, lack of appetite, irritability, and fatigue.
- **Neurologic signs:** Physical signs include confusion, stupor, and coma; seizures; altered mental status; muscle weakness, twitching, or spasticity; tremor or ataxia; or focal neurologic signs such as paresis or abnormal plantar reflexes.

Patients with hypernatremia caused by decreased water intake or excessive water loss in relation to sodium loss (hypovolemic hypernatremia) will have signs and symptoms of dehydration and hypovolemia. These patients will usually report excessive thirst, fatigue, and orthostatic symptoms such as dizziness and lightheadedness.

Treatment

Treatment of hypernatremia includes reduction of ongoing water losses (by treating the underlying cause) and correction of the water deficit. For stable, asymptomatic patients, replacement of fluid by mouth or through a nasogastric tube is effective and safe. In hypovolemic patients the ECF volume is typically restored with normal saline or a 5% dextrose in half-normal saline solution to prevent a rapid fall in the serum sodium concentration. Avoid D_5W; it will reduce serum sodium too rapidly. During rehydration monitor serum sodium closely to ensure a gradual fall (and prevent a rapid fall) in serum sodium.

It is important to remember that sodium abnormalities indicate primarily water problems. The major therapeutic approach is *not* to remove excess sodium but to replace the lost water.

- Most hypernatremic patients are hypovolemic. They have a deficit of free water and sodium, but the free water deficit is more significant than the sodium deficit. Treatment requires careful replacement of both volume and sodium while avoiding a rapid fall in serum sodium and osmolality.
- Too rapid a correction in serum sodium will cause dangerous fluid shifts and risk of cerebral edema or other physiologic derangements.

Calculation of water deficit: Correct the water deficit (usually with normal saline) and stop ongoing water losses by treating the underlying cause. The key step is to calculate the quantity of water needed to correct the water deficit:

Water deficit (in liters)

$$= \frac{\text{plasma Na}^+ \text{ concentration} - 140}{140} \times \text{total body water}$$

Total body water is approximately 50% of lean body weight in men and 40% of lean body weight in women, so to determine total body water, multiply body weight by 0.5 for men or 0.4 for women. For example, if a 70-kg man has a serum Na^+ level of 160 mEq/L, the estimated free water deficit would be

$$\frac{160 - 140}{140} \times (0.5 \times 70) = 5 \text{ L}$$

Rate of replacement: Once the free water deficit is calculated, administer fluid to lower serum sodium at a rate of 0.5 to 1 mEq/h with a decrease of no more than approximately 12 mEq/L in the first 24 hours and the remainder over the next 48 to 72 hours.

Route of replacement: Select the route of replacement of free water based on the patient's clinical status:

- **Stable, asymptomatic:** Give fluids by mouth or through a nasogastric tube.
- **Symptomatic but not significantly hypovolemic:** Typically use 0.45% sodium chloride (half-normal saline) IV.
- **Symptomatic, significantly hypovolemic:** Use 0.9% sodium chloride (normal saline) IV to correct the hypovolemia; then correct the free water deficit with 0.45% sodium chloride (half-normal saline).

Hyponatremia

Normal sodium range: 135 to 145 mEq/L
Hyponatremia is defined as a serum sodium concentration <130 to 135 mEq/L. It represents an excess of water relative to sodium.[20]

Causes

Most cases of hyponatremia are caused by reduced renal excretion of water with continued water intake or by loss of sodium in the urine.[13] Several conditions can impair renal water excretion, including use of thiazide diuretics, renal failure, ECF depletion (eg, vomiting with continued water intake), the syndrome of inappropriate antidiuretic hormone (SIADH), edematous states (eg, CHF, cirrhosis with ascites), hypothyroidism, and adrenal insufficiency. Table 9 presents the most common causes of hyponatremia, grouped in relation to loss or gain of sodium and volume. The most

frequent cause of potentially life-threatening hyponatremia is SIADH.[21]

Most cases of hyponatremia also are associated with low serum osmolality (so-called hypo-osmolar hyponatremia). The one common exception to this is in uncontrolled diabetes, in which hyperglycemia leads to a hyperosmolar state despite a serum sodium concentration that is below normal (hyperosmolar hyponatremia).

Table 9. Common Causes of Hyponatremia

Increased Retention of Free Water (Inadequate Free Water Excretion): Normovolemic Hyponatremia
• Syndrome of inappropriate antidiuretic hormone secretion (SIADH) • Hypoadrenalism (ie, adrenal insufficiency) • Hypothyroidism • Renal failure • Polydipsia (psychogenic
Significant Retention of Free Water (With Moderate Retention of Sodium): Hypervolemic Hyponatremia
• Edematous states: — Congestive heart failure — Hepatic cirrhosis — Nephrotic syndrome (renal failure)
Significant Loss of Sodium (With Moderate Loss of Free Water): Hypovolemic Hyponatremia
• Gastrointestinal losses: vomiting, diarrhea, nasogastric suctioning, fistulas • Renal losses • Third space losses • Excessive sweating • Addison's disease
Miscellaneous Causes
• Sampling error • Pseudohyponatremia: hyperlipemia, hyperproteinemia • Redistributive hyponatremia: hyperglycemia, mannitol

Rapid Response Interventions for Periarrest Hypernatremia	Periarrest hypernatremic patients will be severely hypovolemic and markedly dehydrated with shock. The key for these patients is rapid volume replacement with normal saline: • Give normal saline 500 mL wide open as a *medical bolus* and evaluate clinical response. Repeat every 20 to 30 minutes until the patient is hemodynamically stable. • Alternatively, give 10 to 20 mL/kg over 20 minutes (700 to 1400 mL for a 70-kg person) and evaluate hemodynamic response. Calculate and correct the free water deficit as outlined in the text when the patient is hemodynamically stable.

Syndrome of Inappropriate Antidiuretic Hormone

SIADH can occur in a wide variety of clinical situations common to ACLS patients (see Table 10). SIADH is caused by the nonphysiologic release of vasopressin (antidiuretic hormone, also known as arginine vasopressin [AVP]) from either the posterior pituitary or an ectopic source, such as a malignant tumor. ADH stimulates renal retention of normovolemic free water with continued excretion of sodium. This results in multiple abnormalities: normovolemia combined with low sodium and low osmolality in serum but with high sodium and high osmolality (>100 mOsm/kg) in urine. The hallmark finding of SIADH is a highly concentrated urine with a urine osmolality that is higher than the serum osmolality. This hallmark finding confirms SIADH as the cause of the hyponatremia. Hyponatremia caused by nonrenal sodium losses would be associated with a low urine osmolality (renal sodium retention and thus minimal excretion of sodium in the urine).

Untreated SIADH can be fatal or can result in significant neurologic complications. SIADH should be ruled out when significant hyponatremia develops. The acronym "CONDM" can be used to recall the major causes of SIADH:

C: Central nervous system disease or injury
O: Other (pain, post-op, hypothyroidism)
N: Nonmalignant pulmonary disease (chronic obstructive pulmonary disease, pneumonia)
D: Drugs
M: Malignancy

Diagnosis

Hyponatremia is usually asymptomatic unless it is acute or severe (<120 mEq/L). An abrupt fall in serum sodium produces a free water shift from the vascular to the interstitial space that can cause cerebral edema. In this case the patient may present with nausea, vomiting, headache, irritability, lethargy, seizures, coma, or even death.

Treatment

Treatment of hyponatremia involves administration of sodium and elimination of intravascular free water. If SIADH is present, the treatment is restriction of fluid intake to 50% to 66% of estimated maintenance fluid requirement. Correction of asymptomatic hyponatremia should be gradual: typically increase Na$^+$ by 0.5 mEq/L per hour to a maximum change of about 12 mEq/L in the first 24 hours. Rapid correction of hyponatremia can cause coma, which may be associated with osmotic demyelination syndrome or central pontine myelinolysis, lethal disorders thought to be caused by rapid fluid shifts into and out of brain tissue.

To calculate the amount of sodium to administer per hour for *asymptomatic* hyponatremia, multiply 0.5 mEq/L by the appropriate weight coefficient (0.6 for men, 0.5 for women) and then by body weight (kg).

If the patient develops neurologic compromise, administer 3% saline IV immediately to raise the serum sodium concentration at a rate of 1 mEq/L per hour until neurologic symptoms are controlled (to a maximum of 4 mEq/L over 4 hours). Some experts recommend a faster rate of correction (ie, 2 to 4 mEq/L per hour) when seizures are present. Once neurologic symptoms are controlled, provide 3% saline IV to raise serum sodium at a rate of 0.5 mg/L per hour.

To calculate the amount of 3% saline to administer to patients with neurologic symptoms, use the following formula:

$$\text{Total Na}^+ \text{ dose} = 4 \text{ mEq/L} \times \text{Weight coefficient}^* \times \text{Body weight (kg)}$$

*Use 0.6 for men and 0.5 for women.

After you calculate the total sodium dose, determine the volume of 3% saline (513 mEq/L Na$^+$) needed to reach this dose (divide total dose by 513 mEq/L). Then administer the 3% saline at the appropriate rate (divide the volume of 3% saline by the number of hours over which you wish to administer a total of 4 mEq/L, generally 4). Check serum sodium frequently and monitor neurologic status. Switch to the lower rate (0.5 mEq/L) once neurologic symptoms are controlled.

A stepwise approach taking into account the volume status of the patient can be helpful in determining the rapidity and degree of sodium replacement.

1. **Assess intravascular volume.** Determine if the patient is hypervolemic (edematous states), hypovolemic, or normovolemic.
   — Signs of hypervolemia with volume overload: CHF, peripheral edema, elevated jugular veins, rales, weight gain, S$_3$ heart sound.
   — Signs of hypovolemia with volume depletion: Tachycardia, resting and orthostatic hypotension, dry mucous membranes, poor peripheral perfusion, poor skin turgor.

2. **Plan treatment based on the severity of symptoms and volume status.**
   — Volume depletion: Replace volume with normal saline.
   — Volume overload: Restrict water and initiate diuresis with furosemide. *Note:* Some researchers have reported superior outcomes with IV normal saline or 3% saline administration instead of fluid restriction.
   — Normal or near-normal ECF volume (eg, with SIADH, hypothyroidism, adrenal insufficiency): Restrict fluid intake to one half to one third

Table 10. Common Causes of the Syndrome of Inappropriate Antidiuretic Hormone Secretion (SIADH)

CNS Disease or Injury
• Stroke
• Brain injury, infarction, tumor, abscess
• Meningitis
• Encephalitis

Other
• Pain
• Postoperative complications
• Hypothyroidism

Nonmalignant Pulmonary Disease
• Acute respiratory distress syndrome
• Pneumonia
• Lung cancer
• Tuberculosis
• Lung abscess
• Cystic fibrosis
• Asthma

Drugs
• Vasopressin (exogenous)
• Diuretics
• Chlorpropamide
• Vincristine
• Cyclophosphamide
• Thioridazine

Malignancies
• Pancreatic cancer
• Duodenal cancer
• Oat cell carcinoma
• Lymphoma
• Hodgkin's disease

maintenance fluid requirements and treat underlying cause.

— Asymptomatic: Aim for gradual restoration of serum sodium, limiting the increase in Na^+ to no more than 0.5 mEq/L per hour (maximum increase of 12 mEq/L in the first 24 hours).

— *Note:* Rapid increases in Na^+ can lead to a higher plasma osmolality that can dehydrate and injure the brain. This life-threatening condition, called *osmotic demyelination syndrome* or *central pontine myelinolysis,* is caused by rapid fluid shifts in the brain.

The Periarrest Hyponatremic Patient

Hyponatremic patients will often present with alarming neurologic symptoms, such as seizures or coma, with increased intracranial pressure that can lead to cardiac arrest. Rapid deterioration is more likely with rapid development of hyponatremia.

Calcium (Ca⁺⁺)

Calcium is the most abundant mineral in the body. Many processes depend on intracellular calcium, such as enzymatic reactions, receptor activation, muscle contraction, cardiac contractility, and platelet aggregation. Calcium is essential for bone strength and neuromuscular function. Half of all calcium in the ECF is bound to albumin; the other half is in the biologically active, ionized form. Calcium concentration is normally regulated by parathyroid hormone (PTH) and vitamin D.

Total serum calcium is directly related to the serum albumin concentration. The total serum calcium will increase 0.8 mg/dL for every 1 g/dL rise in serum albumin and will fall 0.8 mg/dL for every 1 g/dL fall in serum albumin.

Although total serum albumin is directly related to total serum calcium, ionized calcium is *inversely* related to serum albumin. The lower the serum albumin, the higher the

Rapid Response Interventions for Life-Threatening Hyponatremia	If neurologic compromise is present, administer 3% saline IV immediately to correct (raise) the serum sodium concentration at a rate of 1 mEq/L per hour until neurologic symptoms are controlled. • After neurologic symptoms are controlled, correct the serum sodium concentration at a rate of 0.5 mEq/L per hour. • Gradual correction is particularly important for treatment of chronic hyponatremia.

Use 3% Saline With Great Caution

Overly aggressive treatment with hypertonic saline can be lethal. Do not use hypertonic saline to *normalize* Na^+; use it only to raise the serum sodium concentration sufficiently to control neurologic symptoms.

Recommended Steps for Using 3% Saline

1. Calculate the amount of 3% saline to administer to increase the sodium concentration to the desired level (generally 1 mEq/L per hour over 4 hours,* for a total increase of 4 mEq/L):

   Total Na^+ dose = 4 mEq/L × Weight coefficient* × Body weight (kg)

   *Use 0.6 for men, 0.5 for women.

2. Calculate the volume of 3% saline (513 mEq Na^+/L) needed to reach this total dose:
   Volume of 3% saline = Total Na^+ dose ÷ 513 mEq/L Na^+

3. Administer the required volume of 3% saline at the appropriate rate (generally 1 mEq/L per hour over 4 hours*):
   Administration rate = Volume of 3% saline ÷ Number of hours
   *Some experts recommend more aggressive correction if the patient is obtunded or comatose (2 mEq/L per hour) or demonstrating seizures (2 to 4 mEq/L per hour). This would require administration of the amount of 3% saline calculated above over 1 to 2 hours instead of over 4 hours.

Clinical Case: Using 3% Saline for Treatment of Life-Threatening Hyponatremia

A 78-year-old woman weighing 70 kg presents with seizures and a serum sodium concentration of 108 mEq/L. To control these neurologic symptoms it will be necessary to give 3% saline. Aim to raise the sodium concentration at a rate of 1 mEq/L per hour for the next 4 hours, for a total of 4 mEq/L.

1. *Calculate the amount of 3% saline to administer to increase the sodium concentration to the desired level:*
   Total Na^+ dose = 4 mEq/L × Weight coefficient* × Body weight (kg)
   $\qquad$ = 4 × 0.5 × 70
   $\qquad$ = 140 mEq
   *Use 0.6 for men, 0.5 for women.

2. Calculate the volume of 3% saline (513 mEq Na^+/L) needed to reach this total dose:
   Volume of 3% saline = 140 mEq ÷ 513 mEq per L of 3% saline
   $\qquad$ = 0.27 L (270 mL) of 3% saline

- *Step 3: Administer 3% saline at the appropriate rate (in this example, increase sodium by 1 mEq/L per hour, or 4 mEq/L over 4 hours*):*
   Administration rate = 270 ÷ 4
   $\qquad$ = 67 mL/h

Monitor neurologic status closely. Check serum Na^+ frequently.

*Some experts recommend administering 3% saline to correct hyponatremia at a rate of **2 to 4 mEq/L per hour** when a patient has ongoing seizures. In the calculations above, you determined the amount of 3% saline to raise the serum sodium 1 mEq/L per hour over 4 hours. If you administer this volume (270 mL) in 1 to 2 hours, it should correct the sodium at a rate of 2 to 4 mEq/L per hour. Begin at the rate of 270 mL/h until seizures stop; then decrease the rate to 67 to 135 mL/h (to raise the sodium at a rate of 1 to 2 mEq/L per hour).

portion of the total calcium that is present in ionized form. In the presence of hypoalbuminemia the total calcium level may be low, but the ionized calcium level may be normal. If the patient is unstable or if symptoms of hypocalcemia are present, request a specific measurement of ionized calcium. Often the widely used "metabolic panels" that present findings of multiple laboratory tests report total serum calcium but not ionized calcium. But the more comprehensive panels include both.

To calculate the true total calcium adjusted for the hypoalbuminemia, use the following formula:

$$\text{True calcium}_{total} = \text{Measured calcium}_{total} + [(0.8) \times (\text{Protein}_{normal} - \text{Protein}_{measured})]$$

Calcium is primarily an extracellular ion. Calcium and sodium are actively pumped out of cells. Because calcium antagonizes the effects of both potassium and magnesium at the cell membrane, it is the agent of choice for treating both severe hyperkalemia and hypermagnesemia. Because of the critical role of calcium, the serum calcium concentration is controlled within a narrow range. This control is chiefly exerted by secretion of PTH from the parathyroid gland in response to low ionized calcium levels. PTH has direct effects on gastrointestinal

(GI) and renal calcium resorption, on the activity of calcitonin on bone osteoclasts, and on the level of the active vitamin D metabolite, calciferol. Figure 2 depicts the body's typical response to a low level of ionized serum calcium. The opposite response occurs with elevated calcium.

Hypercalcemia

Normal total calcium range: 8.5 to 10.5 mg/dL
Normal ionized calcium range: 4.2 to 4.8 mg/dL
Hypercalcemia is defined as a total serum calcium concentration >10.5 mEq/L (or an ionized calcium concentration >4.8 mg/dL). In most forms of hypercalcemia, release of calcium from the bones and intestines is increased, and renal clearance may be compromised.

Gastrointestinal symptoms of hypercalcemia include dysphagia, constipation, peptic ulcer, and pancreatitis. Effects on the kidney include diminished ability to concentrate urine; diuresis, leading to loss of sodium, potassium, magnesium, and phosphate; and a vicious cycle of calcium reabsorption that worsens hypercalcemia.

Foundation Facts **Calcium in ACLS**	Calcium antagonizes the effects of both potassium and magnesium at the cell membrane. For this reason it is extremely useful for treating the effects of hyperkalemia and hypermagnesemia. Indications include <ul><li>Known or suspected hyperkalemia</li><li>Ionized hypocalcemia (eg, multiple blood transfusions)</li><li>Antidote for toxic effects of calcium channel blocker overdose</li></ul>

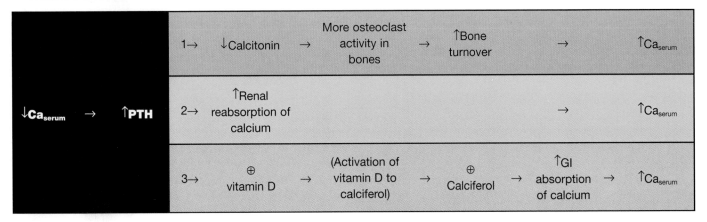

Figure 2. Regulation of serum calcium concentration. This figure illustrates the body's response to an abnormally low level of calcium. Low ionized serum calcium results in increased release of PTH, which has 3 major effects: (1) PTH decreases calcitonin. Because calcitonin inhibits the activity of bone osteoclasts, a decrease in calcitonin allows more bone turnover, resulting in an increase in serum calcium; (2) PTH increases calcium resorption in the kidneys, resulting in a rapid rise in serum calcium; (3) PTH activates vitamin D to the more active metabolite, calciferol, which causes increased GI absorption of calcium. PTH also has a direct effect on calcium absorption in the GI tract.

Causes

The overall incidence of hypercalcemia in the general population is 0.3% to 6%, making it much more common than hypocalcemia. More than 90% of reported cases of hypercalcemia are caused by malignancy or hyperparathyroidism.[22] Some malignancies secrete a PTH-like substance, causing increased calcium release from the bone. Primary hyperparathyroidism causes increased gut resorption of calcium. In the presence of decreased renal clearance, many conditions associated with increased calcium release from the bone or increased calcium absorption from the gut produce hypercalcemia. Table 11 presents the common causes of hypercalcemia.

Table 11. Common Causes of Hypercalcemia

Primary Hyperparathyroidism and Malignancy (>90% of Cases)
• Cancers causing osteolytic bone metastases: Lung, breast, kidney, myeloma, leukemia • Paraneoplastic tumors: Parathyroid hormone–related proteins, bone-resorbing substances, ectopic production of calciferol
Pulmonary and Granulomatous Diseases
• Berylliosis • Adult respiratory distress syndrome • Histoplasmosis • Coccidioidomycosis • Tuberculosis • Sarcoidosis
Drugs
• Lithium • Thiazide diuretics • Hormonal therapy for breast cancer (estrogens) • Hypervitaminosis A and D • Calcium ingestion
Endocrine Disorders (Nonparathyroid)
• Hyperthyroidism • Adrenal insufficiency • Pheochromocytoma • Acromegaly • Vasoactive polypeptide-producing tumors (intestinal)
Miscellaneous Causes
• Immobilization • Paget's disease of bone • Milk-alkali syndrome • Acute renal failure, recovery phase

Diagnosis

A total calcium ≥10.5 mg/dL or ionized calcium >4.8 mg/dL defines hypercalcemia. Symptoms of hypercalcemia usually develop when the total serum calcium concentration is ≥12 to 15 mg/dL. At these levels depression, weakness, fatigue, and confusion may occur. At higher levels (>15 to 20 mg/dL) patients may experience hallucinations, disorientation, hypotonicity, seizures, and coma. Hypercalcemia interferes with renal concentration of urine; the diuresis can cause dehydration. A classic *memory aid* for frequent signs and symptoms of hypercalcemia is: *Stones, bones, moans and groans, and psychologic overtones:*

- Stones: Renal lithiasis
- Bones: Osteolysis releasing calcium (metastatic disease)
- Moans and groans: Abdominal pain in general, plus pancreatitis, peptic ulcers
- Psychologic overtones: Apathy, depression, stupor and coma, irritability, hallucinations

Cardiovascular symptoms of hypercalcemia are variable. Myocardial contractility may initially increase until the calcium level reaches >15 mg/dL. Above this level myocardial depression occurs. Automaticity is decreased and ventricular systole is shortened. Arrhythmias occur because the refractory period is shortened. Hypercalcemia can worsen digitalis toxicity and may cause hypertension. In addition, many patients with hypercalcemia develop hypokalemia. Both of these conditions contribute to cardiac arrhythmias.[23] The QT interval typically shortens when the serum calcium is >13 mg/dL, and the PR and QRS intervals are prolonged. AV block may develop and progress to complete heart block and even cardiac arrest when the total serum calcium is >15 to 20 mg/dL.

Treatment

Treatment for hypercalcemia is required if the patient is symptomatic (typically a total serum concentration of approximately 12 mg/dL or greater) or if the calcium level is >15 mg/dL. Immediate therapy is directed at restoring intravascular volume and promoting calcium excretion in the urine. In patients with adequate cardiovascular and renal function, this is accomplished with infusion of 0.9% saline at 300 to 500 mL/h (saline diuresis) until any fluid deficit is replaced and diuresis occurs (urine output ≥200 to 300 mL/h). Once adequate rehydration has occurred, the saline infusion rate is reduced to 100 to 200 mL/h. During this therapy monitor and maintain potassium and magnesium concentrations closely because the diuresis can reduce potassium and magnesium concentrations.

If the hypercalcemia is due to malignancy, carefully consider the patient's prognosis and wishes before starting treatment. A patient dying of cancer may need no treatment. In all other cases aggressive treatment is needed.

A stepwise approach to hypercalcemia based on serum level and symptoms is useful when treating these patients:

- **Total calcium concentration = 12 to <15 mg/dL:** Begin the treatment outlined below for symptomatic patients.
- **Total calcium concentration = 15 mg/dL:** Begin treatment whether the patient is symptomatic or not. There are 4 components to hypercalcemia therapy. ACLS providers will seldom be responsible for more than the first two: volume restoration and starting calcium elimination through the kidneys.

Treatment Sequence

1. **Restore volume:**

   — Establish vascular access with a large-bore IV.
   — Infuse normal saline (0.9% sodium chloride) at 300 to 500 mL/h until fluid deficits are replaced. Volume replacement promotes increased excretion of calcium by the kidneys.
   — Decrease infusion rate to 100 to 200 mL/h once you establish adequate rehydration.

2. **Increase renal calcium elimination:**

   — The saline diuresis induced by volume restoration will usually decrease the serum calcium concentration by 1.5 to 2.5 mg/dL.

   — Consider furosemide 1 mg/kg, especially for patients in heart failure. But do *not* administer loop diuretics until you have restored intravascular volume. *Note:* Use of furosemide in hypercalcemia is controversial because it can foster reuptake of calcium ions, worsening the hypercalcemia.
   — Some experts recommend empirically adding magnesium (15 mg/h) and potassium (up to 10 mEq/h) during volume restoration because they are excreted during saline diuresis.

3. **Reduce calcium release from bones** by administering drugs that inhibit osteoclast activity. These drugs do not work immediately (onset of action and peak effect may take several hours).

   — Calcitonin inhibits osteoclast activity and promotes calcium deposition in bone, but it produces only modest reductions in serum calcium concentration.
   — Pamidronate (Aredia) and etidronate (Didronel) are 2 currently approved inhibitors of osteoclastic activity.
   — Glucocorticoids, indomethacin, gallium nitrate, and oral phosphates are other options.

4. **Treat the primary disorder** causing the hypercalcemia. For example, discontinue any causative medications; perform parathyroidectomy for hyperparathyroidism due to excess PTH or with vitamin D deficiency and provide specific treatment for paraneoplastic syndromes, nonparathyroid endocrine disorders, or granulomatous diseases.

Rapid Response Interventions for Life-Threatening Hypercalcemia ***Volume Replacement Is Key***	Hypercalcemic patients presenting with the following symptoms require immediate therapy: • Severe neurologic symptoms, such as profound lethargy, confusion, hallucinations, or coma • Cardiac arrhythmias such as complete heart block • Extreme hypovolemia • Cardiac arrest Therapy is directed at restoring intravascular volume and promoting calcium excretion in the urine. Volume expansion is critical to the treatment and reversal of hypercalcemia. • Hemodialysis is the treatment of choice to rapidly decrease serum calcium in patients with heart failure or renal insufficiency.[24] • If volume can be tolerated, begin rapid fluid resuscitation with a normal saline infusion: 500 mL wide open as a *medical bolus*. Evaluate clinical response. Repeat every 20 to 30 minutes until the patient is hemodynamically stable. • Chelating agents (eg, 50 mmol PO_4 over 8 to 12 hours or EDTA 10 to 50 mg/kg over 4 hours) may be used for extreme conditions. • Use of furosemide (1 mg/kg IV) for treatment of hypercalcemia is controversial. In the presence of heart failure administration of furosemide is required, but it can actually foster reuptake of calcium from bone, thus worsening hypercalcemia.

Hypocalcemia

Normal total calcium range: 8.5 to 10.5 mg/dL
Normal ionized calcium range: 4.2 to 4.8 mg/dL
Hypocalcemia is defined as a serum calcium concentration <8.5 mg/dL (or ionized calcium <4.2 mg/dL).

Causes

The incidence of hypocalcemia in the general population is 0.6%. Hypocalcemia may develop with toxic shock syndrome, with abnormalities in serum magnesium, after

Table 12. Common Causes of Hypocalcemia

Insufficient Parathyroid Hormone
• Post-parathyroidectomy for hyperparathyroidism
• Neck surgery (eg, thyroidectomy)
• Post–neck irradiation
• Destruction of parathyroid glands by metastatic carcinoma, infiltrative diseases

Insufficient Vitamin D
• Malnutrition, dietary abnormalities
• Malabsorption
• Congenital rickets
• Chronic liver disease
• Chronic renal disease
• Sunlight deficiency
• Hypo- or hypermagnesemia
• Advanced bone disease

Medications
• Cimetidine (most frequent cause of drug-induced hypocalcemia)
• Phosphates (from enemas, laxatives)
• Dilantin, phenobarbital
• Gentamicin, tobramycin, actinomycin
• Calcitonin, mithramycin
• EDTA (citrate from blood administration)
• Heparin, protamine
• Theophylline
• Glucagon
• Norepinephrine
• Loop diuretics
• Nitroprusside

Miscellaneous Causes
• Pancreatitis
• Shock or sepsis
• Burns
• Toxic shock syndrome
• Magnesium deficiency

thyroid surgery, with fluoride poisoning, and with tumor lysis syndrome (rapid cell turnover with resultant hyperkalemia, hyperphosphatemia, and hypocalcemia). The most important and frequent causes of hypocalcemia are acute pancreatitis, lack of vitamin D, and medications (see Table 12).

Diagnosis

A serum calcium concentration <8.5 mg/dL (or ionized calcium <4.2 mg/dL) defines clinically significant hypocalcemia. Symptoms usually occur when ionized levels fall to <2.5 mg/dL. Symptoms include paresthesias of the extremities and face, followed by muscle cramps, carpopedal spasm, stridor, tetany, and seizures. Hypocalcemic patients show hyperreflexia and positive Chvostek (tap over facial nerve in front of ear produces twitch of eyelid or corner of mouth) and Trousseau signs (carpal spasm of hand and fingers after the blood pressure cuff has been inflated above systolic pressure for 3 minutes; this spasm occurs because cuff inflation induces ischemia of the ulnar nerve). Cardiac effects include decreased myocardial contractility and heart failure. Hypocalcemia can exacerbate digitalis toxicity. ECG changes may include prolongation of the QT interval, terminal T-wave inversion, bradycardias, AV block, and ventricular tachycardia.

Treatment

Treatment of hypocalcemia requires administration of calcium. Calcium exchange depends on adequate serum concentrations of potassium and magnesium. Effective treatment of hypocalcemia often requires administration of all 3 electrolytes.

Treat acute, symptomatic hypocalcemia with 10% calcium gluconate (93 to 186 mg of elemental calcium), giving 10 to 20 mL IV over 10 minutes. Follow this with an IV infusion of 540 to 720 mg of elemental calcium (58 to 77 mL of 10% calcium gluconate) in 500 to 1000 mL D_5W at 0.5 to 2 mg/kg per hour (10 to 15 mg/kg). Alternatively, administer 10% calcium chloride, giving 5 mL (136.5 mg of elemental calcium) over 10 minutes, followed by 36.6 mL (1 g) IV over the next 6 to 12 hours. Measure serum calcium every 4 to 6 hours. Aim to maintain the total serum calcium concentration at 7 to 9 mg/dL. Correct abnormalities in magnesium, potassium, and pH simultaneously. Note that untreated hypomagnesemia will often make hypocalcemia refractory to therapy. For this reason evaluate serum magnesium when hypocalcemia is present, particularly if the hypocalcemia is refractory to initial calcium therapy.

When calcium is administered intravenously, monitor the infusion site closely. Inadvertent tissue infiltration can cause skin necrosis, and some calcium preparations can cause sclerosis of veins. Calcium gluconate tends to be less irritating to tissues than calcium chloride. Patients with hypocalcemia may require continuous IV infusions, so many clinicians prefer calcium gluconate over calcium chloride. Prolonged infusion with calcium chloride is not recommended.

Magnesium

Magnesium is the fourth most common mineral and the second most abundant intracellular cation (after potassium) in the human body. Because approximately half of total body magnesium resides in bone and because extracellular magnesium is bound to serum albumin, magnesium levels do not reliably reflect total body magnesium stores. Magnesium is necessary for the movement of sodium, potassium, and calcium into and out of cells, and it plays an important role in stabilizing excitable membranes. Low potassium in combination with low magnesium is a risk factor for severe arrhythmias. Magnesium balance is closely tied to sodium, calcium, and potassium balance.

Table 13. Common Causes of Hypermagnesemia

Renal Failure (Acute or Chronic) or Increased Magnesium Load
• Laxatives, antacids, or enemas containing magnesium   • Treatment of pre-eclampsia or eclampsia (may affect both mother and neonate)   • Rhabdomyolysis   • Tumor lysis syndrome
Impaired Elimination of Magnesium From GI Tract
• Anticholinergics   • Narcotics   • Chronic constipation   • Bowel obstruction   • Gastric dilatation
Increased Magnesium Absorption by Kidneys
• Hyperparathyroidism   • Hypothyroidism   • Adrenal insufficiency   • Mineralocorticoid deficiency   • Lithium therapy

Hypermagnesemia

Normal magnesium range: 1.35 to 2.2 mEq/L

Hypermagnesemia is defined as a serum magnesium concentration >2.2 mEq/L.

Causes

ACLS providers will rarely encounter hypermagnesemia. When hypermagnesemia does occur, it is almost always associated with significant renal failure since normally functioning kidneys easily excrete large amounts of magnesium. The major causes of hypermagnesemia are increased magnesium load, impaired elimination from the GI tract, and increased renal absorption. Excess intake of magnesium-containing drugs, particularly laxatives and antacids such as Maalox, is an important cause in the elderly and in patients with renal insufficiency. Table 13 lists the most common causes of hypermagnesemia.

Symptoms and Diagnosis

Hypermagnesemia causes neurologic symptoms of muscular weakness, paralysis, ataxia, drowsiness, and confusion. Nausea and vomiting are common GI symptoms. Other symptoms include flushing, transient tachycardia followed by bradycardia, hypoventilation, and cardiorespiratory arrest. ECG changes of hypermagnesemia include increased PR and QT intervals, increased QRS duration, decrease in P-wave voltage, variable degree of T-wave peaking, complete AV block, and asystole.

Symptoms will become more severe as the serum magnesium concentration rises:

- **3 to <4 mEq/L:** Neuromuscular irritability, somnolence, and loss of deep tendon reflexes
- **4 to <5 mEq/L:** Increasing muscle weakness
- **5 to <8 mEq/L:** Onset of severe vasodilation and hypotension
- **≥8 mEq/L:** Onset of cardiac conduction abnormalities, neuromuscular paralysis, hypotension, ventilation failure, and cardiac arrest

Treatment

Hypermagnesemia is treated with administration of calcium, which removes magnesium from serum. It is important

Rapid Response Interventions for Life-Threatening Hypocalcemia	Patients with life-threatening hypocalcemia present with seizures, tetany, laryngospasm, hypotension or shock, profound bradycardias from heart block, acute congestive failure, or coma. For patients in near-arrest and those in cardiac arrest: • Establish IV access with a large-bore catheter and administer a normal saline bolus • Administer 10% calcium gluconate (9.3 mg/mL or 93 mg/10 mL of elemental calcium), giving 30 mL (279 mg) of a 10% solution over 1 to 3 minutes.

to eliminate sources of ongoing magnesium intake. Cardio-respiratory support may be needed until magnesium levels are reduced. Administration of calcium chloride (5 to 10 mEq IV) will often correct lethal arrhythmias. This dose may be repeated if needed.

Treatment Details

- **General treatment for hypermagnesemia:**
  - Stop any oral or parenteral sources of magnesium.
  - Support the ABCDs of ACLS.
  - Dilute the serum magnesium concentration with administration of IV fluids.
  - Antagonize the cellular effects of elevated magnesium with calcium gluconate or calcium chloride.
  - Remove excess magnesium from the body.

- **Antagonize the effects of hypermagnesemia:**
  - Administer *either* calcium gluconate 10 mL IV of a 10% solution or calcium chloride 5 to 10 mL IV of a 10% solution over 5 to 10 minutes.

- **Remove excess magnesium from the body:**
  - Induce diuresis with normal saline IV at 500 mL/h plus furosemide 1 mg/kg if renal function is normal. Saline diuresis will hasten magnesium excretion by the kidneys.
  - *Note:* Saline diuresis may increase calcium excretion, making signs and symptoms of hypermagnesemia worse. Be prepared to administer calcium chloride 10% solution IV.

Hypomagnesemia

Normal magnesium range: 1.3 to 2.2 mEq/L

Hypomagnesemia, defined as a serum magnesium concentration <1.3 mEq/L, is far more common than hypermagnesemia. Hypomagnesemia interferes with the effects of PTH, resulting in hypocalcemia. It may also lead to hypokalemia. Symptoms of low serum magnesium are muscular tremors and fasciculations, ocular nystagmus, tetany, altered mental state, and cardiac arrhythmias such as torsades de pointes (multifocal ventricular tachycardia). Other possible symptoms are ataxia, vertigo, seizures, and dysphagia.

Causes

Hypomagnesemia occurs in 11% of all hospitalized patients and in up to 65% of severely ill patients.[25] Hypomagnesemia usually results from decreased absorption or increased loss of magnesium from either the kidneys or intestines (diarrhea). Alterations in thyroid hormone function and certain medications (eg, pentamidine, diuretics, alcohol) can also induce hypomagnesemia. Multiple neurohumoral mechanisms become activated in patients with decompensated CHF, leading to hypomagnesemia and other acid-base and electrolyte disturbances. These patients face a high risk of deleterious arrhythmias (see Table 14).

Diagnosis

Most patients with hypomagnesemia are asymptomatic. Patients with symptomatic hypomagnesemia most commonly present with one or more of the following symptoms: muscular tremors, fasciculations, vertigo, ataxia, altered mentation, Chvostek's or Trousseau's sign, and various paresthesias. Many of the symptoms indicate the presence of hypocalcemia. Other possible symptoms are ocular nystagmus, tetany, dysphagia, and seizures.

Hypomagnesemia is often associated with hypokalemia or hypocalcemia. Providers should always check the levels of potassium and calcium in patients with low serum magnesium.

ECG changes of hypomagnesemia include prolonged QT and PR intervals, ST depression and T-wave inversion, flattening or inversion of precordial P waves, widening of the

Rapid Response Interventions for Life-Threatening Hypermagnesemia	In urgent situations immediately antagonize the effects of hypermagnesemia at the neuromuscular cellular level:
	
	• Administer calcium gluconate 10 mL IV of a 10% solution given as a slow bolus. Repeat calcium administration every 5 to 10 minutes until patient stabilizes.
	• As the patient stabilizes, begin removal of magnesium with saline diuresis and a diuretic if renal function is normal:
	
	  — Normal saline 500 mL/h IV
	  — Furosemide 1 mg/kg IV bolus
	
	• As treatment continues the patient may require cardiorespiratory support. Provide this support immediately because once the serum magnesium level decreases, the patient should be fine.
	• Dialysis is ultimately the treatment of choice, but ready availability is a problem in some clinical settings.

QRS interval, torsades de pointes, treatment-resistant VF (and other arrhythmias), and worsening of digitalis toxicity.

Treatment

Treatment of hypomagnesemia depends on its severity and the clinical status of the patient. In patients with renal insufficiency, replace magnesium cautiously; there is a significant risk of life-threatening hypermagnesemia.[26]

- **Mild or chronic hypomagnesemia:**
  - Oral replacement is the preferred route for mild hypomagnesemia. (Parenteral magnesium administration is indicated if symptoms are present even if hypomagnesemia is mild.)
  - Give magnesium sulfate ($MgSO_4$) 400 mg PO once or twice a day.
  - Several weeks of therapy may be required to replenish total body magnesium stores.

Table 14. Common Causes of Hypomagnesemia

Decreased Intake
• Alcoholism
• Malnutrition
• Starvation
Increased Loss
• Gastrointestinal loss: Bowel resection, pancreatitis, diarrhea
• Burns
• Lactation
• Renal disease
Miscellaneous Causes
• Drugs: Diuretics, pentamidine, gentamicin, digoxin
• Parathyroid abnormalities
• Hypothermia
• Hypercalcemia
• Diabetic ketoacidosis
• Hyper- or hypothyroidism
• Phosphate deficiency

- **Moderate hypomagnesemia:**
  - Give $MgSO_4$ IV at a rate of 1 to 2 g over 15 minutes, then 6 g in IV fluid per 24 hours. This problem may require 3 to 7 days for correction.
  - Monitor magnesium level and deep tendon reflexes.

- **Significant symptomatic hypomagnesemia:**
  - Start with $MgSO_4$ 1 to 2 g IV over 15 minutes.
  - Add 6 g magnesium to daily IV fluids for the next 3 to 7 days.
  - Check the patient's magnesium levels and reflexes daily.

- **Acute seizures:**
  - Give $MgSO_4$ 2 g IV over 10 minutes.
  - Add calcium chloride 5 to 10 mL of a 10% solution because most patients with hypomagnesemia are also hypocalcemic.

- **Torsades de pointes associated with hypomagnesemia:**
  - Give up to 2 g of $MgSO_4$ over 1 to 2 minutes (over 5 to 60 minutes if pulse is present).

Life-Threatening Acid-Base Abnormalities

Physiology and Definitions

The healthy human body closely regulates serum pH between 7.35 and 7.45. When pH falls below 7.35, *acidosis* is present. When pH rises above 7.45, *alkalosis* is present.

There are 4 main types of acid-base imbalances:
- Metabolic acidosis
- Metabolic alkalosis
- Respiratory acidosis
- Respiratory alkalosis

This classification is actually an oversimplification because there are mixed acid-base disturbances as well. Whenever acid-base imbalances occur, the body attempts to correct the abnormality and bring the pH back toward the normal range. But in mixed disorders the compensatory mechanisms never completely correct the imbalance, so a primary abnormality is offset by a secondary compensation.

Rapid Response Interventions for Life-Threatening Hypomagnesemia	Patients with seizures or unstable ventricular arrhythmias require emergent treatment. For these patients or those in cardiac arrest: • Administer $MgSO_4$ 2 g IV, generally over 10 minutes; give over 1 to 2 minutes for the most urgent cases • Repeat the dose in 10 to 15 minutes if the patient remains unstable or in refractory arrest • Administer calcium gluconate 10 mL of a 10% solution or calcium chloride 5 to 10 mL of a 10% solution, because most patients with hypomagnesemia are also hypocalcemic

Diagnostic Approaches to Acid-Base Abnormalities

Using the ABG: pH, Pco₂, Bicarbonate

To assess a patient's acid-base status, obtain an arterial blood gas (ABG) analysis. The ABG is critical for identifying acid-base abnormalities and the degree of any compensation. In addition to P_{O_2} and O_2 saturation, the following variables appear on a typical ABG report (normal range follows variable):

- pH: 7.35 to 7.45
- P_{CO_2} (partial pressure of carbon dioxide): 35 to 45 mm Hg
- Bicarbonate (HCO_3): 22 to 32 mEq/L
- Base deficit or base excess: −2 to +2

An average P_{CO_2} value of 40 mm Hg is used in calculations to compare the *predicted pH* with the *measured pH*. The magnitude and direction of any difference between predicted and measured pH provide a rough estimate of whether a metabolic or respiratory acidosis or alkalosis is present.

Comparing Predicted pH With Measured pH

When interpreting the ABG, you must evaluate both the P_{CO_2} and the pH to identify any acid-base disorder and metabolic and respiratory components. You make this assessment by first predicting the pH from the P_{CO_2}:

- Step 1: Determine if the pH is acidotic (<7.35), alkalotic (>7.45), or normal (7.35 to 7.45), and note if the patient is hypercarbic (P_{CO_2} >45) or hypocarbic (P_{CO_2} <35). Hypocarbia indicates a respiratory alkalosis, and hypercarbia indicates a respiratory acidosis. Now to identify the primary problem and any compensation, you need to determine the contribution of the P_{CO_2} to any acidosis or alkalosis.
- Step 2: Subtract the patient's measured P_{CO_2} from 40 (estimated normal P_{CO_2}). The result will be either positive (if the patient's P_{CO_2} is low) or negative (if P_{CO_2} is high).
- Step 3: Multiply the result of step 2 by 0.008. Note that the product may be a positive or negative number because Step 2 may result in a positive or a negative number.
- Step 4: Add the positive or negative product obtained in Step 3 to 7.4. This will result in either the addition of a number to 7.4 or subtraction of a number from 7.4. The resulting number is the pH predicted from the P_{CO_2}. Every 1 mm Hg uncompensated rise in P_{CO_2} above 40 mm Hg (more hypercarbic) is predicted to make the pH fall by 0.008 (more acidotic).
- Overall, $(40 - P_{CO_2}) \times 0.008 = \pm\Delta$ in pH from 7.4.

If the patient's measured pH is higher than the calculated pH, *metabolic alkalosis* must be associated with the hypocarbia or hypercarbia. If the measured pH is lower than the calcu-

lated pH, *metabolic acidosis* must be associated with the hypocarbia or hypercarbia.

Example

ABG: pH 7.30, P_{CO_2} 30 mm Hg

Perform the calculation steps noted above:

- Step 1: The pH is acidotic (<7.35). You also note that the P_{CO_2} of 30 mm Hg is hypocarbic, so the patient has a respiratory alkalosis.
- Step 2: Subtract the measured P_{CO_2} (30) from 40. The difference is +10.
- Step 3: Multiply the +10 difference from Step 2 by 0.008. The product is +0.08.
- Step 4: Add the product of step 3 (0.08) to 7.4. This represents the change in pH predicted from the P_{CO_2} alone. Adding +0.08 to 7.4 yields a predicted pH of 7.48.

Interpretation: On the basis of the P_{CO_2} level of 30, this patient's predicted pH is 7.48. But this patient's measured pH is 7.30, which is quite acidotic. The conclusion is that the much lower measured pH is due to the presence of a *primary metabolic acidosis*. The respiratory alkalosis represents partial compensation (the pH is still acidotic), so your conclusion is primary metabolic acidosis with partial respiratory compensation.

Compensation in Acid-Base Disturbances

In the previous example, why is the patient's P_{CO_2} less than the normal range of 35 to 45 mm Hg? The patient is attempting to compensate for the metabolic acidosis by increased ventilation, or "blowing off CO_2." As the CO_2 is "blown off" and the P_{CO_2} falls, the pH rises—what is called a *compensatory respiratory alkalosis*. Provided the patient is alert and has no compromise of the airway, respiratory compensation will be almost immediate. If the acidosis were respiratory, the kidneys would attempt to compensate by retaining bicarbonate (a base). Unlike respiratory compensation, which is immediate, metabolic compensation for underlying respiratory acid-base problems takes 8 to 48 hours to occur. Note that a compensatory mechanism is terminated when the pH approaches normal. A compensatory mechanism will not "overcorrect" the pH (see "The Overcompensation Rule").

Primary Respiratory Acidosis With Compensatory Metabolic Alkalosis

A common example of a primary respiratory acid-base disturbance occurs in chronic obstructive pulmonary disease with CO_2 retention (see "Case Scenario"). As the P_{CO_2} rises, the pH falls, leading to a *primary respiratory acidosis*. Over time the kidneys will retain extra bicarbonate (HCO_3) to neutralize the acid created by the retained CO_2 in an attempt to restore the pH to near-normal. This response is called a *compensatory metabolic alkalosis,* or *metabolic compensation.*

Using the Measured Base Deficit or Base Excess

Another factor to use in interpreting the acid-base balance from the ABG is the base deficit or base excess. It is normally between –2 and +2.

- If the base deficit is more negative than –2, a *metabolic acidosis* is present (base deficit less than –2 indicates metabolic acidosis).
- If a base excess is more positive than +2, *metabolic alkalosis* is present.

Case Scenario

Mr B is a 74-year-old, 40-pack/year smoker with advanced chronic obstructive pulmonary disease. He is a known "CO_2 retainer." He presents to the ED with another in a long series of acute exacerbations. He is tachypneic, cyanotic, and obviously struggling to breathe. He becomes more obtunded as he is being examined. A STAT ABG reveals the following results (patient is on 2 L O_2):

pH 7.30, Pco_2 80, Po_2 58, HCO_3^- 38, base excess +12, oxygen saturation 89%

Perform your analysis of the ABG:

- Step 1: First note that the pH is below the normal range, so *acidosis* is present. Next look at the Pco_2. At 80 it is elevated to twice normal, indicating that respiratory acidosis is present. You know that as Pco_2 rises, the pH falls unless there is metabolic compensation. Now you should determine if there is any compensation.
- Step 2: Subtract the patient's Pco_2 (80 mm Hg) from 40. This yields –40.
- Step 3: Multiply the result of Step 2 (–40) by 0.008. This yields a product of –0.32.
- Step 4: Add the result of Step 3 (–0.32) to 7.4. The pH predicted from the Pco_2 of 80 would be 7.08. Because the pH is 7.3 there must be some metabolic compensation for the respiratory acidosis. This metabolic alkalotic compensation is confirmed by the base excess of +12.

- Then note the HCO_3^-. It is elevated to 38 mEq/L (normal: 22 to 32 mEq/L). This finding shows that the patient's kidneys have resorbed excess bicarbonate to compensate for his respiratory acidosis. The sustained resorption of bicarbonate by the kidneys accounts for the base excess of +12. As noted above, this base excess indicates a *metabolic alkalosis*.
- **Interpretation:** The analysis of Mr B's ABG, then, is primary respiratory acidosis with compensatory metabolic alkalosis (or primary respiratory acidosis with partial metabolic compensation).

The Overcompensation Rule

An additional useful rule to keep in mind with acid-base disturbances is that *compensatory mechanisms are unlikely to **overcompensate** in acid-base abnormalities.* As the pH approaches normal, the compensatory mechanisms shut off. By this rule Mr B's primary problem cannot be a metabolic alkalosis because his pH remained acidotic. His body would not have overcompensated with CO_2 retention to the point of causing an acidosis just to fix a metabolic alkalosis.

If a patient with chronic respiratory failure presents with an *alkalotic* pH, this does not represent metabolic compensation because a compensatory mechanism for respiratory acidosis will not overcorrect the pH to the alkalotic range. You should look for a condition responsible for a metabolic alkalosis. For example, hypochloremic or hypokalemic metabolic alkalosis can develop in patients with chronic respiratory failure. This can occur during diuretic (eg, furosemide) therapy if the patient does not receive adequate potassium chloride supplementation).

Keeping this rule in mind, the ACLS provider can determine which is the primary acid-base disturbance and which is the compensatory mechanism.

Anion Gap

The *anion gap* is another calculated value that can help identify the underlying cause of an acid-base disturbance. The number of positive ions in the body (eg, sodium and potassium) should be approximately equal to the number of negative ions (chloride and bicarbonate). But this balance never occurs because there is always a difference (the gap) caused by unmeasured negative ions such as ketones and lactic acid. This anion gap quantifies the difference between

---

FYI **The Overcompensation Rule**	• A useful rule to keep in mind with acid-base disturbances is that *compensatory mechanisms are unlikely to **overcompensate** in acid-base abnormalities.* As the pH approaches normal, the compensatory mechanisms shut off. • Keeping this rule in mind, the ACLS provider can determine which is the primary acid-base disturbance and which is the compensatory mechanism.

the serum sodium concentration and the serum chloride plus bicarbonate concentrations:

$$\text{Anion gap} = [Na^+] - ([Cl^-] + [HCO_3^-])$$
Normal anion gap: 7 ± 4 mEq/L*

*The normal value of the anion gap was originally listed as 12 ± 4 mEq/L. Newer automated systems are more accurate and the revised normal value has decreased.

With an anion gap in the normal range (7 ± 4 mEq/L), any existing acidosis will be due to the negative ions in the equation, chloride and bicarbonate. A *normal anion gap acidosis* occurs with diarrhea because a fall in serum bicarbonate is balanced by a rise in serum chloride (hyperchloremic metabolic acidosis). With an anion gap that is abnormally high (>11 mEq/L), any existing acidosis is caused by an accumulation of unmeasured negative ions, such as ketones or lactic acid, or a fall in serum bicarbonate that is not balanced by a rise in serum chloride. The classic example of a high anion gap acidosis is diabetic ketoacidosis.

Diabetic Ketoacidosis

Pathophysiology

Diabetic ketoacidosis (DKA) is the most frequent life-threatening acid-base abnormality that ACLS providers will encounter. A relative insulin deficiency is the primary cause of DKA. It is important to understand the major abnormalities in the pathophysiology of DKA because these problems define the therapeutic approach:

- **Hyperglycemia:** Without sufficient insulin, glucose cannot enter the cells, so it reaches higher and higher concentrations in the blood (hyperglycemia). The blood glucose is further elevated by the effects of the hormone *glucagon,* which is released by the liver during insulin deficiency, and catecholamines, which stimulate gluconeogenesis (glucose is made).
- **Dehydration:** The hyperglycemia causes an osmotic diuresis (polyuria), with excretion of glucose-containing urine (glucosuria). Significant volume can be lost during this osmotic diuresis. This volume loss leads to severe dehydration, worsening acidosis, and hypotension.
- **Ketoacidosis:** Without intracellular glucose the body begins to metabolize existing lipids (fat stores). These

lipids are partially oxidized into free fatty acids and acetoacetic acids. The free fatty acids accumulate and the acetoacetic acid is converted into ketones. These processes result in the development of ketoacidosis. These ketones and free fatty acids account for the high-anion-gap metabolic acidosis invariably present in DKA.
- **Hypokalemia:** Total body potassium stores decrease during the osmotic diuresis and dehydrating volume loss of DKA. The serum potassium, however, may be normal or even slightly elevated when the patient presents with DKA. *The ketoacidosis (low pH) results in an acute shift of potassium from the intracellular to the extracellular (including the vascular) space. This explains how the serum potassium may be normal or even elevated despite the total body loss of potassium.* During treatment of DKA and correction of the acidosis, the potassium returns to the intracellular space (from the vascular space). This can result in severe hypokalemia if the ACLS provider fails to anticipate the shift and initiate potassium replacement.

Causes of DKA

Although DKA can develop in patients with insulin-dependent diabetes, it can be the presenting sign of diabetes. If the patient has no history of insulin-dependent diabetes, clinicians can lose valuable time under the mistaken assumption that DKA is a diagnostic impossibility. DKA can be the initial presentation of a person with undiagnosed diabetes. In a study from the 1980s, 20% of all patients admitted for DKA had newly diagnosed diabetes.[27] Furthermore, patients with non–insulin-dependent diabetes may develop insulin dependency that is not recognized until they experience an episode of DKA.[27]

DKA frequently results when a patient with insulin-dependent diabetes stops or reduces insulin therapy. About 15% of patients with DKA are not taking insulin at the time of emergency presentation. The clinical history of many insulin-dependent diabetics qualifies them as "brittle diabetics." The reason for frequent episodes of DKA is unclear: the DKA may develop despite uninterrupted insulin therapy. The risk factors for DKA are well known for most patients with insulin-dependent diabetes. One commonly used memory aid for the more common precipitants of DKA is the so-

---

Critical Concept **DKA Often the Presenting Sign of Diabetes**	If a patient with DKA has no history of insulin-dependent diabetes, do not automatically assume that DKA is a diagnostic impossibility: • DKA can be the initial presentation of a person with undiagnosed diabetes. • Patients with non–insulin-dependent diabetes may develop insulin dependency that is not recognized until they experience an episode of DKA.[27]

called "6 I's": *infection, infarction, ignorance, ischemia, intoxication, and implantation.*

- **Infection:** Pneumonia and urinary tract infections are the infections that most commonly precipitate an episode of DKA.
- **Infarction** (brain): Stroke syndromes, especially those leading to coma, are often associated with rapid deterioration in insulin-dependent diabetics.
- **Ignorance** (poor understanding of diabetes): Noncompliance with insulin regimens or dietary restrictions, and errors of commission and omission in insulin therapy.
- **Ischemia:** Acute myocardial infarction, with its associated stress and hyperadrenaline state, will often induce DKA.
- **Intoxication:** Excessive alcohol consumption is a common offender.
- **Implantation:** This "I" refers to the many complications that diabetic women can experience during pregnancy.

Signs and Symptoms of DKA

The clinical presentation of DKA is highly variable and often nonspecific. All healthcare professionals must maintain the stereotypical "high index of suspicion" in emergency settings, especially when an insulin-dependent diabetic presents with virtually any complaint. The most common symptoms associated with DKA are nausea, vomiting, and vague abdominal pain. The widely repeated clinical axiom that *"any GI complaint in an insulin-dependent diabetic is DKA until proven otherwise"* merits both compliance and repetition.

Treatment of DKA

DKA is a life-threatening condition. The ACLS provider must be able to recognize it and treat it effectively. First, begin general assessment and therapy following the 5 Quadrads Approach of ACLS:

- **Airway patency and breathing effectiveness:** If the obtunded patient demonstrates hypoventilation, intubation may be necessary for airway maintenance and protection and for oxygenation and ventilation.

- **Circulation:** Dehydration and hypovolemia are virtually always present.
- **Diagnosis:** Initially order a 12-lead ECG, serum electrolytes, ABG, and urinalysis.
- **Assess vital signs:** Evaluate temperature, blood pressure, heart rate and rhythm, respirations (rate and pattern), and oxygen saturation (on room air and in response to low-flow oxygen).
- **Oxygen-IV-monitor-fluids:** Provide oxygen, start an IV, attach a cardiac monitor, and initiate fluids.

Then assess the 4 major pathophysiologic abnormalities that may be present in DKA, organize therapy, and plan a strategy. Providers should address the abnormalities in this order of priority:

1. Correct dehydration.
2. Correct hypokalemia.
3. Correct hyperglycemia.
4. Correct ketoacidosis.

Correct Dehydration

Begin with the administration of normal saline (0.9% sodium chloride) IV. Establish IV access with a large-bore catheter and infuse 1 L rapidly; follow with 1 to 2 L over the first and second hours. When volume status is stable, give half-normal saline (0.45% sodium chloride) IV at 150 to 300 mL/h. Ideally urine output should be at least 1 mL/kg per hour after the initial fluid resuscitation. If urine output fails to reach this level by the second hour, more aggressive fluid therapy will be needed, provided the patient has normal renal function. Rather than change to half-normal saline, continue with normal saline at higher rates.

- When serum glucose falls to less than 300 mg/dL, provide dextrose 5% with half-normal saline at 150 to 300 mL/h. This switch to glucose-containing solutions will help prevent the patient from developing hypoglycemia from the IV insulin.
- Determine the effectiveness of fluid resuscitation by close observation of hourly urine output. Most patients with DKA will require insertion of a urinary catheter.

FYI **The 6 I's: Common Precipitants of DKA**	The risk factors for diabetic ketoacidosis are well known for most patients with insulin-dependent diabetes. One memory aid for the more common precipitants of DKA is the so-called "6 I's": • *Infection* • *Infarction (stroke)* • *Ignorance* • *Ischemia (acute myocardial infarction)* • *Intoxication* • *Implantation (complications of pregnancy)*

Correct Hypokalemia

First, DKA patients have severe depletion of total body potassium stores. Because these patients are severely acidotic, they often initially have a false "normal" potassium (as pH falls, potassium moves from intracellular to extracellular space). A normal serum potassium of 3.6 mEq/L in a patient with DKA is likely to represent severe depletion of total body potassium stores. Second, as therapy corrects the acidosis, the serum potassium will fall because the potassium returns to the intracellular spaces (from the extracellular spaces, including from the vascular space). This shift can lead to life-threatening hypokalemia. ACLS providers should anticipate this shift and start IV potassium therapy early.

Add KCl to the above IV fluids at a rate of 10 to 20 mEq/L. Exceptions will be patients with initial hyperkalemia (>6 mEq/L or with ECG signs of high potassium), patients with renal failure, or patients who are not producing urine as confirmed by hourly urine output.

1. For patients with documented hypokalemia on presentation, add KCl at a rate of 40 mEq per *hour*—not per liter!
2. The clinical goal is to maintain potassium levels in the normal range while recognizing 2 major caveats: that DKA patients have severe depletion of total body potassium stores and that as therapy corrects the acidosis, the serum potassium will fall (see above).

A historical side note illustrates the importance of these caveats (see "Relevant Research"). Medical historians speculate that literally decades of unnecessary deaths occurred after the discovery of insulin in 1922.[28,29] Until the early 1950s clinicians failed to recognize both that correction of the acidosis in DKA could produce life-threatening hypokalemia and that intravenous therapy with potassium could be life-saving.[29]

Treat Hyperglycemia

Insulin is needed to help glucose enter the cells. Start with regular insulin 10 U IV push. Then infuse 5 to 10 U/h IV (0.1 U/kg per hour). In terms of treatment priorities, insulin follows initial fluid resuscitation and potassium replacement. The serum potassium should be high enough to prevent hypokalemia (K^+ >3.7 mEq/L) before you initiate the insulin infusion. It is important to reduce the serum glucose concentration gradually. Aim for a gradual reduction of 10% per hour and no faster than 50 to 100 mg/dL per hour.

If the serum glucose concentration is reduced faster than 100 mg/dL per hour, the fall in serum osmolality may be associated with a shift of free water from the vascular to the interstitial space, with the risk of cerebral edema. Remember that severe hyperglycemia increases the serum osmolality and dilutes the serum sodium. As the serum glucose falls, the serum sodium should rise. The risk of cerebral edema is thought to be high if the serum sodium does not rise as the serum glucose concentration falls. For every 100 mg/dL fall in serum glucose, the serum sodium should rise 1.6 mEq/L (see "Cerebral Edema").

- Once glucose drops to <300 mg/dL, change fluids to D_5/0.45% sodium chloride. This switch to glucose-containing solutions will help prevent hypoglycemia from the IV insulin.

Once insulin therapy begins, further ketone formation should cease, the anion gap should lessen, and bicarbonate should increase. IV insulin infusion should continue until bicarbonate is >15 mEq/L, there is no anion gap, the patient can tolerate oral food and liquids, *and* for about 1 hour after the first dose of subcutaneous insulin.

Correct Ketoacidosis

Bicarbonate administration is *not* routine therapy for DKA. The increase in pH from bicarbonate can be severely deleterious, shifting potassium into cells and producing life-threatening hypokalemia[30,31] and cerebral edema, especially in children.[32,33] In addition, the sodium bicarbonate will increase serum osmolality that is already high from the hyperglycemia.

The generally accepted indications for bicarbonate administration in DKA are

- Hyperkalemia producing ECG changes
- Severe acidosis: pH <7.1 (some experts recommend no bicarbonate until pH is <7.0)
- Severe depletion of buffering reserve: bicarbonate <5 mEq/L
- Shock or coma
- Acidosis-induced cardiac or pulmonary dysfunction

Critical Concept

False "Normal" Potassium Levels in Patients With DKA

DKA patients have severe depletion of total body potassium stores. Because these patients are severely acidotic, they often initially have a false "normal" potassium (as pH falls, potassium moves from intracellular to extracellular space).

- A normal serum potassium of 3.6 mEq/L in a patient with DKA is likely to represent severe depletion of total body potassium stores.

If indicated, administer sodium bicarbonate by adding 50 to 100 mEq to 1 L of 0.45% sodium chloride and infusing the 1 L over 30 to 60 minutes. To avoid hypokalemia, some experts recommend the addition of 10 mEq potassium to the 1 L of 0.45% sodium chloride.

- If bicarbonate therapy is initiated, do not try to normalize pH. Just raise the pH enough to *get the patient out of trouble.*

The Periarrest Patient With DKA

Be particularly alert for life-threatening problems in patients with DKA. These problems may include cardiac arrhythmias from hypokalemia or hyperkalemia, shock and lactic acidosis, and cerebral edema (osmotic encephalopathy).

Cardiac Arrhythmias From Hypokalemia or Hyperkalemia

Beware of the false "normal" potassium level in DKA patients as therapy begins. Volume replacement with normal saline and insulin infusion will begin a rapid shift of potassium into the cells. You should expect that the serum potassium will fall as the serum pH rises.

With profound acidosis, potassium can shift outside the cells to such a degree that life-threatening arrhythmias from hyperkalemia may develop before the DKA is treated. In such an event follow the treatment sequence for hyperkalemia outlined in Table 15. Generally the patient will require only urgent addition of calcium chloride or calcium gluconate plus sodium bicarbonate because IV insulin and high levels of glucose are already in place.

Shock and Lactic Acidosis

Shock and lactic acidosis causing tissue hypoxia and abnormalities of cellular metabolism can occur from prolonged dehydration and volume depletion, hypotension, and tissue hypoxia: Suspect these problems in DKA patients who have a persistent anion gap and metabolic acidosis despite appropriate initial therapy. These patients need aggressive fluid resuscitation, and as noted earlier, some may receive sodium bicarbonate administration.

Cerebral Edema (Osmotic Encephalopathy)

The precise mechanism of this complication is not known, but it has been theorized to include rapid correction of hyperglycemia (>100 mg/dL per hour) and a fall in serum osmolality. Suspect the development of cerebral edema in patients with DKA who show signs of increasing intracranial pressure, such as headache, altered mental status, or pupil dilation. Hyponatremia provides an important clue to imminent overhydration and pending cerebral edema. DKA patients will initially have a low serum sodium

concentration, which may be normal in the presence of hyperglycemia.

For every increase in serum glucose of 100 mg/dL above 180 mg/dL, the serum sodium concentration will be reduced by 1.6 mEq/L below 135 mEq/L. For this reason you should watch for a matching rise in serum sodium (ie, 1.6 mEq/L rise for every 100 mg/dL fall in serum glucose) as hyperglycemia is corrected. Failure of serum sodium to rise appropriately as the glucose falls, or an actual fall, is a red flag for cerebral edema. Urgent CT scanning can establish this diagnosis, which should be treated urgently with IV mannitol.

> ## Relevant Research: Recognition of the Importance of Potassium in DKA[29]
>
> It is often said that the introduction of insulin into clinical medicine made a "dramatic" difference in the mortality resulting from diabetic coma. This is true in the sense that before 1922 DKA was almost uniformly fatal, and even in the 1950s the mortality in many large hospitals was as high as 30% to 50%. Often autopsy did not establish a cause of death. Many may have been a result of hypokalemia, a complication that was not recognized until 1946. In that year in the *Journal of the American Medical Association,* Jacob Holler described a patient who developed respiratory paralysis 12 hours into treatment that after several hours in an iron lung was cured by potassium infusion.[28] In the 5 years after Holler's paper there were many reports of deaths resulting from hypokalemia, as well as several "near misses," but clinicians were extremely cautious about early replacement, probably, as an editorialist in *The Lancet* suggested, because "the frightening effects of intravenous injections of potassium made clinicians reluctant to believe in a lack of potassium as a cause of trouble, except in very rare conditions such as familial periodic paralysis." It had been known since 1923 that insulin lowered serum potassium, but this was not of great interest because the symptoms of hypokalemia were not known. Also, potassium was not an electrolyte with which clinicians were familiar. Until the introduction of flame photometry in 1950, it was measured only in research studies because chemical methods took several hours to complete.
>
> —*Reprinted with permission from Tattersall[29]*

Table 15. Life-Threatening Electrolyte Abnormalities With Associated ECG Findings and Recommended Treatment Approaches

Electrolyte Problem and Normal Range	Associated ECG Findings	Recommended Treatment Approach
Hyperkalemia 3.5 to 5 mEq/L	• 5.5 to <6: Tall, peaked T waves • 6 to <6.5: Prolonged PR interval (first-degree heart block), increase in QT interval • 6.5 to <7: Flattened P waves, depressed ST segment • 7 to <7.5: Widened QRS complexes • 7.5 to <8: Deepening S waves, merging of S and T waves • 8 to <10: Sine wave–shaped complexes, idioventricular complexes and rhythms • ≥10: PEA (sine wave look), VT/VF, asystole	Sequence begins with recommendations for the most urgent (arrest) hyperkalemic patient. **Antagonize effects at cellular level:** • Calcium chloride 5 to 10 mL IV 10% solution (500 to 1000 mg) **Shift potassium into cells:** • Sodium bicarbonate 50 mEq (1 ampule) IV bolus or 1 mEq/kg; repeat in 15 min; then 2 ampules (100 mEq) in 1 L D_5W • Regular insulin plus glucose: 10 U regular insulin IV plus 50 mL D_{50} (25 g) glucose; then 10 to 20 U regular insulin with 500 mL $D_{10}W$ IV over 1 hour PRN • Albuterol (nebulized) 10 to 20 mg over 15 min; may repeat PRN **Remove potassium from body:** • Furosemide 40 to 80 mg IV bolus • Kayexalate 15 to 50 g PO or 50 g PR with sorbitol • Peritoneal dialysis or hemodialysis

Hypokalemia 3.5 to 5 mEq/L	• 2.5 to 3: Prominent U waves, flattened T waves, low QRS voltage, prominent P waves
	• 2 to <2.5: More prominent U waves, more ST-segment changes
	• <2: QT interval more prolonged, QRS complex widens, wide-complex tachyarrhythmias, VT, VF
		Rough estimates of total body deficits based on serum K:
		• $[K^+]$ = 3 to <3.5 mEq/L
		  Deficit = 100 to 200 mEq
		• $[K^+]$ = 2.5 to <3 mEq/L
		  Deficit = 200 to 300 mEq
		• $[K^+]$ = 2 to <2.5 mEq/L
		  Deficit = 300 to 400 mEq
		Maximum peripheral IV concentration: KCl approximately 40 mEq in 1 L NS
		Maximum rate: KCl approximately 40 mEq total in 1 hour
		Cardiac arrest (maximum limit):
		• Infuse KCl IV at 2 mEq/min for 10 min (20 mEq)
		• Follow with KCl at 1 mEq/min for 10 min (10 mEq)

Nonketotic Hyperosmolar Syndrome

Pathophysiology

The nonketotic hyperosmolar syndrome (NKHS) is a life-threatening acid-base abnormality that occurs in diabetic patients.[34] DKA occurs predominantly in insulin-dependent (type 1) diabetes mellitus; NKHS occurs almost exclusively in non–insulin-dependent (type 2) diabetes mellitus. NKHS is nonketotic because residual insulin secretion, although insufficient to prevent hyperglycemia, effectively inhibits the breakdown of lipids and the production of free fatty acids and ketones (ketogenesis).

Other than ketoacidosis, all the pathophysiologic abnormalities of DKA occur with NKHS: hyperglycemia with osmotic diuresis develops, leading to dehydration and volume loss and depletion of potassium through increased renal output.

Causes

Most of the same processes that initiate DKA also precipitate NKHS. Patients with NKHS often omit or are unable to take their regular oral antidiabetic agents. Other precipitating factors include infection, infarction (stroke), and indiscretions with medications or diet. NKHS often develops in patients who are manifestly ill and debilitated with near-obtundation.

Diagnosis

Providers should suspect NKHS in any patient who appears to be ill and is known to have type 2 diabetes. Patients will frequently be severely dehydrated and may be obtunded. The syndrome has often been called "nonketotic hyperosmolar coma" because so many of these patients are unconscious and unresponsive on presentation. The laboratory findings are classic and diagnostic:

- Hyperglycemia, often with blood sugar >600 mg/dL
- Hyperosmolality, with plasma osmolality >320 mOsm/L
- Absence of acidosis
- Absence of ketones in the urine and blood

Treatment

For the ACLS provider the initial treatment approach for NKHS is the same as the approach for DKA. These treatment measures include volume replacement with normal saline, potassium replacement, treatment of hyperglycemia with insulin, and close monitoring of electrolytes and pH (usually lactic acidosis in NKHS rather than ketoacidosis), and response to therapy.

The Periarrest Patient With NKHS

Life-threatening NKHS is most likely to occur in elderly patients with known type 2 diabetes. On presentation these patients are often comatose with severe hypotension or overt shock. The mainstay of treatment for the unstable patient with NKHS is rapid volume replacement and consideration of pressor agents for shock.

By definition NKHS patients rarely have the ketoacidosis of DKA with the associated intracellular to extracellular shift of potassium, so the patients are not as likely to develop the intracellular potassium shift (and fall in serum potassium) during therapy.[34] For this reason these patients are less prone to the life-threatening cardiac arrhythmias that may develop in patients with DKA.

The same recommendations noted above for periarrest patients with DKA apply to these NKHS patients. Although cerebral edema can occur in NKHS, it seems to be diagnosed less often. Children with NKHS, like children with DKA, are much more likely than adults to develop cerebral edema during resuscitation.[35,36]

Summary: Electrolyte and Life-Threatening Acid-Base Abnormalities

Electrolyte abnormalities can cause severe physiologic and metabolic derangements, including cardiac arrhythmias and other types of cardiovascular decompensation. Table 15 provides a quick summary of the associated ECG changes and the treatments recommended in this chapter.

Clinicians should maintain a high index of suspicion for possible electrolyte disturbances. Prompt diagnosis and aggressive treatment can often prevent life-threatening complications.

References

1. Jackson MA, Lodwick R, Hutchinson SG. Hyperkalaemic cardiac arrest successfully treated with peritoneal dialysis. *BMJ*. 1996;312:1289-1290.

2. Voelckel W, Kroesen G. Unexpected return of cardiac action after termination of cardiopulmonary resuscitation. *Resuscitation*. 1996;32:27-29.

3. Niemann JT, Cairns CB. Hyperkalemia and ionized hypocalcemia during cardiac arrest and resuscitation: possible culprits for postcountershock arrhythmias? *Ann Emerg Med*. 1999;34:1-7.

4. Allon M. Hyperkalemia in end-stage renal disease: mechanisms and management [editorial]. *J Am Soc Nephrol*. 1995;6:1134-1142.

5. Lin JL, Lim PS, Leu ML, Huang CC. Outcomes of severe hyperkalemia in cardiopulmonary resuscitation with concomitant hemodialysis. *Intensive Care Med*. 1994;20:287-290.

6. Burch GE, Winsor TA. *A Primer of Electrocardiography*. 5th ed. Philadelphia, Pa: Lea & Febiger; 1966:143.

7. Paltiel O, Salakhov E, Ronen I, Berg D, Israeli A. Management of severe hypokalemia in hospitalized patients: a study of quality of care based on computerized databases. *Arch Intern Med*. 2001;161:1089-1095.

8. Higham PD, Adams PC, Murray A, Campbell RW. Plasma potassium, serum magnesium and ventricular fibrillation: a prospective study. *Q J Med*. 1993;86:609-617.

9. Schulman M, Narins RG. Hypokalemia and cardiovascular disease. *Am J Cardiol*. 1990;65:4E-9E, discussion 22E-23E.

10. Gennari FJ. Hypokalemia. *N Engl J Med*. 1998;339:451-458.

11. Adrogue HJ, Madias NE. Aiding fluid prescription for the dysnatremias. *Intensive Care Med*. 1997;23:309-316.

12. Fraser CL, Arieff AI. Epidemiology, pathophysiology, and management of hyponatremic encephalopathy. *Am J Med*. 1997;102:67-77.

13. Adrogue HJ, Madias NE. Hyponatremia. *N Engl J Med*. 2000;342:1581-1589.

14. Gross P, Reimann D, Neidel J, Doke C, Prospert F, Decaux G, Verbalis J, Schrier RW. The treatment of severe hyponatremia. *Kidney Int Suppl*. 1998;64:S6-S11.

15. Menashe G, Borer A, Gilad J, Horowitz J. Rhabdomyolysis after correction of severe hyponatremia. *Am J Emerg Med*. 2000;18:229-230.

16. Laureno R, Karp BI. Myelinolysis after correction of hyponatremia. *Ann Intern Med*. 1997;126:57-62.

17. Soupart A, Decaux G. Therapeutic recommendations for management of severe hyponatremia: current concepts on pathogenesis and prevention of neurologic complications. *Clin Nephrol*. 1996;46:149-169.

18. Brunner JE, Redmond JM, Haggar AM, Kruger DF, Elias SB. Central pontine myelinolysis and pontine lesions after rapid correction of hyponatremia: a prospective magnetic resonance imaging study. *Ann Neurol*. 1990;27:61-66.

19. Ayus JC, Krothapalli RK, Arieff AI. Treatment of symptomatic hyponatremia and its relation to brain damage: a prospective study. *N Engl J Med*. 1987;317:1190-1195.

20. Anderson RJ, Chung HM, Kluge R, Schrier RW. Hyponatremia: a prospective analysis of its epidemiology and the pathogenetic role of vasopressin. *Ann Intern Med*. 1985;102:164-168.

21. Miller M. Syndromes of excess antidiuretic hormone release. *Crit Care Clin*. 2001;17:11-23, v.

22. Barri YM, Knochel JP. Hypercalcemia and electrolyte disturbances in malignancy. *Hematol Oncol Clin North Am*. 1996;10:775-790.

23. Aldinger KA, Samaan NA. Hypokalemia with hypercalcemia. Prevalence and significance in treatment. *Ann Intern Med*. 1977;87:571-573.

24. Edelson GW, Kleerekoper M. Hypercalcemic crisis. *Med Clin North Am*. 1995;79:79-92.

25. Elisaf M, Milionis H, Siamopoulos KC. Hypomagnesemic hypokalemia and hypocalcemia: clinical and laboratory characteristics. *Miner Electrolyte Metab*. 1997;23:105-112.

26. al-Ghamdi SM, Cameron EC, Sutton RA. Magnesium deficiency: pathophysiologic and clinical overview. *Am J Kidney Dis*. 1994;24:737-752.

27. Faich GA, Fishbein HA, Ellis SE. The epidemiology of diabetic acidosis: a population-based study. *Am J Epidemiol*. 1983;117:551-558.

28. Holler JW. Potassium deficiency occurring during the treatment of diabetic acidosis. *JAMA*. 1946;131:1186-1189.

29. Tattersall RB. A paper which changed clinical practice (slowly): Jacob Holler on potassium deficiency in diabetic acidosis (1946). *Diabet Med*. 1999;16:978-984.

30. Viallon A, Zeni F, Lafond P, Venet C, Tardy B, Page Y, Bertrand JC. Does bicarbonate therapy improve the management of severe diabetic ketoacidosis? *Crit Care Med*. 1999;27:2690-2693.

31. Kannan CR. Bicarbonate therapy in the management of severe diabetic ketoacidosis. *Crit Care Med*. 1999;27:2833-2834.

32. Glaser N, Barnett P, McCaslin I, Nelson D, Trainor J, Louie J, Kaufman F, Quayle K, Roback M, Malley R, Kuppermann N. Risk factors for cerebral edema in children with diabetic ketoacidosis. The Pediatric Emergency Medicine Collaborative Research Committee of the American Academy of Pediatrics. *N Engl J Med*. 2001;344:264-269.

33. Dunger DB, Edge JA. Predicting cerebral edema during diabetic ketoacidosis. *N Engl J Med*. 2001;344:302-303.

34. Magee MF, Bhatt BA. Management of decompensated diabetes. Diabetic ketoacidosis and hyperglycemic hyperosmolar syndrome. *Crit Care Clin*. 2001;17:75-106.

35. Gottschalk ME, Ros SP, Zeller WP. The emergency management of hyperglycemic-hyperosmolar nonketotic coma in the pediatric patient. *Pediatr Emerg Care*. 1996;12:48-51.

36. Ellis EN. Concepts of fluid therapy in diabetic ketoacidosis and hyperosmolar hyperglycemic nonketotic coma. *Pediatr Clin North Am*. 1990;37:313-321.